Clinical Radiology of the Horse

Clinical Radiology of the Horse

Third Edition

JANET A. BUTLER
Willesley Equine Clinic Ltd, Tetbury, UK

CHRISTOPHER M. COLLES BVetMed, PhD,
Hon FWCF, MRCVS
Avonvale Veterinary Practice Ltd., Banbury, UK

SUE J. DYSON MA, VetMB, PhD, DEO, FRCVS
Centre for Equine Studies, Animal Health Trust, Newmarket, UK

SVEND E. KOLD DVM, Dr Med Vet, CUEW, RFP, MRCVS
Willesley Equine Clinic Ltd, Tetbury, UK

PAUL W. POULOS JR, DVM, PhD, DipACVR
Poulos Veterinary Imaging, Ukiah, California, USA

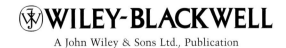

A John Wiley & Sons Ltd., Publication

This edition first published 2008
© 1993, 2000 by Blackwell Science Ltd, a Blackwell Publishing Company
© 2008 by Janet Butler, Christopher Colles, Sue Dyson, Svend Kold and Paul Poulos

Blackwell Publishing was acquired by John Wiley & Sons in February 2007. Blackwell's publishing programme has been merged with Wiley's global Scientific, Technical, and Medical business to form Wiley-Blackwell.

Registered office
John Wiley & Sons Ltd, The Atrium, Southern Gate, Chichester, West Sussex, PO19 8SQ, United Kingdom

Editorial office
9600 Garsington Road, Oxford, OX4 2DQ, United Kingdom
2121 State Avenue, Ames, Iowa 50014-8300, USA

For details of our global editorial offices, for customer services and for information about how to apply for permission to reuse the copyright material in this book please see our website at www.wiley.com/wiley-blackwell.

The right of the author to be identified as the author of this work has been asserted in accordance with the Copyright, Designs and Patents Act 1988.

Library of Congress Cataloging-in-Publication Data

Clinical radiology of the horse / Janet
    A. Butler . . . [et al.]. – 3rd ed.
        p. ; cm.
    Includes bibliographical references and index.
    ISBN-13: 978-1-4051-7108-3 (hardback : alk. paper)
    ISBN-10: 1-4051-7108-1 (hardback : alk. paper)   1. Horses–Anatomy–Atlases.
    2. Veterinary radiography–Atlases.   I. Butler, Janet A.
[DNLM: 1. Horse Diseases–radiography.   2. Horses–anatomy & histology. SF 951 C641 2008]
    SF765.C56   2008
    636.1′0891–dc22

                                        2008002416

A catalogue record for this book is available from the British Library.

Set in 10.5 on 14 pt Times
by SNP Best-set Typesetter Ltd., Hong Kong
Printed in Spain
by GraphyCems, Navarra, Spain

1   2008

Contents

Contents

About the Authors

Janet A. Butler

Jan has specialized in equine radiography and has 30 years' experience in this field. In 1975 she joined the Animal Health Trust in Newmarket where she gained considerable experience working with many internationally renowned veterinary surgeons. Since 1997 she has been working in private practice at the Willesley Equine Clinic in Gloucestershire.

Christopher M. Colles

Chris qualified from the Royal Veterinary College, London in 1971. After three years in mixed practice (where he obtained a Part I Diploma in Radiology) he joined the Animal Health Trust as a clinician in 1975. He was awarded a PhD for work on Navicular Disease in 1981, and has carried out research in many areas of equine orthopaedics and radiology, having a particular interest in the horse's foot. In 1988 he returned to practice, where he is a senior partner in Avonvale Veterinary Practice, specializing in equine orthopaedics. He is recognized by the Royal College of Veterinary Surgeons as a Specialist in Equine Orthopaedic Surgery. Chris was awarded an Honorary Fellowship of the Worshipful Company of Farriers in 2000 in recognition of his research into conditions of the foot, and involvement with farriery education.

Sue J. Dyson

After qualifying from the University of Cambridge in 1980, Sue worked for a year at New Bolton Center, University of Pennsylvania, and then spent a year in private practice in Pennsylvania. Sue then joined the Centre for Equine Studies of the Animal Health Trust, Newmarket, where she has specialized in lameness diagnosis and diagnostic imaging. Sue is recognized as a Specialist in Equine Orthopaedics by the Royal College of Veterinary Surgeons and holds the RCVS Diploma in Equine Orthopaedics. She has published widely on lameness, radiography ultrasonography, nuclear scintigraphy and magnetic resonance imaging.

Svend E. Kold

Svend qualified in 1981 in Copenhagen. He then spent over 10 years at the Animal Health Trust in Newmarket, where he completed his thesis on femoro-tibial subchondral bone cysts. After a sabbatical year at Colorado State University he joined the Willesley Equine Clinic, Gloucestershire, where he is now a partner. He specializes in lameness and orthopaedic surgery and is recognized as a Specialist in Equine Orthopaedic Surgery by the Royal College of Veterinary Surgeons. His time is spent mostly at the clinic seeing first opinion and referral cases. He has published regularly on orthopaedic subjects.

Paul W. Poulos

Following graduation from the University of California at Davis in 1960, Paul founded a private practice. In 1972 he returned to Davis to specialize in radiology where he was awarded Diplomate of the American College of Veterinary Radiology. He moved to the Royal Veterinary College of Stockholm, Sweden and was awarded a Veterinary Medicine Doctorate (PhD) for his thesis on osteochondrosis in 1977. He was Associate Professor at Radiology at the University of Utrecht, and on return to the USA, was Professor of Radiology at University of Florida. From 1983, he was chairman of the Department of Radiology. In 1990 Paul left academe to establish his own consulting practice, Poulos Veterinary Imaging, based in Ukiah, California. He has published widely on osteochondrosis, navicular disease and diseases of the fetlock.

Preface

As the knowledge of equine radiology and radiography progressed, the need for a textbook specifically in this field became more obvious. We set out with the intention of creating such a book, but more particularly a book that would be of practical help to general practitioners, as well as providing specialist information. The authors all practise equine radiography and radiology daily, and we have pooled our knowledge to write a book by consensus, rather than a multiauthor text with chapters contributed by different people. There is no doubt that writing this way has tested the patience and endurance of us all, but we hope that it has enhanced the value of the book to the reader.

This third edition of the book has been significantly enlarged to include new information, to provide additional illustrations and line diagrams, and to incorporate the most recent relevant literature references. The authors have collectively gained considerably more experience in a variety of clinical situations, and in some instances have changed their opinions in the light of new knowledge; the text has been updated accordingly. Technology has advanced with the development of computed and digital radiography and a new chapter is now devoted to this subject. We believe that digital techniques can potentially enhance our ability to obtain high-quality radiographs and to provide more diagnostic information. However, unless attention is paid to the basic details of radiography, image quality may in fact be inferior.

We have replaced some of the original illustrations by digital images to demonstrate the quality that can be achieved. It was not possible to substitute digital images of all lesions, nor did we feel that this was appropriate, because we hope this book will be used by veterinarians both with and without digital or computerized equipment.

The authors recognize that there have also been advances in other complementary imaging techniques such as nuclear scintigraphy, diagnostic ultrasonography, computed tomography and most particularly magnetic resonance imaging. Where appropriate, brief references have been made to these techniques, but the authors have continued to focus the text on radiography and radiology, and advise the reader to consult other more specialized texts for information on these methods. Appropriate references are listed in the Further Reading lists.

We would particularly like to thank J. G. Lane, BVetMed, DES, FRCVS, and I. G. Mayhew, BVSc, DipOVC, PhD, MRCVS, DACVIM, for their assistance in reading and providing specialist advice on parts of the text for the first edition.

Radiographs for the first and second editions were provided primarily from the Animal Health Trust, and the Faculty of Veterinary Medicine,

University of Florida. Additional images for the third edition have also been provided by Willesley Equine Clinic and Avonvale Veterinary Practice. We also thank the School of Veterinary Science, University of Bristol, for several radiographs of the head, and the College of Veterinary Medicine, Swedish University of Agricultural Sciences, Uppsala, for a number of radiographs of the thorax and feet. We thank J. Weaver, S. Stover and T. O'Brien and the *Equine Veterinary Journal* for figures illustrating soft tissue attachments in the fetlock and pastern regions and B. Maulet, I. Mayhew, E. Jones and T. Booth and the *Equine Veterinary Journal* for figures illustrating soft tissue attachments in the stifle. Finally we must thank D. R. Ellis, BVetMed, DEO, FRCVS, D. Hawkins DVM, M. Nowak DVM, P. Dixon MVB, PhD, MRCVS, R. Pilsworth VetMB, MRCVS, M. Ross DVM, A. Rucker, DVM, E. Santschi, DVM and T. Weinberger DVM for providing radiographs of a number of conditions that other archives could not provide.

We also thank Antonia Seymour of Blackwell Publishing for facilitating the production of this third edition. Her boundless enthusiasm for the project was a source of inspiration for us all.

Without the willing support of all the above, our many other colleagues within the profession from whom we have learnt, and our wives, husbands, partners, families and friends, this book could never have been written.

Jan Butler, Chris Colles,
Sue Dyson, Svend Kold
and Paul Poulos

Chapter 1
General principles

INTRODUCTION

There are many books that describe the principles of radiographic imaging. This book does not attempt to provide detailed information in this area, and readers who do not have a working knowledge of radiography are advised to consult one of the standard texts in order to obtain the necessary understanding of radiographic physics. This book does aim to provide up-to-date information specific to the horse. As various forms of competitive and pleasure riding become more popular, the demand on veterinarians to provide the highest quality of treatment is increasing. Radiography of the horse in sickness as well as in health, for insurance and purchase examinations, is increasing. The book is intended for all who radiograph horses, be they equine specialist, general practitioner or student. It gives information on radiographic techniques, equipment, positioning and views required to examine the various areas of the horse adequately. It also provides information on the normal radiographic anatomy of the immature and skeletally mature horse, variations, and incidental findings. Finally it gives information on the types of lesion that may be detected, with examples of as many of the more common problems as practicable, as well as brief clinical remarks where appropriate. The 'Further Reading' lists at the end of each chapter are not intended to be complete lists of every paper written on the subject of the chapter. They list references that the authors consider of particular interest, and that are complementary to the text. Many of these references give more detailed information in specific areas than can be justified in a textbook of this type.

Interpreting the clinical significance of radiographic changes is always difficult. We set out to indicate certain lesions that may always be regarded as clinically significant, and some that are known to have no clinical significance. The section in each chapter on 'Normal variation and incidental findings' attempts to differentiate between variations that have no clinical significance at any time (e.g. unossified radiolucent lines in the fibula, that represent remnants of separate centres of ossification) and those that may be clinically significant for a specific but limited period of time, and therefore require further clinical investigation to determine their significance (e.g. entheseophyte formation). The radiograph is only a reflection of the state of the tissues at the fraction of a second when they were radiographed. There are many findings which indicate a past event that has 'left its mark', but which is no longer clinically significant. For example, entheseophyte formation at the insertion of a ligament may indicate a sprain to that ligament at some time in the past. As entheseophytes take time to form, once they are visible on radiographs they no longer represent an acute injury, but are the result of an incident that occurred at least several weeks previously.

Radiography is a continually developing science, and as more powerful and sophisticated equipment becomes generally available, the diagnostic possibilities for veterinary practitioners become ever greater. It is hoped that this book will enable veterinarians to get the best out of their equipment, to obtain diagnostic radiographs, and to give a correct and meaningful diagnosis from the radiographs. The information in the text has been collated from the literature where possible, and complemented by the authors' experience. In some areas, however, there is no published work, or published information is contradictory. In these circumstances the authors have relied on their own collective experience, but have only presented information if all the authors are in agreement. (For example, reported physeal closure times for some physes vary widely between texts. The times given are based on the authors' experience of radiographic closure, in some cases backed up by radiographic examinations of animals specifically to aid completion of this text.) The authors are experienced clinicians who routinely obtain and read equine radiographs, and it is hoped that the broad range of experience that they offer to the reader will prove to be of practical value. It is important to remember that, as radiography is a developing science, 'new' lesions and radiographic views are continually being found and described, and no text can hope to be complete when published, let alone as time progresses.

This text has made use of current terminology. *Nomina Anatomica Veterinaria* (5th edition, 2005) was consulted for anatomical names. Radiological views are described using the method advocated by the American College of Veterinary Radiologists. Reference to Figure 1.1 may help to elucidate

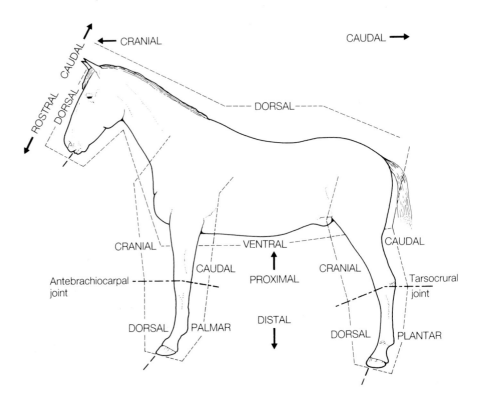

Figure 1.1 Correct nomenclature to describe various aspects of the horse.

the current terminology used. While at first sight this may appear cumbersome, it does provide a specific description of the views, which allows them to be reproduced accurately. Terminology in common usage is included in parentheses and serves only to maintain continuity with other texts and references. A glossary (Appendix C) is also included and lists former and current scientific terminology as well as common lay terms.

We have not set out to provide radiographs of every variation of all lesions. Rather we have given typical examples of lesions, and in the text have indicated how these may vary. We also hope that the reader will use this text as a basis to understand why certain types of lesions form, and the processes that are likely to cause them, so that an inexhaustible supply of radiographic variations would be superfluous. Although we have done our utmost to find radiographs that reproduce well, we ask the reader to remember that inevitably some detail is lost in the process of transferring radiographs to print, and in some cases the lesions depicted are far easier to detect on original films.

PRINCIPLES OF RADIOLOGY

The following paragraphs serve only as a reintroduction to the subjects of image production and differentiation. For more detailed information the reader is referred to the standard radiology texts. It is important that any radiograph is of maximum quality and yields sufficient detail to allow subtle radiographic lesions to be detected.

Production of x-rays

An x-ray beam consists of high-energy electromagnetic radiation. It is produced by accelerating a beam of electrons into a tungsten target. This results in the production of a beam of x-rays, and the liberation of considerable energy as heat. A smaller target area produces a narrower beam of x-rays, and better definition on the resultant radiograph than a larger area of the target. The area of the target struck by electrons is called the 'focal spot'. Ninety-nine percent of the energy from the electron beam is given off as heat, not x-rays, and so there is a risk of the target being melted. Dissipating this heat and keeping the target as small as possible are major factors in design of x-ray tubes. For generators with a large output, the target in the tube is the edge of a disc. By rotating the disc at very high speeds during x-ray production, the area being heated is continually being changed, allowing a small focal spot in spite of high output. This is standard in large static x-ray generators. Smaller mobile or portable generators generally have fixed targets, which does limit the output possible. Any x-ray beam is made up of photons of mixed wavelengths. The older half- and full-wave rectification in small x-ray generators resulted in very marked variations in the energy of the individual photons of the x-ray beam. The high-frequency generators currently available have greatly improved the consistency of the x-ray beam produced, causing less scatter and a better resultant image.

[3]

Production of a radiographic image

An image is created by detecting the differential absorption of x-rays that pass through an object placed in the path of the primary x-ray beam. The x-rays that pass right through the object are either detected using conventional x-ray film, or digital images are created (see Chapter 2). The number of x-rays that are absorbed by a given thickness of a specific tissue varies between tissues, and thus affects the number of x-rays passing through to form the image. For example it is more difficult to penetrate bone than air, and therefore less x-rays reach the film if they have to penetrate bone rather than air. The areas of the image relating to relatively unobstructed x-rays are black, whereas the areas protected by bone, which absorbs or deflects a proportion of the x-rays, are paler or white. Intermediate densities of tissues produce variable shades of grey. Fat is the least dense tissue, and gives relatively black tones, with muscle and bone giving increasingly light tones. It is the juxtaposition of these tissues of varying densities that allows differentiation of form and structure.

Exposure factors

Exposure factors affect the *opacity* and *contrast* of the radiographic image. The quantity of photons (x-rays) reaching the film (or digital sensor) affects opacity (blackness). This is primarily controlled by the milliampere (mA), higher mA resulting in a greater number of photons being produced in the x-ray beam. By lengthening the time for which the beam is produced, the total number of photons is increased in proportion, i.e. doubling the time, doubling the number of photons reaching the film. This is normally recorded for any exposure as mAs, i.e. mA times time (milliampere seconds).

A major factor influencing the number of photons reaching the film is the distance of the film from the focal spot. This is known as the focus–film distance (FFD), or the source–image distance (SID). Because the x-ray beam spreads out to cover a two-dimensional area, the number of photons reaching the film falls as a square of the distance. This means that changing the distance by a relatively small amount can have a marked affect on image opacity, although it has only a minor affect on contrast, because all areas experience a similar percentage drop in numbers of photons reaching the film.

The kilovoltage (kV) governs the energy of the x-rays and their ability to penetrate through tissue. The higher the kV, the greater the energy of the x-rays, and the greater their ability to penetrate tissues. This has some affect on opacity, but more importantly affects contrast. Soft tissues such as fat and muscle absorb limited numbers of x-rays, even of low kV. Bone however absorbs far more x-rays of low kV than high kV, so there is a relatively large difference in numbers of x-rays passing through the soft tissues compared to the bone using low kV, giving relatively high contrast. Increasing the kV allows relatively more x-rays to penetrate through the bone, and so affects both opacity and contrast. A low kV produces a high-contrast image but has low exposure latitude; therefore the exposure values are critical for a diagnostic image. In contrast a high kV results in low contrast, but has wider exposure latitude and the exact exposure levels are less critical.

To obtain a radiograph with the same opacity as an original but decreased contrast, halve the mAs and increase the kV by 15% (approximately 10 kV). Conversely, to increase contrast levels, double the mAs and reduce the kV by 15% to achieve the same opacity. Normally for good bone detail the kilovoltage should be less than 70 kV. Attenuation of the x-ray beam is heavily dependent on the atomic number of the tissues, and it is desirable that photoelectric absorption predominates. Increasing the kV also results in more forward scatter (see Scatter below).

X-ray film and image intensifying screens

Details of the structure of film, image intensifying screens and chemistry cannot be covered here, but are readily available in other radiographic textbooks. The principle however is important to an understanding of radiography. In simple terms a film consists of a cellulose acetate sheet coated with a light- (or x-ray-) sensitive emulsion (a layer of complex silver halide crystals). When these crystals are subjected to x-rays (or light), they undergo partial chemical reduction, creating a latent image. Submersion in developer completes the chemical reduction. Subsequently when immersed in fixer, the reduced crystals are insoluble and remain on the film, but the unexposed crystals are dissolved, leaving the visible image. To make the system more sensitive, it is usual for the film to be placed in a cassette, which places an image intensifying screen on either side of the film. The screens fluoresce when stimulated by x-rays, and because the film is much more sensitive to light than x-rays, an image can be produced with a reduced x-ray exposure.

Important variables include the type of film being used and the compatibility of the screens, which intensify the image. It is important to match the spectral output of the screen with the spectral sensitivity of the film (see Appendix B). The large number of film and screen combinations available is beyond the scope of this book. The clinician should rely on a veterinary radiologist or knowledgeable sales person to help decide which film–screen combination is best suited to the x-ray machine and the practice, although Appendix B gives some guidelines. With a high-output x-ray machine (100 kV, 100 mAs), it is worthwhile investing in high-definition screens for use with single emulsion, relatively slow film, for distal extremity work. This gives excellent detail, but is unsuitable for low-output machines, because long exposure times result in loss of definition through movement blur. Rare earth screens are essential for obtaining high-quality images proximal to the carpus and tarsus. Old screens are like old horses, they collect scars and lose performance as they age, and therefore should be replaced on a regular basis in order to maintain the optimum level of performance. It is also important that screens are cleaned regularly, to prevent the build-up of dust and extraneous materials within the cassette, which can result in white spots and lines on processed films.

Film processing

Good darkroom practice is an important consideration in the final quality of the radiograph but is often overlooked. Correct processing, whether manual or automatic, plays a major role. Standard darkroom procedures are available in any standard radiology text and are not covered here. There are however some processing errors that often cause film artefacts (see Appendix B) and thus affect interpretation. The following is a brief review of some of the basics principles that most often affect film quality and interpretation, especially when hand processing.

Film fogging

The most common darkroom problem whether using hand or automatic processing is fogging of the film either by light leaking into the darkroom, or improper darkroom lighting. Regardless of whether blue- or green-sensitive films are used, never rely on red or ruby bulbs as the source of darkroom lighting. For blue-sensitive film use a Wratten Series 6B filter with a 7–10 Watt bulb and for green-sensitive film use a Kodak GS1 filter with a 7–10 Watt bulb. In general the Kodak GS1 works with both blue- and green-sensitive film. The safelight should be a least 1 metre from the working area. There are two methods to check film for possible fogging:

1 In the darkroom place a sheet of film on the counter, then place an object on the film. Turn on the darkroom safelight and wait for approximately 30 seconds. This is the time it normally takes to place a film in a processor or on a hanger. Process the film as normal. If the darkroom is adequately dark and the safelight is suitable for the film, the film will be perfectly clear after developing. If the filter is incorrect or there is light leakage in the room, there will be fogging of the film around the object and the area covered by the object will be clear.

2 Expose a film in the cassette to an x-ray beam of 1–2 mAs and 40–50 kVp. This increases the sensitivity of the film. In the dark room place the exposed film on the counter and cover two thirds of the film with cardboard. Turn on the safelight for 30 seconds then move the cardboard over another third and continue the exposure for an additional 30 seconds. Process the film normally and compare the areas for fogging as described above.

Processing

There are three stages in the processing cycle that affect the final quality of the radiograph:
- Developer – converts exposed silver halide grains to metallic silver
- Fixer – converts unexposed, undeveloped silver halides into a form that can be removed from the emulsion and clear the film
- Washing – removes residual chemicals from film emulsion

Important factors are the temperature and dilution of the chemicals and the time the film is in the developer and fixer.

1 Prepare the chemicals to the correct working dilution and agitate to ensure even mixing. Temperature is absolutely correlated with processing time. Deviation from time and temperature guidelines results in under- or over-development and loss of detail. At the optimal temperature of 20°C (68°F) developing time should be 5 minutes. A variation in time should be calculated for other temperatures. The temperature of the solutions should be checked after the rinse water has been on for at least 15 minutes. The darkroom should be kept at a constant temperature to assist in maintaining the solutions at the ideal temperature.

2 During development, fixing and washing, agitate the film several times to remove any air bubbles that cling to the emulsion. Air bubbles cause light or dark spots, or circular artefacts on the film, depending upon which solution the bubbles occurred in. Care must be taken to prevent films touching or being scraped by the hangers during agitation in order to prevent scratches of the wet (swollen) emulsion, or the development of kissing defects. A kissing defect occurs when two films cling to each other during any phase of the developing process, resulting in an area of incorrect processing. This can also occur when two films overlap each other in an automatic processor. When processing several films, all films should be loaded into hangers prior to being processed in order to maintain optimal timing.

3 Chemical levels must be high enough to cover the film in the hanger. Low chemical levels result in portions of the films being undeveloped which can result in loss of important information. To avoid chemical carry-over, in order to maintain developer and fixer strengths, fluid should drain from the film and hanger prior to placement in each solution, including the rinse tank. Loss of strength of developer results in underexposed film, while loss of fixer strength results in yellowing with age. Developer should be replenished after every session of processing to maintain it at correct working strength.

4 Developer deteriorates when not in use, therefore it must be changed regularly. If not kept covered the developer oxidizes. In either case this results in underdevelopment.

5 If it is essential to examine a wet film, wait until fixing is complete then quickly rinse the film and view it. Remember that wet films have swollen emulsion and detail is lost until the film is dry, when the halide crystals will have coalesced into a more definitive image!

6 The final wash is an important part of the processing cycle to remove residual chemicals from the emulsion. This prevents discolouration and fading of the image.

AUTOMATIC PROCESSING

The advantages of an automatic processor over manual processing are considerable. There is absolute consistency of processing, which enables a consistent estimate of exposure values, and results in marked improvement in film quality. There are also benefits of economy and speed. With automatic

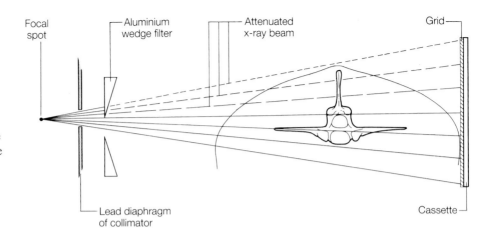

Focal spot — Aluminium wedge filter — Attenuated x-ray beam — Grid — Lead diaphragm of collimator — Cassette

Figure 1.2 Use of an aluminium wedge filter placed between the x-ray machine collimator and the object to be radiographed. The upper leaves of the filter placed in the x-ray beam reduce the exposure of the upper part of the beam.

processing a dry film is available to read within 60–90 seconds compared with approximately 1 hour for manually processed film. Both manual and automatic processing require proper upkeep and maintenance of equipment to ensure diagnostic quality films. Regular maintenance of the processor is important as is making sure that processing fluids are fresh and in adequate supply. The most common problems with an automatic processor occur when upkeep is not maintained.

Radiographic practice

In several parts of the following text, reference is made to an aluminium wedge filter (Figure 1.2). This is placed immediately in front of the x-ray tube, and absorbs a proportion of the x-rays. It allows the intensity of the beam to be reduced in specific areas. It is of particular value when radiographing parts of the horse that show a marked change in soft-tissue thickness from one side of the film to the other, e.g. the thoracolumbar spine or stifle, but may be of less value when used with digital systems.

Exposure chart

It is advantageous to record the exposure settings used for each image, and gradually build an exposure chart. This should include a record of the size and age of the horse, the area radiographed, and the exposures and the film–screen combination used. This allows better and more consistent radiographs to be obtained, and also provides a basis for estimating the required exposures for animals of different sizes and ages. When creating this chart, it is important to maintain a constant FFD. A reduction in FFD increases the radiation reaching the screen by a square of the change in distance (necessitating a reduction in the exposure factors). An increase in distance has the opposite effect. Generally in equine radiography a FFD of 75–100 cm is used. Note that single emulsion film is particularly sensitive to changes in radiation dose; a slight change in FFD can therefore have a relatively big effect on exposure.

Grids

Most of the radiation during an exposure passes through the subject and exposes the film, or is absorbed by the tissues. Some radiation however is deflected (termed 'scatter') and this results in a low background exposure over the entire film, causing reduced film contrast. Good collimation of the primary beam reduces the amount of scatter. The effect of scatter can be reduced by placing a grid in front of the cassette to absorb the scattered radiation. As a rough guide, grids are generally only needed if the area being radiographed exceeds 11 cm in thickness. Thus equine extremities below the carpus and tarsus usually do not require the use of a grid. Grids are generally not required for soft-tissue evaluation, and may be contraindicated in this situation. There are numerous types of grid, and advice on the best one for any specific situation is beyond the scope of this text. The disadvantages of a grid are that they increase the exposure required and produce lines on the films, which are sometimes found objectionable when reading the radiograph. If a focused grid is used, the x-ray beam must be perpendicular to the grid, centred on it, and at the correct FFD. When grids are of value, this is noted in the discussion of the projections described in the following text. Grids used with digital radiography have particular problems, and can cause serious image artefacts. The reader is advised to obtain specialist advice before acquiring grids for use with digital systems.

Preparation and positioning

Preparation of the patient is essential to good radiography. Quiet and careful handling reduces movement, and sedation is often beneficial. Blinkers, blocking the horse's line of vision, may make it less apprehensive. Cotton wool earplugs or background music may make the horse less aware of the noise of the x-ray machine. Areas to be radiographed should be brushed to remove mud from the coat, which can produce confusing artefacts. For radiographs of the feet, the shoes normally need to be removed and the feet trimmed to remove loose horn and dirt.

It is important to ensure correct positioning of the horse before acquiring the radiograph. A small deviation in limb position can result in poor quality images with misleading information, making accurate interpretation difficult (Figure 1.3). In a well positioned radiograph, the x-ray beam is perpendicular to the cassette to minimize image distortion.

Radiation safety

Radiation safety, i.e. ensuring that personnel around the horse do not receive doses of radiation, is extremely important. There are codes of practice available in different countries, but the basic principles can be summarized as follows:

1 Keep the number of people present when radiographing a horse to the absolute minimum required for its safe handling.

2 Use appropriate restraint of the horse to keep it still during exposures (so that repeat exposure to radiation is not necessary). Sedation may be required.

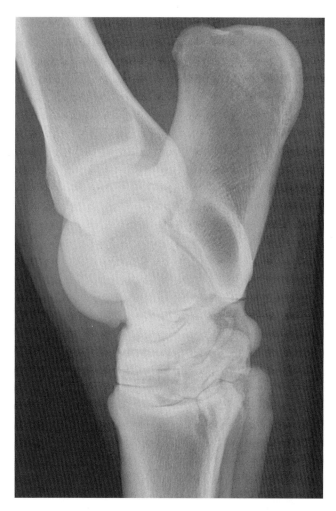

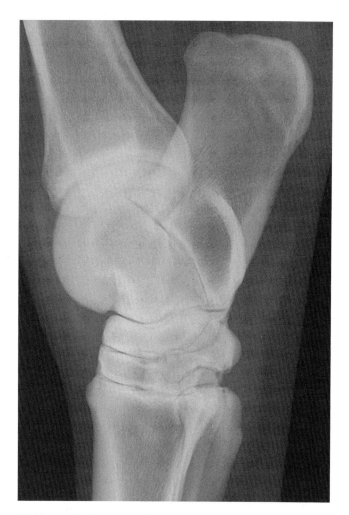

Figure 1.3(a) Lateromedial radiographic view of a hock of a 7-year-old riding horse with distension of the tarsocrural joint. This radiograph is not of diagnostic quality. The horse was standing base wide during image acquisition and as a result this is not a true lateromedial view. There is considerable overlap of the joint spaces of the talocalcaneal-centroquartal, centrodistal and tarsometatarsal joints. The trochleas of the talus are not superimposed.

Figure 1.3(b) Lateromedial radiographic view of a hock of a 7-year-old riding horse, the same hock as in Figure 1.3a. This is a well positioned image and the joint spaces of the talocalcaneal-centroquartal, centrodistal and tarsometatarsal joints are clearly defined. The trochleas of the talus are superimposed.

3 Use cassette holders whenever possible. Certain views, where 'patient tolerance' is low, may prompt the hand holding of cassettes. This may be justified if it reduces the repetition of radiographs or prevents the horse panicking. If it is essential to hand hold a cassette, then large cassettes should be used, with the x-ray beam well collimated, and the holder's gloved hands as far from the primary x-ray beam as possible.

4 The primary x-ray beam should be well collimated, and a light beam diaphragm used to enable maximum collimation. *No part of any attending person, even if covered with protective clothing, should be placed in the primary beam.* Protective lead clothing protects from scattered radiation only, not the primary beam. Remember that the primary beam continues through the patient and cassette, and personnel standing on the opposite side of the patient are at risk.

[10]

5 All personnel who must remain present during radiography must wear protective gowns, and if near the primary beam should also wear gloves or similar hand and arm protection, and a thyroid protector.

6 All personnel working with and around x-ray machines should be monitored using a film badge or dosemeter system.

Examination for purchase

Because of the general acceptance of this text world wide, it is impossible to write a comprehensive section that covers all areas of the radiographic examination included as part of a pre-purchase examination in all countries. When making such an examination, it is necessary to take into account many variable factors such as the breed and intended use, as well as considering both the country of origin and the country to which an animal is being sold. This carries many different legal implications and is therefore well beyond a text that is limited to radiology. Guidelines regarding this have been published, and the reader is referred to 'Further Reading', page 35.

As a general guide, the radiographic portion of a pre-purchase examination must first take into account the general health, age and condition of the horse. It is important that the previous and intended use(s) of the horse are considered, with special emphasis on conditions prevalent in the relevant breed or use of the horse. The radiographic evaluation should follow the physical examination, to include areas that might be expected to face the greatest stress in the performance of the expected use, and to investigate potentially significant findings discovered during the physical examination.

As always it is essential that if adequate interpretation is to be made, film quality is good, and an adequate number of views is obtained to evaluate the specific area(s) of concern. No simple guide can be given for this, except to say that as a general rule there must be at least two views of a suspected lesion, and it is clinically better to have too many views than too few, bearing in mind the overriding importance of radiation safety. When imaging apparently normal joints (such as hock or fetlock) it is generally necessary to obtain dorsopalmar, lateromedial and two oblique views of each joint. If the horse is to be insured, the insurance company may have specific minimum requirements for views to be obtained. Sales companies for Thoroughbred racehorses in training frequently specify what views of which joints are required. Some countries have a designated set of radiographs that are obtained as part of a pre-purchase examination. If a client is purchasing a horse abroad they should be advised that the radiographs obtained may not be the same as in their own country, where additional views may be considered necessary to provide a comprehensive examination.

A report on pre-purchase radiographs should begin with a clear identification of the animal examined. This must be followed by sections on each area examined, stating the views obtained and giving a clear and concise description of the radiographic findings, starting with the most significant finding. Finally an opinion on the potential significance of any abnormalities should be provided, relative to the intended use of the horse. If for any reason the radiographic study is limited, this should be clearly stated in a disclaimer. For example, 'The owner refused to allow sedation and therefore the examination of the foot is incomplete'; or, 'The study is compromised by the presence of shoes which could not be removed due to permission being refused'. In extensive reports it is useful to finish with a clear summary of significant findings relevant to the potential use of the horse if purchased.

Records and labelling

Radiographic images and reports are part of medical records, and should be stored carefully with patient records. In the United States both radiographs and radiographic reports must be kept for legal reasons for a minimum of 7 years, and this is a good principle to apply. The quality of the films will reflect on the quality of the practice, and this becomes particularly important when films may be viewed by other practitioners, for example in a pre-purchase examination. All films and digital images should be clearly identified with permanent labels at the time of acquisition.

With the increasing use of radiography, and the rise in litigation involving veterinarians worldwide, it is essential that radiographs are carefully labelled. This should be done photographically on the film, either by the use of one of the special tapes produced for this purpose, attached to the cassette when the film is exposed, or by a labelling light-box system in the darkroom. Labels should include as a minimum:
1 The identity of the horse and owner
2 The limb radiographed
3 The date
4 Lateral or medial markers where relevant should be placed on the cassette
Ideally the veterinary practice and view employed should also be identified. Digital systems usually produce such labelling automatically.

It is essential that a complete examination is carried out, with an adequate number of views of each area involved. The exposures must be correct to demonstrate any lesions present, and the radiographs must be of diagnostic quality. An inadequate examination may be at best inconclusive and at worst totally misleading. Such examinations in the hands of the legal profession may prove devastating!

PRINCIPLES OF RADIOGRAPHIC INTERPRETATION

It is important to read radiographic films when they are dry. The emulsion swells when wet and detail cannot be appreciated on wet films.

It is helpful if radiographs are always viewed using the same orientation, i.e. with the horse facing to the viewer's left, medial on the left, and when appropriate the left side on the right. This aids interpretation, as only one image need be remembered for each area radiographed. (This varies slightly from the convention that any film should be viewed as if the examiner was looking at the patient face on, e.g. the left forelimb is viewed with medial to the left, and the right forelimb with medial to the right.) The number of views required for any area varies, and is mentioned in the text. It is important to obtain an adequate number of views to ensure that no lesion is missed, and an attempt to compromise with fewer views is a false economy. The use of 'special' views, e.g. obliques and skyline views, of suspected lesions can be very rewarding.

Adequate radiographic interpretation is dependent on complete and systematic evaluation of all of the information that is found on the image. Films should be viewed on a viewing box, in a room with subdued light. This optimizes the ability of the reader to differentiate structures and to obtain the maximum information from a film. The darker the film, the more important it becomes that the conditions under which it is read are ideal.

Initially the film should be evaluated from a distance of several feet before viewing closely, in order to get an overall impression before concentrating on details. Areas of diffuse, subtle change in radiopacity are usually more readily identified from a distance than close up. Masking the light around the edge of the radiograph also improves the ability to read a film, as do high-intensity illumination devices.

Digital images should be viewed on high-definition flat screens, again in a room with subdued light. As with film, it is helpful to mask the image to remove light areas around the point of interest. In many systems it is then possible to select the area of most relevance, and to adjust contrast and brightness of the region concerned to aid evaluation of a wide range of tissue densities. Most systems also allow for enlargement of the whole image, or of specific regions of interest (see Chapter 2).

With film or digital images, start by assessing the image itself:
- Is the quality of the image adequate for interpretation?
- Is the view correctly positioned to allow correct interpretation?
- Are there any processing or other artefacts (e.g. mud on the horse) that will influence interpretation?

Then move on to assess the area radiographed:
- Is there any soft-tissue swelling?
- Is there any alteration of opacity of the soft tissues?
- What is the approximate age of the patient?

Finally look at the outline of the bones and their detailed internal structure:
- If an 'abnormality' is identified, ensure that it is real – can it be seen on another view? Can it be explained by positioning or overlap of other bones or soft-tissue structures? Is it a variation rather than an abnormality, e.g. the position and shape of a nutrient foramen can vary considerably. Could a radiolucent zone be explained by introduction of air during a previously performed local analgesic technique (Figure 1.4)? Intra-articular gas appears as a semicircular or more diffuse radiolucent area, often in the proximal part of a joint, whereas extra-articular gas appears as a linear radiolucency. These lucencies may persist for up to 48 hours after injection. Would additional views aid or complete adequate evaluation?

[13]

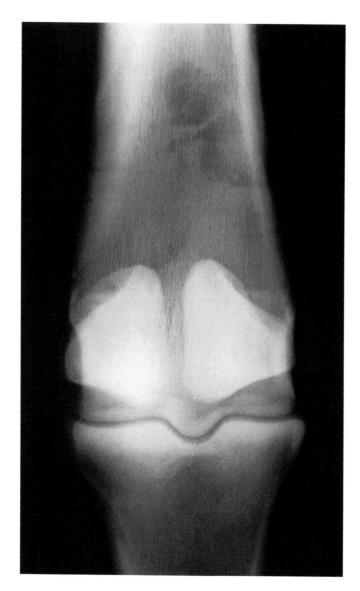

Figure 1.4 Dorsopalmar view of the distal metacarpal region and metacarpophalangeal joint of a mature horse. There are radiolucent areas superimposed over the third metacarpal bone. These gas shadows are the result of inadvertent introduction of air into the metacarpophalangeal joint while performing intra-articular analgesia. Such lucent areas may persist for up to 48 hours.

● If it is a true radiographic lesion, describe it in radiographic terms. In this process of description it is often possible to determine if it is an active or inactive process. In general, terms like smooth, regular and well margin-ated (defined) lead towards a conclusion of normal, benign or long-standing lesions. Terms such as roughened, irregular, sharp, poorly demarcated or destructive, lead to a conclusion of active disease. If the process is consid-ered to be pathological, then think what pathological process could cause this change and then consider what diseases could cause this type of pathology.

If films are obtained to confirm the presence of a specific disease or disease process and are not completely evaluated, the severity of the condi-tion, complications of the process or other concurrent lesions may be over-looked. Thus to read radiographs successfully, it is important to relate the changes seen to known behaviour of the tissues under consideration, rather than relating the radiographic appearance to a clinical condition seen before. The latter method relies heavily on experience and does not allow interpretation of changes that have not been previously encountered. It is important to remember that each radiograph can only represent a fraction of a second in the life of the patient, and the development of a disease process. It is a static image of a dynamic process. When a radiograph is read, all the changes from the normal should be considered and used to build up an impression that can then be related to disease processes known to occur in the region. For accurate interpretation it is important to take into account factors such as the period of time for which the clinical signs have been present, the age, sex and breed of the patient, and the validity of the history and possible complicating factors. A working diagnosis can then be formed, which will complement any laboratory findings and other imaging techniques, and help to confirm a clinical diagnosis. There is no substitute for a good clinical history and examination, and radiographs should only be used as an aid to the clinical diagnosis.

It is beneficial to have bone specimens available when reading radiographs, particularly oblique views. An anatomy book and a library of normal radiographs of each anatomical area at different ages are invaluable. If problems are encountered in evaluating an area, it is often helpful to obtain a similar radiograph of the contralateral limb for comparison, thus providing a perfect age-, sex- and breed-matched radiograph. Remember that, in the neonate, some structures are not ossified and therefore cannot be visualized. More confusing is the appearance of partially ossified structures (e.g. incompletely ossified subchondral tissues have an irregular opacity, which may seem similar to the radiographic appearance of infection). The normal radiographic appearance of the structures of immature animals is therefore described in each chapter.

Radiographs are only one part of a jigsaw puzzle and may be used for several purposes:
- To confirm, refute or suggest a diagnosis
- To give information on progression and severity of a condition, and aid formation of a prognosis
- To add information regarding size, shape, position, alignment and possibly duration of a lesion

When reading a radiograph the result must be fitted into the general picture presented to the clinician. It is one aid to diagnosis that the clinician has available. In some cases special views or contrast studies may provide valuable additional information. There are many other complementary imaging techniques (e.g. ultrasonography, nuclear scintigraphy, computed tomography and magnetic resonance imaging) and other sources of clinical information that are available. The radiograph is an aid to diagnosis and not the ultimate diagnosis in itself.

One of the most difficult questions to answer is how long a lesion has been present. This is often of importance, but can seldom be answered with any degree of certainty. Minimum times for certain lesions to develop can be estimated, but the time for which a lesion has been present often remains uncertain. The following pointers may be of value:
- Osteophyte formation of any type is not normally visible, even under optimum conditions, in less than 3 weeks.

- Treatment after injury may delay osteophyte formation.
- Incomplete or fissure fractures may take up to 2 weeks to become visible.
- Active bone changes are characterized by lesions with irregular or fuzzy margins, which may be less opaque than the parent bone.
- Inactive bone changes are generally smooth, regular and uniformly opaque.
- Large productive changes may take months to form and become smooth in outline.
- An old inactive bone lesion may not indicate current disease, although it may be present in the same region as a current problem.
- Bone models due to the stress applied to it (Wolff's law). Non-stressed bone does not model.
- Scars in bone, as in any other tissue, do not model.

It should be noted that the terms remodel and model are frequently used incorrectly in radiology (see Appendix C: Glossary). In this text, the term remodel is frequently employed because of its common usage. Modelling is, however, a more correct term, compatible with changes detectable radiographically (and histologically).

RADIOLOGICAL APPEARANCE OF PHYSIOLOGICAL CHANGES AND SOME COMMON PATHOLOGICAL LESIONS

Bone changes

The basic ability of bone to respond to stimuli is affected by various factors, such as diet, disease and the physiological state of other organs such as the lungs, kidneys and gastrointestinal tract.

It is important to remember that the normal bone status varies throughout life. During the period of skeletal growth, there is increased bone formation relative to resorption. The skeleton of the young individual lacks density and is more pliable (35% mineral to 65% matrix and cells). As the individual matures, the density gradually increases (approaching 65% mineral and 35% matrix and cells). With advancing age the bone–mineral balance changes towards decreased formation and increased resorption.

Although it is common to think of bone as being largely calcium, the mineral content of bone is roughly 35% calcium, 17% phosphorus and 12% copper and other minerals. Radiologically it is not possible to detect a decrease in mineralization of less than approximately 30% of the total mineral content, and therefore changes in bone mineralization may be undetectable radiographically early in a disease process. Diagnostic ultrasonography may be helpful in early detection of some bony changes, e.g. periosteal new bone formation.

It is important to remember that some changes reflect past history, rather than the response to current stimuli; thus some radiographic lesions may no longer have clinical significance, but persist as incidental findings.

[16]

Wolff's law states that bone models in relation to the stresses placed on it, and modelling is dependent upon bone function and the distribution of the load. Forces are applied to bone at the sites of attachment of ligaments and tendons or through the joints. Application of a load may deform the part concerned. Deformity is dependent upon the degree of the stress and the number of loading cycles.

When evaluating radiographs it should be remembered that bone is a living dynamic tissue that can only respond in a finite predictable way to an infinite number of outside stimuli or insults.

Demineralization of bone

GENERALIZED DEMINERALIZATION

Generalized demineralization or osteoporosis may be recognized by: thinning of the cortices; coarser, more obvious trabecular pattern; apparent radiographic overexposure due to reduced bone density (check the FFD, exposure values and processing technique). With digital imaging, exposure differences are more difficult to detect, and evaluation of the cortices and the trabecular pattern becomes more important.

Generalized demineralization (Figure 1.5) may result from a mobilization of minerals because of a need elsewhere in the body, e.g. in pregnancy, dietary inadequacy or metabolic imbalance (e.g. secondary nutritional hyperparathyroidism), or renal disease. Alternatively the lack of mineral may indicate that the patient is very young or very old.

LOCALIZED DEMINERALIZATION

Loss of mineral in a single limb indicates a process limited to that area, e.g. the loss of mineral in one leg may relate to disuse osteopenia (Figure 1.6). Mineral is lost due to muscular inactivity and/or reduction in weight bearing. It should be compared with the contralateral limb if a generalized disease might be implicated.

FOCAL DEMINERALIZATION

Focal loss of bone (Figure 1.7) may indicate the presence of infection, neoplastic invasion, or replacement of bone by fibrous tissue as a result of a previous disease process (this may be considered to be equivalent to a scar in bone). It is also seen: as an osteochondral defect in osteochondrosis (although this may actually represent delayed mineralization rather than demineralization); in osseous cyst-like lesions; as subchondral bone loss in degenerative joint disease; in association with vascular abnormalities; and along fracture lines. It may also result from continuous pressure on bone, as in chronic proliferative synovitis or other space-occupying mass.

[17]

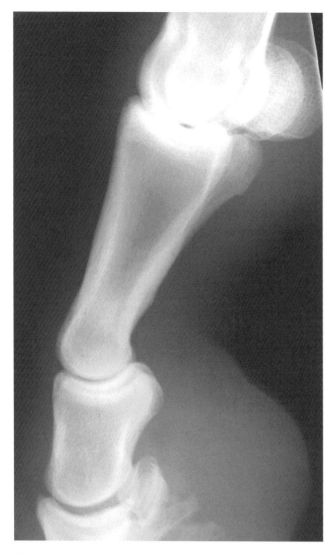

Figure 1.5 Slightly oblique lateromedial view of the distal limb of a mature pony, showing generalized demineralization due to secondary nutritional hyperparathyroidism. Note the thin poorly defined cortices and the very prominent trabecular pattern (compare with Figure 3.78c–f, pages 159–162, of a normal metacarpophalangeal joint).

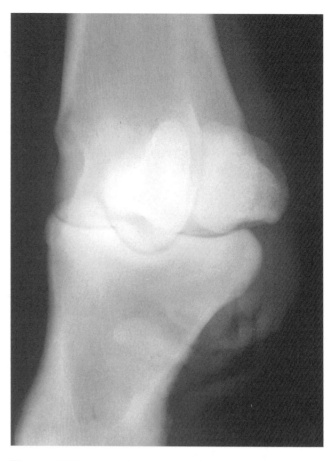

Figure 1.6 Dorsolateral-plantaromedial oblique view of a metatarsophalangeal joint of a mature horse. Note the extremely obvious trabecular pattern in the lateral proximal sesamoid bone due to disuse osteopenia. The horse had not borne full weight on the left hindlimb for the preceding 6 months due to severe navicular disease and adhesions between the deep digital flexor tendon and the navicular bone. Note also the opacities on the plantar distal aspect of the joint, which represent the ergot.

Increased bone production

Increased bone production may result in increased bone density and thus radiopacity.

A generalized increase in bone density may be due to fluorine poisoning or a hereditary disease such as osteopetrosis. In some species, but as far as is known not the horse, mineral deposition could indicate hypervitaminosis A.

CORTICAL THICKENING

Wolff's law states that bone models in relation to the stresses placed on it, and is dependent on its function and the distribution of the load. Cortical

[18]

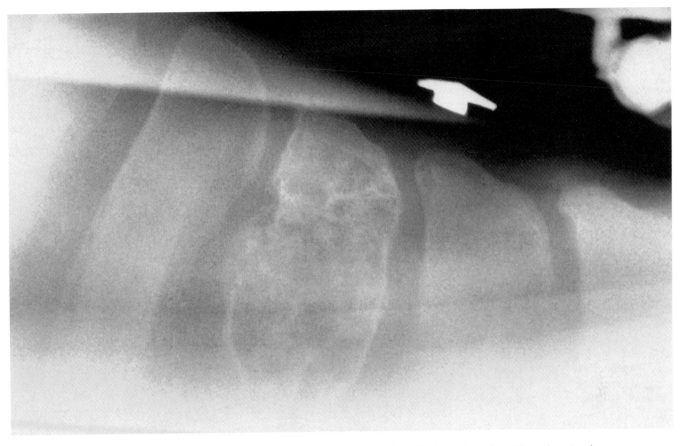

Figure 1.7 Lateral view of the summits of the dorsal spinous processes in the mid-thoracic region. There is extensive demineralization of the dorsal spinous process of the ninth thoracic vertebra. The cortex is also irregular in outline.

thickness, particularly of the third metacarpal and metatarsal bones, changes from a young, skeletally immature, untrained horse to a mature trained horse. The dorsal cortex becomes significantly thicker than the palmar cortex. If a horse has a marked conformational abnormality, such as 'off set knees', the distal limb bones will model accordingly, resulting in increased thickness of the cortices of the regions of the bones carrying increased load.

FOCAL NEW BONE FORMATION

An osteophyte is a small spur of bone on a joint margin. Osteophyte formation occurs in response to various stimuli. The time for osteophyte development after a stimulus varies between individuals and depends upon the inciting cause. It may take as little as 2 weeks, or may take several weeks. Osteophyte formation with uniform opacity and a smooth outline is likely to be longstanding and inactive. More lucent osteophyte formation, or a formation with a more lucent tip, is likely to be actively developing. *Periarticular osteophytes* may be associated with intra-articular pathology, and develop at the margins of articular cartilage and periarticular bone (Figure 1.8). They also develop as a consequence of joint instability.

[19]

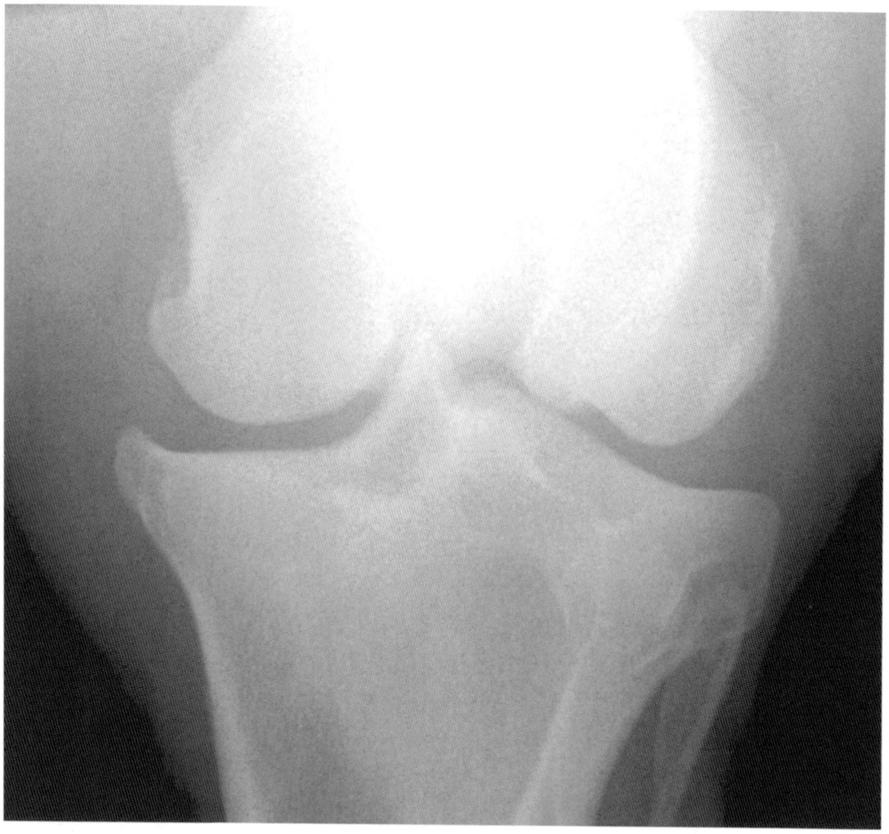

Figure 1.8 Caudocranial radiographic view of a stifle of a 14-year-old Welsh Section D Cob. Medial is to the left. There is a moderately sized osteophyte on the proximomedial aspect of the tibia, reflecting osteoarthritis. Lameness was improved by intra-articular analgesia of the femorotibial and femoropatellar joints. Arthroscopic evaluation revealed a tear of the medial meniscus and severe fibrillation of the cranial ligament of the medial meniscus.

Entheseophytes are spurs of bone that develop where tendons, ligaments or joint capsules attach to bone. They represent the response of bone to stress applied through these structures, whether it is tearing of a portion of a ligament, chronic stress applied by a tendon, capsular traction, or chronic capsular distension. It may be difficult to differentiate between osteophytes and entheseophytes in some areas.

PERIOSTEAL OR ENDOSTEAL NEW BONE

Periosteal or endosteal new bone formation results from inflammation of the periosteum or endosteum. This may result from a fracture (the callus forming endosteal and periosteal new bone), trauma, infection, abnormal stress at a soft tissue attachment, or tumour formation.

SCLEROSIS

Sclerosis is a localized increased opacity of the bone due to increased bone mass within existing bone. It is most readily recognized in trabecular bone, and occurs in response to several stimuli including:
- Stress (e.g. subchondral sclerosis in degenerative joint disease)
- An attempt to wall off infection (e.g. in the medullary cavity adjacent to an area of osteomyelitis, in response to osteitis of cortical bone adjacent to the site of infection, or adjacent to sequestration)

• To support or protect a weakened area (e.g. sclerosis surrounding an osseous cyst-like lesion)

Bone lesions

Physitis (epiphysitis)

Physitis (or physeal dysplasia) is the term that should be used to describe abnormal widening and bony irregularity at the epiphyseal and metaphyseal margins of the growth plate in skeletally immature horses. The metaphysis of the bone is broadened and asymmetrical. There is sclerosis of the metaphysis adjacent to the physis, which may be more irregular in appearance than normal, reflecting retained cartilage cones. The cortices of the metaphysis may be abnormally thick. Soft-tissue swelling over the area of involvement is usually present, and there may be an associated angular limb deformity. These changes are secondary either to rapid cartilage production or to defects in mineralization within the primary spongiosa.

Although any physis may be involved in this process, physitis is most commonly associated with the distal radial (see Figure 5.19, page 262) and distal metacarpal/metatarsal physes. Focal osteochondral defects have been noted histologically and result from repeated haemorrhage and/or microfractures that interfere with the blood supply to the mineralizing cartilage. Osteochondrosis-like defects have also been described.

Widened metaphyseal and physeal bone that is produced during the acute stage of the disease may persist through life, resulting in an irregular or flared appearance at the location of the physeal scar.

Neoplasia

Primary tumours and metastatic malignancy of the long bones of horses are rare. The majority of tumours that involve bone occur in the skull (see Chapter 9, pages 443, 466 and 477) or occasionally the spine (see Chapter 10, page 533). Tumours result in space-occupying lesions that may be radiopaque or radiolucent. Adjacent bone may be distorted in outline, and there may be associated new bone production. It is frequently not possible to differentiate specific tumour types by their radiographic appearance. A malignant tumour may be similar radiographically to the result of infection, and differentiation is based on history, clinical signs, laboratory tests and biopsy.

Osteitis and osteomyelitis

Osteitis is inflammation of bone, and osteomyelitis is inflammation of cortical bone and its myeloid cavity. In bones that do not have a myeloid cavity (e.g. the distal phalanx), it is not appropriate to use the term osteomyelitis. Osteitis is usually the result of trauma or inflammation in adjacent soft tissues. It is characterized by new bone formation and sometimes bone resorption. Differentiation should be made between aseptic osteitis and infectious osteitis (see below).

Infectious osteitis and infectious osteomyelitis

Infectious osteitis (inflammation of bone due to infection) and infectious osteomyelitis (inflammation of the bone involving the myeloid cavity) are common in the horse. In an adult, infectious osteitis is more common and is usually seen at a single site, often related to trauma such as wire cuts or puncture wounds. The hallmarks of infection are:

- Soft-tissue swelling with bone destruction and new bone formation
- An attempt to wall off infection resulting in radiopaque bone being laid down adjacent to the area of bone infection and destruction
- Infection of bone may result in the formation of a sequestrum (a piece of dead radiopaque bone) surrounded by an involucrum (an area of lucent granulation tissue) (see Figures 4.19b and 4.19c, page 215). A radiolucent tract may be visible extending from the infected area (a sinus)
- The distal phalanx, navicular bone and skull show a slightly different reaction to infection. In these bones, infection tends to cause destruction of bone with little evidence of new bone formation
- In the foal, osteomyelitis is more common and may occur simultaneously at several sites, often extending into adjacent joints. The converse is also true, and septic arthritis commonly extends into adjacent bone causing an osteomyelitis. Osteomyelitis in the foal tends to be very destructive and there is usually very little response by the bone to wall off the infection.

A useful classification of infection of bone and joints has been devised by Firth (see 'Infectious arthritis', pages 32–33).

Hypertrophic osteopathy

Hypertrophic osteopathy was formerly known as Marie's disease, hypertrophic pulmonary osteoarthropathy or hypertrophic osteoarthropathy. It is now termed hypertrophic osteopathy because it has been shown that pulmonary involvement is not a prerequisite for the development of the disease, as was once thought, although pulmonary lesions may be present. Hypertrophic osteopathy principally affects the metaphyses and diaphyses of the long bones, while sparing the joints. The disease is typified by periosteal new bone that often appears to be perpendicular to the cortices of the bone and irregular in outline in the acute stage (Figure 1.9). In the early stages, soft exposures must be used to avoid overexposure of this relatively lucent new bone. Later the margins of the new bone become more opaque and smoother, and the appearance of the original cortex of the bone becomes less clear. The bony lesions develop secondarily to a primary lesion, usually in the thorax or occasionally the abdomen, such as a tumour, an abscess or diffuse granulomatous disease. The cause and distribution of the bony lesions are not understood, however, the bone changes may regress and remodel if the primary disease can be identified and successfully treated.

Enostosis-like lesions and other circumscribed opacities

An enostosis is defined as bone developing within the medullary cavity or on the endosteum, resulting in a relatively sclerotic region. In the horse

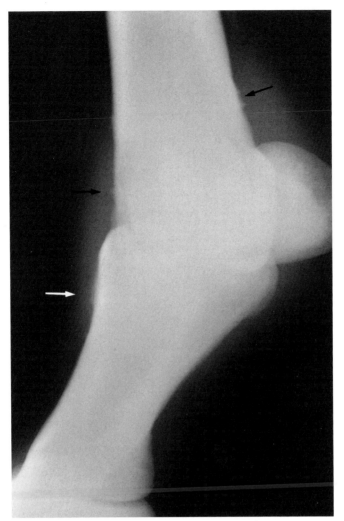

Figure 1.9 Dorsolateral-palmaromedial oblique view of a metacarpophalangeal joint of a 3-year-old Thoroughbred with a history of raised plasma fibrinogen for the preceding 4 months, and very recent onset forelimb stiffness associated with diffuse oedematous painful swellings of the distal limbs. There is soft-tissue swelling and active periosteal new bone on the distal diaphysis of the third metacarpal bone (black arrows) and the proximal metaphysis/diaphysis of the proximal phalanx (white arrow). Note its palisade-like appearance perpendicular to the cortex. This is typical of hypertrophic osteopathy. The horse had a dissecting aneurysm of the thoracic aorta. Diagnosis: hypertrophic osteopathy.

enostosis-like lesions have been described as focal or multifocal, intramedullary sclerosis. They are usually in the diaphyseal region of long bones, near the nutrient foramen, often developing on the endosteal surface of the bone. The most common sites are the tibia, radius, humerus and third metacarpal and metatarsal bones (Figure 1.10). The aetiology and clinical significance of the lesions are unknown. However, they may be associated with lameness, which usually resolves with rest. Enostosis-like lesions are frequently associated with focal increased radiopharmaceutical uptake, whether or not they are causing lameness. Such sclerotic reactions should be differentiated from endosteal callus secondary to a fatigue or stress fracture. Small focal opacities in the proximal metaphyseal or diaphyseal region of the tibia have been recognized. Their aetiology and clinical significance are unknown.

Fractures

A fracture is a discontinuity of the bone seen radiographically as a lucent line or lines. Radiography is performed to establish the type, severity and degree of displacement of the fracture, and to assess the damage to adjacent

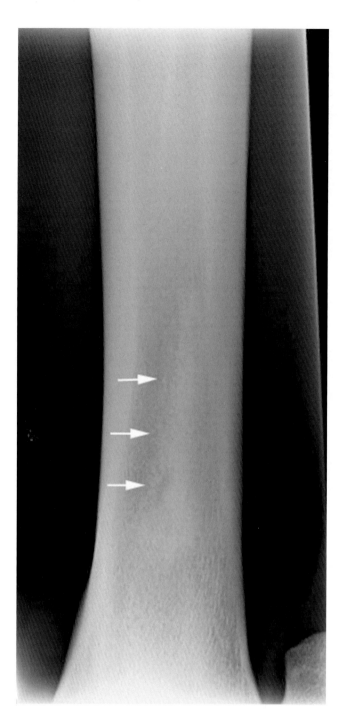

Figure 1.10 Craniolateral-caudomedial oblique radiographic view of a tibia. There is a vertical linear band of increased opacity in the middle of the distal aspect of the tibial diaphysis (arrows). This is an enostosis-like lesion.

joints and surrounding soft tissues. Later radiographs may be obtained to assess the degree of reduction achieved and to monitor healing. In order to establish the presence of a fracture, at least two projections, preferably obtained at right angles to each other, are essential. Many more views may be necessary to establish the exact configuration of the fracture.

Fatigue (stress) fractures and other non-displaced and/or incomplete fractures can be extremely difficult to detect in the acute stage. Mach lines due to edge enhancement should not be confused with fractures. For best visualization of a fracture, the x-ray beam must be parallel to the plane of the fracture, and thus detection may necessitate obtaining many views at 5°

angles to each other. Two radiolucent lines often represent a single complete fracture, which traverses through two cortices, e.g. dorsal and palmar, and should not be confused with two fractures. During the normal healing process there is osteoclasis along the fracture line within 5–10 days, resulting in apparent broadening of the lucent fracture line (see Figures 4.24a and 4.24b, page 222). Thus a fracture line that was not readily apparent in the initial radiographs may be detected on follow-up films obtained 5–10 days later. In the acute stage, nuclear scintigraphy may be a better method of detecting the presence of an incomplete fracture or a fatigue fracture. Some fractures are never visible radiographically, despite there being strong evidence of a fracture from nuclear scintigraphic evaluation. Some radiographically detectable stress (fatigue) fractures may be preceded by the development of sclerosis (see page 20) before the fracture becomes apparent.

A fracture should be evaluated to establish whether it is simple, multiple or comminuted, whether there is articular involvement, the degree of displacement of the fracture fragments and to identify any concurrent pathology which may adversely influence the prognosis.

Fractures involving the physis of a bone may be classified according to Salter-Harris, based upon the configuration and relationship of the fracture plane to the growing cells of the metaphyseal growth plate. Salter-Harris classifies the fractures as follows (Figure 1.11):

Type I Fracture through the zone of hypertrophied cells without involvement of the adjacent epiphysis or metaphysis.

Type II Fracture through the physis across part of the width of the bone and through the metaphysis, leaving a segment of the metaphysis attached to the epiphysis.

Type III Fracture through the physis across part of the width of the bone and through the epiphysis, entering the joint.

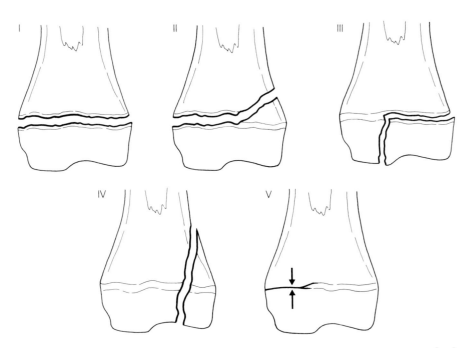

Figure 1.11 Salter-Harris classification of physeal fractures.

[25]

Type IV Fracture across the epiphysis, physis and a portion of the metaphysis, perpendicular to the plane of the physis.

Type V Compression fracture of the physis with minimal displacement. Although this classification has now been further extended, we feel that the above classification is adequate for practical clinical purposes.

Fracture healing should be monitored radiographically to determine the progression of healing. The time interval between re-examinations depends on the severity of the fracture, the type of repair and the clinical reassessment of the patient. Following initial mineral resorption along the fracture line, and formation of a fibrous callus, calcified periosteal and endosteal callus develops. The amount and quality of callus that develops depends upon the degree of stability at the fracture site (Figure 1.12) and the presence or absence of concurrent infection. Endosteal callus is more difficult to visualize radiographically, but ultimately results in disappearance of the fracture line. Stability of the fracture may develop long before the fracture line disappears radiographically. Some bones (e.g. the proximal and distal sesamoid bones and the accessory carpal bone) tend to heal by fibrous union, resulting in a persistent lucent line. The rate of healing varies and is dependent on many factors, including the age of the horse, its nutritional and metabolic status, the degree of stability of the fracture, the site of the fracture, the presence or absence of periosteum, the blood supply to the bone, and the presence or absence of infection. Infection is likely to be progressive and impair osseous union unless there is stability at the fracture site.

If a fracture is repaired by internal fixation, and there is adequate stability at the fracture site, healing should be predominantly by primary union, with minimal periosteal callus. Instability at a fracture site results in secondary union by the production of periosteal callus (Figure 1.13), or may result in fibrous union or malunion of the fracture.

If a fracture has been repaired by internal fixation, the implants and surrounding bone should be examined carefully on follow-up radiographs. The development of localized lucent zones around the implants indicates loosening of the implant, or infection, and it may be necessary to remove one or more selected portions of the implant. Diagnostic ultrasonography may be helpful in early detection of osteomyelitis in some cases, e.g. detection of fluid around a screw head.

If implants are removed when there is stability at the fracture site, radiolucent tracts will persist for 8–12 weeks. These tracts may act as stress points until adequate remineralization has occurred, and are potential sites for fracture to recur. Such stress points, of course, are also present with the implants in place.

Whether a fracture is treated conservatively or surgically, once initial mineral resorption along the fracture line has occurred, there should be progressive narrowing of the fracture line or lines, and they should gradually disappear. Healing may be complete within 6–12 weeks, but some fractures take considerably longer. A horse may be sound and be able to withstand work, despite the persistence of a radiolucent fracture line. In some locations (e.g. third metacarpal condylar fractures) the long-term persistence of

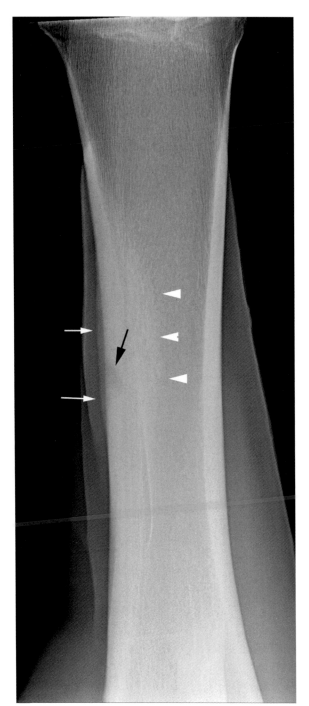

Figure 1.12 Craniocaudal radiographic view of a radius of a 6-year-old Irish Sports Horse obtained 4.5 weeks after a kick injury. Lameness was not apparent until 3 days after the injury and progressively deteriorated over the following week. Medial is to the left. There is marked endosteal reaction of the medial cortex of the mid-diaphyseal region (arrow heads), extending proximal and distal to an ill-defined radiolucent line through the cortex, an incomplete fracture (black arrow). There is smoothly marginated periosteal new bone, callus, extending proximal and distal to the radiolucent line and mild overlying soft tissue swelling (white arrows).

a lucent line is commonly associated with recurrent lameness. If a fracture line persists beyond 6 months it can be considered to be a delayed union. There may be sclerosis of the bone adjacent to the fracture line, and the ends of the bone may become slightly flared (Figure 1.14). Although delayed union is not uncommon in the horse, non-union (complete failure of osseous

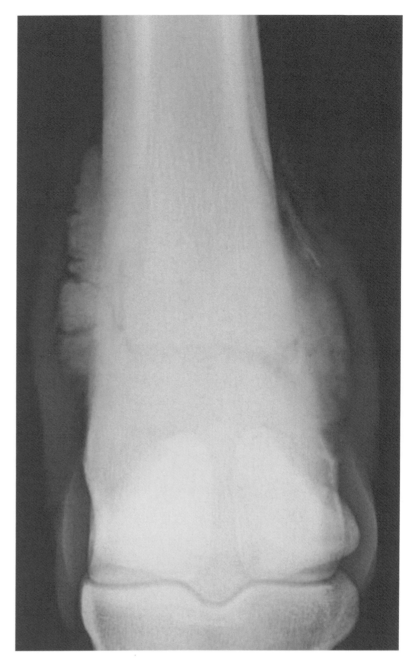

Figure 1.13 Dorsopalmar radiographic view of the distal metacarpal region of a 3-year-old Thoroughbred racehorse with sudden onset of left forelimb lameness 6 weeks previously. Medial is to the left. There is an approximately horizontal radiolucent line traversing the distal metaphyseal region, representing a complete fracture and very extensive irregularly marginated periosteal callus extending along the medial and lateral cortices, reflecting a secondary healing response to an unstable fracture.

union after 12 months) is rare, except in the areas previously mentioned where healing is frequently by fibrous union. If there is apparent healing by fibrous union, it is usually impossible to state when the original fracture occurred. Fractures of the navicular bone usually heal by fibrous union, and frequently lucent zones develop adjacent to the fracture line. These lucent zones are indicative of a fracture of at least 6–8 weeks' duration.

Joint lesions

Swelling

Soft-tissue swelling in and around joints may be classified as shown below.

[28]

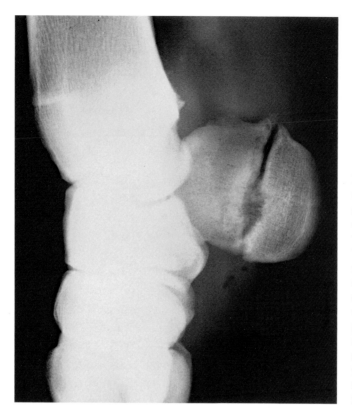

Figure 1.14 Lateromedial view of the carpus of a mature Thoroughbred steeplechaser, 8 months after the onset of acute lameness. There is a delayed union fracture of the accessory carpal bone. Note the flaring of the fracture margins proximally and the sclerosis along the fracture edges, especially distally. There is no evidence of osseous union proximally. Note also the periosteal new bone on the distal caudal radius, of questionable clinical significance. The horse made a functional recovery, although bony union was not achieved. Diagnosis: delayed union fracture of the accessory carpal bone.

INTRA-ARTICULAR SWELLING

With intra-articular swelling the joint capsule is distended and in a non-weight-bearing patient there may be a widened joint space. In some locations (e.g. the carpus) the normal dorsal lucent fat pad may disappear due to compression. Joint distension is usually associated with inflammation and may be septic or aseptic. If several joints are involved in a neonatal animal, septic arthritis should be considered. If several joints are involved in older animals, immune-mediated disease should be considered, especially if the occurrence is cyclical in nature.

PERIARTICULAR SWELLING

Periarticular swelling does not involve the joint space, but may involve the joint capsule as is seen in sprains. Periarticular swelling may also be caused by conditions that are more obvious on examination of the patient than on the radiograph, such as wire cuts, puncture wounds and external trauma. With cuts and wounds, gas may be evident within the soft-tissue swelling.

GENERALIZED PERIARTICULAR SWELLING

Generalized periarticular swelling may result in the inability to differentiate between intra-articular and extra-articular fluid accumulation. The inability to differentiate may result from massive swelling or the loss of soft-tissue fat which is normally found in the pericapsular, peritendonous and periligamentous areas.

Table 1.1 Classification of sprains.

Type of tissue damage	Radiographic finding
Ligament strain or partial rupture	Soft-tissue swelling
Ligament rupture	Soft-tissue swelling
Ligament avulsion	Soft-tissue swelling and the presence of a bone fragment

Trauma

Joint trauma may be classified as follows:

SPRAIN

Joint sprain is the wrenching of a joint with partial rupture or other injury of its attachments, and without luxation of bones. There is usually rapid swelling, heat and pain. Sprains must be differentiated from fissure fractures and other causes of acute joint swelling. Sprains may be classified as shown in Table 1.1.

If ligament rupture or avulsion is suspected, stressed radiographs (Figures 1.15a and 1.15b; see below) should be obtained to assess the integrity of the joint and the possibility of subluxation. Ultrasonography may yield additional information.

SUBLUXATION AND LUXATION (DISLOCATION)

Luxation is the complete loss of contact between the articular surfaces of a joint. Subluxation of a joint is partial loss of contact between joint surfaces, and may be intermittent. Luxation and subluxation in the horse are usually the result of trauma, although congenital luxation of the patella occurs rarely. Subluxation of the proximal interphalangeal joint may develop without an obvious cause. Luxation is usually easily identified radiographically, but multiple radiographic views are required in order to assess whether or not there is a concurrent fracture that may adversely influence the prognosis. If luxation is incomplete (i.e. subluxation), radiographic assessment is more difficult. Radiographs should be obtained in the weight-bearing position and compared carefully with the normal anatomy. When luxation or subluxation is suspected clinically, so-called 'stress radiographs' may be helpful to determine the integrity of the periarticular soft tissues such as the collateral ligaments. Stress radiographs are obtained with the limb not weight bearing, with force applied to the joint in either a mediolateral or dorsopalmar direction to determine whether the bones may be moved abnormally in relation to each other (Figures 1.15a and 1.15b). Ultrasonography may yield additional information.

INTRA-ARTICULAR FRACTURES

Intra-articular fractures exist when there is a break in the articular surface. Unless there is some degree of displacement, damage to the articular carti-

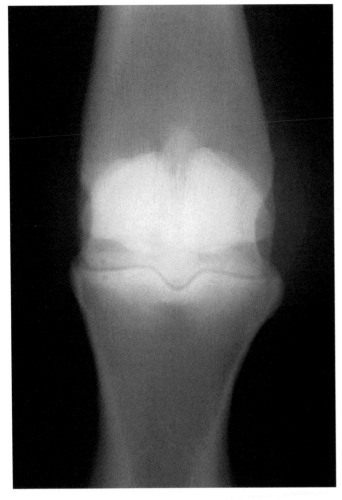 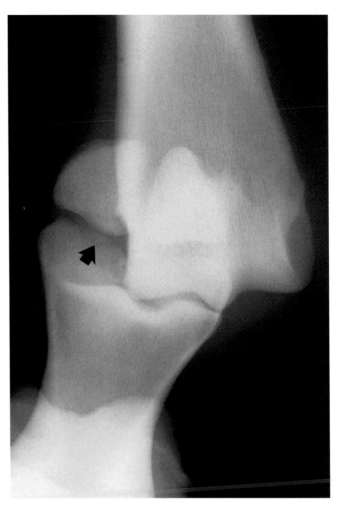

Figure 1.15(a) Dorsoplantar view of a metatarsophalangeal joint of an event horse with acute onset severe lameness 3 weeks previously. The horse was bearing full weight on the limb without discomfort. The bones are in normal alignment.

Figure 1.15(b) Stressed dorsoplantar view of the same horse as in Figure 1.15a. There is luxation of the metatarsophalangeal joint, and disruption of the proximal articular margin of the proximal phalanx (arrow).

lage may not be seen, but should be assumed to exist. A small degree of displacement is indicated by the presence of a slight 'step' in the two sides of the articular portion of the fracture line. Fissure fractures are not displaced and many views may be required in order to visualize the fracture, as the x-ray beam must be exactly aligned in the plane of the fissure.

Fractures of the articular margin are termed chip fractures. Radiographs should be carefully inspected for evidence of additional chips, pre-existing degenerative joint disease, or other concurrent pathology, which may adversely affect the prognosis. Differentiation between chip fractures, ectopic mineralization and separate centres of ossification may not be possible. The position of the mineralized body relative to the articular margin, the size and shape of the body, and the contour of the articular margin should all be assessed carefully. A recent chip fracture may have a sharp edge, and a fracture 'bed' may be discernible. Separate centres of ossification, or old chip fractures, may be very well rounded uniformly opaque bodies, and a fracture bed is usually not detectable. Ectopic mineralization may be present within the joint capsule.

[31]

A slab fracture is a fracture extending from one joint surface to another, e.g. from the proximal to distal articular surface of the third carpal or tarsal bones. These fractures may be extremely difficult to detect radiographically in the acute stage if not displaced. Oblique views are invaluable in the carpus. In the tarsus it may be necessary to re-radiograph the joint after 7–10 days when some demineralization has occurred along the fracture line.

Infectious arthritis

Infectious arthritis is most commonly seen in young foals, and frequently involves several joints. It may occur in an adult, usually associated with trauma, but may be iatrogenic. Radiographic features of joint infection include:

- Periarticular soft-tissue swelling
- Joint capsule distension, with or without apparent widening of the joint space
- Irregularity of outline of the subchondral bone
- Lucent zones in the subchondral bone, with or without sclerosis
- Periarticular osteophyte formation, due to secondary joint disease
- Partial collapse of the subchondral bone

The presence of bony abnormalities indicates that the disease is advanced and warrants a guarded prognosis. The absence of detectable radiological abnormalities does not preclude a diagnosis of infection. The speed of development and degree of cartilage and bone destruction depend on the causative organism.

In a neonate, care should be taken to differentiate the radiographic appearance of incompletely ossified bones, which may have an irregular outline and granular opacity, similar to that seen in infection. Reference should be made to the text in the subsequent chapters, which describes the appearance of incomplete ossification where it is a normal feature at birth. In a foal, joint infection may develop secondarily to infection of an adjacent physis, or may spread from a joint to an adjacent epiphysis.

Firth classified infectious polyarthritis of foals into several syndromes as follows:

1 Physeal type P osteomyelitis. There are areas of irregularity and focal widening in the physis. At this point the term physitis may appear more appropriate than physeal osteomyelitis; however, once the changes have advanced sufficiently far to be seen radiographically, there is usually also involvement of the metaphyseal or epiphyseal bone adjacent to the site of origin. Infection may continue to extend into the epiphysis or metaphysis, where the infection is characterized by relatively opaque areas of bone surrounded by lucent areas. These are frequently triangular in shape. As the condition progresses, soft-tissue swelling associated with the joints may be seen, and this may develop into infectious arthritis secondary to underlying osteomyelitis.

2 Type E osteomyelitis begins in the epiphysis and progression is similar. The classification is only used to denote where the nidus of infection was established.

3 Type S osteomyelitis actually begins in the synovium, and extends from there, rapidly becoming septic arthritis.

4 Type T osteomyelitis is limited to the tarsus and must be differentiated from aseptic necrosis of the central and third tarsal bones. Type T cases usually present because of generalized tarsal enlargement or tarsocrural joint capsule distension. Although the central and third tarsal bones are occasionally involved, the majority of pathology is noted in the distal tibial physis and or tarsocrural joint. The main radiographic findings include soft-tissue swelling, distension of the tarsocrural joint and irregularity of the distal tibial physis (type P osteomyelitis). When the central and third tarsal bones are involved, they are normal in shape but have a mottled lucent appearance.

5 Type C osteomyelitis. Recently osteomyelitis of the carpal bones has been described, and appears similar in many respects to tarsal osteomyelitis. It may therefore be appropriate to include a fifth category in Firth's classification – osteomyelitis identical to type T, but localized to a single carpal bone (Figure 5.18, page 260).

Osseous cyst-like lesions (bone cyst)

Osseous cyst-like lesions (OCLLs) are usually solitary, circular lucent areas in a bone, which may be surrounded by a narrow rim of sclerosis. They are usually unicameral (single chambered) but may be multicameral. They are often close to the articular surface of the bone and sometimes a 'neck' connecting the cyst-like lesion with the joint surface can be identified. Some OCLLs ultimately fill in radiographically, but others persist virtually unchanged. Osseous cyst-like lesions occurring near the articular surface in young horses may appear to migrate progressively away from the joint surface, as normal endochondral ossification occurs.

The aetiology of OCLLs is obscure. Some are true subchondral bone cysts and have a fibrous cystic lining, but there are probably a number of causes, despite their similar radiographic appearance. It has been suggested that they are part of the osteochondrosis syndrome, but the evidence for this is limited. There is increasing evidence that some OCLLs are traumatic in origin.

Osseous cyst-like lesions may or may not be associated with lameness. Cyst-like lesions which occur deep within bone, such as in the carpal bones, are rarely associated with lameness, whereas those close to an articular surface, such as in the medial femoral condyle, are frequently associated with lameness, although lameness may resolve despite radiographic persistence of the lesion.

An OCLL may first be identified as a small lucent depression in the articular surface (see Chapter 8, page 385). This progressively enlarges and a sclerotic margin may develop around the cyst-like lesion. The radiographs should be carefully examined for evidence of concurrent secondary degenerative joint disease.

Osteochondrosis

Osteochondrosis is considered to be a disturbance of endochondral ossification, but there is increasing evidence to show that there may also be primary subchondral bone lesions. The disease may be generalized, although only evident radiographically in certain joints. The femoropatellar, tarsocrural, fetlock and scapulohumeral joints are the most commonly affected in the horse (see Chapters 8, 7, 3 and 6, respectively). The radiographic appearance of osteochondritic lesions is variable between individuals, and the joints involved, but the changes normally include:

- Discrete osteochondral fragments
- Alterations in the contour of the articular surface, e.g. flattening or a depression
- Irregularly shaped lucent zones in the subchondral bone
- Sclerosis surrounding the lucent zones
- Secondary remodelling of joints

Lesions are not always of clinical significance but must be interpreted in the light of the clinical signs. Some lesions remodel gradually and become increasingly sclerotic. Clinical signs are generally recognized in horses less than 3 years of age, but occasionally horses remain asymptomatic until later in life, especially if the horse does not work until a later age.

Degenerative joint disease

Degenerative joint disease (DJD), osteoarthrosis, osteoarthritis and secondary joint disease are often used synonymously in veterinary medicine, yet distinctions can be made in some cases.

Arthritis simply means inflammation of a joint, and if recognized radiographically is seen as joint capsule distension without evidence of new bone involvement. There is inflammation of the synovial lining and changes in the quantity and quality of synovial fluid. Osteoarthritis or osteoarthrosis indicate that bone has become involved and that an inflammatory soft-tissue component may (itis) or may not (osis) be present. The term secondary joint disease is used when the primary cause is known, such as in osteochondrosis or intra-articular fracture. Degenerative joint disease is used to refer to any number of causes that affect the joint and its supporting structures. In the horse, the degenerative process, which results in DJD, may be associated with poor conformation and/or hard use. Advanced DJD, however, is sometimes seen in immature horses, less than 3 years of age, with no identifiable predisposing cause. Any condition that damages cartilage directly, causes joint instability, or subjects the joint to abnormal directional forces, can cause DJD. Immune-mediated joint disease should be considered whenever there is polyarthritis and sepsis can be ruled out.

Radiographic abnormalities associated with DJD include:

- Periarticular osteophyte formation
- Subchondral bone sclerosis, and loss of trabecular pattern
- Ill defined small lucent zones in the subchondral bone
- Small well defined osseous cyst-like lesions

- Narrowing of the joint space
- Joint capsule distension
- Periarticular soft-tissue swelling

One or more of the above may be seen in association with DJD in any joint. If possible, periarticular osteophyte formation should be differentiated from entheseophyte formation. Small periarticular osteophytes are not necessarily synonymous with clinically significant DJD. It must also be borne in mind that the absence of detectable radiographic abnormalities does not preclude the presence of cartilage degeneration. As DJD progresses, radiographic abnormalities become more obvious. Ultrasonography may give useful information about the integrity of the articular cartilage.

Dystrophic and metastatic mineralization (calcification)

Calcium is seldom deposited alone. Even in bone the opacity seen on radiographs is due to a mixture of calcium, phosphorus, zinc, manganese and magnesium, and therefore dystrophic and metastatic calcification is more correctly termed mineralization.

Mineralization in soft tissue can occur in association with inflammation, neoplasia, trauma or metabolic disease. The most reliable indication of the cause of the mineralization is the location in which it occurs, combined with knowledge regarding the organs or structures located in the area. Knowledge of what diseases result in mineralization of a particular organ provides valuable information, and occasionally a definitive diagnosis. The size, shape and pattern of mineralization may vary, and therefore are poor indications of a specific aetiology.

Soft-tissue mineralization has been classified as being metastatic or dystrophic. Metastatic mineralization is the deposition of minerals in tissues that have not previously been damaged. It is associated with hypercalcaemia, hypercalciurea and hyperphosphataemia.

Dystrophic mineralization is the process whereby mineral is deposited in injured, degenerating or necrotic tissue, and is more commonly seen in the horse. It can occur secondary to any injury to soft tissue, e.g. in tumours that have become necrotic, at the site of fat necrosis, subsequent to infarction, and in association with inflammation or haemorrhage. Either type of mineralization may eventually result in the formation of mature bone.

FURTHER READING

Armstrong, S. (1990) *Lecture Notes on the Physics of Radiology.* Clinical Press Ltd., Bristol

Bushong, S. (2001) *Radiologic science for technologists: Physics, biology and protection,* 7th edn, Mosby, St. Louis

Garret, K. and Berk, J. (2006) How to properly position Thoroughbred repository radiographs. *Proc. Am. Assoc. Equine Pract.,* **52**, 600–608

Greet, G. and Greet, T. (1966) The use of specific radiographic projections to demonstrate three intra-articular fractures. *Equine vet. Educ.,* **8**, 208–211

Harrison, L. and Edwards, G. (1996) Radiographic investigation of osteochondrosis. *Equine vet. Educ.,* **8**, 172–176

[35]

Holmes, M. and Pilsworth, R. (2007) *Radiation safety in equine practice.* DVD British Equine Veterinary Association, Newmarket

Kirberger, R., Gottschalk, R. and Guthrie, A. (1996) Radiological appearance of air introduced during regional limb anaesthesia. *Equine vet. J.*, **28**, 298–305

Lavin, L. (2006) *Radiography in Veterinary Technology*, 4th edn, W.B. Saunders

Mair, T., Dyson, S., Fraser, J. *et al.* (1996) Hypertrophic osteopathy (Marie's disease) in Equidae: a review of twenty-four cases. *Equine vet. J.*, **28**, 256–262

May, S. (1996) Radiological aspects of degenerative joint disease. *Equine vet. Educ.*, **8**, 114–120

Meredith, W.J. and Massey, J.B. (1971) *Fundamental Physics of Radiology*, 2nd edn, John Wright, Bristol

Morgan, J. and Silverman, S. (1993) *Techniques of Veterinary Radiography*, 5th edn, Iowa State University Press

Phillips, T. (1998) The use of radiography in the pre-purchase examination. In: *British Equine Veterinary Association Manual The Pre-Purchase Examination* Ed. Mair, T. pp 154–160. *Equine vet. J.*, Newmarket

Poulos, P. (1992) Radiological evaluation of the horses relevant to purchase. *Vet. Clin. N. Amer.: Equine Pract.*, **8**, 319–328

Smallwood, J., Shiveley, M., Rendano, V. and Habel, R. (1985) A standard nomenclature for radiographic projections used in veterinary medicine. *Vet. Radiol.*, **26**, 2–9

Thrall, D. (2007) *Textbook of Veterinary Diagnostic Radiography*, 5th edn, Saunders Elsevier, St. Louis

Chapter 2
Computed and digital radiography

Digital radiography is a generic term that has been widely used to describe both computerized (computed) radiography and direct capture digital radiography. Both techniques result in a radiographic image captured electronically and displayed as a digital image on a computer monitor. The image can be archived digitally and/or transferred into a 'hard copy' using a laser printer. The generation of the x-ray beam remains unchanged and, just as with conventional film–screen radiography, the quality of the digital image is greatly affected by the quality of the x-ray generator, the radiographer's technique and the ability of the radiographer to choose correct exposure factors.

New terms have come into common usage. DICOM is an acronym for Digital Imaging and Communication in Medicine and is a standardization of image format to facilitate exchange of images. A DICOM file contains a header, which gives the patient information and image data, giving information about the image. The term PACS, Picture Archiving and Communication System, applies to the combined hardware and software used for digital imaging, allowing communication between computers. As with any computer-based system, training in the use of both hardware and software and in information technology, and maintenance support for the system are invaluable.

COMPUTERIZED RADIOGRAPHY

Computerized or computed radiography has similarities to conventional film–screen radiography, despite the absence of film and chemical processing. The phosphor plate, otherwise known as an imaging plate, is stored in a cassette, allowing existing x-ray equipment to be used, but replacing a traditional film cassette with a computed radiography cassette.

Computed radiography uses photostimulable phosphors (storage phosphors); trace amounts of impurities have been added to their crystalline structure to alter their physical properties. The storage phosphors are coated on to either a flexible or rigid plate (dependent on the system), much like screens used in conventional radiography. The storage phosphors come from the barium fluorohalide family and are deposited on to a substrate (backing plate) in powder form. The size of the phosphor grain used influences the resolution of the screen. Low-resolution screens use a larger phosphor grain than a high-resolution screen. Most screens are designed to be around 10–20 phosphor grains thick.

Computed radiography storage phosphors differ from traditional screen phosphors because instead of emitting light in response to the incident radiation, they store the energy as a latent image. This is subsequently stimulated optically and released in an image plate reader. The amount of energy released is directly proportional to the intensity of radiation reaching the imaging plate during exposure.

Imaging plate reading

In most commercially available systems a flying spot readout system is used. In this system a laser spot scans the exposed plate using a mirror in a point to point raster pattern. This causes the phosphor to release the stored energy as a violet blue glow. The intensity of the phosphor glow is directly proportional to the amount of energy stored from the exposure made. The glow is captured by the system and enhanced using photomultiplier tubes. The resultant optical signal is converted into a digital signal using an analogue to digital converter. The digital signal is processed within the control computer using algorithms predetermined for different body parts. The total processing time currently takes between 40 and 90 seconds, depending on the system, and only one imaging plate can be read at a time. The systems are developing rapidly, and readers are advised to seek up-to-date information if considering purchase of any digital system.

The resultant image should be transmitted to a high-resolution monitor for image reading. With the larger stationary readers the image is displayed on an adjacent work station monitor on which the image can be checked for appropriate positioning and exposure. However, the image is displayed at a much lower resolution than the information captured and this image should not be used for diagnostic purposes.

The laser scan does not release all the energy stored in the phosphor. After scanning the plate goes through an erase cycle in which the phosphor plate is exposed to a bright fluorescent light. This removes any remaining residual energy, enabling the plate to be re-used. This process takes up to 30 seconds.

The latent image can be stored for up to 24 hours, but generally it is best to 'read the plate' as soon as possible after exposure. Just as with conventional film screen radiography, it is possible for dust and other foreign bodies to get into the cassette holding the imaging plate, therefore regular cleaning using the manufacturer's recommended procedure (e.g., pure alcohol and lint-free wipes) is essential. The imaging plate must be allowed to dry before it can be reused, so this is a procedure to be carried out at the end of a day. Ideally there should be a regular system of cleaning and a log maintained.

The plates can be subject to physical damage, either during exposure or in the plate reader, both of which can result in artefacts. Correct handling of the plates is therefore important.

DIRECT DIGITAL CAPTURE RADIOGRAPHY

Direct to digital, or direct digital capture, or direct radiography or digital radiography are synonymous terms used to describe a system which converts the x-ray photons to a digital signal without the use of a phosphor plate. This saves considerable time and energy. As with computed radiography, direct radiography is used in conjunction with conventional x-ray machines. There are two types of plate currently in use. In both types the image is captured by an electronic array, and transmitted directly to a computer to generate the required image. The image is initiated by a thin layer of scintillation material made of cesium iodide, which emits light when stimulated by x-rays. Under this layer of scintillant is the recording layer. In a charge-coupled device (CCD plate) under the scintillation layer are myriad chips, electronically coupled together. The more reliable, but more expensive plates use a layer of amorphous silicon as a detector (like one huge computer chip), converting the light into digital data. In direct digital systems the digital data are transmitted directly via a cable attaching the detecting plate to the processing computer, the image appearing on the monitor in a few seconds.

The initial purchase price of a direct digital radiography system is currently more expensive than computed radiography. Currently only small imaging plates are routinely available, largely because of the very expensive price of large (24 × 30 cm) plates, limiting the use of direct digital radiography to the distal limbs. The cable connection to the computer which processes the image may be of some concern when dealing with a horse that is difficult to restrain, with inherent risk of damage to the equipment. However, since images can be read within a few seconds there are potential time savings compared with either conventional radiography or computed radiography.

IMAGE RESOLUTION

Images are comprised of pixels and the pixel size determines spatial resolution, the ability to define two objects close together. To increase resolution the number of pixels is increased without changing the field of view (the physical area being examined), thus decreasing the matrix size. A 2048 × 2048 (2-K) matrix or higher is recommended for digital radiography. Dynamic range refers to the number of shades of grey that can be represented. Each pixel has a bit depth which determines the number of shades of grey that can be represented. Eight bits represents a grey scale range of 256 (2^8), ranging from 0 (white) to 255 (black). The human eye can only resolve a limited number of shades of grey, therefore excessive bit depth results in large file sizes without providing additional useful information. The dynamic range of most digital x-ray systems is determined by the computer and software. Most use an 8-, 10- or 12-bit dynamic range (i.e., 2^8, 2^{10} or 2^{12}). The American College of Radiologists recommends a minimum of 10-bit depth.

EXPOSURE FACTORS

When choosing exposure factors for computed radiography it is important to recognize the change in technology from conventional film–screen

[39]

radiography and how to optimize exposure factors, which will not be the same. In film–screen radiography mAs controls the opacity of the image. This is because the same medium is used for detection of the photons and for the display of the resulting image, making them intimately linked. In computed radiography the image display and image detection are now separated. The mAs still determines the number of photons absorbed into the imaging plate, which affects the density and the noise in the stored image, but these data are now also subjected to image processing in the form of algorithms. These algorithms control the display of the signal and hence the image opacity.

kVp controls contrast in both film–screen and computed radiography. With conventional film–screen radiography the response is non-linear, which means that matching of subject contrast to kVp and film–screen combination is important. With computed radiography the response is linear and it can therefore compensate for loss of subject contrast through image processing and algorithms. Thus computed radiography offers higher contrast resolution or exposure latitude compared with conventional film–screen radiography.

When choosing an exposure it is still important to adjust kVp and mAs to body part and size of the individual, but it is equally important to choose the correct algorithm. It is not necessarily straightforward to determine whether the imaging plate has been under- or overexposed, because the displayed image is not a true representation of the exposure due to the image processing. With conventional film–screen radiography an overexposed image appears relatively black throughout and an underexposed image appears relatively white (assuming there are no development problems). With computed radiography the digital image is selected from a portion of the black/white spectrum. Overexposure may take the image out of the part of the spectrum being read by the computer, thus the image appears light, white, or pale. Similarly an underexposed image may appear dark. It will usually however have a grainy, mottled appearance. Each manufacturer's system produces a figure which gives an estimation of whether or not the exposure was appropriate. Each system uses different terminology for this figure and has a different range which is considered appropriate. Terminology includes exposure index, S value, DDI and REX. To determine whether an image needs to be repeated the exposure index (or equivalent) should be consulted. If this figure is within reasonable limits (according to the manufacturer's guidelines), the image should be manipulated on the display rather than repeated.

The speed of the imaging plates may be different from conventional film–screen combinations and will influence the exposures that are required. If the imaging plate has a slower speed than the conventional film–screen combination then the exposure factors will need to be increased, whereas if it is faster the exposure factors may be reduced.

Algorithms can be modified in some instances by the user; however, it is vital that appropriate training by the manufacturer has been given. If this is inappropriate and algorithms for specific body parts are not performing to a good standard, the applications consultant from the service provider should be consulted to help modify algorithms and improve image quality.

Imaging an area within which there are tissues of widely differing densities potentially poses some difficulties, and it may result in the more dense area appearing completely white and without detail and more lucent areas being black and 'burnt out'. The image histogram has too many extreme pixel values. Most systems can display a histogram of pixel density across different areas, and/or have other features to indicate areas that are outside the readable densities. It is important to recognize these areas, and if they contain potentially important information, then an additional exposure is required, with exposure factor adjusted accordingly.

Grids can be used with both computed and digital radiography, but may cause problems, and the manufacturer of the system should be consulted for advice. Grid lines that have a similar frequency (lines/cm) as the laser reader cause a wavy (moiré) pattern of lines (Figure 2.1) that may destroy image quality. Other combinations can also be a problem. Generally grids should have at least 60 lines/cm and grid lines should preferably run perpendicular to the plate reader's laser scan lines. However some systems have grid line removal software that may eliminate this problem. In the authors' experience, while grids remain important for radiography of thick areas such as the thoracolumbar region, they can often be dispensed with for imaging

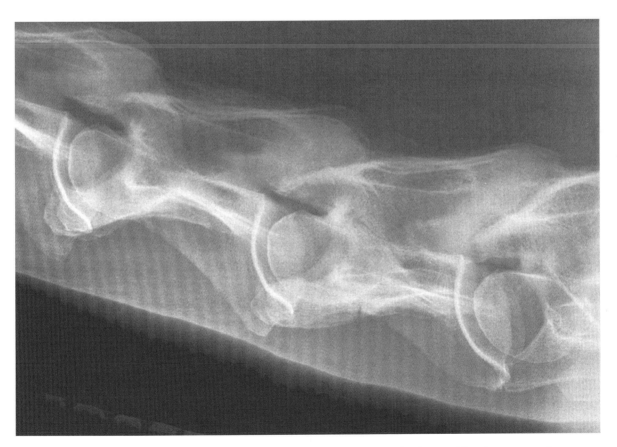

Figure 2.1 Lateral radiographic view of the mid-cervical vertebrae obtained using a grid and a computed radiography system. There are repetitive light and dark bands extending from the top of the image to the bottom. These are moiré lines.

the feet. It may be necessary to borrow several grids from the manufacturer to determine which is most appropriate.

Appropriate collimation of the x-ray beam and standard focus–image plate distances (source–image distances) are particularly important with digital imaging in order to achieve optimal image quality. Lack of collimation can affect the algorithm and the appearance of an image because the system processes the whole of the image as one exposure. This can be aided in some systems by selecting the area to be processed. However, the better the initial image, the better will be the end result, despite all processing applied to the image. Collimation is particularly important in areas with marked changes in density of tissues within the exposed area. The system looks for unexposed black and grey areas and tries to subtract white areas so that only useful information is processed. The system effectively looks for collimation lines.

MONITORS

When reviewing digital images it is important to consider the monitor that the image is displayed on. There are currently two basic types of monitor to choose from: cathode ray tubes (CRTs) or active-matrix liquid crystal displays (AMLCDs). For the diagnostic workstation, it is important to choose the highest-resolution monitor that is affordable.

Resolution of monitors is measured by the number of pixels displayed on the screen at any one time. This is displayed as two numbers multiplied together which is often abbreviated, e.g., a 1028 × 768 pixel monitor and a 1600 × 1200 pixel monitor are referred to as 1 Meg (megapixel) and 2 Meg monitors respectively. With 3 Meg and 5 Meg monitors widely available, the limiting factor is cost. Display monitor specification includes spatial resolution and contrast resolution. Spatial resolution is described as either pixels/mm or line pairs/mm. Three millimetres/pixel is equivalent to 6 mm/line pair. Contrast or depth resolution is described as grey values or bits. An 8 bit image has 256 grey levels; a 12 bit image has 4096 grey levels. However the human eye can only resolve approximately 100 scales of grey. The American College of Radiologists has recommended that computed radiography image capture should be digitized to at least 2.5 line pairs/mm and that the image should be digitized to 10 bits per pixel or more.

The monitor ideally should be a true DICOM monitor and not just a DICOM compatible monitor. The DICOM compatible monitor only shows a representation of a DICOM image; the grey scale is reduced, and greatly affects the image quality. The high-resolution DICOM compatible monitors on the market should be able to display digital images in varying degrees of luminance with various background colour settings that are similar to film choices. This should aid user preference being accommodated when viewing radiographs, and allow adjustment for the lack of grey scale.

Imaging plate artefacts

Flexible imaging plates are found in many table top/compact computed radiography systems and are very susceptible to cracking. The imaging plates generally start to crack around the edges, which does not interfere with image quality. However, as the imaging plates are continually used the cracks will begin to spread into the more central areas of the plate, overlying the image being examined. These artefacts may appear on radiographs as linear radiopacities or radiolucencies. If this occurs it is imperative that the plate is replaced.

Back scatter from dense objects behind the imaging plate can cause the plate to be exposed from behind creating a 'ghost-like' image over the radiograph. This is more likely with large exposures. It can be prevented by placing a piece of rubberized lead or equivalent behind the cassette to absorb the scattered radiation.

Hair stuck on the imaging plate results in a linear curved white artefact, because anything blocking the imaging plate's emission of light will be blocked when scanned by the laser in the reader. Other debris causes a white artefact of variable shape. A linear black line on one side of the image can be the result of back scatter transmitted through the cassette hinge.

Plate reader artefacts

Imaging plates are automatically erased after they are read, to prepare them for the next exposure. If imaging plates have not been used for a period of time (according to the manufacturer's guidelines) they should be manually erased. Imaging plates are not only sensitive to x-rays but also to other electromagnetic radiation (ultraviolet and gamma rays) and particulate radiation (alpha and beta radiation). These are present as natural background radiation. Thus imaging plates are susceptible to background noise creating black dots (Figure 2.2a), unless manually erased shortly before use (Figure 2.2b). Most computed radiography readers have a dedicated erase cycle and manufacturers will provide guidelines on the maximum recommend period of time between erasure and usage.

Some manufacturers provide more than one erasure setting; if an incorrect exposure is made it is vital to choose the correct setting to ensure the plate is fully erased. If this does not happen it could result in a 'ghost' image from the previous exposure appearing on the next radiograph.

Dirt and dust that get into the plate reader can attach to the reader optics or the mirror in the reader, which can cause horizontal or vertical white lines on images depending on the orientation of the cassette. If lines are seen it is important to have the cassette reader serviced to clean the particles from the optics or mirror. To prevent this from happening it is important to keep the reader in a dust-free environment, to keep it as clean as possible, to clean imaging plates on a regular basis (as directed by the

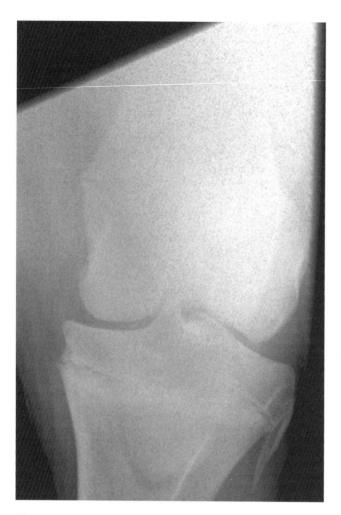

Figure 2.2(b) Background noise, the result of processing a computed radiography imaging plate that had not been cleared for several days.

Figure 2.2(a) A poor-quality caudocranial radiographic view of an immature stifle obtained using a computed radiography system. Superimposed over the denser tissues of the femur and surrounding musculature is a dark speckled pattern, an artefact created by the digital system. This can occur when there are tissues of greatly varying opacity within the area being examined.

manufacturer), and to clean the cassette housing if dust or dirt are visible before submitting plates to be read. Multiple lines may appear across an image which represent an artefact during image acquisition or processing (Figure 2.3).

Operator-induced artefacts

Operator errors may be more frequent in instances where a new computed radiography machine has been installed as a replacement for conventional screen–film combinations. It is important to store the imaging plates correctly. They must be protected from direct heat and extremes of humidity to prevent environmental damage to the imaging plate, and should also be stored where they will not be subjected to inadvertent exposure either from

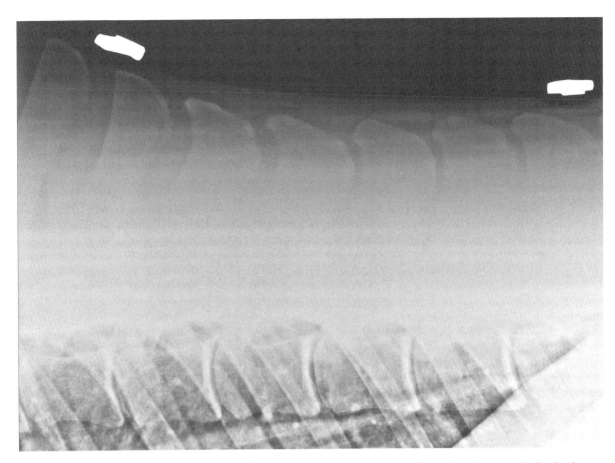

Figure 2.3 Lateral radiographic view of the 12th to 18th thoracic vertebrae of a 620 kg Warmblood horse, obtained using a computed radiography system. The image is not ideally collimated; both the dorsal spinous processes and vertebral bodies have been exposed. There are multiple horizontal lines across the image, which are artefacts.

a direct exposure or from scatter. They are much more sensitive to scattered radiation than a conventional film–screen cassette.

As with film–screen systems, it is also important to identify the correct side of the cassette for exposure. This should be easily recognisable, and is often marked with a sticker stating 'tube side'. If an exposure is made with the wrong side up there will be a distinctive pattern across the image, resulting in the need for a repeat.

IMAGE READING

The angle of the monitor can influence the information that can be obtained from the image. The image should be viewed from perpendicular to the monitor because contrast ratios can change rapidly (10:1) for a change in viewing angle from 90° to 85°. Ambient light is also critical to minimize reflections on the monitor. If using a laptop computer it should have an antireflective or antiglare screen. The monitor should be viewed in dim light; ideally the reading room should be illuminated at 2–25 lux (sunlight is 105 lux). A room fitted with blinds to obscure direct sunlight is ideal.

[45]

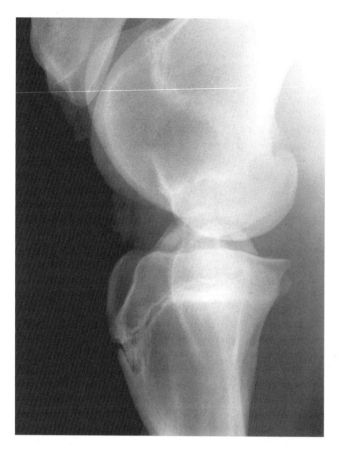

Figure 2.4(a) Lateromedial radiographic view of an immature stifle obtained using a computed radiography system. Cranial is to the left. The image has been windowed for optimal evaluation of the internal osseous architecture.

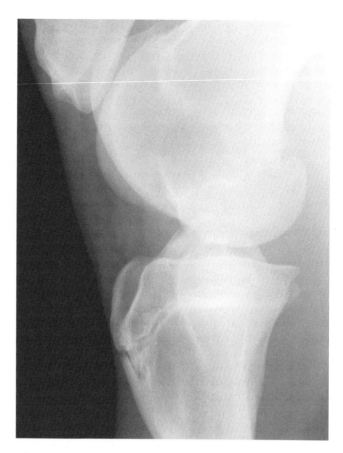

Figure 2.4(b) Lateromedial radiographic view of an immature stifle obtained using a computed radiography system. This is the same as Figure 2.4(a), obtained as the same exposure (i.e. identical exposure factors and algorithm), but the image has been windowed to permit better evaluation of both the soft tissues and some of the bone margins cranially.

Image manipulation

The image can be manipulated in a variety of ways, including alteration of brightness and contrast, magnification, and by edge enhancement. Alteration of brightness and contrast should enable thorough examination of the internal architecture of bone, the bone margins and the surrounding soft tissues on a single image, if these were not evident on the original image (Figures 2.4a and 2.4b). Thus potentially more information can be gained with appropriate manipulation. Maximal information will always be obtained from a well positioned, appropriately exposed image, and digital imaging and image manipulation are not a substitute for poor technique. Digital imaging provides the opportunity to enhance good radiographic technique.

It is necessary to learn how to examine a digital image. With a conventional film–screen image it is important to view the image from a distance and close up, and to use high-intensity illumination to examine bone margins more closely. With a digital image the reader should examine the entire image making use of the windowing facility to alter brightness and contrast

[46]

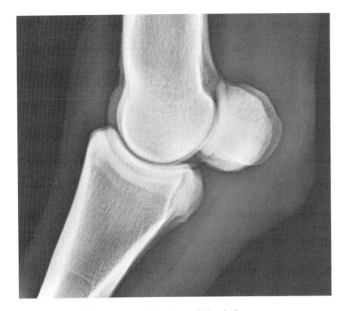

Figure 2.5(a) Lateromedial view of the left metatarsophalangeal joint of a 4-year-old Thoroughbred flat racehorse with bilateral hindlimb lameness associated with fetlock region pain. The image was acquired using computed radiography. There is sclerosis of the plantar aspect of the condyles of the third metatarsal bone.

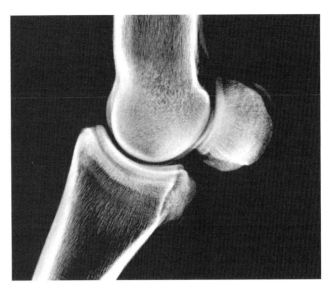

Figure 2.5(b) The same image as Figure 2.5(a) windowed, thus changing the appearance of the trabecular architecture. The relatively greater opacity of the condyles of the third metatarsal bone compared with the metaphyseal region of the proximal phalanx is clearly apparent, and sclerosis of the plantar aspect of the condyles is more obvious than in Figure 2.5(a).

as necessary (Figures 2.5a and 2.5b), to evaluate all the structures in the image. However, with optimal exposure factors and algorithms, little image manipulation should be necessary. The use of edge enhancement may or may not help image interpretation, by increasing the contrast between areas of different densities. Incorrect use of edge enhancement may produce confusing artefacts. For example it may create the impression of increased bronchial wall opacity in a thoracic image. Enlarging the image is often useful, but excessive enlargement results in the image becoming more pixellated and potentially more difficult to interpret. It is also important to recognize that when examining large bones, such as the distal aspect of the femur, windowing the image by alteration of the brightness and contrast may result in the apparent development of radiolucent areas (Figure 2.6) which should not be misinterpreted as a pathological lesions. Because the brightness and contrast of images can be manipulated easily, detection of conditions such as osteoporosis or increased lung density becomes more difficult.

The size of the displayed image is scaled according to the screen size, so real size may be more difficult to determine. Many images have a scale at the side of the image, and if this is present then very accurate measurements can be made much more easily than on conventional radiographs. Some software allows 'true' size measurement calibration. Angle measurements can also be obtained.

It should be possible to show more than one image on the monitor simultaneously in order to compare different views of the same area, or to compare images obtained on two different occasions. This facility is a feature

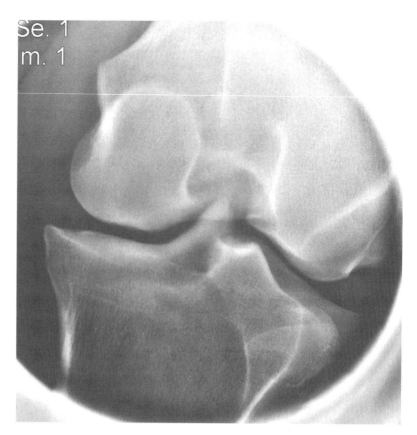

Figure 2.6 Coned caudocranial view of the right stifle of a 12-year-old Welsh Cob mare with left hindlimb lameness associated with the femorotibial joint. The image was acquired using computed radiography. Medial is to the left. The potentially superior image quality of a digital radiograph can lead to over-interpretation. There is a relatively radiolucent, oval-shaped area in the medial femoral condyle. This should not be misinterpreted as a subchondral bone cyst.

of the software provided with the system. The ease with which previous images can be recalled for viewing depends on the system and method of archiving.

IMAGE ARCHIVING AND TRANSMISSION

Digital radiography removes the necessity for hard copy. It can also make image retrieval much easier. All images can be stored electronically and the method used depends on the number of images acquired daily. The retrieval systems vary considerably and it is important to establish how images can be searched, e.g., patient name, owner, case number, area examined. Whatever system is used for image storage, it is vital that it is backed up as for any computer system, to ensure data are not irretrievably lost. Some systems have an automatic back-up system (e.g., CD burn and autorun), but others require a regular back-up protocol to be instituted. (Images can be stored on magnetic disk (hard disk), DVDs (digital versatile discs), optical discs or magneto optical discs.) A DICOM server can be used for data storage in a multisite practice that can be accessed via a telemedicine network allowing any authorized and connected user to view and handle files from many sites.

[48]

Additional software may be required to function fully with some management systems.

Although in theory digital images can be readily e-mailed, they do create large data files, which may not be suitable for transmission, unless specialized software is used. The reader should refer to their system advisers for up-to-date details of this rapidly changing field. Images can readily be saved to CDs, allowing transfer of information between users. It is necessary however to ensure that if DICOM files are used, the recipient of the disc has the necessary software to read the information. Many manufacturers now provide a software viewing package that is loaded on to the disc with the digital images.

Conversion to a compressed format allows more efficient storage and transmission. The original DICOM image can be compressed using, for example, Lossy compression. Such images retain all the original information, and can be more readily sent electronically. The word 'Lossy' appears on each image, identifying it as a compressed image. Such images are safe and cannot be fraudulently tampered with. When viewing the images the brightness and contrast can be altered, but such changes cannot be saved. Alternatively a DICOM image can be compressed by conversion to another format (e.g., jpeg). However, the receiver then has to open each file individually, which can be time consuming and laborious. The receiver also has to record the identity of each file (e.g., lateromedial view of the left front foot), which is often completely anonymous other than a jpeg number. Such jpeg files can easily be altered by changing brightness and contrast, and these changes can be saved. Alternatively the image could be imported into an image manipulation programme, e.g., Adobe Photoshop, and lesions obliterated and the image resaved. Thus it is potentially possible to mask a lesion by image manipulation. It may be possible to determine whether an image is an original or has been manipulated by looking at the storage data which should state the date and time of the original acquisition and details about when it was altered. Use the right mouse click on the image and then scroll down to 'Properties' which will give the dates and times of the original image creation and when it was modified. This is obviously a time-consuming process and would not be done routinely unless there was a suspicion of fraudulent manipulation. Alternatively large files can be sent off site using file transfer protocol (FTP), or a customized teleradiology system.

A potential problem with digital radiography is the different file formats in which images may be saved which can be difficult to open by a remote user. Although some systems load viewer software with the images on to a CD, this is not universal. This can present problems when images are saved on a CD and sent to another veterinarian for their interpretation. The files may not open with standard Windows applications and the header information (patient details) is inaccessible. Some systems open automatically in their own format, but for others a special piece of software, a DICOM viewer is required. Many modern veterinary computer systems running with Windows already have a DICOM viewer installed, but in order to view images on your PC or laptop computer a DICOM viewer must be installed. Many internet sites offer free software that can be downloaded and can be found by searching for 'DICOM viewer' using an appropriate search engine.

Software and software tools for viewing DICOM images are unfortunately not standardized. Some are more intuitive to understand than others. As with most Windows software, placing the mouse arrow over the tool symbol, will usually produce a short text describing the function of the tool. If images have been sent from another country, this is likely to be in the language of the country of origin of the images, and so may be of limited assistance. In this case, it may be necessary to resort to trial and error. If the result is not what was wanted, the operation can be cancelled and the image returned to the original stored image.

The way in which images are presented also varies. Some are presented in stack mode, so that by selecting forward and back arrows each can be viewed sequentially in maximum size. Others present the images in tile mode i.e. the images side by side in a grid pattern.

ADVANTAGES OF DIGITAL RADIOGRAPHY COMPARED WITH CONVENTIONAL FILM–SCREEN RADIOGRAPHY

The capital costs of digital equipment can be weighed against the absence of costs of conventional film and the chemicals required for processing. Digital systems eliminate the potential health and safety and environmental issues of darkroom processing, and eliminate the need for a darkroom. They also eliminate the environmental hazard of disposal of processing chemicals. Digital imaging should also reduce the number of images acquired, because fewer repeat x-rays are needed due to inappropriate exposures, and fewer repeat images are needed with different exposures to visualize specific lesions. There is reduced storage area needed for both processing chemicals and archiving of x-rays. The risk of processing artefacts is reduced. The time taken to obtain images can be reduced, especially with direct digital radiography. For a practitioner in the field, acquisition of images with digital radiography is no longer limited by the number of available cassettes. Images can be viewed on a laptop computer in the field, and although this may not have the same resolution as a better monitor, the images can be assessed for suitability of positioning and a preliminary diagnosis made.

Images are readily archived, and retrieval should be easier and more reliable than with conventional radiographs. Images are less likely to be lost (assuming that files are backed up), or misfiled. Image quality should also be stable over time. Images can easily be transmitted electronically making it much easier to obtain a second opinion on interpretation. Images acquired on behalf of a prospective purchaser can easily and rapidly be sent to their own veterinary surgeon for independent review.

Although theoretically film–screen radiographs contain more detailed information than computed or digital radiographs, given equivalent standards of radiography, in practice we have found that image quality and diagnostic capabilities have actually increased using computed systems. For example, the recognition of osseous fragments distal to the medial and lateral angles of the distal border of the navicular bone has increased. The potential for increased detail means relearning what is normal and not over-interpreting normal findings as pathological lesions. Over-interpretation is a common problem when first using a digital system. (Figure 2.6)

FURTHER READING

American College of Radiology (2005) *ACR Technical Standard for Teleradiology*, American College of Radiology

Armbrust, L. (2007) Digital images and digital radiographic image capture. In: *Textbook of Veterinary Diagnostic Radiology*, 5th edn, Ed. Thrall, D., pp 22–37, Elsevier, St. Louis

Cesar, L., Scheler, B., Zink, F. *et al.* (2001) Artefacts found in computed radiography. *Brit. J. Radiol.*, **74**, 195–202

www.idoimaging.com

Chapter 3
Foot, pastern and fetlock

The foot is a complex area, involving several bones as well as the hoof wall. This chapter has therefore been subdivided into anatomical areas in order to make description easier. Although several of these areas may be obtained on a single radiograph, radiographs centred on the area of interest are required for accurate appraisal.

Except where stated otherwise, the text refers to both front and hind feet.

Distal phalanx (pedal bone)

RADIOGRAPHIC TECHNIQUE

Equipment

Radiographs of the distal phalanx (third phalanx, pedal bone) can be obtained with low-output (minimum 15 mA) portable x-ray machines. Slow, high-detail screens with compatible film are recommended to obtain maximum definition. If machines with an output of 100 mA or less are used, slow, high-detail rare earth screens are appropriate.

Prior to obtaining radiographs, the shoe should be removed and the sole and hoof wall must be cleaned of mud and dirt. Loose flakes of horn from the sole, bulbs of the heel and frog should be trimmed. Particular care should be taken if the frog clefts are deep. A sharp pointed instrument, such as a searching knife, a hoof pick or rat tail file, is helpful for removal of packed debris. The clefts should finally be cleaned using a stiff brush. Radiographs of the distal phalanx do not normally require the foot to be packed, although packing around the point of the frog will eliminate air shadows from the foot and may avoid confusion in some cases, especially if a fracture is suspected. Care must be taken to ensure that the sole is packed evenly, as the low exposures required to visualize the solar margin of the distal phalanx can also result in images of uneven packing. Loose packing may mimic, or mask, fractures; excessive packing may create radiopaque artefacts. These packing artefacts are particularly evident on digital radiographs. Previous paring of the foot in search of a sub-solar abscess may result in confusing radiolucent areas superimposed over osseous structures.

Lateromedial and dorsopalmar or plantarodorsal views of the distal phalanx may be obtained using a grid (see relevant view for details), although this is not essential. Oblique views, particularly palmaroproximal-palmarodistal oblique and dorsoproximal-palmarodistal oblique views of the palmar processes, and soft exposures, e.g. radiographs to visualize separation of the hoof wall from the distal phalanx, lucent lines in the dorsal hoof wall, or subtle remodelling of the extensor process, are best obtained without a grid. When using digital systems, grids may cause moiré lines on the image, and so radiographs of areas such as the distal phalanx may be better obtained without the use of a grid.

Positioning

Any examination of the foot should always include lateromedial and dorsoproximal-palmarodistal oblique views. Mediolateral views have a similar appearance to lateromedial views and may be used if preferred. For hind feet it may be easier to obtain plantarodorsal rather than dorsoplantar views.

Lateromedial view

Lateromedial views of the distal phalanx normally require the foot to be raised on a block of sufficient height to bring the solar surface of the foot level with the centre of the x-ray beam. This also allows the bottom of the cassette to be placed lower than the solar surface of the foot, so that it is included on the film. The cassette can be supported on the floor, or on a second block, to minimize the risk of movement blur. The x-ray beam should be horizontal, and centred on the distal phalanx. Care must be taken when assessing the hoof–pastern axis with this technique, since this will be altered if the horse is not fully weight bearing on a level surface. An 8:1 ratio grid will give the best results for this view when using film, but acceptable results can be obtained without the use of a grid. Digital images are probably best obtained without a grid.

A survey lateromedial view of the entire foot and pastern may be obtained. In this case the maximum information will be obtained if the x-ray beam is centred on the navicular bone – the beam should be centred approximately 1 cm below the coronary band, and midway between the most dorsal and most palmar aspects of the foot at the level of the coronary band. The x-ray beam should be aligned parallel with a line drawn tangential to the bulbs of the heel. The importance of a true lateromedial view for accurate interpretation cannot be overemphasized. This may be difficult to obtain in horses with marked distortion of the hoof capsule, obvious toe-in or toe-out conformation, or if there is a poor medial–lateral hoof balance. If specific lesions of the distal phalanx are anticipated, the x-ray beam should be centred on the lesion, or on the distal phalanx, at approximately the region of insertion of the deep flexor tendon – a point approximately midway between the coronary band and the ground surface at the junction of the dorsal and middle thirds of the hoof. The beam should be aligned parallel with a line drawn tangential to the bulbs of the heel.

Dorsoproximal-palmarodistal oblique view

For hind feet it is often preferable to obtain a plantarodorsal view rather than a dorsoplantar projection of the foot. This gives good visualization of the structures within the foot and makes little difference to interpretation of radiographs of the distal phalanx.

A dorsoproximal-palmarodistal oblique view gives good visualization of the body, solar margin and palmar processes (wings) of the distal phalanx, and is suitable for use as a routine view. It may be obtained in one of two ways. The technique giving least distortion is the 'upright pedal' view. The toe of the foot is placed on a wooden block with a groove cut along its top surface (referred to as a 'navicular block', see Figure 3.38c, page 104), and the limb is manipulated until the sole of the foot is vertical. A horizontal x-ray beam is centred on the coronary band and aligned perpendicular to the sole of the foot (Figure 3.1a). A low-ratio grid (6:1) is ideal for this view when using film, but acceptable results can be obtained without the use of a grid (Figure 3.1b). For digital images, better results may be obtained without using a grid.

A similar view, a dorsoproximal-palmarodistal (high coronary) oblique, may be obtained with the horse standing on a tunnel containing the cassette. The x-ray beam is angled in a dorsoproximal-palmarodistal oblique direction, at approximately 65° to the horizontal, centred on the coronary band (Figure 3.2a). This technique has the disadvantage that the beam is oblique to the cassette, and therefore results in some distortion. It may be useful for visualizing fractures, and is helpful in some horses that resent placing the foot in a 'navicular block'. A parallel 6:1 ratio grid is used if the x-ray beam can be aligned with the grid lines; otherwise a better result is obtained without a grid (Figure 3.2b). For radiation safety reasons, this technique may be preferable.

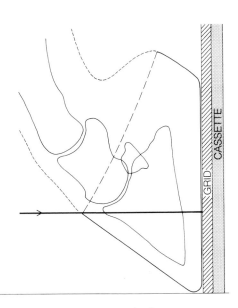

Figure 3.1(a) Positioning to obtain a dorsoproximal-palmarodistal oblique ('upright pedal') view of the distal phalanx. The x-ray beam (arrow) is centred on the coronary band.

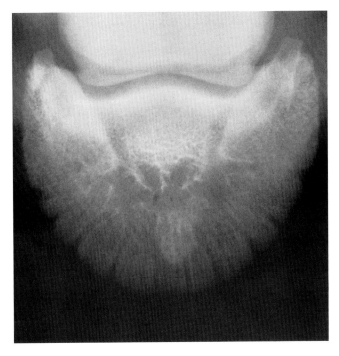

Figure 3.1(b) Dorsoproximal-palmarodistal oblique radiographic view of the distal phalanx of a normal adult horse, obtained using the 'upright pedal' technique.

[55]

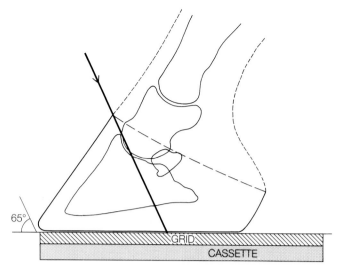

Figure 3.2(a) Positioning to obtain a dorsoproximal-palmarodistal oblique ('high coronary') view of the distal phalanx. The x-ray beam (arrow) is centred on the coronary band.

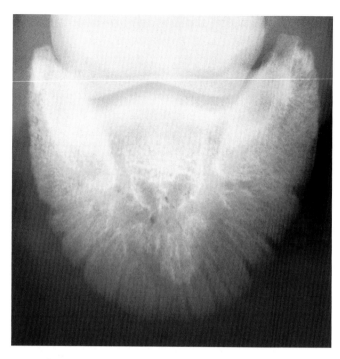

Figure 3.2(b) Dorsoproximal-palmarodistal oblique radiographic view of the distal phalanx of a normal adult horse (the same horse as Figure 3.1b), obtained using the 'high coronary' technique. Note the apparent elongation of the bone (compare with Figure 3.1b).

Dorsopalmar (weight-bearing) view

A dorsopalmar weight-bearing view is useful in selected cases, e.g. identification and assessment of a sagittal fracture of the distal phalanx, assessment of width of the distal interphalangeal joint and lateromedial foot imbalance, assessment of ossification of the cartilages of the foot and identification of changes in opacity of the submural soft tissues. The horse stands weight bearing on the limb, on a flat block, so that the cassette may be placed lower than the solar surface of the foot. A horizontal x-ray beam is centred midway between the coronary band and the ground surface, at the midline of the hoof (Figure 3.3). It should be aligned at right angles to a line drawn across the bulbs of the heel. This ensures a straight dorsopalmar view of the foot. If it is desired to record medial or lateral deviation of the limb distal to the fetlock, the beam should be aligned dorsoplantar to the metacarpal region. A 6:1 ratio grid is preferred.

Palmaroproximal-palmarodistal oblique view

This view is used to give good visualization of the palmar processes of the distal phalanx, particularly for identification of separation of the laminae of the heel of the foot, or a frontal plane fracture of a palmar process that may not be detectable in any other view.

[56]

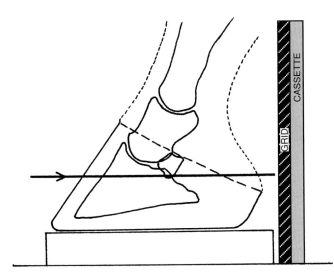

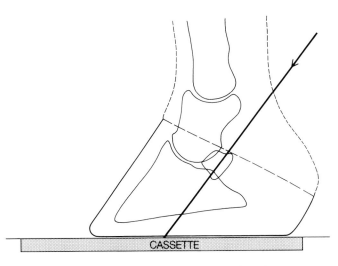

Figure 3.3 Positioning to obtain a dorsopalmar (weight-bearing) view of the distal phalanx and navicular bone (see Fig. 3.8c, page 64). The x-ray beam (arrow) is centred midway between the coronary band and the ground surface of the hoof.

Figure 3.4 Positioning to obtain a palmaroproximal-palmarodistal view of the distal phalanx (see Fig. 3.8d, page 65). The x-ray beam is centred between the bulbs of the heel.

The horse stands on a cassette tunnel, flat on the floor. The foot to be radiographed is positioned as far caudally under the horse as is consistent with the horse standing flat on the foot. The x-ray machine is placed ventral to the thorax of the horse and the x-ray beam centred between the bulbs of the heel (Figure 3.4). The angle of incidence of the x-ray beam to the cassette is 45–70°, dependent upon the slope of the pastern and the positioning of the foot. The beam is angled so that the image of the fetlock is not superimposed over the palmar processes of the distal phalanx. If the foot is positioned too far forward, it is impossible to avoid superimposition of the image of the fetlock over the foot, especially if the ergot is prominent. This view is obtained without a grid. An alternative technique to obtain this view is described on page 106.

Other oblique views

Oblique views of the distal phalanx and hoof wall are often required. These are particularly valuable if fractures involving the body or palmar processes of the distal phalanx are suspected, if new bone is present on the dorsal wall of the distal phalanx, or there is mineralization in the dermal laminae. They also help to identify periarticular modelling or entheseophytes on the dorsomedial and dorsolateral aspects of the distal interphalangeal joint. Obliquity is determined by one of two factors:
1 An attempt to align the x-ray beam parallel with the line of a fracture.
2 Positioning the x-ray beam so that new bone will be 'skylined' (i.e. the beam will form a tangent to the surface of the distal phalanx). For this purpose, reduced exposures should be used, and a grid is unnecessary.

Osteophyte or entheseophyte formation on the dorsolateral or dorso-medial aspects of the distal phalanx is often best seen on flexed oblique

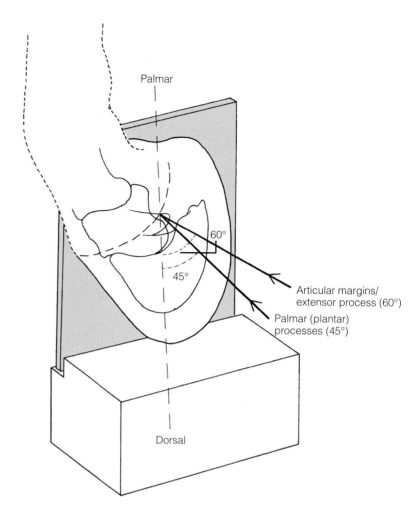

Figure 3.5 Positioning to obtain a dorsolateral-palmaromedial oblique (flexed) view of the distal phalanx and interphalangeal joints. The x-ray beam (arrow) is centred on the coronary band. An angle of 45° from dorsal highlights the lateral palmar process of the distal phalanx (see Fig. 3.8f, page 68). The dorsal margins of the interphalangeal joints are best imaged with an angle of 60° from the dorsal plane (see Fig. 3.8e, pages 66–67).

views, which open the distal interphalangeal joint. The toe of the foot is placed in a navicular block with the sole of the foot approximately vertical. Dorsal 60° lateral-palmaromedial oblique and dorsal 60° medial-palmarolateral oblique views are obtained. A horizontal x-ray beam is used, centred on the coronary band (Figure 3.5). To highlight the lateral and medial palmar processes, dorsal 45° lateral-palmaromedial oblique and dorsal 45° medial-palmarolateral oblique views respectively should be obtained.

Alternatively, to image the palmar processes, stand the horse on a tunnel containing the cassette. Angle the beam at 45° proximally and centre on the coronary band on the lateral or medial aspect of the foot (Figure 3.6). A lateral 45° proximal-mediodistal oblique highlights the lateral palmar process, a medial 45° proximal-laterodistal oblique images the medial side.

[58]

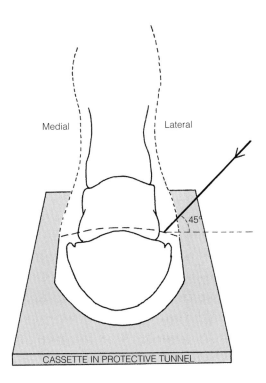

Medial   Lateral

45°

CASSETTE IN PROTECTIVE TUNNEL

Figure 3.6 Technique to obtain a lateral 45° proximal-mediodistal oblique view of the distal phalanx to skyline the lateral palmar process. The x-ray beam is centred on the coronary band. See also Figure 3.8(g), page 69.

The frog clefts should be carefully cleaned and packed to avoid radiolucent artefacts mimicking a fracture.

NORMAL ANATOMY

The front and hind distal phalanges have a similar appearance, but the bones of the hind feet are slightly narrower mediolaterally than those of the fore feet.

Immature horse

The distal phalanx develops from a single centre of ossification, which is present at birth (Figures 3.7a and 3.7b). It continues to enlarge and model until at least 18 months of age. The palmar processes are not evident at birth, and gradually ossify over 12 months, but may not obtain their full length until about 18 months.

Skeletally mature horse

Lateromedial view

The dorsal surface of the distal phalanx is smooth and opaque (Figure 3.8a). The cortex is of variable thickness. It may be slightly dorsally convex from

[59]

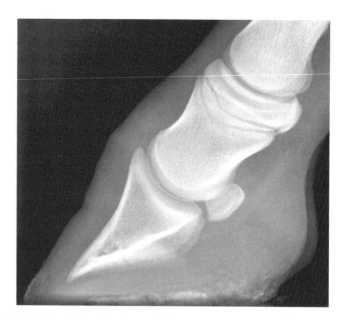

Figure 3.7(a) Slightly oblique lateromedial radiographic view of the foot of a normal foal of approximately 2 months of age. Note the rounded extensor process of the distal phalanx and the rounded shape of the navicular bone. The proximal physis of the middle phalanx is open. The foot shape is more upright than in an adult.

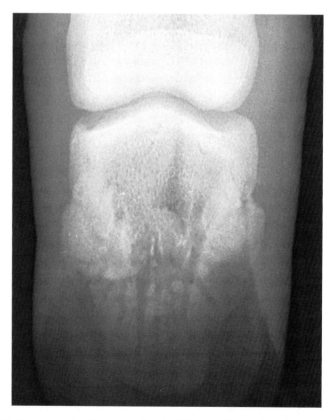

Figure 3.7(b) Dorsoproximal-palmarodistal oblique radiographic view of a foot of a normal foal of approximately 1 month of age. The medial and lateral borders of the distal phalanx are rather poorly defined. The triangular-shaped relatively radiolucent area to the right of the midline in the proximal half of the distal phalanx is a packing artefact.

the solar margin to the base of the extensor (pyramidal) process, especially in the hindlimbs, and should meet the solar margin at a sharp angle. In horses with a large crena marginis solearis (Figure 3.9a, page 70), a radiolucent indentation or a double line may be seen at the junction of these margins (Figure 3.9b). There are considerable variations in the shape of the extensor process, but they are usually bilaterally symmetrical (see Figure 3.11, page 72).

The solar surface of the distal phalanx is smooth in outline and is said to be normal if at a 3–10° angle to the sole, sloping proximally toward its palmar aspect. There are significant breed differences, with Thoroughbreds generally having a smaller angle than Warmbloods. The solar canal of the distal phalanx (through which runs the terminal arch of the digital arteries) is seen between the solar surface of the bone and the distal interphalangeal joint. It is seen with a variable degree of clarity, depending on the exposure factors used and the direction of the x-ray beam. It may appear as a very distinct radiolucent zone in the middle of the bone, proximal to the solar surface, but in some bones it is barely evident. Palmar to the solar canal is a sharply defined, smoothly outlined relatively sclerotic band of bone, the facia flexoria. The deep digital flexor tendon attaches to the palmar aspect (Figure 3.8a).

The articular surfaces of the middle and distal phalanges are reasonably congruous. There is sometimes a smoothly outlined V-shaped notch in the articular margin of the distal phalanx (Figure 3.9c, page 70). The middle of the articular margin of the middle phalanx may be slightly flattened. The width of the joint space depends on the amount of weight being borne on the foot, and the presence of any effusion within the joint.

Dorsoproximal-palmarodistal oblique view

The appearance of the distal phalanx on dorsoproximal-palmarodistal oblique upright pedal and high coronary views is essentially the same (Figure 3.8b). The solar margin is well defined, describing a regular curved outline. Some irregularity may be present. The distal phalanges of the hind feet are narrower and have a slightly more pointed outline at the toe than those of the front feet.

A distinct somewhat blunted V-shaped notch (crena marginis solearis) may be present in the midline in the dorsal aspect of the solar margin of the bone. This is usually present bilaterally, and is variable in size (up to 1.5 cm in depth) (Figure 3.9a).

Vascular channels are evident as radiolucent lines, radiating between the solar canal and the solar margin. They are variable in number and width, and may appear to narrow or widen slightly close to the solar margin.

The solar canal is evident as an irregular, roughly U-shaped lucency running through the centre of the distal phalanx, extending from the level of the distal interphalangeal joint to approximately midway between the joint and the solar margin of the bone.

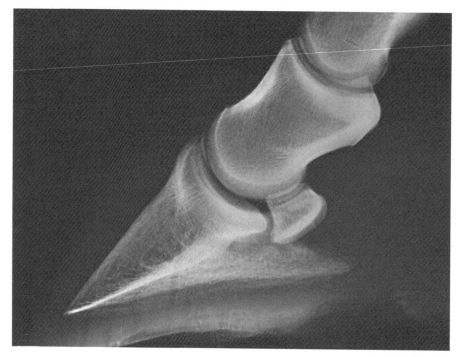

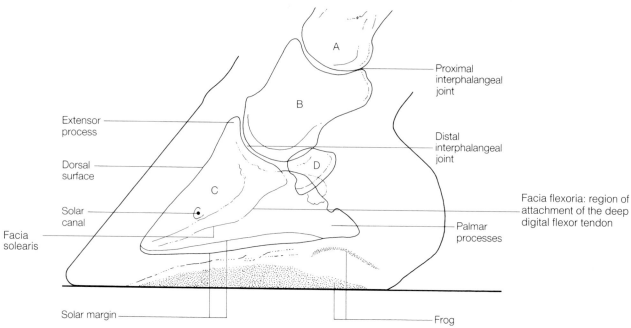

Figure 3.8(a) Well positioned lateromedial radiographic view and diagram of a normal adult foot. A = proximal phalanx, B = middle phalanx, C = distal phalanx, D = navicular bone. The toe of the foot has been cut off.

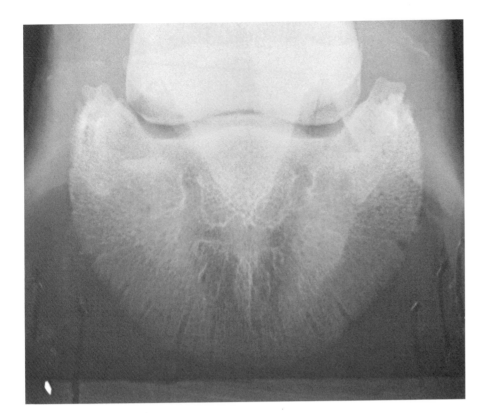

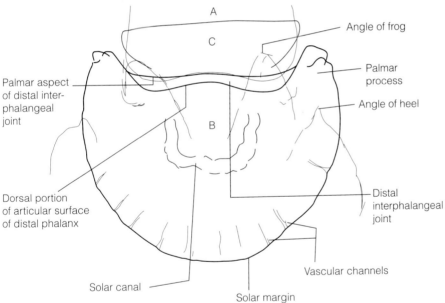

Figure 3.8(b) Dorsoproximal-palmarodistal oblique (upright pedal) radiographic view and diagram of a normal adult distal phalanx. Lateral is to the right. A = middle phalanx, B = distal phalanx, C = navicular bone. There is an oblique radiolucent line crossing the distal interphalangeal joint laterally, which represents a packing defect. There is mild modelling of the proximolateral aspect of the navicular bone.

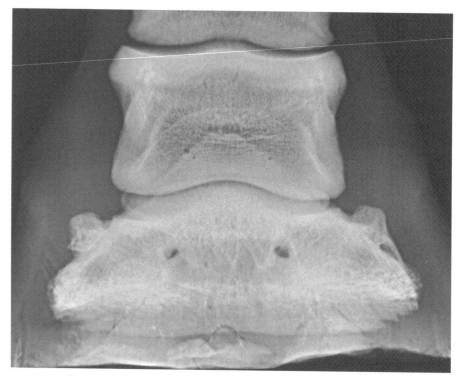

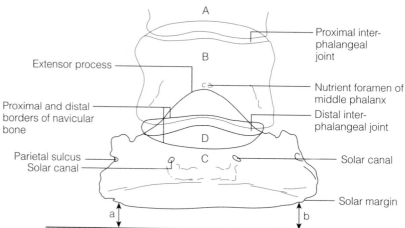

Figure 3.8(c) Dorsopalmar radiographic view and diagram of a normal adult foot. The radiographic image has been collimated so that the medial and lateral extremities of the hoof wall cannot be seen. Medial is to the left. The sole is thicker medially than laterally. Arrows a and b indicate the height between the distal border of the distal phalanx and the ground surface. A = proximal phalanx, B = middle phalanx, C = distal phalanx, D = navicular bone.

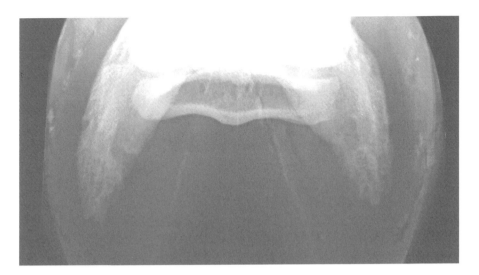

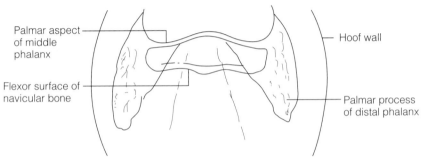

Palmar aspect of middle phalanx

Flexor surface of navicular bone

Hoof wall

Palmar process of distal phalanx

Figure 3.8(d) Palmaroproximal-palmarodistal oblique radiographic view and diagram of a normal adult foot. Medial is to the left. The slightly irregular margins of the palmar processes of the distal phalanx are normal. The horse had very deep frog clefts, so these were difficult to pack completely. Note also the radiolucent areas in the hoof wall medially and laterally, representing nail holes and the circumferential radiolucent area in the palmar lateral aspect of the hoof wall, representing an area of hoof wall separation.

The distal interphalangeal joint is evident as two distinct lines, the uppermost representing the palmar aspect of the articulation of the distal phalanx with the middle phalanx, close to its articulation with the distal sesamoid (navicular) bone. The lower of the two lines represents a more dorsal portion of the articular surface of the distal phalanx, its exact position depending on the angulation of the bone when radiographed.

Approximately oval-shaped radiolucent areas in the proximolateral and proximomedial aspects of the distal phalanx are seen with variable clarity at the insertions of the collateral ligaments of the distal interphalangeal joint (Figure 3.10, page 71). These should not be confused with osseous cyst-like lesions.

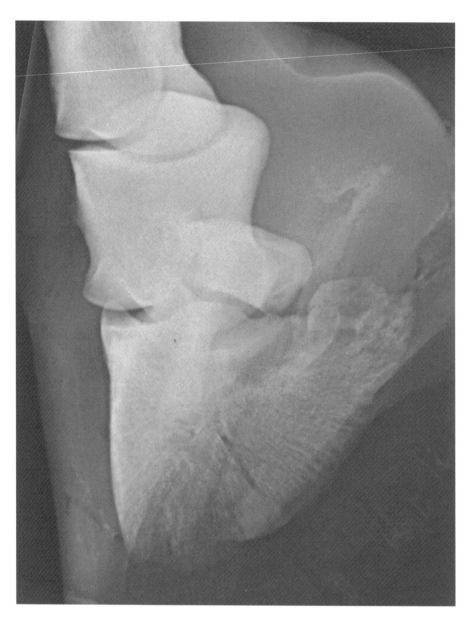

Figure 3.8(e) A flexed dorsal 60° lateral-palmaromedial oblique view and diagram of the pastern and foot of a normal adult horse. A = proximal phalanx, B = middle phalanx, C = distal phalanx, D = navicular bone.

Dorsopalmar (weight-bearing) view

In a dorsopalmar (weight-bearing) view (Figure 3.8c, page 64), the openings of the solar canal are seen as two distinct circular foramina distal to the articular surface. The extensor process may be difficult to examine, as it is superimposed over the distal end of the middle phalanx and the navicular bone. The parietal sulci (dorsal grooves) of the distal phalanx are seen as notches on the lateral and medial aspects of the bone. Occasionally these appear as a complete foramen rather than a notch. The solar margin of the bone should be an equal distance from the ground surface of the foot laterally and medially.

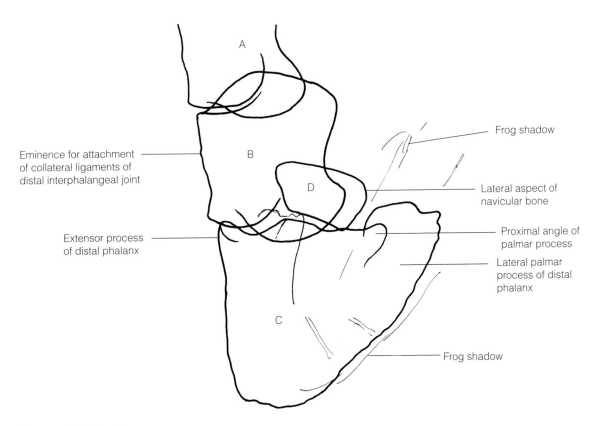

Eminence for attachment
of collateral ligaments of
distal interphalangeal joint

Extensor process
of distal phalanx

Frog shadow

Lateral aspect of
navicular bone

Proximal angle of
palmar process

Lateral palmar
process of distal
phalanx

Frog shadow

Figure 3.8(e) *Cont'd*

This is the best view to assess mediolateral foot balance (see page 99). The degree and symmetry of ossification of the cartilages of the foot (sidebone) are also best evaluated in this projection.

Palmaroproximal-palmarodistal oblique view

The palmar aspects of the palmar processes of the distal phalanx are seen on either side of the navicular bone (Figure 3.8d, page 65). The axial and abaxial surfaces have a relatively smooth appearance, although some irregular radiolucencies within the body of each process are often present. An oval opaque ring may be present in the processes, representing mineralization in the base of the hoof cartilage (collateral cartilage) (see also 'Ossification of the hoof cartilages', page 80). A lucent 'halo' is evident in the hoof wall immediately adjacent to the bone, representing the dermal tissue and laminae of the hoof.

Flexed dorsal 60° lateral-palmaromedial oblique and dorsal 60° medial-palmarolateral oblique views

The contour of the extensor process of the distal phalanx is smoothly curved. Depending on the degree of flexion, one of the condyles of the middle phalanx may be partially superimposed over the extensor process. The

[67]

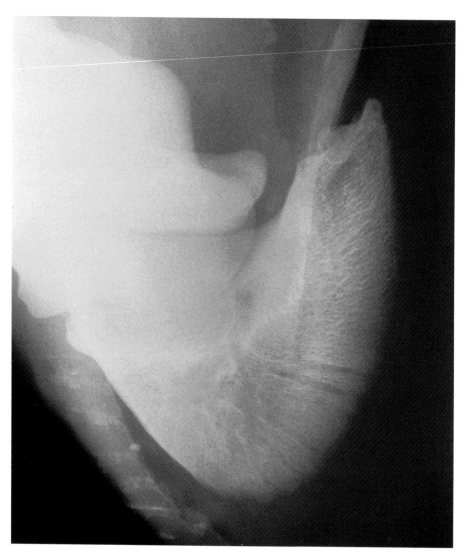

Figure 3.8(f) Dorsal 45° lateral-palmaromedial oblique (flexed) view of a pastern and foot of a normal adult horse.

eminence for the attachment of a collateral ligament on the distal aspect of the middle phalanx on the opposite side is also seen (Figure 3.8e). These eminences tend to be more prominent in heavier breeds of horses and cob-types compared with Thoroughbred-types. A lucent line courses obliquely across the distal phalanx. This may be either an edge effect created by the superimposition of the contralateral palmar process, or a frog shadow, depending on the projection angle. It should not be confused with a fracture. There is a variably sized notch or foramen on the palmar aspect of the palmar process, the parietal incisure or foramen of the palmar process, leading to the parietal sulcus (dorsal groove).

The dorsal 60° lateral-palmaromedial oblique view (Figure 3.8e, page 66) allows better evaluation of the proximal and distal interphalangeal joint margins than the dorsal 45° lateral-palmaromedial oblique view (Figure 3.8f). The lateral 45° proximal-medial distal oblique view permits more assessment of the lateral palmar process (Figure 3.8g).

[68]

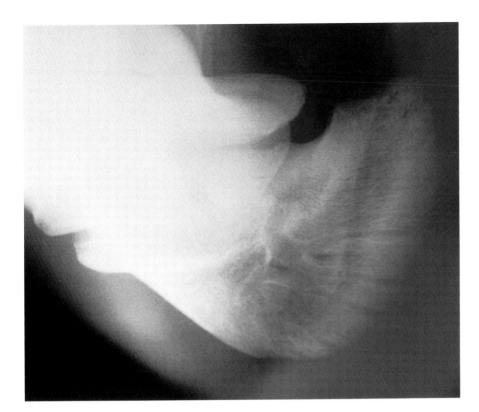

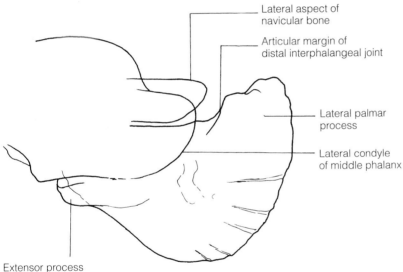

Lateral aspect of
navicular bone

Articular margin of
distal interphalangeal joint

Lateral palmar
process

Lateral condyle
of middle phalanx

Extensor process

Figure 3.8(g) Lateral 45° proximal-medial distal oblique view to highlight the lateral palmar process of the distal phalanx.

NORMAL VARIATIONS AND INCIDENTAL FINDINGS

A small circumscribed bony 'fragment' palmar to the palmar processes of the distal phalanx may represent a separate ossification centre or possibly a fracture sustained early in life. When present they are usually evident palmar to both palmar processes of both feet, although they may only occur in one foot or only at one process. Their diameter may vary between approximately 1 and 10 mm. These are best seen in lateromedial or dorsal 60° lateral-palmaromedial oblique or dorsal 60° medial-palmarolateral oblique

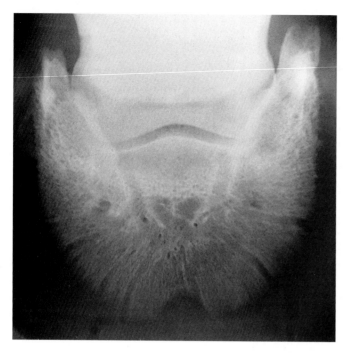

Figure 3.9(a) Dorsoproximal-palmarodistal oblique view of a normal adult horse. There is a large notch at the toe of the distal phalanx, the crena solearis.

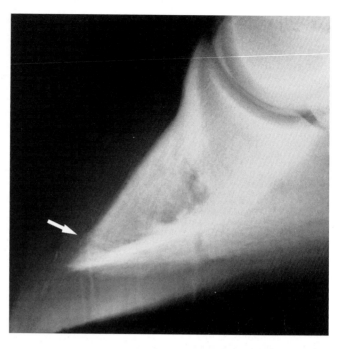

Figure 3.9(b) Lateromedial view of a distal phalanx of a normal adult horse, the same horse as Figure 3.9(a). Note the irregular appearance of the dorsal margin of the bone at the toe (arrow). This is created by the large crena solearis.

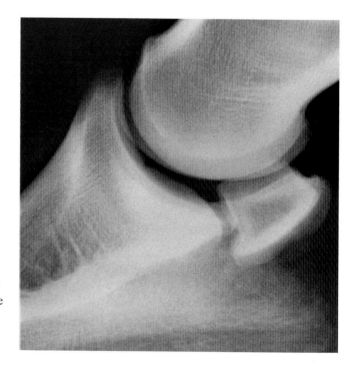

Figure 3.9(c) Lateromedial view of a distal interphalangeal joint of an adult horse. There is a V-shaped notch in the middle of the articular surface of the distal phalanx, of questionable clinical significance. Note also the smoothly outlined depression in the sagittal ridge of the navicular bone.

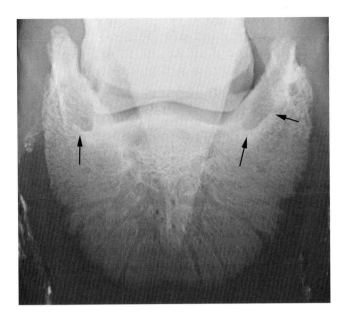

Figure 3.10 Dorsoproximal-palmarodistal oblique radiographic view of a normal distal phalanx. Medial is to the left. There are quite clearly demarcated smoothly outlined radiolucent areas medially and laterally (arrows) at the insertion sites of the collateral ligaments of the distal interphalangeal joint. These are normal and are seen with variable clarity, depending on the shape of the foot and its position during image acquisition. There are some irregularities of the solar margin of the distal phalanx at the quarters, medially and laterally, and a smoothly outlined depression, a crena, at the toe of the distal phalanx. These are normal variants. There is a moderately sized entheseophyte on the proximolateral aspect of the navicular bone.

views, but may also be seen in a dorsoproximal-palmarodistal oblique view. There may be slight sclerosis at the palmar aspect of the palmar process and at the dorsal aspect of the separate centre of ossification (Figure 3.12). These fragments should not be confused with clinically significant fractures of the palmar process, which are usually larger, and tend to have a sharper division from the body of the bone (see pages 87 and 88). A small radiopaque 'fragment' less than approximately 6 mm in diameter is sometimes present proximal to the extensor process (Figure 3.13). This is usually present in the midline, and may represent a separate centre of ossification, a fracture, or dystrophic mineralization within the common digital extensor tendon. They may be present bilaterally. Many of these fragments have a smooth outline, but trabeculation of the fragment may be seen. They may be of no clinical significance, although some may cause lameness (see 'Significant findings', pages 72–90).

Some degree of ossification of the hoof cartilages may be regarded as normal. Fusion between the ossified cartilage and the distal phalanx may not be present, may be incomplete or be complete. One or several ossification centres may be present, proximally, midway or distally in the cartilage. In most horses the cartilages of the foot are approximately symmetrically ossified medially and laterally, and there is symmetry between the front feet. Although ossification may extend slightly more proximally in one cartilage, usually the lateral one, this is usually not of clinical significance (see page 80).

Occasionally, on the dorsoproximal-palmarodistal oblique view, there may be a smoothly marginated, concave defect in the solar margin of the

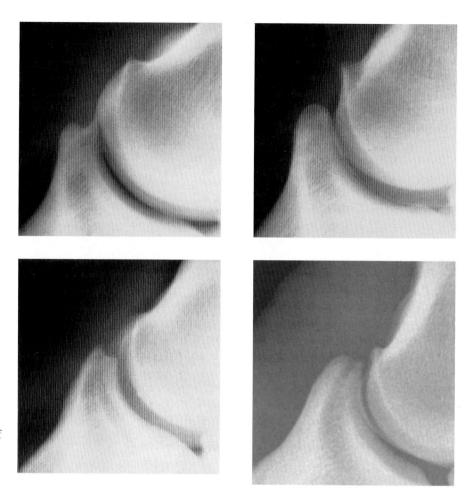

Figure 3.11 Lateromedial radiographs of the extensor process of normal distal phalanges, showing the variation in shape that may occur.

distal phalanx. These may extend 10–20 mm around the border, and be up to 5–6 mm in depth. They probably represent areas of resorption of bone resulting from pressure on the bone, secondary to infection or severe bruising. As long as there is a well defined margin to the bone, and no associated hoof wall distortion, these defects usually have no clinical significance. Once formed, they do not progress or regress over time.

In some horses one or both of the the parietal sulci of the distal phalanx appear as a foramen rather than a notch. Occasionally a well demarcated osseous cyst-like lesion is identified axially, distal to the articular surface of the distal phalanx; the overlying proximal cortex may have a smoothly demarcated indentation, but is clearly intact. Small cyst-like lesions may also be present at the medial or lateral margins of the joint within the distal phalanx. Magnetic resonance imaging suggests that the prevalence of asymptomatic osseous cyst-like lesions is probably much higher than previously recognized. Their significance must be assessed for each individual case, as they may be asymptomatic or associated with lameness.

SIGNIFICANT FINDINGS

Pedal osteitis

The term *pedal osteitis* strictly means inflammation of the distal phalanx, and has been widely used to describe a broad spectrum of radiographic

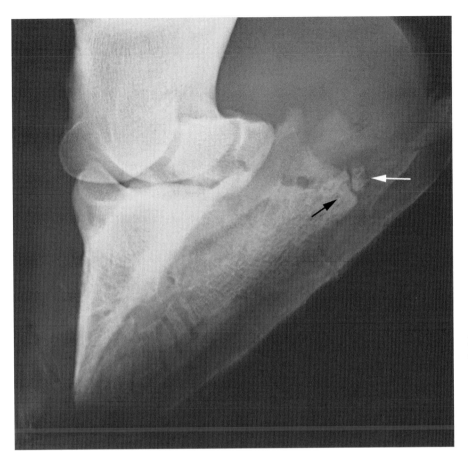

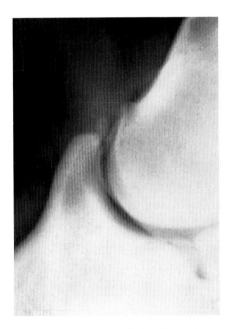

Figure 3.12 Dorsolateral-palmaromedial oblique view of a foot, highlighting the lateral palmar process of the distal phalanx, which has a separate centre of ossification palmarly (white arrow). The palmar aspect of the main part of the palmar process is sclerotic (black arrow). These are normal variants.

abnormalities of the distal phalanx. It is likely that there are both septic and aseptic forms of what has become known as 'pedal osteitis', but there is currently a dearth of information concerning the aetiology of some of the radiographic changes described. The authors acknowledge that there is a wide variation in the radiographic appearance of the distal phalanx in apparently normal horses, and that any radiographic changes that develop in the distal phalanx tend to persist. Because of the present lack of knowledge, the authors have elected to describe several discrete radiographic findings and their associated clinical signs under the general heading of 'pedal osteitis complex', without ascribing a specific name or aetiology to them. Other conditions with a known aetiology are then discussed under separate subheadings.

Pedal osteitis complex

The most common change referred to as part of the pedal osteitis complex is modelling of the solar margin of the bone. Changes are most obvious on dorsoproximal-palmarodistal oblique views (Figure 3.14a). The solar margin of the bone loses its relatively smooth, opaque outline due to demineralization. In mild cases the bone near the solar margin may have some increased radiolucency, making its visualization difficult. In more severe or long-standing cases, larger areas of bone may be resorbed from the solar margin of the bone, resulting in apparent widening of the vascular channels primarily at the solar margin.

Figure 3.13 Lateromedial radiograph showing a radiopaque body proximal to the extensor process of the distal phalanx (these fragments are of variable clinical significance – see pages 88–90).

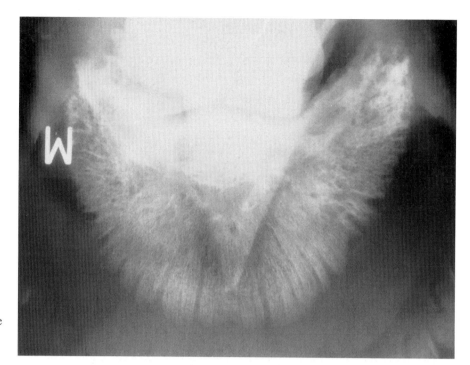

Figure 3.14(a) Pedal osteitis complex. Dorsoproximal-palmarodistal oblique ('upright pedal') view of a distal phalanx, showing demineralization of the solar margin and discrete circular lucent areas in the palmar processes.

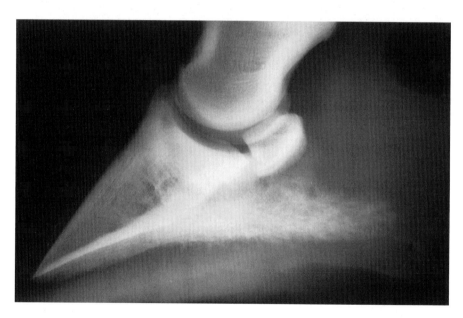

Figure 3.14(b) Lateromedial view of a distal phalanx of a 12-year-old Selle Francais with low, collapsed heels and foot pain. There is modelling and irregularity in outline of the solar margin of the distal phalanx. Nuclear scintigraphic examination confirmed increased bone activity in this area. Note also the small radiolucent zone immediately distal to the extensor process.

On lateromedial views these changes may be evident as remodelling of the tip of the bone, the solar margin no longer showing a straight outline but curving proximally towards the dorsal aspect of the bone. This change appears to be exaggerated if the radiograph is not a true lateromedial projection. In more advanced cases new bone may be laid down on the dorsal surface of the bone at the toe. This change is frequently seen in animals that,

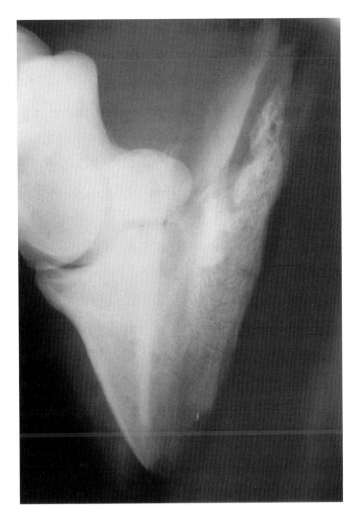

Figure 3.14(c) Dorsal 60° medial-palmarolateral (flexed) oblique view of a distal phalanx of a 10-year-old Dutch Warmblood with low, collapsed heels and foot pain. There is modelling and elongation of the medial palmar process of the distal phalanx. Nuclear scintigraphic examination confirmed increased bone activity in this region.

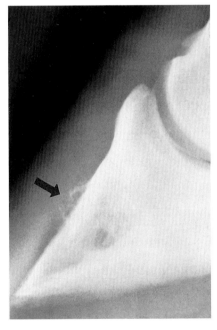

Figure 3.14(d) Pedal osteitis complex. Lateromedial radiograph of the dorsal surface of a distal phalanx, showing mineralization (arrow) in the dermal laminae. (N.B. This is a slightly oblique view.)

over a period of time, have taken an increased pressure on the sole, e.g. after laminitis or in horses with flat soles. Active bone formation along the distal portion of the dorsal cortex is nearly always considered abnormal. Slight new bone formation seen in oblique views along the middle portion of the dorsal cortex is sometimes seen in horses not displaying lameness and may not be of clinical significance.

A second change associated with the pedal osteitis complex is seen in the palmar processes of the distal phalanx. It is best visualized on dorso-proximal-palmarodistal oblique or palmaroproximal-palmarodistal oblique radiographs. Discrete circular radiolucent areas, 2 mm or 3 mm in diameter, are present in the palmar processes of the bone, and these may be associated with new bone, particularly on the axial surfaces of the palmar processes (Figure 3.14a). Modelling changes of the palmar processes may also be seen

[75]

in a lateromedial view. The solar aspect of the palmar processes may have an irregular outline (Figure 3.14b). There may be a change in shape with elongation of the palmar processes, seen also in a flexed dorsolateral-palmaromedial (or dorsomedial-palmarolateral) oblique view (Figure 3.14c). These changes are sometimes seen in association with an abnormally thin sole and/or abnormal orientation of the solar surface of the distal phalanx seen in a lateromedial view (the solar surface of the distal phalanx may be horizontal, or the palmar processes may be lower than the toe) (see also 'Long-toe, low-heel syndrome', page 97).

These changes, and those described above, are probably associated with concussion of the bone and may be related to poor foot conformation and shoeing imbalances. They may be associated with lameness that is most marked on hard surfaces. Treatment is by corrective trimming and shoeing. Although the condition may resolve clinically, the radiological changes usually remain throughout life. Nuclear scintigraphy may help to determine the significance of these radiographic changes within the distal phalanx. Focal intense or moderate increased radiopharmaceutical uptake in one (most commonly the medial) or both palmar processes may occur with or without detectable radiographic abnormality, although generally in association with altered signal intensity on magnetic resonance images. This may indicate acute or chronic bone trauma.

Mineralized lesions on the dorsal wall of the distal phalanx may be seen (Figure 3.14d). These are usually approximately midway between the proximal border and solar margins of the bone on its dorsal surface, either in the midline or slightly to either side of it. These lesions are best visualized on a lateromedial or slightly oblique lateromedial view. Slight irregularities associated with the parietal sulci may be normal. The aetiology of this lesion is uncertain. It may represent new bone on the dorsal surface of the distal phalanx, or mineralization within the dermal tissue or dermal laminae. Although slight roughening of the dorsal cortex may be an incidental finding, mineralization in the laminae is usually associated with lameness.

Infectious osteitis

The pedal bone has no medullary cavity and therefore infection of this bone is, strictly speaking, an infectious osteitis, not osteomyelitis. It has only a single layer of fibrous periosteum, which thins distally, therefore new bone formation associated with infection is less obvious than at other locations. Infections of the foot are common, but only infrequently do they involve the distal phalanx, with a resultant infectious osteitis. When present, infection most commonly involves the dorsal or solar surfaces of the distal phalanx, where it may cause focal demineralization (this may appear on a dorsoproximal-palmarodistal oblique view as a defect in the solar margin of the bone; Figure 3.15a). The lucent lesion usually has an irregular margin and there is seldom surrounding sclerosis, although new bone may be present at its margins (most easily seen on tangential views). There may be signs of chronic bone inflammation including a focal or generalized loss of radiopacity and widening of the vascular channels. Early lesions are more difficult to detect and are seen as an irregular margin or ill defined lucent area in the solar margin of the distal phalanx. High-quality radiographs are essential. In more advanced cases a radiopaque sequestrum is sometimes seen, surrounded by a lucent border.

Infectious osteitis is extremely painful and usually requires surgical treatment. The prognosis following surgery is fair to good, depending on the extent of tissue that has been involved. Supportive shoeing may be required until complete solar strength has eventually been regained (see also 'Infection', page 100).

Penetrating wounds through the sole of the foot may result in infectious osteitis of the solar surface of the distal phalanx. Initially this appears as a lucent area of bone on a dorsoproximal-palmarodistal oblique view. Occasionally antibiotic treatment of these lesions will result in a pocket of inspissated pus being walled off within the distal phalanx. This may result in a well defined radiolucent zone appearing as an osseous cyst-like lesion (Figure 3.15b). These lesions may cause intermittent lameness when the horse is worked on a hard surface. Close examination of these lesions reveal no connection with the distal interphalangeal joint, which may help to differentiate them from other osseous cyst-like lesions.

Osseous cyst-like lesions

Osseous cyst-like lesions not connected to the distal interphalangeal joint may be associated with infectious osteitis (see above).

Solitary osseous cyst-like lesions (see Chapter 1, page 33) close to or associated with the distal interphalangeal joint are occasionally seen. Care should be taken not to confuse this with a lucency created by a cavity frequently seen in the centre of the frog. They are generally most easily visualized on the dorsopalmar or dorsoproximal-palmarodistal oblique views (Figure 3.16a). When cysts are present, the distal interphalangeal joint should be carefully inspected for evidence of secondary degenerative joint disease. Lameness associated with osseous cyst-like lesions in the midline rarely resolves with conservative treatment. Surgical treatment of the cyst has proved successful in some cases, especially in horses less than 3 years of age. Small osseous cyst-like lesions (1–3 mm diameter) may occur at the lateral or medial border of the distal interphalangeal joint, and a better prognosis may be given for conservative treatment in these cases. Osseous cyst-like lesions may occasionally be seen at a pre-purchase examination in a clinically sound horse. Their significance is unpredictable.

A poorly or well defined osseous cyst-like lesion may be seen in the axial aspect of a palmar process of the distal phalanx at or close to the insertion of one of the collateral ligaments of the distal interphalangeal joint (Figure 3.16b). These vary in size and occur more commonly medially than laterally. These osseous cyst-like lesions reflect bone necrosis at the ligament's insertion and may or may not be associated with desmitis of the body of the ligament.

Occasionally an ill defined radiolucent line is seen within the dorsoproximal aspect of the distal phalanx on a lateromedial view, approximately

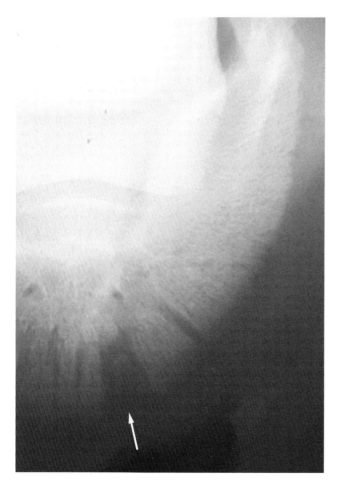

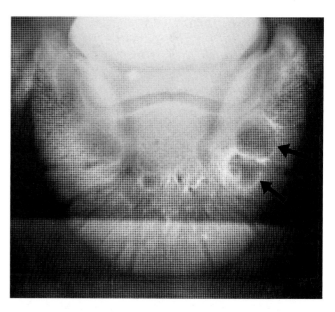

Figure 3.15(b) Infection of the distal phalanx. Dorsoproximal-palmarodistal oblique view of a distal phalanx, showing lucent areas (arrowed) surrounded by sclerosis. These represent inspissated pus within the distal phalanx. (The increased opacity at the toe of the bone is due to superimposition of the block supporting the foot.)

Figure 3.15(a) Infection of the distal phalanx; infectious osteitis. Collimated dorsoproximal-palmarodistal oblique radiographic view of a distal phalanx. Medial is to the left. Lateral to the toe there is a large radiolucent defect in the distal phalanx, the result of infection (arrow). Within the radiolucent area is an ill defined opacity, which may represent necrotic bone.

1–2 cm palmar to the apex of the extensor process (Figure 3.16c). The presence of an osseous cyst-like lesion has been confirmed at arthroscopic evaluation of the joint, and generally the surrounding bone and cartilage are also abnormal. Response to surgical debridement has been poor.

Tumours

The most common tumour to involve the distal phalanx is a keratoma. Typically it is seen on a dorsoproximal-palmarodistal oblique view. Additional oblique views may be required for better visualization. Pressure from the tumour on the dorsal wall of the distal phalanx causes resorption of bone. This is most easily seen at the solar margin of the bone, where a distinct semicircular notch is evident. This has a smooth outline, the bone underlying the keratoma frequently being sclerotic, which helps to differentiate this lesion from infection. There is usually no new bone associated with the lesion (Figure 3.17a).

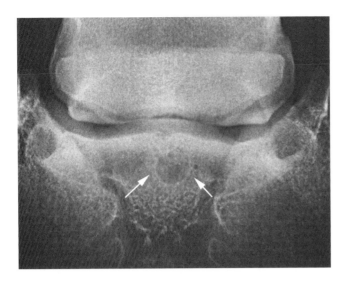

Figure 3.16(a) Osseous cyst-like lesion. Dorsoproximal-palmarodistal oblique view of a distal phalanx. There is a central osseous cyst-like lesion in the distal phalanx (white arrows), surrounded by a narrow rim of sclerosis. There is a small, smoothly outlined depression in the subchondral bone of the distal phalanx proximal to the lesion, but no communication with the distal interphalangeal joint could be identified. The osseous cyst-like lesion was not believed to be contributing to lameness. The radiolucent zones in the distal phalanx medially and laterally represent the depressions in which the collateral ligaments of the distal interphalangeal joint insert.

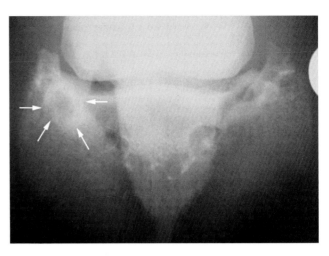

Figure 3.16(b) Osseous cyst-like lesion at the insertion of a collateral ligament of the distal interphalangeal joint. Dorsoproximal-palmarodistal oblique view of a foot. Medial is to the left. There is a broad sclerotic rim around a relatively radiolucent area medially (arrows), which represents a lesion at the insertion of the medial collateral ligament of the distal interphalangeal joint, which was confirmed using magnetic resonance imaging.

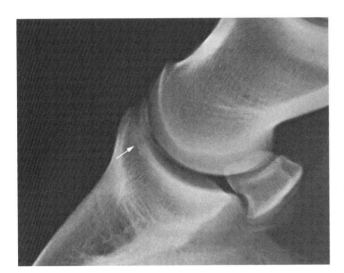

Figure 3.16(c) Collimated lateromedial view of the right front foot of a Warmblood showjumper, with lameness improved by intra-articular analgesia of the distal interphalangeal joint. There is an ill defined osseous cyst-like lesion in the dorsoproximal aspect of the distal phalanx (arrow), which communicated with the distal interphalangeal joint. The lesion was treated by surgical debridement, however lameness persisted.

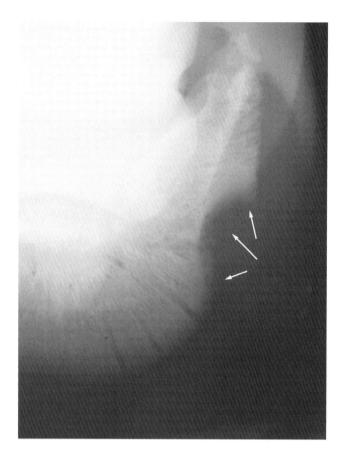

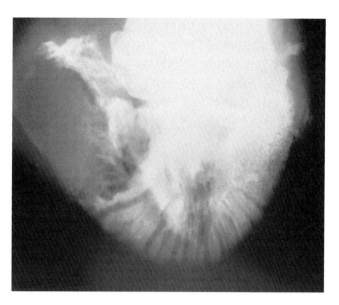

Figure 3.17(b) Fibrosarcoma. Dorsolateral proximal-palmaromedial distal oblique view of the distal phalanx, showing modelling of the bone resulting from a fibrosarcoma.

Figure 3.17(a) Keratoma. Dorsoproximal-palmarodistal oblique view of a distal phalanx. There is a large, smoothly outlined defect in the distal phalanx (arrows) resulting from resorption of bone due to pressure caused by a keratoma.

Keratomas may occur at any point in the hoof wall. Although initially causing little distortion of adjacent tissues, they cause deformation of the wall, sole and white line as they progress. Keratomas in the hoof wall are most commonly seen in the dorsal half of the foot, but have also occasionally been recorded in the solar horn. A keratoma may cause lameness as it enlarges, and may be associated with secondary infection. Treatment is by surgical removal of the keratoma and carries a reasonable prognosis, although the tumour may recur up to several years later.

Other tumours have been recorded infrequently (e.g. fibrosarcoma, neurofibroma, haemangioma, squamous cell carcinoma and malignant melanoma). They tend to be associated with remodelling of adjacent bone (Figure 3.17b). Non-neoplastic focal fibroplasia may also occur, resulting in a smoothly marginated defect anywhere in the margin of the distal phalanx.

Ossification of the cartilages of the foot (side bone)

A degree of mineralization of the cartilages of the foot is a very common finding, particularly in heavy breeds and large British native ponies, and is frequently not associated with clinical signs, although extensive ossification may result in slight shortening of the stride. Ossification, or mineralization

[80]

progressing from the distal aspect of the cartilage proximally to the level of the proximal border of the navicular bone, may be considered a normal process in any animal of 2 years of age or more (Figure 3.18). Ossification may commence in the proximal half of the cartilage and spread outwards. This is usually asymptomatic (Figure 3.19).

The proximal half of the cartilage is directed slightly axially, and where ossification occurs from the base and from the proximal half of the cartilage simultaneously, a radiolucent line may be apparent at the point where the two meet (Figure 3.20), frequently at the level where the axial deviation in the cartilage occurs. This may be difficult to differentiate from a fracture of the ossified cartilage. Nuclear scintigraphy may be helpful. The junction between separate ossification centres usually has no radiopharmaceutical uptake, or uptake similar to the regions of ossification, whereas a fracture or trauma to the union between ossification centres is associated with increased radiopharmaceutical uptake and eventually formation of a callus. Fracture of an ossified cartilage is rare, but causes acute onset of lameness which normally resolves with rest. Fractures usually occur in the distal part of the ossified cartilage. Horses with moderate to extensive ossification of the cartilages of the foot are at higher risk than horses with mild or no ossification of both fracture of the ossified cartilage or bone trauma at the junction of the cartilage with the distal phalanx. Bone trauma can only be identified using nuclear scintigraphy and magnetic resonance imaging. Completely ossified cartilages are rarely seen, and may extend proximally to the level of the proximal interphalangeal joint (Figure 3.21).

The degree of ossification is usually approximately bilaterally symmetrical within a foot and between front feet; if there is asymmetry within a foot, the lateral cartilage is usually more extensively mineralized. Marked asymmetry of ossification is unusual (Figure 3.22) and may be associated with lameness.

Entheseophytes on the extensor process of the distal phalanx

The common digital extensor tendon inserts on the extensor process of the distal phalanx. Tearing of the insertion may result in lameness, and entheseophyte formation on the dorsal aspect of the extensor process, rather than at its apex (Figure 3.23). This change must be distinguished from the normal variation in shape of the extensor process (see Figure 3.11, page 72). The outline caused by formation of entheseophytes is irregular, and there may be alteration in the opacity and trabecular structure of the underlying bone. Its significance must be interpreted in the light of clinical signs, since the radiographic changes persist despite resolution of lameness.

Entheseophytes at the insertion of the deep digital flexor tendon

The deep digital flexor tendon inserts on the facia flexoria of the distal phalanx, in a smoothly outlined concavity (Figure 3.8a, page 62). The cortex of the bone at this site should be smooth and regular as it meets the more

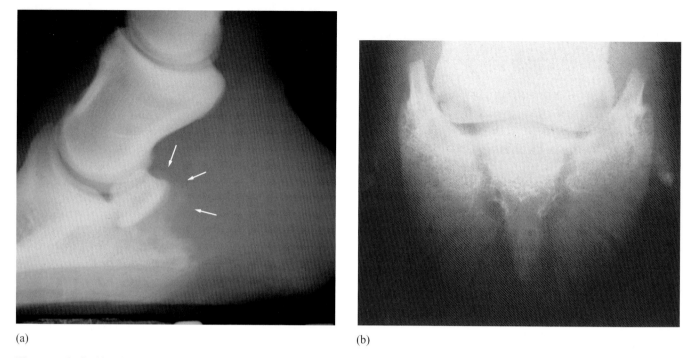

(a)

(b)

Figure 3.18 Ossification of the cartilages of the foot. Ossification from the distal aspect (arrows) of the cartilages: (a) lateromedial view; (b) dorsoproximal-palmarodistal oblique view.

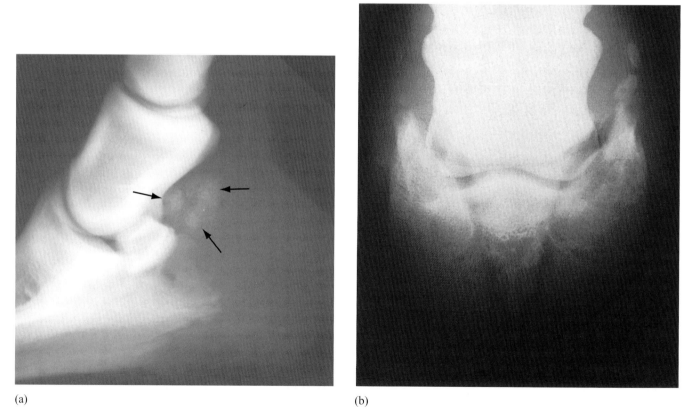

(a)

(b)

Figure 3.19 Ossification of the cartilages of the foot. Separate centres of ossification in the proximal half of the cartilages and in the distal aspect of the cartilages: (a) slightly oblique lateromedial view – note that the proximal areas of ossification are seen as poorly defined radiopaque areas (arrowed) proximal to the navicular bone; (b) dorsoproximal-palmarodistal oblique view.

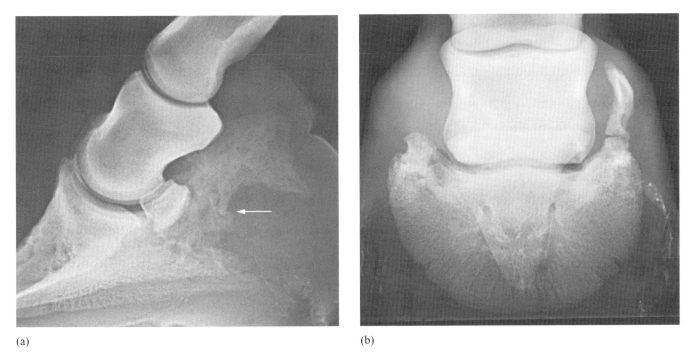

(a)   (b)

Figure 3.20 Ossification of the lateral cartilage of the foot. Separate centres of ossification in the proximal and distal aspects of the cartilage have met to give almost complete ossification of the cartilage. (a) Lateromedial view. There is a radiolucent line (arrow) between the two ossification centres, note also modelling of the dorsal articular margins of the distal interphalangeal joint; (b) dorsoproximal-palmarodistal oblique view of a different horse. Lateral is to the right. There is a separate ossification centre of the lateral ossified cartilage.

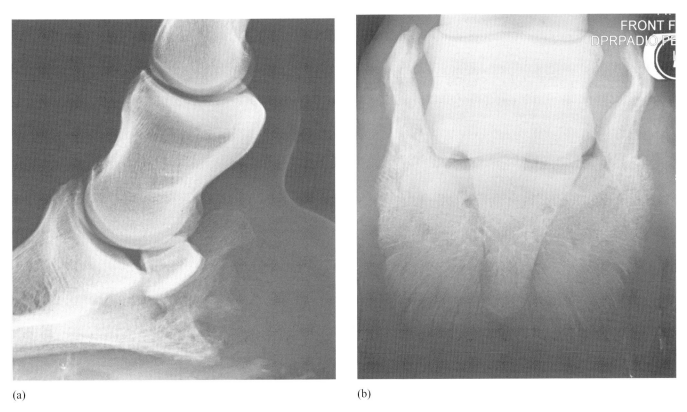

(a)   (b)

Figure 3.21 Complete ossification of the cartilages of the foot: (a) lateromedial view; (b) dorsoproximal-palmarodistal oblique view.

[83]

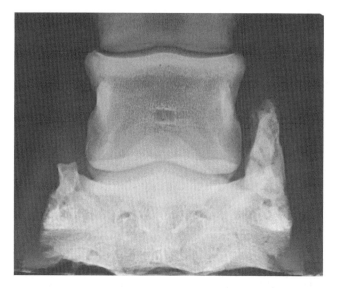

Figure 3.22 Dorsopalmar radiographic view of a foot of a 7-year-old Irish Sports Horse. Medial is to the left. There is mild ossification of the medial cartilage of the foot and extensive ossification of the lateral cartilage of the foot. The lateral ossified cartilage has rather heterogeneous opacity. Such marked asymmetry of ossification may be a risk factor for lameness. This horse was unilaterally lame in association with evidence of bone trauma of the distal phalanx distal to the lateral ossified cartilage and desmitis of the ipsilateral collateral ligament of the distal interphalangeal joint.

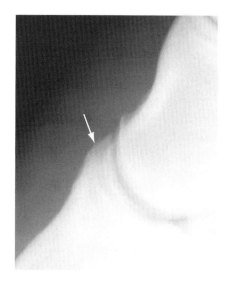

Figure 3.23 Entheseophytes on the extensor process of the distal phalanx (arrow) (slightly oblique lateromedial view).

proximal site of the insertion of the distal sesamoidean impar ligament. Tearing of the attachment of the deep digital flexor tendon may result in irregular new bone formation, or ill defined lucent areas in the normally uniformly opaque bone. This may be associated with lameness. Transcuneal ultrasonography may provide additional information.

Degenerative joint disease of the distal interphalangeal joint

Degenerative joint disease of the distal interphalangeal joint is a common cause of lameness, although frequently associated with little, if any, radiographic change. Radiographic abnormalities are seen most easily on lateromedial (Figure 3.24a) and flexed oblique views (Figure 3.24b). Modelling of the extensor process of the distal phalanx is commonly, but not invariably, associated with degenerative joint disease (see 'Entheseophytes on the extensor process of the distal phalanx' above), and its presence should alert the clinician to examine the joint carefully. It is important to distinguish between modelling, modelling with loss of trabeculation and cortex and modelling with fragmentation. Arthroscopic assessment of the extensor process often reveals poor quality bone despite relatively normal radiographs. Radiographic changes of degenerative joint disease include periarticular and periosteal osteophytes on the proximal articular margin of the distal phalanx, on the distodorsal and/or distal palmar aspects of the middle phalanx, and slight irregularity and incongruity of the joint surfaces,

[84]

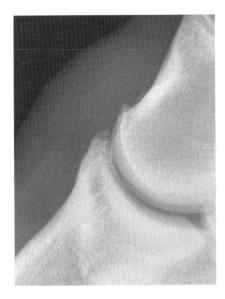

Figure 3.24(a) Lateromedial radiographic view of the distal phalanges of a 7-year-old showjumper with lameness substantially improved by intra-articular analgesia of the distal interphalangeal joint. There is modelling of the extensor process of the distal phalanx and the distal dorsal aspect of the middle phalanx, consistent with degenerative joint disease. Note that the spur on the apex of the extensor process of the distal phalanx is less opaque than the parent bone.

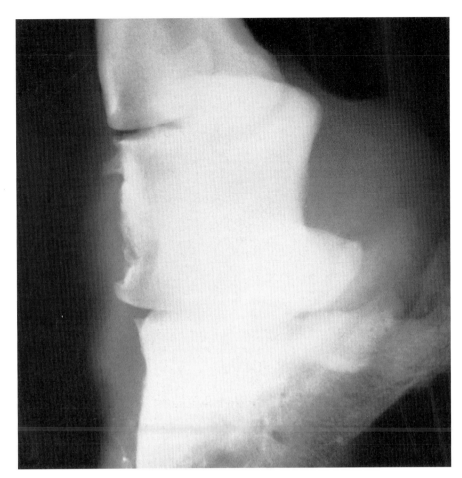

Figure 3.24(b) Flexed dorsolateral-palmaromedial oblique view of a pastern and foot of a 6-year-old Warmblood with degenerative joint disease of the proximal and distal interphalangeal joints. There is osteophyte formation on the dorsoproximal medial aspects of the middle and distal phalanges. The distal dorsomedial aspect of the middle phalanx is also modelled. Note also the rather irregular contour of the entire dorsomedial aspect of the middle phalanx and the distal palmarolateral aspect of the proximal phalanx. This may suggest that trauma was the inciting cause of degenerative joint disease.

particularly the articular surface of the extensor process. Periarticular osteophytes on the dorsoproximal articular margin of the navicular bone may also be an indicator of osteoarthritis, but should not be confused with entheseophyte formation, which occurs more palmad. Non-articular new bone on the dorsal diaphysis of the middle phalanx (see page 141 and Figure 3.65, page 144) should not be confused with periarticular osteophyte formation, and is not necessarily associated with degenerative joint disease. In more advanced cases some subchondral bone lucency may be visible at the dorsal aspect of the joint, or there may be altered trabecular architecture. There may also be narrowing or unevenness of the joint space visible on a dorsopalmar (weight-bearing) view (Figure 3.25). (Genuine narrowing of the joint space reflects advanced osteoarthritis, but should not be confused with the distal interphalangeal joint space being widened on one side due to a hoof imbalance. A mediolateral hoof imbalance may result in this appearance on dorsopalmar views, despite the horse bearing full weight on the

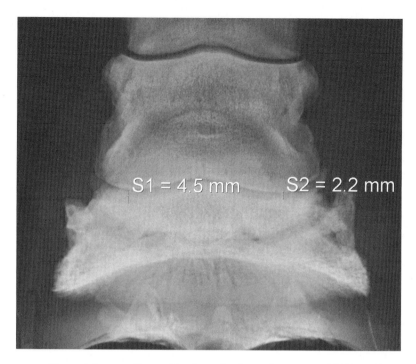

Figure 3.25 Dorsopalmar radiographic view of a foot of a 5-year-old Warmblood gelding with severe lameness. Medial is to the left. The lateral aspect of the distal interphalangeal joint ($S_2 = 2.22$ mm) is considerably narrower than the medial aspect ($S_1 = 4.5$ mm). This is consistent with advanced degenerative joint disease. Compare with the much more consistent joint space width of the proximal interphalangeal joint. There is also a large entheseophyte on the proximal lateral aspect of the navicular bone.

limb, and this is not synonymous with degenerative joint disease. A medio-lateral hoof imbalance may also make it difficult to obtain true lateromedial views.)

Degenerative joint disease carries a poor prognosis once radiographic changes are present, although modelling of the extensor process alone need not be associated with current lameness. Some cases will respond to careful balancing of the feet, the use of anti-inflammatory drugs and/or intra-articular medication. Modelling changes of the distal interphalangeal joint are sometimes seen in association with navicular disease.

Subluxation of the distal interphalangeal joint

Dorsopalmar subluxation of the distal interphalangeal joint is usually the result of partial or complete disruption of the deep digital flexor tendon. It is best identified on a lateromedial projection. There is widening of the joint space and the middle phalanx is displaced in a palmar direction. Mediolateral subluxation of the joint occasionally occurs as a result of disruption of a collateral ligament of the distal interphalangeal joint. This can be difficult to recognize in radiographs obtained with the foot bearing weight evenly. 'Stressed' dorsopalmar radiographs obtained with the horse standing on a wedge-shaped block may reveal abnormal widening of the joint space.

Agenesis or hypoplasia of the distal phalanx

Agenesis (congenital absence of) or hypoplasia of the distal phalanx is a rare radiographic finding in foals, usually associated with malformation of the hoof capsule.

Fractures

Common fracture sites of the distal phalanx are shown in Figure 3.26. A fracture through the body or a palmar process of the distal phalanx may initially be difficult to visualize on radiographs, but after 7–10 days some rarefaction adjacent to the fracture occurs making identification easier. An acute fracture appears as a well defined narrow radiolucent line (or lines) with normal adjacent trabecular architecture. Sagittal, parasagittal and marginal fractures are normally best visualized on a dorsoproximal-palmarodistal oblique view (Figure 3.27a), although a fracture of a palmar process may first be suspected on the lateromedial view (Figure 3.27b). When a fracture is suspected it may be necessary to obtain a number of oblique views in order to visualize the fracture clearly.

A fracture of a palmar process may require a number of oblique views in order to demonstrate the fracture line and to ascertain if the fracture is articular or non-articular. A significant proportion of these fractures are not detectable in a standard dorsoproximal-palmarodistal oblique projection, especially in the acute stage. If a fracture is suspected (either on clinical grounds or as the result of nuclear scintigraphic examination), but it is not detectable on the standard radiographic views, a palmaroproximal-palmarodistal oblique view, weight-bearing or flexed lateral 45° proximal-medial distal oblique, or medial 45° proximal-lateral distal oblique view should be obtained. In racehorses in Australia and the United States of America palmar process fractures occur most commonly on the lateral aspect of the left front foot and the medial aspect of the right front foot, associated with counter-clockwise racing. In sports horses, however, medial palmar process fractures are more prevalent. Frontal plane fractures of a palmar process are usually only detectable in lateromedial or palmaroproximal-palmarodistal oblique views of the distal phalanx.

A fracture is best seen as a lucent line when the x-ray beam is in line with the plane of the fracture (Figure 3.27c). Frequently it appears as two lines, representing the exit points through dorsal and palmar surfaces of the bone. By careful comparison of a number of slightly different oblique views, it is possible to establish whether a fracture is simple or comminuted. It should also be remembered that more than one fracture may be present. Some palmar process fractures of the distal phalanx occur as the result of repetitive trauma, rather than a single event. In these cases the surrounding trabecular architecture is disrupted. Precise ageing of such a fracture is difficult.

Clinically, a fracture of the distal phalanx presents as acute lameness, with pain to pressure and concussion of the hoof. In some horses with a palmar process fracture there is no reaction to hoof testers and lameness is

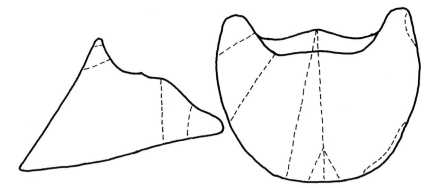

Figure 3.26 The common fracture sites of the distal phalanx.

mild. Fractures of the distal phalanx which enter the distal interphalangeal joint, occurring in animals more than 18 months old, respond best to internal fixation, although this is not necessary in all cases. Fractures which do not enter the distal interphalangeal joint, fractures of the palmar processes of the bone and fractures in animals of less than 18 months of age have a good prognosis with conservative treatment, shoeing the affected foot with a broad-webbed bar shoe, and ensuring correct mediolateral balance. Some horses never develop complete bony union radiographically, even though clinically sound. Non-union palmar process fractures can therefore be seen as an incidental finding.

Non-articular osseous fragments on the abaxial margin of one or both palmar processes may occur in foals from a few weeks to 1 year of age. These are often associated with a club foot appearance and lameness, but are occasionally seen without associated clinical signs. These are believed to be the result of fractures and not secondary centres of ossification. They appear as a triangular-shaped bone fragment of the distal angle of the palmar process, or an oblong bone fragment extending from the incisure of the palmar process to the solar margin. These fractures heal by osseous union, with rapid resolution of lameness.

A fracture of the solar margin of the bone (running parallel and adjacent to the margin of the bone) is best visualized on the dorsoproximal-palmarodistal oblique view (Figure 3.28). This fracture frequently occurs in animals that are flat footed and suffer repeated bruising of the sole. These horses are frequently footsore and several sources of pain may contribute to the lameness. There is seldom a history of acute onset of lameness. Many of these fracture fragments persist radiographically, although some heal and others appear to be resorbed. Treatment is usually by shoeing with a broad-webbed seated-out shoe, to give increased protection to the sole. Occasionally the fracture may become secondarily infected and may require surgical removal of the fragment. A reasonable outcome can be given for these fractures, but their presence often indicates that the foot is prone to concussion and this must be taken into account when giving a prognosis.

A fracture of the extensor process is best visualized on a lateromedial radiograph. A small radiopaque fragment proximal to the extensor process

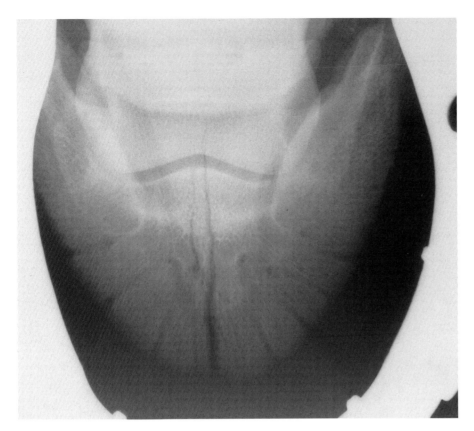

Figure 3.27(a) Sagittal fracture of the distal phalanx (dorsoproximal-palmarodistal oblique view). Note the separate lucent lines which represent the fracture through the dorsal and solar cortices. The shoe was left in place to give support to the foot until the injury was fully assessed.

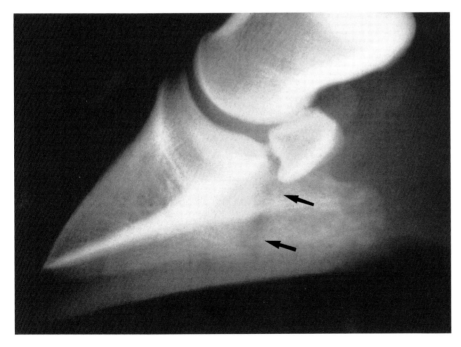

Figure 3.27(b) Palmar process fracture (arrows) of the distal phalanx (lateromedial view).

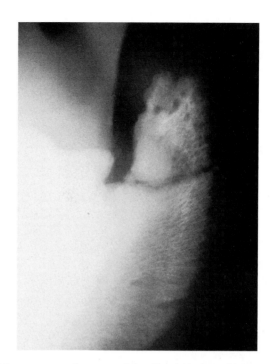

Figure 3.27(c) Palmar process fracture of the distal phalanx (dorsoproximal lateral-palmarodistal medial oblique view).

may represent a recent fracture, a fracture sustained early in life, a separate ossification centre, or dystrophic mineralization within the extensor tendon (see Figure 3.13, page 73). A fragment may be homogeneously radiopaque, with a smooth outline or have a cortex and medullary pattern. However, it is often not possible to determine radiographically the significance of such fragments. Local analgesic techniques should be used to determine their clinical significance. Lameness associated with a fragment less than approximately 5 mm in diameter, or not involving the joint surface, frequently resolves with conservative treatment, although the fragment may persist radiographically. Lesions approximately 5–10 mm in diameter, which are shown clinically to be causing lameness, may require surgical removal. The radiographs should be inspected carefully for evidence of osteoarthritis of the distal interphalangeal joint, which may adversely influence the prognosis (Figure 3.29a). A fracture of the extensor process more than 10 mm from its proximal border carries a poor prognosis. A large discrete osseous fragment proximal to the extensor process, often occurring bilaterally, may be seen as an incidental finding.

Large extensor process fragments involving up to one-quarter to one-third of the articular surface of the distal phalanx are sometimes seen either unilaterally or bilaterally in young horses starting work and are associated with acute onset of lameness. There is usually extensive sclerosis of the distal phalanx palmar to the fragment, indicating chronicity despite the recent onset of clinical signs (Figure 3.29b). It has been suggested that such fragments could be secondary to an osseous cyst-like lesion in the extensor process and an associated abnormal ossification centre. The prognosis for long-term full athletic function is guarded with either conservative or surgical management.

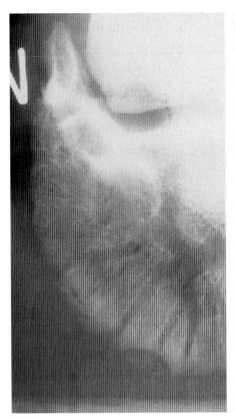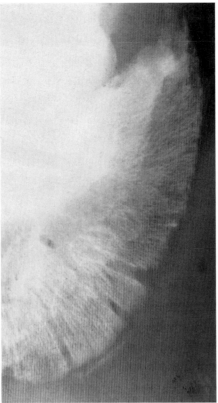

Figure 3.28 Fracture of the solar margin of the distal phalanx of two horses (dorsoproximal-palmarodistal oblique view).

Hoof

RADIOGRAPHIC TECHNIQUE

The radiographic views for examination of the hoof wall are similar to those for the distal phalanx (see page 53); however, the exposures should be considerably reduced in order to visualize the hoof wall, and it is preferable not to use a grid. The wide latitude available using digital radiography may allow the distal phalanx and hoof wall to be examined simultaneously, but further radiographs may be required. It is frequently useful to place a radiodense marker on the hoof wall in order to mark its outer surface. This can be done using tape and a piece of wire, or with barium paste. The barium is difficult to remove completely if plain radiographs are required subsequently. In cases where separation of the distal phalanx from the hoof wall is suspected, the use of a small screw or thumb tack to mark a precise location on the hoof wall may be beneficial.

For assessment of hoof conformation on radiographs, care must be taken to ensure that exact lateromedial and dorsopalmar radiographic views are obtained. In particular, dorsopalmar (weight-bearing) views must be obtained with the horse standing squarely and bearing weight evenly on the foot to be radiographed. To evaluate foot imbalance the x-ray beam should be perpendicular to the foot, whereas to assess distal limb deviation the x-ray beam should be perpendicular to the antebrachium or parallel to the spine.

[91]

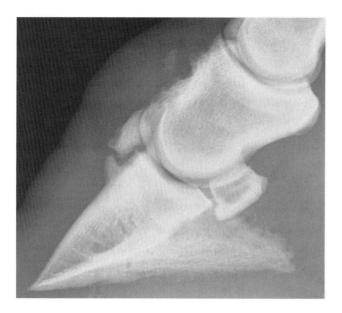

Figure 3.29(a) Slightly oblique lateromedial radiographic view of the left front foot of a 10-year-old Thoroughbred with left forelimb lameness. There is a large, articular, displaced fracture of the extensor process of the distal phalanx, with extensive periarticular new bone on the dorsal aspect of the middle phalanx, entheseophyte formation at the insertion of the common digital extensor tendon on the distal phalanx, and mineralization in the soft tissues on the dorsal aspect of the diaphysis of the middle phalanx. There is also periarticular modelling of the dorsoproximal aspect of the middle phalanx and a small periarticular osteophyte on the dorsoproximal aspect of the navicular bone. The horse had been examined radiographically 2 years previously, and no abnormality had been detectable.

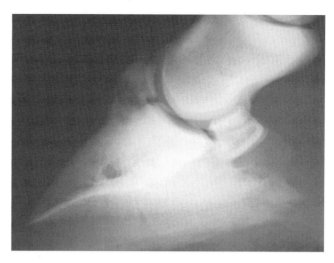

Figure 3.29(b) Slightly oblique lateromedial view of the left front foot of a 3-year-old Warmblood gelding with sudden onset, acute, bilateral forelimb lameness. Lunge work had recently commenced as part of the breaking process. There is a large, displaced, articular fracture of the extensor process of the distal phalanx and entheseophyte formation at the insertion of the commond digital extensor tendon. The palmar two-thirds of the distal phalanx is profoundly sclerotic. Clearly these radiographic abnormalities predated the onset of lameness.

NORMAL ANATOMY

Hoof shape and conformation are dependent upon hoof trimming, and feet which are incorrectly trimmed (out of balance) may result in intermittent lameness, due to foot pain or pain elsewhere in the limb caused by uneven weight bearing. Assessment of hoof conformation on lateromedial and dorsopalmar (weight-bearing) radiographs is possible, but more information is usually available from clinical evaluation. On lateromedial views, the solar border of the distal phalanx is closer to the bearing surface of the foot at the toe than at the heels, sloping 3–10° (Figure 3.30). The centre of the radius of curvature of the distal interphalangeal joint should be vertically above the middle of the bearing surface of the foot. The horn at the toe should be virtually parallel to that of the heels (this is often easier to assess clinically than on radiographs). On dorsopalmar (weight-bearing) views, the solar margin of the distal phalanx should be the same height from the ground on the lateral and medial aspects of the foot (Figure 3.8c, page 64), although a recent study demonstrated that in 63% of feet the medial distance was significantly smaller than the lateral. This probably reflects the horse's ability to compensate for minor imbalances.

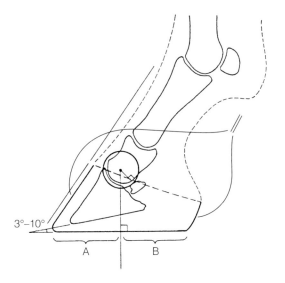

Figure 3.30 Normal hoof conformation. Lateromedial view. Note that A = B.

The tissues of the dermal laminae are slightly less dense than the horn of the hoof wall. For this reason a halo effect is always seen immediately around the distal phalanx on correctly exposed radiographs.

NORMAL VARIATIONS AND INCIDENTAL FINDINGS

Slight variation in hoof conformation is acceptable. The normal thickness of the dorsal wall varies, with a mean of 16 mm in Thoroughbreds and a mean of 18 mm in Warmbloods. There is also considerable individual variation in the thickness of the sole. No other normal variations have been recognized.

DIGITAL VENOGRAPHY

Digital venography is described in Chapter 14 (pages 693–694).

SIGNIFICANT FINDINGS

Laminitis

The primary radiographic changes detected in laminitis (other than in angiographic examinations) relate to separation of the distal phalanx from the hoof wall, and/or thickening of the dorsal hoof wall, because of inflammation and separation of the laminae. Most commonly this is evident as a rotation of the bone, with the toe moving distally and away from the hoof wall. This results in the dorsal wall of the hoof ceasing to be parallel to the dorsal wall of the distal phalanx. However in some horses there is no rotation, only increased thickness of the hoof wall. As the condition progresses, a faint radiolucent line may appear between the distal phalanx and the sole or hoof wall. This initially represents serum collected between the dermal and epidermal laminae, and is visible because of the slight difference between

[93]

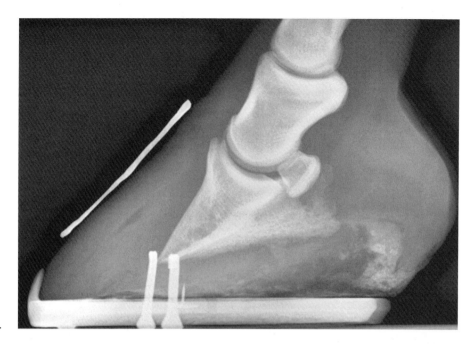

Figure 3.31(a) Lateromedial radiographic view of the left front foot of a 6-year-old Arab gelding with chronic laminitis. The radiograph was obtained with a shoe on, a linear radiodense marker on the dorsal hoof wall and a drawing pin at the apex of the frog. The toe of the foot is excessively long. There is rotation of the distal phalanx. There are linear radiolucent areas in the dorsal hoof wall.

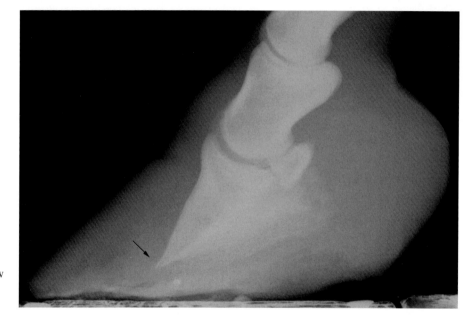

Figure 3.31(b) Laminitis. Lateromedial view of a case of chronic laminitis, showing rotation of the distal phalanx. Note the mottled lucent areas in the separated laminae at the toe of the foot and new bone formation on the dorsal aspect of the toe of the distal phalanx (arrow). There is new horn growth below the coronary band with divergence of the horn distally.

fluid and horn densities. This can only be seen on very high-quality radiographs. Subsequently this area may become more lucent, mimicking the appearance of gas. This may not develop until 12–18 days after an initial laminitis episode. This line represents necrotic laminar tissue. The lucent lines move distally relative to the coronary band with hoof wall growth (Figure 3.31a). However, increasing width of this lucent line is indicative of progressive rotation or laminar necrosis. With extension of the lucent line to the sole, a portal for infection may be established (see also 'Infectious osteitis', pages 76–77), but this is also a common site to which haematological spread of infection may occur.

[94]

The degree of rotation may be important in assessing prognosis, but this is subject to dispute. It is a subjective measurement and recent trimming of the dorsal hoof wall will make the degree of rotation appear less. If the toes are excessively long with distortion of the hoof wall this may make the degree of rotation appear greater. It may be helpful to place a radiodense marker on the dorsal hoof wall in order to delineate its position in relation to the distal phalanx, and in particular to mark the position of the coronary band. Since laminitis may affect all four feet, lateromedial radiographs of all feet may be required. If progressive rotation is suspected, radiographs obtained at regular intervals may be valuable to monitor progress. The more marked the rotation and the more rapidly it progresses, the worse the prognosis. Attention should also be paid to the toe of the distal phalanx. Radiographic changes include increased lucency of the solar margin at the toe, followed by new bone formation on the dorsal surface of the bone (Figure 3.31b). The presence of these changes justifies a more guarded prognosis for return to full athletic function. Occasionally there is new bone along most of the dorsal cortex of the distal phalanx. Extensive solar margin fragmentation may occur following laminitis with rotation of the distal phalanx. Chronic deformation of the dorsal aspect of the distal phalanx due to demineralization occurs with increasing chronicity. It is best demonstrated on softly exposed dorsoproximal-palmarodistal oblique views. Infection of the laminar tissues may be a complication of laminitis, which may result in gas shadows, evident as areas of increased lucency between the distal phalanx and hoof wall, or the distal phalanx and the sole. Infection of the distal phalanx may also occur in chronic cases.

In 'sinker syndrome' (a very severe form of laminitis, sometimes referred to as founder), the entire distal phalanx sinks within the horny capsule. This is difficult to visualize on a single radiographic examination, as the dorsal wall of the hoof and distal phalanx may remain parallel. Assessment of the vertical distance between the coronary band and the extensor process of the distal phalanx compared with the contralateral limb, or previous radiographs, may allow a more objective assessment to be made (Figure 3.32a). There may be soft-tissue swelling at the coronary band, which appears more opaque at its dorsal aspect. This is followed by the development of a distinct depression immediately above the coronary band (Figure 3.32b). A small screw placed in the dorsal hoof wall in these cases will help in the comparison of repeat radiographs obtained on successive days. Further dropping of the distal phalanx can be assessed by measuring from the marker to a set point on the distal phalanx (usually the proximal border of the extensor process); however, care must be taken to reproduce positioning and magnification factors accurately when measurements are made.

Radiographic evidence of previous laminitis is sometimes seen in a clinically normal horse. This includes increased thickness of the dorsal hoof wall (>18 mm in a horse; >15 mm in a pony) (Figure 3.33), with or without a radiolucent line, and modelling of the toe of the distal phalanx. Uncorrected rotation of the distal phalanx may also be evident.

Treatment of laminitis must include systemic treatment followed by corrective farriery. Lateromedial radiographs are helpful to the farrier when

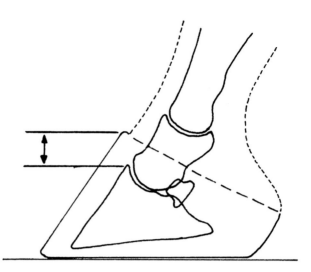

Figure 3.32(a) Diagram to show a method to evaluate 'sinking' of the distal phalanx. Monitor the distance between horizontal lines drawn at the levels of the coronary band and the proximodorsal aspect of the extensor process of the distal phalanx.

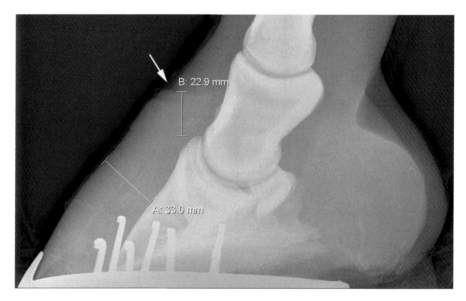

B: 22.9 mm

A: 33.0 mm

Figure 3.32(b) Slightly oblique lateromedial radiographic view of a foot of a 14-year-old Warmblood with severe laminitis. There is marked sinking of the distal phalanx. The distance between the coronary band (arrow), above which is a depression, and the extensor process of the distal phalanx is B, 22.9 mm. The dorsal hoof wall is abnormally thick, A, 33.0 mm. The toe of the distal phalanx is obscured by the shoe.

dressing the dorsal wall of the hoof parallel with the dorsal surface of the distal phalanx and to assist correct placement of corrective shoes.

Venography and laminitis

The technique of venography is described in Chapter 14 (pages 693–694). In a normal horse the lateral and medial digital veins, capillaries and arteries are filled retrograde, permitting visualization of the terminal arch, coronary

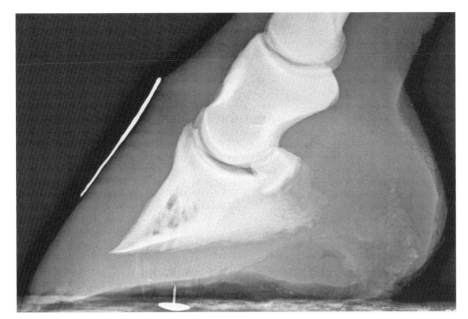

Figure 3.33 Lateromedial radiographic view of a foot of a 7-year-old pony with chronic foot soreness associated with chronic laminitis. There is a linear radiopaque marker on the dorsal aspect of the hoof wall, extending from the coronary band distally. There is a drawing pin at the apex of the frog. The dorsal hoof wall is abnormally thick and there is modelling of the toe of the distal phalanx.

plexus, dorsal lamellar vessels, circumflex vessels and vessels of the heel region (Figure 3.34a). A second lateromedial view can demonstrate the contrast agent diffusing into the soft tissues, and may delineate an abnormality. In chronic laminitis, displacement of the distal phalanx, morphological changes in the laminae and compression of vessels can all contribute to alterations of the vasculature, notably in the coronary plexus, dorsal lamellar vessels and circumflex vessels (Figure 3.34b). Such abnormalities may have some influence on treatment and prognosis.

Long-toe low-heel syndrome

On lateromedial radiographs of a normal foot, the centre of the radius of curvature of the distal interphalangeal joint should be vertically above the centre of the bearing surface of the foot (see Figure 3.30, page 93). If the joint is over the palmar third of the bearing surface, this indicates poor dorsopalmar hoof balance which may contribute to lameness. On a weight-bearing lateromedial radiograph it is also important to assess the position of the solar margin of the distal phalanx relative to the ground. If the palmar processes of the distal phalanx are closer to the ground than the toe (sometimes referred to as 'reverse inclination'), this indicates extremely poor hoof balance and is usually associated with lameness (Figure 3.35a). Palmaroproximal-palmarodistal oblique views of the distal phalanx should be obtained in these cases, to look for increased lucency around the palmar processes indicative of separation of the laminae at the heels (Figure 3.35b). New bone formed on the axial or abaxial surfaces of the palmar processes of the distal phalanx is suggestive of repeated trauma to this area (see also 'Pedal osteitis complex', pages 73–76).

[97]

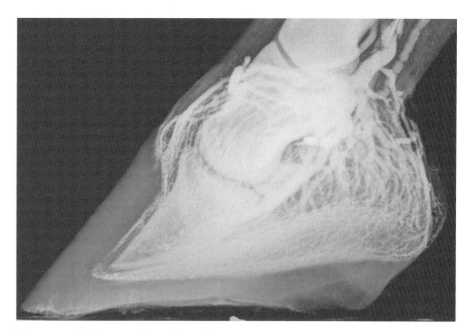

Figure 3.34(a) A normal lateral venogram. Note that the circumflex vasculature is several millimetres distal to the toe of the distal phalanx. The anastomosis of the circumflex vasculature and the dorsal lamellar vasculature has a normal triangular appearance. The coronary plexus is filled normally. The solar and coronary papillae are parallel to the dorsal aspect of the distal phalanx.

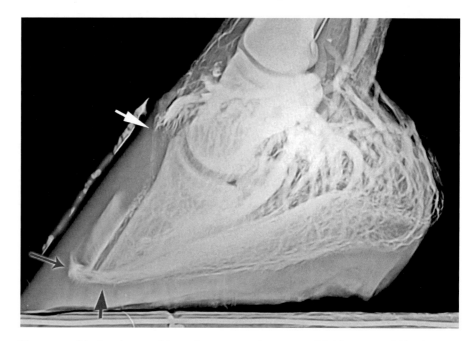

Figure 3.34(b) An abnormal lateral venogram (compare with Figure 3.34(a)) of an 18-year-old American Saddlebred with laminitis of 7 days' duration. Plain radiographs revealed no evidence of rotation of the distal phalnx. Note the lack of filling of the vessels at the dorsal aspect of the coronary band (white arrow); perfusion of the coronary plexus is truncated at the proximal aspect of the extensor process of the distal phalanx. There is rectangular pooling of radiographic contrast medium in the dorsal lamellar vasculature extending 12 mm proximally on the dorsal aspect of the distal phalanx. The apex of the distal phalanx is ventral to the circumflex vasculature (large black arrow), causing distortion of both the circumflex/lamellar anastomosis (small black arrow) at the toe and the terminal solar papillae. These vascular changes are secondary to distal displacement or sinking of the distal phalanx.

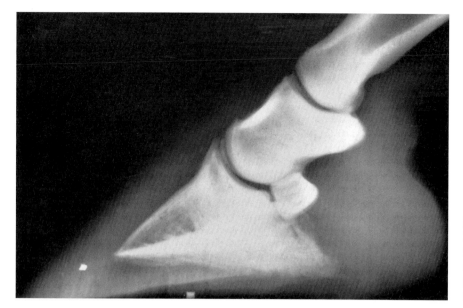

Figure 3.35(a) Low heel conformation. Lateromedial view. The solar surface of the distal phalanx is abnormally aligned with the ground (compare with Figure 3.8a). Note two clenches left in the hoof when the shoe was removed.

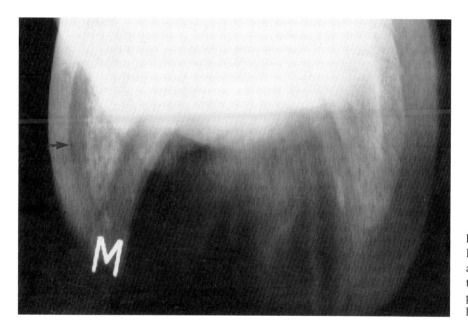

Figure 3.35(b) Low heel conformation. Palmaroproximal-palmarodistal view of a distal phalanx, showing separation of the laminae around the medial palmar process seen as an area of increased lucency (arrow).

Mediolateral foot imbalance

Mediolateral foot balance can be assessed on weight-bearing dorsopalmar radiographs of the feet, provided that the horse is loading the foot squarely with the limb vertical. The relative distance of the medial and lateral solar margins of the distal phalanx from the ground can be assessed (Figure 3.36). In addition the alignment and congruity of the distal and proximal interphalangeal joints should also be noted. This assessment is most accurately made with the horse standing with both feet on a relatively low (5 cm) wooden block. Uneven load bearing makes interpretation difficult. The authors believe that careful clinical assessment of the distal aspect of the limb is also essential for assessment of mediolateral imbalance, because other aspects of conformation must also be taken into account.

[99]

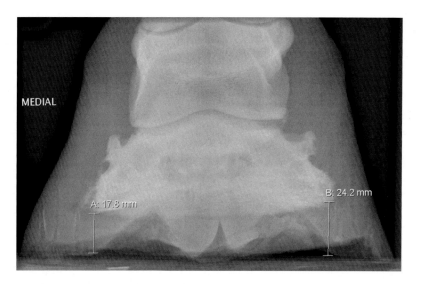

Figure 3.36 Dorsopalmar radiographic view of a front foot of a 3-year-old French Thoroughbred. Medial is to the left. There is marked mediolateral hoof imbalance. The distance between the distal medial aspect of the distal phalanx and the ground (17.8 mm) is considerably less than laterally (24.2 mm).

Infection

Infection of the foot is usually diagnosed clinically, but the extent of the area involved can be difficult to assess. Radiographically lucent zones may be seen within the hoof. These vary in shape and size, but with the careful use of oblique views the extent of hoof separation can be determined. They must be distinguished from the lucent lines seen with separation of the hoof wall in laminitis (see pages 93–94). The margin of the distal phalanx should be inspected carefully for evidence of infectious pedal osteitis (see pages 76–77), particularly if infection is recurrent.

In some cases, clinical signs may indicate the presence of infection, but a discharging sinus may be slow to occur. This is most common if the sole is hard or unusually thick. In these cases radiographs may reveal a lucent zone beneath or adjacent to the distal phalanx, indicating infection.

Infection is occasionally seen in conjunction with the presence of a radiopaque foreign body.

Penetrating injuries

Penetrating injuries of the foot are common and can have catastrophic consequences if not recognized early and treated appropriately. If a radiopaque foreign body has penetrated the sole and is still *in situ* then lateromedial and dorsopalmar radiographs should be obtained in order to determine the depth and direction of penetration. It is important to establish whether it is likely that a synovial cavity has been punctured, or if either a bone or the deep digital flexor tendon have been traumatized or contaminated. If the foreign body is absent or has been removed a metal probe inserted into the tract can help to determine the extent of the penetration.

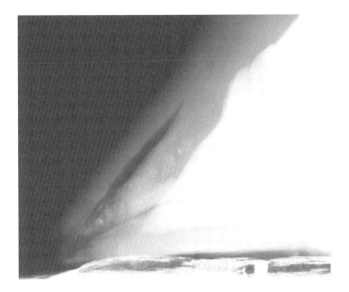

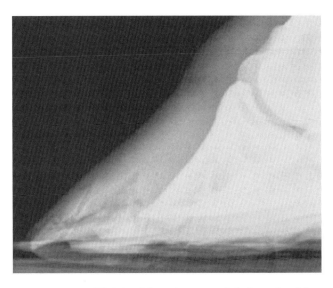

Figure 3.37(a) Laminar separation at the toe. Lateromedial view, showing separation of the hoof wall at the toe of the foot. This extends up the dorsal wall and laterally around the toe. The granular opaque material is dirt packed into the separated area. The radiograph is deliberately underexposed to demonstrate the laminar abnormalities.

Figure 3.37(b) Slightly oblique lateromedial view of a right front foot with an excessively long toe, resulting in apparent rotation of the distal phalanx. There is a radiolucent defect extending from the toe of the foot, reflecting necrotic material in the white line, so called seedy toe. There is also a radiolucent line distal to the distal phalanx, parallel with the sole.

Fistulography or *sinography* (see Chapter 14, page 706), as well as ultrasonography, can also be helpful.

Hoof wall separation

Separation of the hoof wall may occur for a number of reasons other than laminitis (see page 93) and infection (see page 100). Excessive length of horn at the toe may result in the dorsal aspect of the hoof wall lifting away from the distal phalanx. A radiolucent area will be evident under the hoof wall (Figure 3.37a). Separation can also occur as a result of an acute traumatic incident, e.g. jumping on hard uneven ground.

The term 'seedy toe' is used to describe a condition in which there appears to be separation of the dermal and epidermal laminae, or there is poor horn formation from the dermal laminae. The aetiology of this condition is uncertain. It may initially be detected proximally and, as the horn grows down, the separated area moves distally. Seedy toe can be seen radiographically as a lucent area in the laminar portion of the hoof wall (Figure 3.37b). It may have no apparent opening through the hoof wall or white line when first detected. When the distal margin of the separated area reaches the bearing surface, trimming the foot will open into the separation, which may then act as a portal for infection. If the lesion is extensive, the increased loading on the adjacent laminae may result in lameness, particularly on hard ground. The extent of the lesion may be determined by the careful use of oblique views. (The term seedy toe is sometimes used to refer to the separated laminae seen in the hoof after rotation of the distal phalanx in laminitis. These two conditions should be distinguished from each other, as they have different aetiologies and require different treatments.)

Navicular bone

RADIOGRAPHIC TECHNIQUE

In this chapter the distal sesamoid bone is referred to as the navicular bone.

Equipment

Adequate radiographs of the navicular bone can be obtained using portable x-ray equipment, but a minimum output of 15 mA at 80 kV is required. With machines of low output (less than 40 mA at 80 kV), rare earth screens and appropriate films (or digital systems) are essential to avoid movement blur. Machines with a high milliamperage output allow short exposure times, and therefore fine-grain high-definition screens and compatible films can be used to obtain more detail. Dorsoproximal-palmarodistal oblique radiographs of the navicular bone obtained using traditional x-ray technique should be acquired with a grid (8:1 or 6:1 ratio). However, with digital systems a grid may not be necessary and if used should be appropriate for the individual digital system, to avoid moiré lines. Careful collimation of the x-ray beam will also enhance the quality of the radiographs.

It is essential that the shoes are removed and the feet carefully cleaned prior to radiography. Loose horn in the sole and irregular growth of the frog should be removed. Scrubbing the feet with water can result in artefacts due to loose packing in the frog clefts (see below).

The frog clefts need to be packed to eliminate air shadows being cast over the navicular bone for at least one dorsoproximal-palmarodistal view, and for the palmaroproximal-palmarodistal oblique view. This can be achieved using Playdoh or equivalent, Vaseline or soft soap. The latter two may trap air bubbles creating artefacts which may mimic pathology. There is also the danger of the horse slipping. Packing should be kept to a minimum, to avoid creating artefacts. The use of a water bath is not recommended as this increases scatter, resulting in reduced contrast on the final radiograph.

Positioning

For complete evaluation of the navicular bone it is recommended that lateromedial, dorsoproximal-palmarodistal oblique and palmaroproximal-palmarodistal oblique views should be obtained. A second dorsoproximal-palmarodistal oblique may be required to rule out artefacts, or to verify the presence of a distal border fragment. In some cases a dorsopalmar (weight-bearing) view should also be obtained.

Lateromedial view

A lateromedial radiograph is obtained with the foot to be examined placed on a flat block. It is preferable, but not essential, for the foot to be bearing weight. The x-ray beam should be horizontal and centred on the end of the navicular bone (approximately 1 cm below the coronary band at a point midway between the most dorsal and most palmar aspects of the coronary band). The beam is aligned parallel to a line drawn across the bulbs of the heel, so that it traverses the navicular bone through its long axis. A true lateromedial view is essential to evaluate the thickness of the flexor (palmar) cortex, the junction between the cortex and the trabecular bone of the spongiosa and the trabecular architecture, and to identify periarticular osteophytes and modelling of the proximal and distal aspects of the bone, which may reflect entheseous new bone at the attachments of the collateral sesamoidean ligament and the distal sesamoidean impar ligament.

Dorsoproximal-palmarodistal oblique views

Two dorsoproximal-palmarodistal oblique views are helpful to aid recognition of artefacts. These views can be obtained using either of two techniques, the choice of which is used being largely a matter of personal preference.

DORSOPROXIMAL-PALMARODISTAL OBLIQUE ('UPRIGHT PEDAL') VIEW

The least distorted radiographs are obtained using the dorsoproximal-palmarodistal oblique (upright pedal) view. The toe of the foot is placed on a navicular block (see below), and the dorsal wall of the foot and the pastern angled forwards at approximately 85° to the horizontal (Figure 3.38a). The x-ray beam is kept horizontal and centred 2–3 cm proximal to the coronary band at the midline of the foot. The beam should be well collimated. The cassette is placed behind and as close as possible to the foot. If the navicular block is placed too close to the horse, the fetlock and pastern joints will flex too much and the x-ray beam will traverse too great a distance through the middle phalanx, with resultant loss of quality of the radiograph. If positioned too far in front of the horse, the dorsal wall of the hoof and the pastern become too upright and the distal border of the navicular bone is superimposed over the distal interphalangeal joint.

A second dorsoproximal-palmarodistal (upright pedal) oblique view may be helpful to aid interpretation and to differentiate artefacts. This view is obtained in a similar manner to the first, but with the dorsal wall of the hoof and the pastern vertical and the x-ray beam centred on the coronary band (Figure 3.38b).

The first of these two views gives good visualization of the distal border of the bone. The second view gives good visualization of the proximal border and the body of the navicular bone.

A 'navicular block' can take a number of forms, but is basically a solid block of wood with a groove cut in the top in which the toe of the foot can

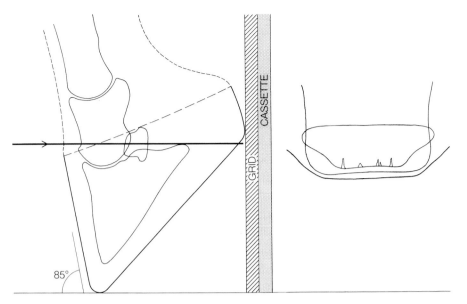

Figure 3.38(a) Positioning to obtain a dorsoproximal-palmarodistal oblique view of the navicular bone (85° upright pedal view). Inset diagram shows resultant radiographic positioning of the distal border of the navicular bone proximal to the distal interphalangeal joint.

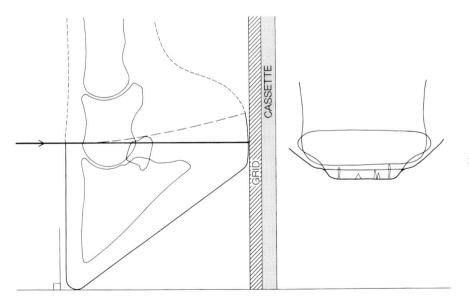

Figure 3.38(b) Positioning to obtain a dorsoproximal-palmarodistal oblique view of the navicular bone (90° upright pedal view). Inset diagram shows resultant radiographic positioning of the distal border of the navicular bone superimposed over the distal interphalangeal joint.

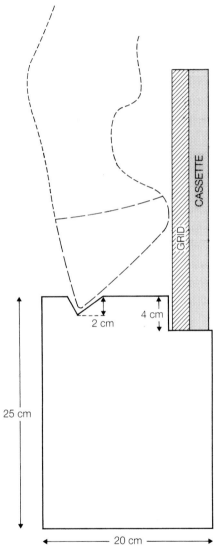

Figure 3.38(c) A 'navicular block' (used to position the foot for radiographs of the navicular bone and distal phalanx in the 'upright pedal' position).

be rested (Figure 3.38c) while the limb is held by an assistant. By moving the block forward or backward relative to the horse, the dorsal wall of the hoof can be positioned at different angles. A horse will normally stand quietly if the limb is raised on a block about 25 cm high. With a smaller block the horse will continually try to straighten the limb and stand on it. It is also important to have a block that feels solid, to give the horse confidence.

DORSOPROXIMAL-PALMARODISTAL OBLIQUE ('HIGH CORONARY') VIEW

The 'high coronary' technique has the disadvantage that the x-ray beam is not at right angles to the film, nor is the film parallel to the flexor surface of the navicular bone (see Figure 3.2a, page 56). This results in some distortion of the image. Nonetheless, in some horses ease of handling the animal may outweigh other considerations, and some workers prefer to use this technique routinely. The cassette is placed in a suitable tunnel on the floor, and the horse stands on it. The x-ray beam is centred 2 cm above the coronary band in the midline, and angled distally, at an angle of at least 60° to the horizontal (i.e. a dorsal 60° proximal-palmarodistal oblique view). It is recommended that two views should be obtained with 10–15° difference in angle of the beam.

The radiographic image is normally improved by the use of a parallel grid. A grid ratio of 6:1 is preferable to 8:1 because of the difficulty of aligning the foot, grid lines and x-ray beam. If using digital systems, then experimentation will be required to determine the best grid to avoid moiré lines. Alignment of the grid with the x-ray beam and the foot is more difficult than with the upright pedal view.

Palmaroproximal-palmarodistal oblique view

The palmaroproximal-palmarodistal oblique view provides good visualization of the medulla, flexor cortex and flexor surface of the navicular bone.

The foot to be radiographed is positioned caudal to the contralateral forelimb, on a cassette tunnel containing the cassette. The heel should be flat on the ground, but the weight of the horse should be forward on the contralateral limb. The x-ray machine is placed ventral to the thorax of the horse. The x-ray beam is centred between the bulbs of the heel at the base of the pastern at an angle of approximately 45° to the horizontal (Figure 3.39a), getting the x-ray beam as near to parallel to the flexor cortex as possible.

Alternatively, the horse stands on a cassette tunnel which is placed on a wedge-shaped block, which has a slope raising the toe of the foot approximately 10–15°. The contralateral limb can be lifted to restrict movement. The x-ray beam is angled at approximately 30° from the horizontal, centring as above (Figure 3.39b). In both techniques it is important to avoid superimposition of the palmar aspect of the fetlock over the navicular bone.

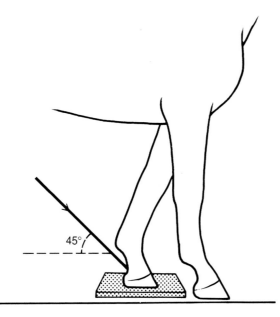

Figure 3.39(a) Positioning to obtain a palmar 45° proximal-palmarodistal oblique view of the navicular bone. The heel of the foot to be examined should be on the ground, caudal to the contralateral foot, with the weight of the horse forward on the opposite limb. The x-ray beam (arrow) is centred on the midline between the bulbs of the heel, at the distal aspect of the pastern.

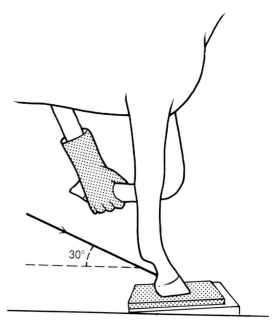

Figure 3.39(b) Positioning to obtain a palmar 30° proximal-palmarodistal oblique view of the navicular bone, with the foot on a wedge-shaped block, with the toe elevated. The x-ray beam (arrow) is centred on the midline, between the bulbs of the heel.

The angle of the x-ray beam should be parallel to the flexor surface of the navicular bone. Both foot conformation and limb placement have an effect on the optimum angle of the x-ray beam. An upright foot conformation will require a larger (more upright) angle, whereas if the heel is low the angle should be reduced. The lower limb conformation of some horses occasionally makes this extremely difficult to achieve. Poor technique can create artefacts and mimic pathology, in particular resulting in poor corticomedullary definition and loss of medullary trabeculation (Figure 3.42c,d, page 113).

This view can be difficult to acquire in a small pony, especially if fat, because the x-ray machine cannot physically be placed in the optimum position. It can also be difficult to acquire in a horse with severe palmar foot pain, because this results in unwillingness to extend the distal interphalangeal joint as it increases the load on the podotrochlear apparatus and deep digital flexor tendon. Use of sedation and analgesia may facilitate positioning. Obtaining this view in hindlimbs may also be more difficult than in forelimbs.

Dorsopalmar (weight-bearing) view

A true dorsopalmar radiograph is obtained with the horse bearing weight on the limb (see Figure 3.3, page 57). The x-ray beam is kept horizontal, and centred approximately 2 cm below the coronary band at the dorsal aspect of the foot. It is aligned perpendicular to a line tangential to the bulbs of the heel. The cassette is placed vertically behind the foot, at a right angle to the x-ray beam.

This is not recommended as a standard view for examining the navicular bone, but can give valuable additional information about a fracture of the navicular bone, and about new bone on its proximal border.

Dorsoplantar views of the hind feet

It is normally easier to obtain plantarodorsal rather than dorsoplantar views of the hind feet. The positioning of the limb for these views is the same as for the dorsoproximal-palmarodistal oblique view of the forefeet, except that a low flat block (5 cm) is recommended for supporting the toe. The cassette is placed in front of the foot and the x-ray beam is centred in the midline of the bulbs of the heel, level with the dorsal aspect of the coronary band. It does result in relatively greater magnification of the navicular bone than a dorsoplantar view.

NORMAL ANATOMY

Immature horse

The navicular bone usually ossifies from a single centre, and at birth has an oval outline on dorsopalmar views. It continues to ossify until about 18 months of age, at which time it has acquired its adult shape.

Skeletally mature horse

Lateromedial view

Lateromedial radiographs of the navicular bone show the joint surfaces which articulate with the middle and distal phalanges (Figures 3.40a-d). The flexor surface is visualized as two lines, the more palmar representing the sagittal ridge of the bone, and the more dorsal representing the main flexor surface. A smooth-edged depression is frequently seen in the central part of the sagittal ridge (Figure 3.40c). The dorsal third of the distal border of the bone articulates with the distal phalanx. At the distal palmar aspect is a smoothly defined ridge which is the region of origin of the distal sesamoidean impar (interosseous) ligament. There is usually a notch of variable depth between the articular surface and the ridge on the distal border of the bone, which has been referred to as a synovial fossa. Lucent zones (also referred to as nutrient foramina and synovial invaginations of the distal interphalangeal joint) extending proximally from this notch are generally not evident in a normal horse on a lateromedial view. A clear linear trabecular pattern is seen within the medulla. The medulla and cortices of the bone are distinct. In the majority of horses the outline of the deep digital flexor tendon is seen as a faint opacity palmar to the navicular bone.

[107]

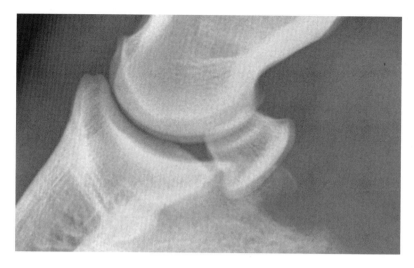

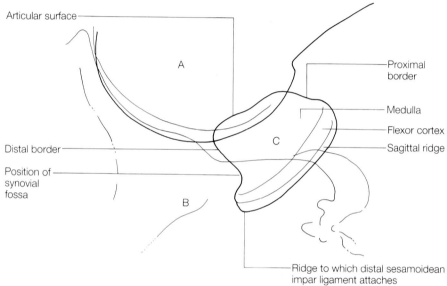

Articular surface

A

Proximal border

Medulla

Flexor cortex

C

Sagittal ridge

Distal border

Position of synovial fossa

B

Ridge to which distal sesamoidean impar ligament attaches

Figure 3.40(a) Lateromedial radiographic view and diagram of a normal adult navicular bone. Note that the flexor cortex of the navicular bone is thickest proximally. A = middle phalanx, B = distal phalanx, C = navicular bone. The joint space between the distal aspect of the navicular bone and the distal phalanx is convergent.

Dorsoproximal-palmarodistal oblique views

DORSOPROXIMAL-PALMARODISTAL OBLIQUE ('UPRIGHT PEDAL') VIEW

The outline of the navicular bone varies considerably between animals, but is normally a mirror image of that of the contralateral limb (Figures 3.41a and 3.41b). Several triangular-shaped lucent zones are often visible along the distal horizontal border of the bone (see page 114). The distal border is visualized as two lines: one (the more prominent and more proximal) represents the articulation of the bone with the distal phalanx; the other represents the distal border of the ridge from which the distal sesamoidean impar ligament originates. On poorly positioned views the proximal border of the bone may also be evident as two lines representing the palmar and dorsal margins. Three different shapes of the proximal border have been

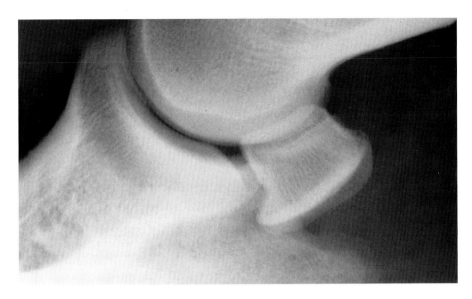

Figure 3.40(b) Lateromedial view of a normal adult navicular bone with a parallel joint space between the navicular bone and the distal phalanx (compare with Figure 3.40a).

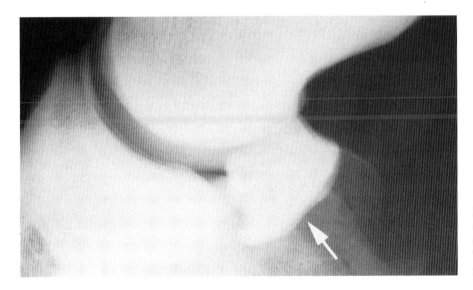

Figure 3.40(c) Lateromedial view of an adult navicular bone, showing a smooth depression in the sagittal ridge (arrow). The radiograph is deliberately underexposed to demonstrate this.

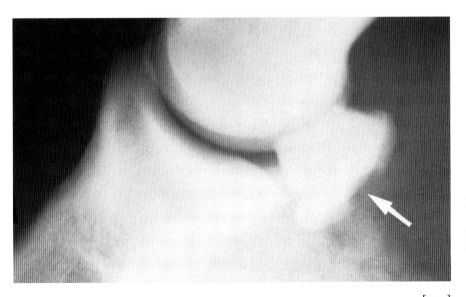

Figure 3.40(d) Lateromedial view of an adult navicular bone, showing a penetrating lesion of the flexor surface of the bone (arrow). The radiograph is deliberately underexposed to demonstrate this.

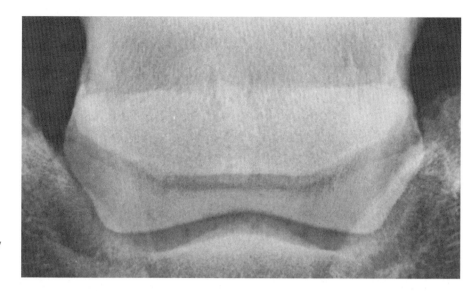

Figure 3.41(a) Dorsoproximal-palmarodistal oblique radiographic view of a normal adult navicular bone (upright pedal view).

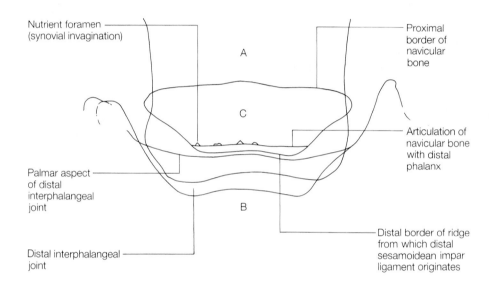

Nutrient foramen (synovial invagination)

Proximal border of navicular bone

A

C

Articulation of navicular bone with distal phalanx

Palmar aspect of distal interphalangeal joint

B

Distal interphalangeal joint

Distal border of ridge from which distal sesamoidean impar ligament originates

Figure 3.41(b) Diagram of a dorsoproximal-palmarodistal oblique view of a normal adult navicular bone (upright pedal view). A = middle phalanx, B = distal phalanx, C = navicular bone.

described in Warmblood horses, straight, undulating and convex, and it is suggested that shape may be heritable and possibly related to risk of disease.

DORSOPROXIMAL-PALMARODISTAL OBLIQUE ('HIGH CORONARY') VIEW

The image seen using this technique (Figure 3.41c) is distorted when compared with the upright view (Figure 3.41d), the navicular bone appearing longer in a proximodistal direction.

Palmaroproximal-palmarodistal oblique view

In a well positioned and exposed palmaroproximal-palmarodistal oblique view the dorsal articulation of the navicular bone with the middle phalanx

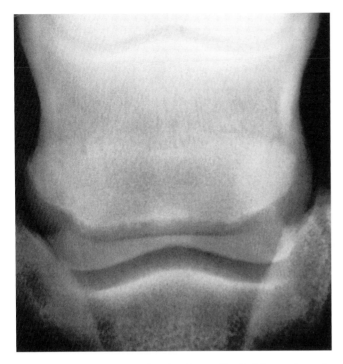

Figure 3.41(c) Dorsoproximal-palmarodistal oblique view of a normal navicular bone obtained using the 'high coronary' technique. Note the slight elongation of the navicular bone in a proximodistal plane compared with Figure 3.41(d) and loss of definition of its margins.

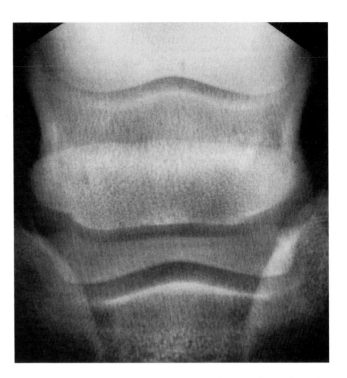

Figure 3.41(d) Dorsoproximal-palmarodistal oblique view of the same foot as Figure 3.41(c), obtained using the 'upright pedal' technique.

should be clearly seen and the palmar aspect of the flexor cortex should be seen as a distinct single line. If these cannot be seen then an additional radiograph should be obtained. The navicular bone has two distinct cortices separated by a less dense medulla, which has a distinct trabecular pattern (Figures 3.42a and 3.42b). The lucent zones seen on the distal border of the bone in dorsoproximal-palmarodistal views are visible within the medullary cavity as circular or oval lucencies. The flexor cortex has an even thickness, but a small, crescent-shaped or oval lucency may be evident in the sagittal ridge. The thickness of the cortex may vary between breeds and between individuals, but a sharp margin between the cortex and the medulla should always be present. In horses with upright foot conformation the flexor cortex is usually thinner than in horses with more normal foot conformation.

The crescent-shaped lucent zone in the sagittal ridge of the navicular bone is rarely seen in very young horses. It represents early navicular bone modelling in response to stress and is of unknown clinical significance. A relatively sclerotic reinforcement line develops in the subchondral bone parallel with the flexor cortex in the region of the sagittal ridge. The intervening bone is relatively radiolucent and is projected in the palmaroproximal-palmarodistal oblique view as the crescent-shaped lucent zone in the sagittal ridge. If the bone between the reinforcement line and the flexor cortex becomes compacted, then the lucent zone becomes less clear and may be obliterated.

[111]

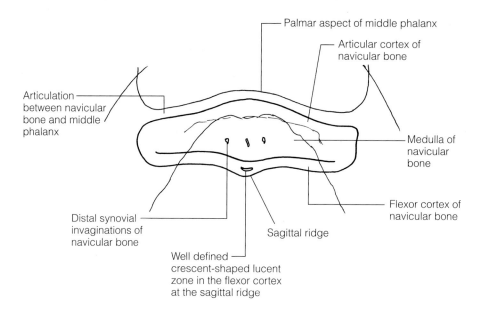

Figure 3.42(a) Palmaroproximal-palmarodistal oblique view of a normal adult navicular bone. Note the well defined lucency in the sagittal ridge, which may or may not be present.

Palmar aspect of middle phalanx

Articular cortex of navicular bone

Articulation between navicular bone and middle phalanx

Medulla of navicular bone

Distal synovial invaginations of navicular bone

Flexor cortex of navicular bone

Well defined crescent-shaped lucent zone in the flexor cortex at the sagittal ridge

Sagittal ridge

Figure 3.42(b) Diagram of a palmaroproximal-palmarodistal oblique view of a normal adult navicular bone.

Dorsopalmar (weight-bearing) view

The navicular bone is largely obscured by the extensor process of the distal phalanx. The medial and lateral margins of the bone are seen clearly, as is its proximal border (see Figure 3.8c, page 64).

NORMAL VARIATIONS AND INCIDENTAL FINDINGS

The outline of the navicular bone is extremely variable. Occasional cases have been reported where the navicular bone was absent, bipartite or tripartite. The significance of these findings is uncertain.

Lateromedial view

The navicular bone may be trapezoid in shape (Figure 3.8a, page 62), but frequently the flexor cortex has proximal and/or distal elongations (Figure 3.40a). Such proximal and distal elongation may reflect modelling as the

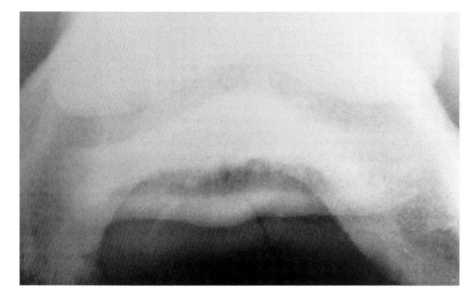

Figure 3.42(c) Palmar 45° proximal-palmarodistal oblique view of the navicular bone of a normal horse with an upright foot conformation. The medulla of the navicular bone is partially obliterated by the distal phalanx. The dorsal cortex of the navicular bone cannot be assessed. There is apparent sclerosis of the medulla and poor corticomedullary demarcation. The x-ray beam was not parallel to the flexor surface of the navicular bone and the foot had been positioned too far forward. Compare with Figure 3.42(d).

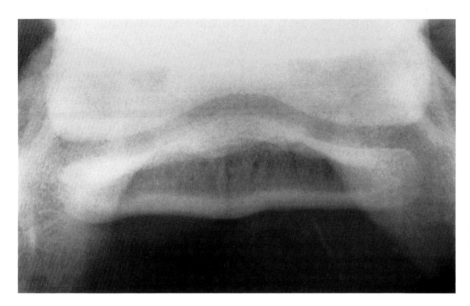

Figure 3.42(d) Palmar 50° proximal-palmarodistal oblique view of the navicular bone of the same horse as in Figure 3.42(c). There is a clear trabecular pattern within the medulla and excellent corticomedullary demarcation. Note also that the flexor cortex appears narrower than in Figure 3.42(c). The sagittal ridge is relatively flat, a normal variation.

result of chronic stress at the insertion of the collateral sesamoidean ligament or the origin of the distal sesamoidean impar ligament respectively. The joint space between the navicular bone and the distal phalanx may be parallel (Figure 3.40b) or convergent (Figure 3.40a). The thickness of the flexor cortex of the navicular bone is variable. It tends to be thinner in horses with an upright foot conformation. Marked increase in thickness may reflect disease. A small, shallow smooth-edged depression is present in the centre of the sagittal ridge of many normal horses (Figure 3.40c, page 109).

Smooth opaque entheseophytes on the proximal border of the navicular bone may be evident at the insertions of the collateral sesamoidean ligaments. These are best seen on the dorsopalmar views (see below and also 'Navicular disease', pages 115–122).

Dorsopalmar ('upright pedal') view

The number and size of the lucent zones along the distal border of the navicular bone vary between individuals and between breeds. It is probably normal to have up to seven lucent zones in the bone, and these are normally conical, and taller than they are wide. The hind feet generally have two or three fewer than the front. There may be a double contour along the proximal border of the navicular bone. This may be due either to elongation of the flexor cortex proximally, or entheseophyte formation.

New bone on the proximal border of the navicular bone may be present in clinically normal horses. This is entheseophyte formation in the insertion of the collateral sesamoidean ligaments. It is normally most prominent at the medial and lateral aspects of the proximal border, where it is sometimes referred to as spurs. Spurs are more common on the lateral aspect of the navicular bone than the medial. The clinical significance of these spurs is equivocal, but they indicate previous stress to the ligaments. They are unlikely to indicate 'navicular disease' *per se*, although they may indicate a foot imbalance. Spurs or new bone along the proximal border may accompany other changes in the navicular bone, and are associated with 'navicular disease', especially if extensive. (On plantarodorsal views the navicular bone appears slightly larger relative to the middle phalanx.)

A double contour along the distal border of the bone represents the distal articular margin proximally and the distal aspect of the flexor cortex distally. Discrete mineralized fragments are sometimes detectable distal to the navicular bone (see also pages 118 and 119). Although these occur more commonly in association with navicular disease, they are sometimes present as an incidental finding, if not associated with other abnormalities of the navicular bone.

Occasionally a bipartite or tripartite navicular bone occurs, sometimes bilaterally. In contrast to a fracture, the radiolucent line between the separate bone sections is broad with or without lucent areas adjacent to it, and the bone margins tend to be smooth and rounded.

Palmaroproximal-palmarodistal oblique view

Large nutrient foramina or synovial invaginations along the distal border of the navicular bone appear as large oval-shaped lucencies within the medulla. The thickness of the flexor cortex varies considerably between horses and is generally thinner in Thoroughbreds than in Warmbloods. It is usually bilaterally symmetrical unless there is disparity in foot shape. It tends to be thinner in horses with upright foot conformation. The prominence of the sagittal ridge varies between horses. It sometimes appears flattened.

A small well defined crescent-shaped or oval lucency may be evident in the sagittal ridge (Figures 3.42a and 3.42b).

Structures overlying the navicular bone on radiographs are easily misinterpreted as radiographic lesions. The following should be borne in mind:

1   There is a variable sized depression in the palmar aspect of the middle phalanx, proximal to the articular surface, which may appear relatively lucent, and is easily superimposed over the navicular bone.

2   The clefts and central sulcus of the frog are superimposed over the navicular bone on the dorsoproximal-palmarodistal oblique ('upright pedal') view. They can mimic radiolucencies or fractures, especially if poorly filled with packing or if the packing becomes loose.

3   Excess and poorly distributed packing in the frog clefts can appear as an opacity proximal to the navicular bone, mimicking entheseophyte formation. If there is difficulty in differentiating lesions from artefacts, it is recommended that the foot be re-packed and the view repeated using a slight change in angle.

4   The marrow cavity in the middle phalanx, when present, is variable in size. It is easily superimposed over the navicular bone and care should be taken, when assessing radiographs, not to confuse it with a lucent lesion in the navicular bone.

5   There is a row of nutrient foramina in the proximal end of the middle phalanx running across the shaft of the bone, immediately distal to the transverse prominence or tuberosity. These foramina are visualized to varying degrees on the dorsoproximal-palmarodistal oblique ('upright pedal') view, depending on the angle of the projection. If the pastern is angled too far forward during radiography, these foramina may be superimposed over the navicular bone giving the appearance of abnormal proximal nutrient foramina.

6   A radiolucent lesion in the middle phalanx may be superimposed over the navicular bone and mimic an osseous cyst-like lesion in the navicular bone.

Navicular disease

There is no universally accepted definition of navicular disease based on pathological or radiological findings. There is, however, a clinically recognizable condition which is frequently termed navicular disease. For the purposes of this book, the term is used to describe a clinical condition, causing a bilateral (or occasionally unilateral) progressive forelimb lameness which is not permanently alleviated by rest or corrective shoeing alone. It is acknowledged that there are horses which show clinical signs typical of navicular disease which may have pain arising from the navicular bone or its associated soft-tissue structures, but the condition can be alleviated by rest or shoeing. The term navicular syndrome can be used to encompass these horses since they may at a later stage progress towards a less responsive disease. They must be differentiated from horses which have pain in the palmar aspect of the foot due to other causes (see 'Long-toe low-heel syndrome', page 97).

Recent advances in knowledge with the advent of magnetic resonance imaging and pathological investigation of less chronic cases of navicular disease indicate that there is a variety of different pathological changes that may affect the navicular bone, and thus confirm that the term navicular disease may be over simplistic.

Considerable controversy exists over the significance of radiographic changes in the navicular bone. To relate them to the clinical situation, it is probably best to use the description given on pages 112–114 as being indicative of a normal bone, and accept that a number of apparently normal horses do show radiographic changes in the navicular bones. When these changes are present in sound horses, their significance is equivocal. Some workers consider that they may predispose the horse to developing navicular disease at a later date, but this is by no means certain. Repeat radiographs are sometimes obtained after a period of 4–6 months, to assess the progression of such lesions. Progression, however, can occur in animals which remain clinically normal, and those that become lame may show no such progression. Bilateral radiographic abnormalities are frequently seen in horses with unilateral lameness, and unilateral changes may be seen in horses that are bilaterally lame.

It is probably best, therefore, to accept that the more changes present, and the greater the degree of change, the more likely the horse is to have navicular disease. In the absence of radiographic abnormality, navicular disease should only be diagnosed with extreme caution. However, significant abnormalities of the navicular bone have been detected using magnetic resonance imaging in horses in which the navicular bone has been radiographically normal. These abnormalities have been verified histologically. Radiographic abnormalities of the navicular bone are frequently accompanied by lesions of the collateral sesamoidean ligament and/or the distal sesamoidean impar ligament and/or the deep digital flexor tendon which may adversely influence prognosis.

Although navicular disease is generally assumed to be a disease of the front feet, it can occur in hind feet, either unilaterally or bilaterally.

Lateromedial view

There are contradictory reports about changes in the shape of the navicular bone in navicular disease. It is however known that the bone models because of chronic stress on the collateral sesamoid ligaments and distal sesamoidean impar ligament, resulting in proximodistal elongation of the bone.

In some cases the synovial fossa may become more prominent. In advanced cases some lucency of the bone proximal to this notch may be seen. In the later stages of the disease the trabecular bone may appear more opaque and the cortex may increase in thickness. There is also reduced corticomedullary demarcation. Irregular endosteal new bone may be seen dorsal to the flexor cortex of the navicular bone (Figure 3.47a).

When a radiolucent lesion is present in the body of the bone, it can frequently be seen on the lateromedial view. It is generally accepted as confirming some form of pathological process in the navicular bone (Figure

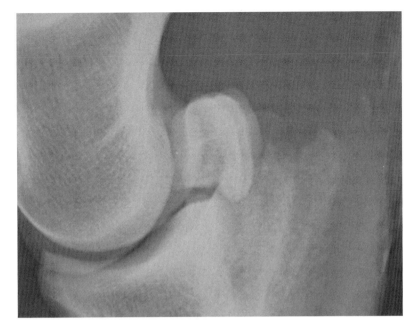

Figure 3.43(a) Oblique lateromedial view of the left hind navicular bone of a 5-year-old general purpose Thoroughbred cross horse with lameness improved by perineural analgesia of the plantar digital nerves or intrathecal analgesia of the navicular bursa. There is distal extension of the flexor cortex of the navicular bone. Compare with Figure 3.43(b).

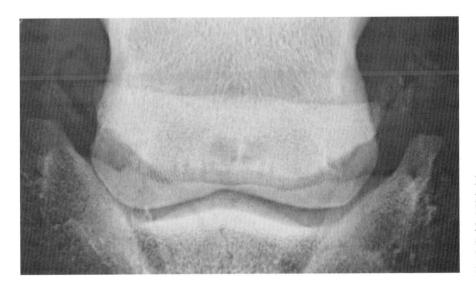

Figure 3.43(b) Dorsoproximal-plantarodistal oblique view of the left hind navicular bone seen in Figure 3.43(a). There are two large radiolucent areas abaxial to the sagittal midline in the distal half of the spongiosa of the navicular bone.

3.43b). If it penetrates the flexor surface of the bone, it may be evident as a sharp-edged lesion in the flexor surface (see Figure 3.40d, page 109). This lesion must be differentiated from the previously described depression in the sagittal ridge (see Figure 3.40c, page 109).

Entheseophytes can be seen on the lateromedial view on the proximal and distal borders of the bone (Figure 3.43a). These are described in more detail under 'New bone formation' (see page 122).

Irregularity of the bone at the origin of the distal sesamoidean impar ligament is an indication that the dorsoproximal-palmarodistal oblique view should be carefully examined. This irregularity may be due to either entheseophyte formation in the distal sesamoidean impar ligament or to a mineralized opacity distal to the bone.

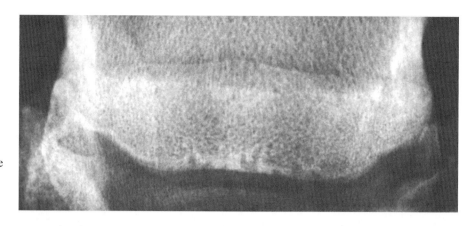

Figure 3.44(a) Dorsoproximal-palmarodistal oblique view of a navicular bone of a 5-year-old Quarterhorse gelding. There are multiple variably shaped and sized radiolucent zones along the horizontal distal border of the navicular bone.

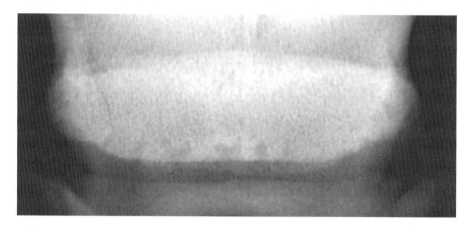

Figure 3.44(b) Dorsoproximal-palmarodistal oblique view of a navicular bone of a 7-year-old crossbred gelding. Medial is to the left. There are multiple large variably shaped lucent zones along the distal horizontal and medial sloping borders of the navicular bone.

New bone, an osteophyte, on the dorsoproximal margin of the navicular bone is an indicator of degenerative joint disease of the distal interphalangeal joint, and does not reflect navicular disease, although it may be seen in association with it.

Dorsoproximal-palmarodistal oblique ('upright pedal') view

The distal lucent zones frequently show a change in shape from the normal described above (Figure 3.41a, page 110; Figures 3.44a–c). It has been suggested that lucent zones of certain shapes have a greater significance than others, but this is still a subjective assessment. There is evidence that the greater the number of abnormally shaped lucent zones, the more likely are clinical signs of navicular disease to be present. Similarly an increased number of lucent zones (more than seven), and the radiographic appearance of lucent zones on the lateral, medial or proximal borders of the bone (Figure 3.44d), are all indicators of abnormality. An irregular appearance of lucent zones, i.e. of many different shapes and sizes, and lucent zones surrounded by a halo of sclerosis should also be viewed with suspicion.

If there is a lucent area at the medial or lateral angle of the distal border of the navicular bone (at the junction between the horizontal and medial and lateral sloping borders), it is likely that there is an associated distal border fragment (Figure 3.45). The frequency of recognition of such fragments has increased with better-quality radiographs obtained with digital

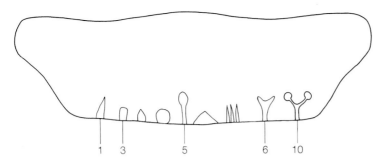

Figure 3.44(c) Diagram of a dorsoproximal-palmarodistal oblique view of a navicular bone showing distal nutrient foramina of different shapes (after Colles, 1982). The numbers refer to the scoring system of MacGregor (1986). Larger numbers may indicate foramina of greater diagnostic significance.

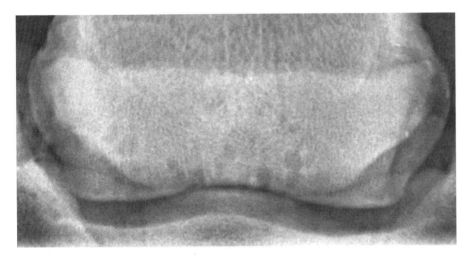

Figure 3.44(d) Dorsoproximal-palmarodistal oblique view of a navicular bone of a 7-year-old Warmblood gelding. Medial is to the left. There are multiple large lucent zones along the distal medial sloping and distal horizontal borders of the navicular bone and ill defined lucent zones in the spongiosa of the bone. The lateral proximal border of the bone is modelled.

or computerized radiography. A distal border fragment seen in association with a radiolucent area at the ipsilateral angle of the distal aspect of the navicular bone is likely to be of clinical significance. However, mineralized fragments in isolation with no other abnormality of the navicular bone may be seen unassociated with clinical signs.

Distinct areas of radiolucency within the navicular bone (Figure 3.46a) which are not associated with the distal border of the bone should always be regarded with extreme caution. Although clinical signs may not be present at the time of examination, lameness is likely to develop. The majority of these lucent lesions occur in the central one-third of the bone, but the entire bone should be inspected carefully. If these lesions are detected on dorsoproximal-palmarodistal oblique views, it is important to inspect latero-medial and palmaroproximal-palmarodistal oblique views carefully to ascertain whether they are contained within the body of the bone or penetrate the flexor surface (Figure 3.46b). If the lesion progresses to penetrate through the flexor surface of the bone, adhesion of the deep digital flexor tendon will result. Adhesions may also occur in the absence of other radiological changes in the navicular bone. Once adhesions are present, a very poor prognosis must be given.

In advanced stages of the disease there may be an appreciable increase in opacity of the bone, with or without thickening of the flexor cortex and loss of definition between the cortex and the medulla. This is best assessed on the lateromedial or palmaroproximal-palmarodistal oblique views.

[119]

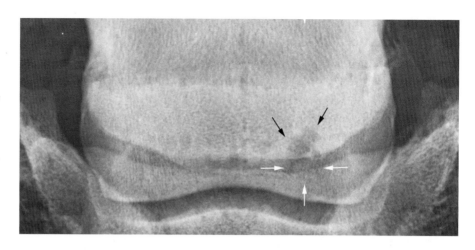

Figure 3.45 Dorsoproximal-palmarodistal oblique radiographic view of the navicular bone of an 8-year-old Thoroughbred cross gelding. Medial is to the left. There are several variably shaped and sized lucent zones along the distal border of the navicular bone. There is a large radiolucent zone at the lateral angle of the navicular bone (black arrows), distal to which is an osseous fragment (white arrows).

Palmaroproximal-palmarodistal oblique view

On a palmaroproximal-palmarodistal oblique view, alterations in the shape of the lucent zones on the distal border of the bone cannot be identified, but increased size and numbers are sometimes evident early in the course of navicular disease.

This view may help to determine whether lucent lesions are present in the medulla or flexor cortex of the bone, or both (Figure 3.46b). A palmaroproximal-palmarodistal oblique view may not highlight the entire flexor cortex of the bone from its proximal to distal border, and a focal defect which does penetrate the flexor cortex may not be detectable radiographically, either because the x-ray beam is not tangential to that portion of the bone, or as a result of summation of surrounding normal dense bone. In some horses significant radiolucent zones are seen in the flexor cortex of the navicular bone only in this view, but in all other views the navicular bone appears normal (Figure 3.46c).

Localized thinning or reduced radiopacity of the cortex is associated with fibrocartilage degeneration, which may ultimately be associated with tendon adhesions.

The flexor cortex may become uniformly thicker, encroaching into the medulla (Figure 3.47a), or endosteal new bone may develop (Figure 3.47b). The trabecular pattern of the medulla may become less obvious due to sclerosis, resulting in loss of corticomedullary definition (Figure 3.46b). Apparent poor corticomedullary demarcation may be an artefact (Figure 3.42c, page 113) due to inappropriate radiographic technique; it is therefore important to compare the lateromedial and palmaroproximal-palmarodistal oblique views, and to be critical of the positioning of both the lateromedial and the palmaroproximal-palmarodistal oblique views.

Occasionally new bone is seen on the flexor cortex (Figure 3.48). This may be seen in the absence of other radiographic abnormalities, emphasizing the importance of this radiographic view in horses with suspected navicular pathology. Such new bone warrants a poor prognosis for future soundness.

A distal border fragment may be seen superimposed over the spongiosa in some horses, resulting in an area of relatively increased opacity. This is

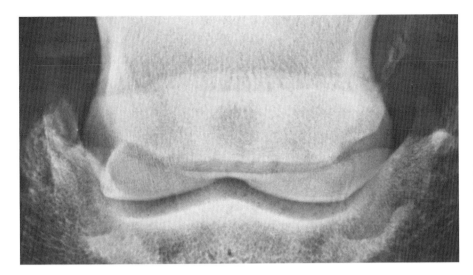

Figure 3.46(a) Dorsoproximal-palmarodistal oblique radiographic view of a navicular bone of a 6-year-old Warmblood gelding. There is a large circular radiolucent zone in the centre of the bone, which penetrated the flexor cortex of the bone. See Figure 3.46(b).

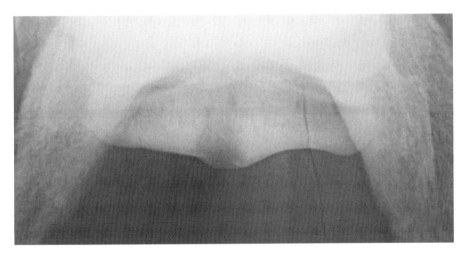

Figure 3.46(b) Palmaroproximal-palmarodistal oblique radiographic view of the same navicular bone as in Figure 3.46(a). There is a large radiolucent defect in the flexor cortex at the sagittal ridge. The flexor cortex is markedly thickened and there is extensive sclerosis of the spongiosa of the navicular bone. There was an adhesion of the deep digital flexor tendon to the flexor cortex defect.

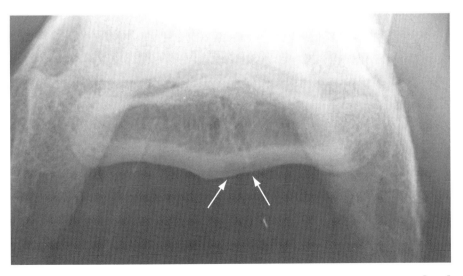

Figure 3.46(c) Palmaroproximal-palmarodistal oblique radiographic view of a navicular bone of a 6-year-old Warmblood cross gelding. Medial is to the left. There is a large radiolucent defect in the flexor cortex of the navicular bone lateral to the sagittal ridge (arrows). There are also two large oval-shaped radiolucent zones in the spongiosa. No significant abnormalities were detected in other radiographic projections.

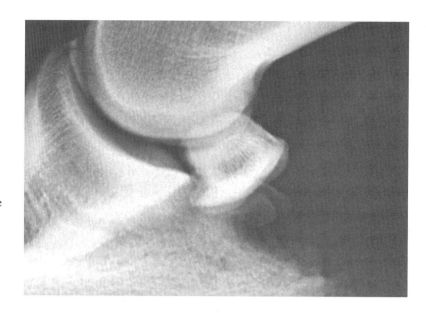

Figure 3.47(a) Lateromedial radiographic view of the navicular bone of a 4-year-old Warmblood mare with bilateral forelimb lameness. The flexor cortex of the navicular bone is abnormally thick and there is distal extension of the flexor cortex of the bone.

Figure 3.47(b) Palmaroproximal-palmarodistal oblique radiographic view of a navicular bone of a 7-year-old general-purpose riding horse. The flexor cortex of the navicular bone is thick and there is considerable endosteal new bone.

usually apparent when there is an extensive radiolucent region in the distal aspect of the navicular bone seen in a dorsoproximal-palmarodistal oblique view, which highlights the potential presence of a fragment.

A magnifying glass may be useful to study the flexor cortex in fine detail.

Positive contrast studies of the navicular bursa may enhance the interpretation of flexor cartilage changes. Defects may also be identified using transcuneal ultrasonography.

New bone formation

The clinical significance of new bone along the margins of the navicular bone is questionable; however, large amounts of new bone accompanied by other changes may be significant.

Entheseophyte formation is frequently seen in the collateral sesamoidean ligaments. This is seen on the proximal border of the bone on dorsopal-

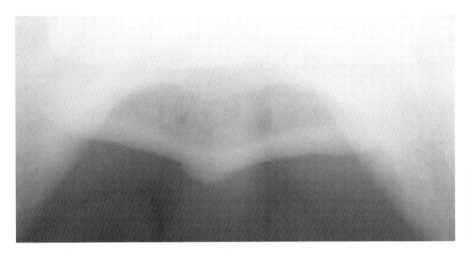

Figure 3.48 Palmaroproximal-palmarodistal oblique radiograph of a navicular bone. Note the irregular outline of the sagittal ridge due to new bone formation.

mar and dorsoproximal-palmarodistal oblique views, and on the palmar aspect of the proximal border of the bone on lateromedial views (see page 117). Entheseophytes are believed to be evidence of abnormal tension in the suspensory apparatus of the navicular bone, and should be differentiated from osteophytes (see below). There is a significantly higher incidence on the lateral side of the foot. Larger entheseophytes are more likely to be of clinical significance than small entheseophytes.

Dystrophic mineralization or ossification can occur within the navicular collateral ligaments as a discrete opacity proximal to the lateral or medial border of the bone. It is often, but not always, associated with lameness (Figure 3.49).

Periarticular osteophytes are occasionally seen along the dorsal margin of the proximal border on lateromedial views (Figure 3.50). They are frequently seen in association with degenerative joint disease of the distal interphalangeal joint and warrant a poor prognosis.

Entheseophytes on the distal margin of the navicular bone at the origin of the distal sesamoidean impar ligament tend to be smaller than on the proximal border, and are thought to be more significant.

Discrete radiopaque bodies may be seen along the distal border of the bone (Figure 3.51). These are of variable aetiology, but cannot be differentiated radiographically. They may be located within a depression in the distal border of the bone and are more common at the medial and lateral borders of the bone. They may result from avulsion fractures, fractures of entheseophytes or dystrophic mineralization in the distal sesamoidean impar ligament. Their significance is discussed on pages 118–119.

Mineralization in the deep digital flexor tendon

Focal mineralization occasionally occurs in the deep digital flexor tendon palmar to the middle phalanx or the navicular bone (Figure 3.52). The cause of this is unknown, but probably reflects chronic tendon injury (see Chapter 1, page 35). It carries a poor prognosis. It is most easily seen on a lateromedial view, but should not be confused with ossification of the cartilages of the foot, which can be differentiated on a dorsopalmar (weight-bearing)

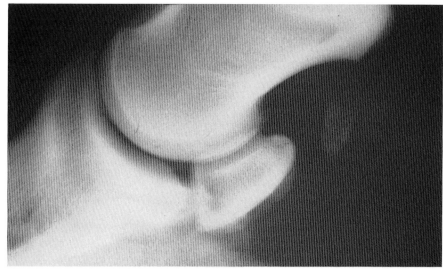

(a)

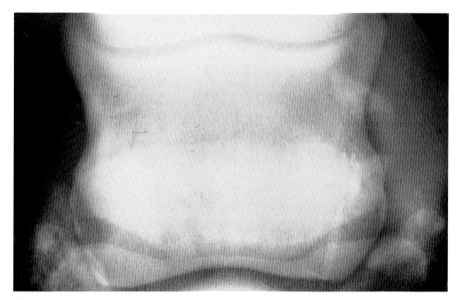

(b)

Figure 3.49 Radiographs of a navicular bone, showing dystrophic mineralization in the lateral collateral sesamoidean ligament: (a) lateromedial view; (b) dorsoproximal-palmarodistal oblique ('upright pedal') view (lateral is to the right). Note that there is some dirt in the frog clefts and modelling of the proximal border of the navicular bone. There are a number of enlarged lucent zones along the distal border of the bone, some of which also show a change in shape.

view. Dystrophic mineralization, in or close to the navicular bursa, or palmar to the deep digital flexor tendon, has also been seen as a sequel to repetitive medication of the navicular bursa (region) with corticosteroids.

Infection

Infection of the navicular bursa or bone usually occurs subsequent to a penetrating wound or after an injection into the navicular bursa. Plain radiographs obtained at the time of injury may reveal no abnormality, but if a draining sinus is present, contrast radiography may be of value (see 'Fistulography', page 706). Use of a radiodense probe can also be useful to determine the depth and orientation of a penetrating injury. Lateromedial and palmaroproximal-palmarodistal oblique views should be obtained. Follow-up radiographs may be helpful if lameness persists. Extensive ill

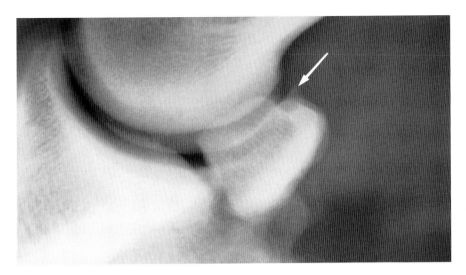

Figure 3.50 Lateromedial view of a navicular bone, showing periarticular osteophytes (arrow) on the dorsoproximal border.

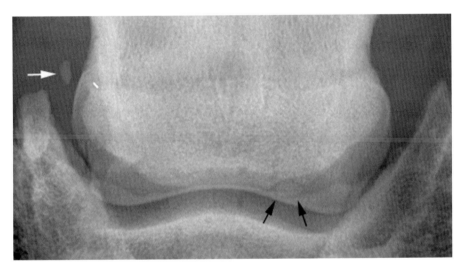

Figure 3.51 Dorsoproximal-palmarodistal oblique radiographic view of a navicular bone. Medial is to the left. There is a well defined osseous opacity distal to the navicular bone at the lateral angle (black arrows). The opacity of the navicular bone is relatively normal. Note also the discrete mineralized opacity proximomedial to the navicular bone (white arrow), probably dystrophic mineralization within the collateral sesamoidean ligament.

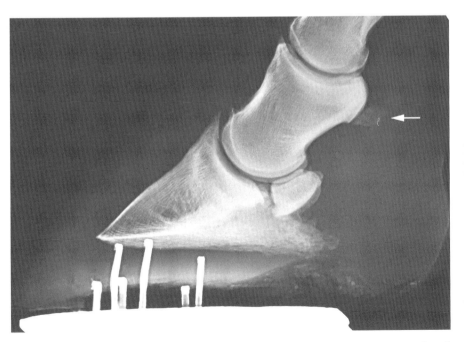

Figure 3.52 Lateromedial radiographic view of a foot of a 9-year-old Warmblood pleasure horse. There is mineralization in the deep digital flexor tendon (arrow). There is modelling of the proximal border of the navicular bone and periarticular osteophyte formation, together with periarticular osteophyte formation involving both the proximal and distal interphalangeal joints. The distal solar margin of the distal phalanx slopes downwards from dorsal to palmar.

defined lucent lesions, and occasionally sclerosis of the flexor cortex of the navicular bone, warrant a very poor prognosis. If a penetrating wound has occurred, immediate and extensive flushing of the navicular bursa and antimicrobial treatment are required.

Fractures

Small radiopaque bodies in the distal sesamoidean impar ligament, adjacent to the distal border of the bone, are discussed previously (see pages 118–119, 123 and Figure 3.51). They are very difficult to demonstrate clearly on any radiographic view, but are most easily detected on the dorsoproximal-palmarodistal oblique view. Occasionally a fracture occurs at the insertion of the collateral sesamoidean ligament.

Fractures through the body of the navicular bone normally occur parallel to the sagittal ridge of the bone, or slightly obliquely to it, and at varying distance from it (Figure 3.53a). There is normally little or no displacement, and the fracture may be very difficult to visualize, particularly in the acute stage. After 2–4 weeks the fracture line becomes more obvious due to bone demineralization. Subsequently lucent zones develop along the fracture line (Figure 3.53b) and an increased number of lucent zones along the distal border of the bone may be seen, especially in the bone immediately adjacent to the fracture. Frequently several dorsopalmar views of slightly varying obliquity as well as palmaroproximal-palmarodistal views are required to confirm the presence of a fracture, and to differentiate it from overlying artefacts (such as lucent lines caused by the frog). A parasagittal fracture should remain in the same position relative to the medial or lateral margin of the bone, should not extend beyond the bone margins and should be seen in both dorsoproximal-palmarodistal oblique and palmaroproximal-

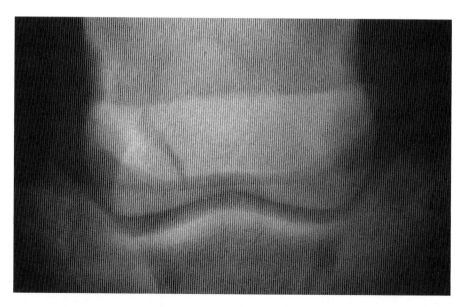

Figure 3.53(a) Dorsoproximal-palmarodistal oblique view of a navicular bone showing a sagittal fracture of the body of the bone (the fracture is of 3 weeks' duration).

palmarodistal oblique views. It may also be necessary to adjust the packing in the frog clefts. There may also be damage to the adjacent deep digital flexor tendon.

Surgical fixation of an acute fracture (less than 10 weeks' duration) should be considered. More longstanding fractures may respond to surgery, but the success rate becomes poorer the longer the fracture has been present. Radiolucencies along the length of the fracture line and adjacent to it generally start to develop 6–8 weeks after the fracture occurs. If a fracture appears chronic radiographically at the time of onset of lameness (i.e. a broad radiolucent line with multiple lucent zones along the fracture line), the fracture

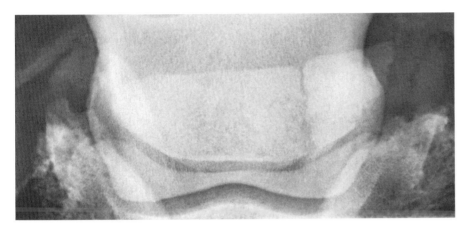

Figure 3.53(b) Dorsoproximal-palmarodistal oblique radiographic view of the navicular bone of a 9-year-old general purpose riding horse with recent onset lameness improved by perineural analgesia of the palmar digital nerves. Medial is to the left. There is a chronic parasagittal fracture of the navicular bone laterally. The fracture line is quite wide and there are lucent areas adjacent to it. There is modelling of the lateral aspect of the navicular bone. Radiopharmaceutical uptake in the bone was normal and lameness was due to a core lesion of the deep digital flexor tendon.

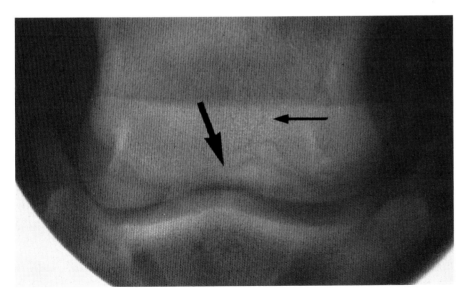

Figure 3.53(c) Dorsoproximal-palmarodistal oblique view of a navicular bone, showing a recent fracture of the distal border of the bone (large arrow). Note that there is also a vertical component to the fracture (small arrow).

may not be the cause of lameness. Nuclear scintigraphy may be helpful to determine if it is an active lesion.

Fractures occasionally occur horizontally across the bone, close to and parallel with its distal border (Figure 3.53c). It is important to remember that more than one fracture may occur simultaneously.

Fractures, especially in the forelimb, carry a poor prognosis for return to work without internal fixation. A good prognosis, however, can be given for breeding purposes. In very small ponies a slightly better prognosis for return to work can be given with conservative management.

Proximal displacement of the navicular bone

Complete disruption of the distal sesamoidean impar ligament results in proximal displacement of the navicular bone. There may or may not be associated avulsion fragments of the distal aspect of the bone. This unusual injury occurs more in hindlimbs than in forelimbs. Some horses have returned to full work (steeplechasing) following prolonged rest. Proximal displacement of the navicular bone occasionally occurs subsequent to ligament disruption by a deeply penetrating foreign body.

Proximal and middle phalanges

The proximal aspect of the proximal phalanx is also discussed under 'The metacarpophalangeal joint' (see page 150).

RADIOGRAPHIC TECHNIQUE

Equipment

Radiographs of the proximal and middle phalanges (pastern region) can easily be obtained using portable machines. High-definition screen and appropriate film combinations can be used even with portable equipment, since movement blur is seldom a problem. It is unnecessary to use a grid even in large horses.

Positioning

Survey radiographs of the proximal and middle phalanges are often obtained as part of the examination of the foot or fetlock. Specific views of this area are best obtained with the horse bearing weight on the limb, and should include lateromedial, dorsopalmar and two oblique views. When evaluating the dorsal joint margins, flexed oblique views may be more useful (see pages 57–58). The x-ray beam is kept horizontal, and centred midway between the fetlock and coronary band. The x-ray beam should normally be aligned with reference to the bulbs of the heel in order to obtain correct lateromedial or dorsopalmar views. Dorsal 5–10° proximal-palmarodistal oblique views may be obtained with the x-ray beam aligned at right angles to the dorsal surface of the pastern, and angling the cassette accordingly. This view results in less distortion, and is particularly useful for assessment of the middle phalanx and the proximal interphalangeal joint.

Chip fractures of the phalanges are best visualized on oblique views. Fractures of the phalanges are frequently spiral, and a series of oblique radiographs may be required to determine their course. Fractures, separate centres of ossification or osteochondritic lesions of the proximal palmar aspect of the proximal phalanx may best be evaluated (and/or detected) using dorsal 30° proximal 70° lateral-palmarodistomedial oblique or dorsal 30° proximal 70° medial-palmarodistolateral oblique views (see page 151).

Subtle osteophyte formation is sometimes best evaluated on flexed oblique (dorsolateral-palmaromedial and dorsomedial-palmarolateral oblique) views. These are obtained with the toe of the foot placed in a navicular block, with the sole of the foot approximately vertical (see pages 57–58).

NORMAL ANATOMY

Immature horse

The proximal and middle phalanges both ossify from three centres. In both bones the distal epiphysis unites with the shaft before birth. In foals that are skeletally immature at birth, a lucent crescent is occasionally noted in the distal metaphysis of the bone, which represents a non-mineralized cartilage remnant of the physeal plate. The proximal physis closes at about 1 year of age in the proximal phalanx, and at 8–12 months in the middle phalanx.

Skeletally mature horse

There is an area relatively devoid of trabeculae in the central part of the proximal and middle phalanges. This is a marrow or fat cavity, and is of variable size. It appears as a lucent zone, best seen on dorsopalmar views, although the clarity with which it is seen will depend upon a number of radiographic factors. It may not be visible radiographically in the middle phalanx. On dorsopalmar views there are relatively sclerotic lines on the medial and lateral aspects of this lucent area, which extend proximally and distally. These are the areas of insertion of the oblique (middle) distal sesamoidean ligaments (Figures 3.54a and 3.54b; 3.55a and 3.55b).

On dorsopalmar radiographs, the ergot may be recognized as a circumscribed opacity superimposed on the proximal aspect of the proximal phalanx.

Both the proximal and middle phalanges have a row of nutrient foramina across the shaft of the bone at their proximal and distal ends. These may be seen to varying degrees on dorsopalmar views depending on the angle of projection, and are a normal finding. Care should be exercised, when interpreting radiographs of the navicular bone, that the foramina of the middle phalanx are not superimposed over the navicular bone giving the appearance of abnormal proximal nutrient foramina.

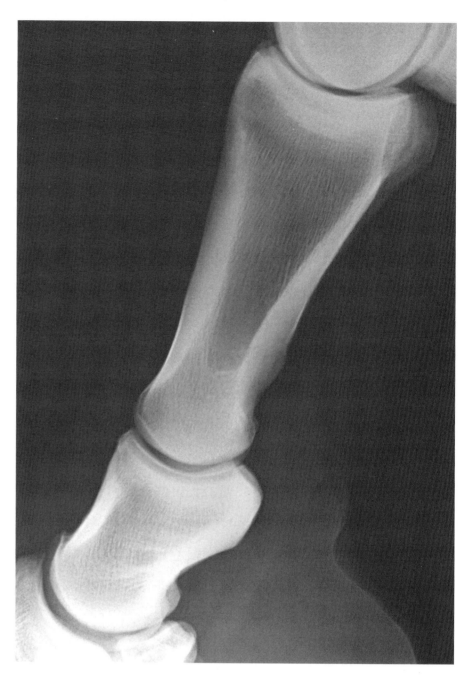

Figure 3.54(a) Lateromedial view of the proximal and middle phalanges of a normal adult horse.

On lateromedial views of the proximal phalanx, a small irregularity may be evident on the palmar aspect of the bone at approximately one-third of the length of the bone from the distal end. This is the apex of the area of insertion of the oblique (middle) distal sesamoidean ligaments. The irregular bone may extend proximally in an oblique lateral and/or medial direction following the line of insertion of the ligaments, and is seen more readily on oblique radiographic views. This finding tends to be more prominent in older and/or large horses.

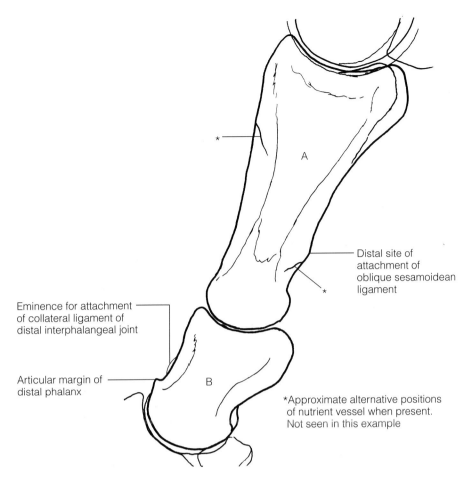

Eminence for attachment
of collateral ligament of
distal interphalangeal joint

Articular margin of
distal phalanx

Distal site of
attachment of
oblique sesamoidean
ligament

*Approximate alternative positions
of nutrient vessel when present.
Not seen in this example

Figure 3.54(b) Diagram of a lateromedial radiograph of the proximal and middle phalanges of a normal adult horse. A = proximal phalanx, B = middle phalanx.

There may be a circular lucency or a slightly oblique radiolucent line in the centre of the middle or proximal phalanx on dorsopalmar and oblique views. This represents the normal nutrient foramen of the bone.

The middle phalanx is approximately half the length of the proximal phalanx. There are two prominent bony ridges, either side of the distal dorsal aspect of the bone, where the collateral ligaments of the distal interphalangeal joint originate. These are particularly obvious on slightly oblique views. The bony eminences at ligament insertions tend to be more prominent in large horses.

The articular surface of the distal end of the middle phalanx normally has a smooth curved outline, which extends dorsally into a point (Figure 3.54). The central third of the articular surface may be relatively flatter than the more dorsal and palmar aspects. The articular surfaces of the proximal and middle phalanges in the proximal interphalangeal joint are otherwise reasonably congruous (Figure 3.54).

NORMAL VARIATIONS AND INCIDENTAL FINDINGS

There is often new bone formation (entheseophytes) at the site of the ligament insertions on the distal dorsal aspect of the middle phalanx, and the

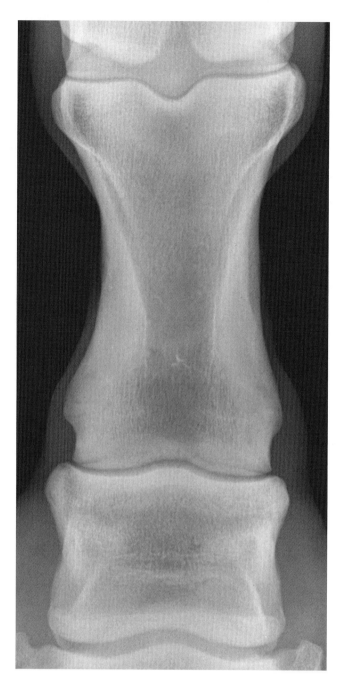

Figure 3.55(a) Dorsopalmar view of the proximal and middle phalanges of a normal adult horse.

palmar distal third of the proximal phalanx. This is of no long-term significance, but indicates that the ligaments have undergone acute or chronic trauma at some time prior to radiography. Entheseophytes should alert the clinician to a potential soft-tissue problem.

A small mineralized opacity may occasionally be present at the dorsal aspect of the proximal articular surface of the middle phalanx. Local analgesia may be required to assess its clinical significance.

Occasionally there are one or two small smoothly outlined, discrete opacities on the palmar proximal aspect of the proximal phalanx. These are

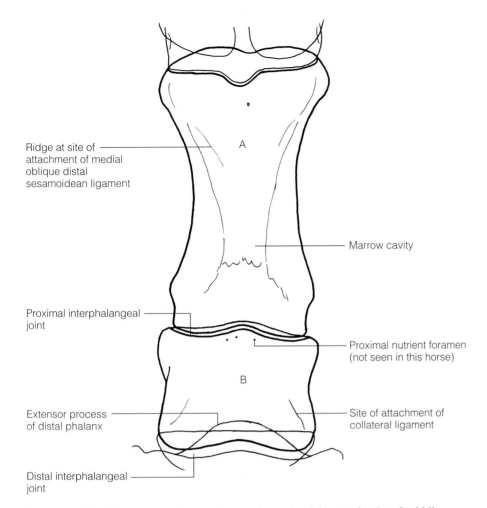

Ridge at site of
attachment of medial
oblique distal
sesamoidean ligament

Marrow cavity

Proximal interphalangeal
joint

Proximal nutrient foramen
(not seen in this horse)

Extensor process
of distal phalanx

Site of attachment of
collateral ligament

Distal interphalangeal
joint

Figure 3.55(b) Diagram of a dorsopalmar radiograph of the proximal and middle phalanges of a normal adult horse. A = proximal phalanx, B = middle phalanx.

present within the sesamoidean ligaments, and their origin is uncertain. They may represent fabellae, small chip fractures sustained early in life, or mineralization within the ligaments. Provided that they are smooth and opaque and do not involve the joint surface, they may be regarded as an incidental finding. They should not be confused with so-called Birkeland fractures (see page 169).

A small rounded osseous opacity is sometimes seen at the dorsoproximal aspect of the proximal phalanx. This may be unilateral or bilateral. If small (less than approximately 2 mm in diameter) and uniformly opaque, they may be an incidental finding (see Figure 3.90, page 178). They may require selective local analgesia to establish their significance.

On lateromedial radiographs, the distal end of the proximal phalanx may appear to be displaced dorsally relative to the proximal aspect of the middle phalanx. Although this can give the impression of subluxation, it has not been associated with any clinical abnormalities, and is most commonly seen in horses with upright conformation. The impression of subluxation of this joint may also be seen in radiographs obtained with the limb non-weight-bearing (see also 'Subluxation of the proximal interphalangeal joint').

[133]

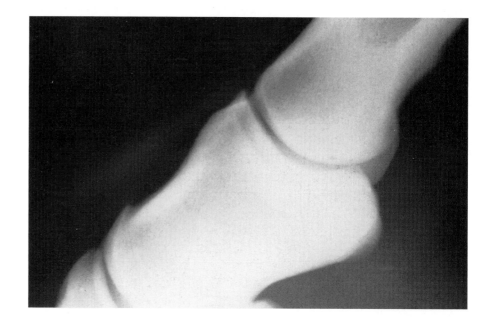

Figure 3.56 Lateromedial view of a pastern, showing a periarticular osteophyte on the dorsoproximal aspect of the middle phalanx.

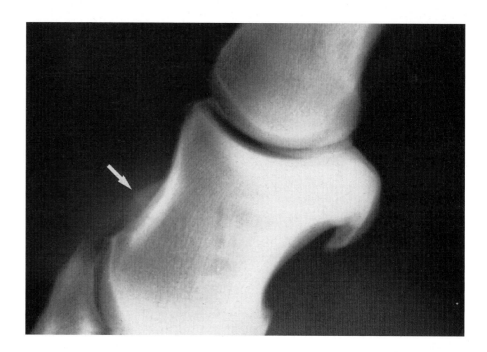

Figure 3.57 Lateromedial view of a pastern showing a 'spur' on the palmaroproximal aspect of the middle phalanx. Note the pronounced bony ridge at the region of origin of the collateral ligaments of the distal interphalangeal joint on the dorsal aspect of the middle phalanx (arrow).

Small periarticular osteophytes are frequently seen on the dorsoproximal aspect of the middle phalanx. Because this joint is relatively immobile, small changes may not have any clinical significance, but they cannot be differentiated from the early signs of degenerative joint disease and so should be viewed with suspicion (Figure 3.56).

A smoothly outlined spur may be present on the palmar aspect of the proximal end of the middle phalanx, pointing distally. The significance of this is uncertain, and it has been seen in lame and sound horses (Figure 3.57).

The position of the nutrient foramen is variable: in some horses it is seen on lateromedial views to enter dorsoproximally or palmarodistally.

[134]

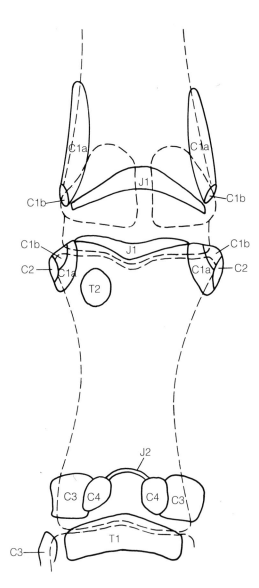

Figure 3.58(a) Diagram of a dorsal 15° proximal-palmarodistal oblique view of the fetlock and pastern regions, to illustrate the sites of attachment for those soft-tissue structures attaching to surfaces seen from the dorsal aspect. Refer to Table 3.1. (Adapted figure courtesy of *Equine vet. J.*)

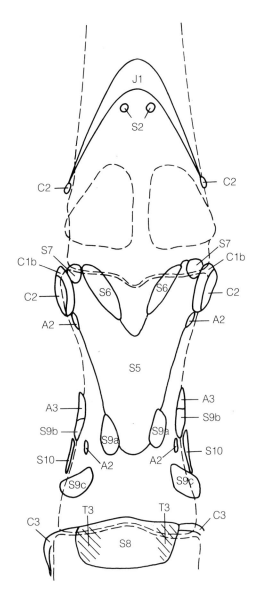

Figure 3.58(b) Diagram of a dorsal 15° proximal-palmarodistal oblique view of the fetlock and pastern regions, illustrating the site of soft-tissue attachments seen from the palmar aspect. See Table 3.1. (Adapted figure courtesy of *Equine vet. J.*)

It is important to be aware of the sites of attachment of tendons, ligaments and joint capsules (Figures 3.58 and 3.59; Table 3.1) in order to be able to interpret the significance of new bone formation at particular sites.

There is a depression between the condyles on the palmar distal aspect of the proximal phalanx that can appear as a radiolucent zone on dorsopalmar views and should not be confused with a lesion. Osseous cyst-like lesions in the distal aspect of the proximal phalanx or the proximal or distal aspects of the middle phalanx are occasionally seen as incidental findings, but should be evaluated very carefully as they may be the cause of lameness (see also page 139).

[135]

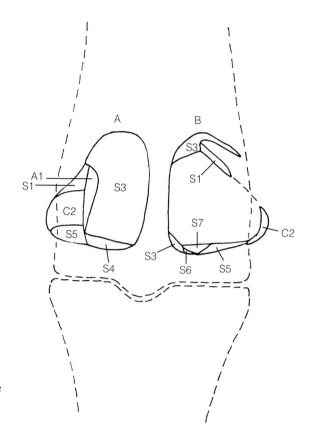

Figure 3.58(c) Diagram of a dorsal 15° proximal-palmarodistal oblique view of a fetlock joint illustrating the sites of attachment of soft-tissue structures to the palmar (A) or dorsal (B) aspects of the proximal sesamoid bones. See Table 3.1. (Adapted figure courtesy of *Equine vet. J.*)

Table 3.1 Legends for the soft tissue structures indicated in Figures 3.58 and 3.59

J1	Fetlock joint capsule
J2	Pastern joint capsule
C1a	Superficial part of the collateral ligaments of the metacarpophalangeal joint
C1b	Deep part of the collateral ligaments of the metacarpophalangeal joint
C2	Collateral sesamoidean ligaments of the proximal sesamoid bones
C3	Collateral ligaments of the proximal interphalangeal joint
C4	Collateral sesamoidean ligaments of the distal sesamoidean (navicular) bone
S1	Suspensory ligament
S2	Metacarpointersesamoidean ligament
S3	Intersesamoidean ligament; proximal scutum; palmar ligament of the metacarpophalangeal joint
S4	Straight sesamoidean ligament
S5	Oblique sesamoidean ligaments
S6	Cruciate sesamoidean ligaments
S7	Short sesamoidean ligaments
S8	Middle scutum
S9a	Axial palmar ligaments of the proximal interphalangeal joint
S9b	Superficial abaxial palmar ligaments of the proximal interphalangeal joint
S9c	Deep abaxial palmar ligaments of the proximal interphalangeal joint
S10	Ligaments to the cartilage of the distal phalanx
A1	Palmar annular ligament
A2	Proximal digital annular ligament
A3	Distal digital annular ligament
T1	Common digital extensor tendon
T2	Lateral digital extensor tendon
T3	Superficial digital flexor tendon

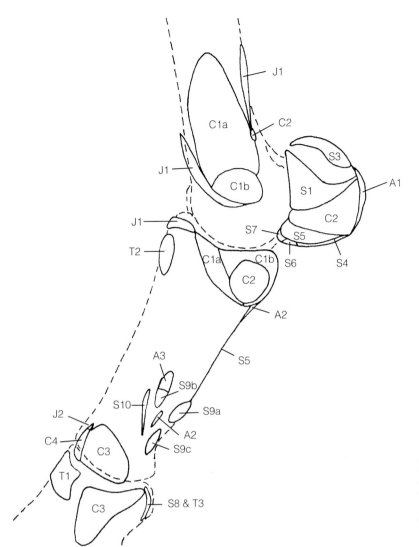

Figure 3.59(a) Diagram of a lateromedial view of the fetlock and pastern regions showing the sites of attachment of soft-tissue structures. See Table 3.1. (Adapted figure courtesy of *Equine vet. J.*)

In heavy cob-type and draught horses there are often thick folds of skin on the palmar aspect of the pastern. These can create potentially confusing opacities when superimposed over the phalanges in dorsal and oblique projections.

SIGNIFICANT FINDINGS

A number of the findings mentioned above as incidental may at some time have been significant. These include small discrete opacities close to the joint margins, small osteophytes (lipping) at the dorsal aspect of the proximal interphalangeal joint, and new bone formation (entheseophytes) at the attachments of ligaments (Figure 3.60). All of these findings probably result from trauma which occurred at least 3–6 weeks prior to radiography. An active osteophyte or entheseophyte may be less opaque than the parent bone and have an irregular or 'fuzzy' outline (Figure 3.66, page 145). It is not possible to age smoothly outlined and uniformly opaque osteophytes or entheseophytes. These lesions may be regarded as an indicator of potential problems, but in chronic lameness should only be incriminated if they can be shown by other techniques to be causing lameness.

[137]

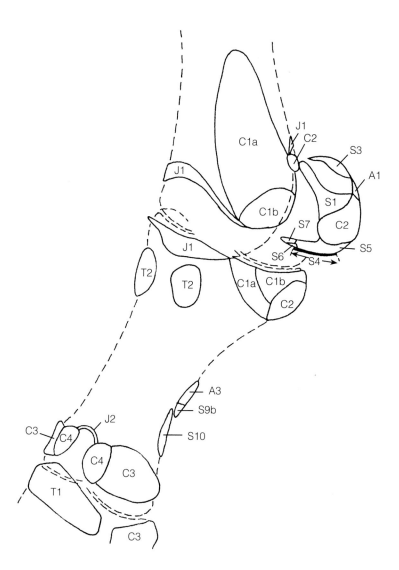

Figure 3.59(b) Diagram of an oblique view of the fetlock and pastern regions to illustrate soft-tissue attachments seen from the dorsomedial or dorsolateral aspects. See Table 3.1. (Adapted figure courtesy of *Equine vet. J.*)

Subluxation of the proximal interphalangeal joint

Subluxation of the proximal interphalangeal joint occurs most commonly in hindlimbs and may be unilateral or bilateral. It is generally seen in young horses (up to 5 years of age), but is occasionally seen in older horses. The horse may superficially appear normal at rest, although in some horses the contour of the proximal interphalangeal joint appears abnormal when viewed from the side. At the walk abnormal dorsal displacement of the distal end of the proximal phalanx may be apparent. At faster gaits usually no gait abnormality can be seen. Lateromedial radiographic views confirm slight dorsal displacement of the distal aspect of the proximal phalanx (Figure 3.61). Other radiographic abnormalities are occasionally seen in older horses in which subluxation develops secondary to injury of the straight sesamoidean ligament or palmar ligaments of the proximal interphalangeal joint; entheseous new bone may be seen at their attachments on the proximal and middle phalanges. In some horses the condition resolves spontaneously, but assessment of foot balance and tone in the flexor muscle groups may aid in treatment. Desmotomy of the accessory ligament of the deep digital flexor

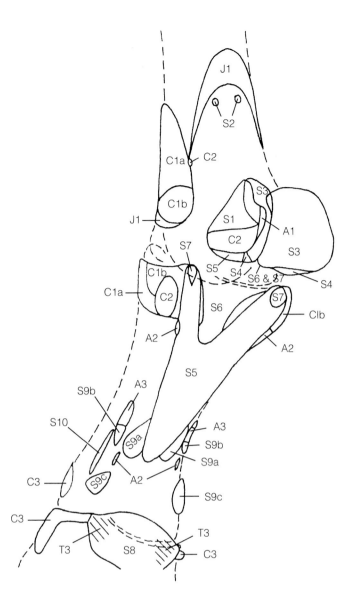

Figure 3.59(c) Diagram of an oblique view of the fetlock and pastern regions illustrating the site of soft-tissue attachments seen from the palmarolateral or palmaromedial aspects. See Table 3.1. (Adapted figure courtesy of *Equine vet. J.*)

tendon has been successful in young horses that did not respond to conservative management.

Osseous cyst-like lesions

Single osseous cyst-like lesions occur in both middle and proximal phalanges, usually close to the proximal interphalangeal joint and sometimes respond to either conservative or surgical treatment.

Multiple small osseous cyst-like lesions may be associated with degenerative joint disease in the proximal interphalangeal joint and warrant a poor prognosis. This has been described as juvenile degenerative joint disease following osteochondrosis in young horses. Despite the relative immobility of this joint, the prognosis is poor without surgical intervention and guarded with surgical arthrodesis, albeit better in the hindlimb than in the forelimb.

An osseous cyst-like lesion is occasionally seen adjacent to the origin of a collateral ligament of the distal interphalangeal joint in association with ipsilateral collateral desmitis.

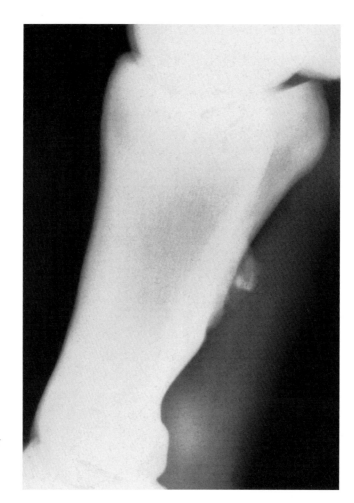

Figure 3.60 Lateromedial view of a pastern (slightly oblique), showing entheseophyte formation on the palmar aspect of the proximal phalanx at the region of insertion of the distal sesamoidean ligaments.

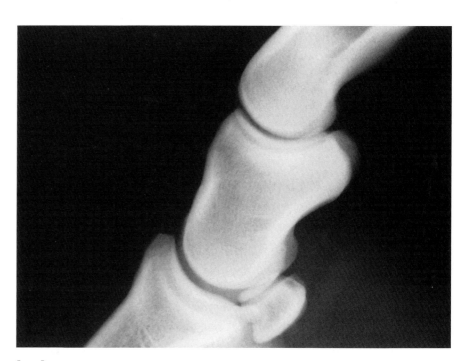

Figure 3.61 Lateromedial view of a pastern and foot of a hindlimb of a 5-year-old Arab, with a history of an audible click associated with the pastern of approximately 8 months' duration. The horse occasionally stumbled, but no lameness was detectable. The distal aspect of the proximal phalanx is positioned slightly dorsal relative to the middle phalanx, i.e. there is subluxation of the proximal interphalangeal joint.

Degenerative joint disease of the proximal interphalangeal joint

In early cases of degenerative joint disease of the proximal interphalangeal joint, there may be small osteophytes on the dorsoproximal aspect of the middle phalanx. These are evident on lateromedial and dorsolateral-palmaromedial and dorsomedial-palmarolateral oblique radiographs, and careful examination of the dorsopalmar view often reveals other subtle changes at the joint margins. In some cases, osteophyte formation may be best evaluated in flexed oblique (dorsolateral-palmaromedial and dorsomedial-palmarolateral oblique) views (see pages 57–58 and Figure 3.24b, page 85). With more advanced disease there may be narrowing of the joint space, subchondral sclerosis and more extensive marginal osteophyte formation.

These latter changes are most easily seen on dorsopalmar radiographs (Figure 3.62). In advanced cases, there may be extensive new bone forming from the proximal aspect of the middle phalanx and the distal aspect of the proximal phalanx, attempting to bridge the proximal interphalangeal joint and create ankylosis.

Once radiographic changes are established the prognosis for spontaneous resolution of lameness and the response to intra-articular medication are poor. Surgical arthrodesis is an option, but the prognosis for this is guarded in competition horses.

New bone formation

The term ringbone is widely used to describe any new bone formed distal to the fetlock. It is an imprecise term, and should be avoided.

There are many causes of new bone formation in the pastern region. These include degenerative joint disease (see page 141), a sagittal fracture of the proximal or middle phalanx (see page 144), localized trauma, entheseophytes, localized infection and hypertrophic osteopathy (see page 22).

Extensive modelling of the dorsal articular margins of the proximal interphalangeal joint can be seen alone, or in association with chronic oblique sesamoidean desmitis (Figure 3.63). It is not synonymous with degenerative joint disease, and although dramatic in radiographic appearance may be asymptomatic.

Entheseophyte formation may be seen at the dorsomedial or dorsolateral aspect of the middle phalanx at the origin of the collateral ligaments of the distal interphalangeal joint in association with ipsilateral collateral desmitis.

Focal, usually unilateral, new bone seen in localized areas on the diaphysis of the proximal or middle phalanges at sites unrelated to ligament or joint capsule attachments is probably due to periostitis as a result of trauma. This may be associated with lameness. The bone normally remodels and the lameness resolves, unless the bone is forming in a position prone to repeated trauma, e.g. on the medial aspect of the limb where it is constantly struck by the contralateral limb (Figure 3.64).

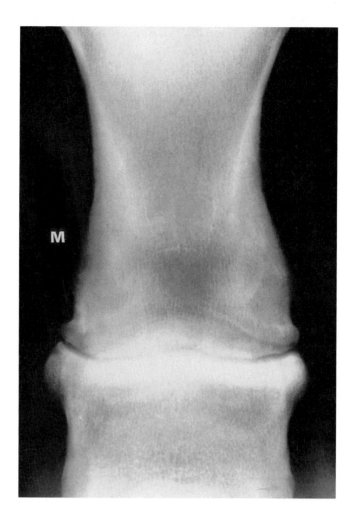

Figure 3.62 Dorsopalmar view of a pastern, showing degenerative joint disease of the proximal interphalangeal joint. Note the narrowing of the medial aspect of the joint and modelling of the articular margins. There is sclerosis of the proximal end of the middle phalanx and mottled opacity of the distal end of the proximal phalanx, due to new bone on the dorsal aspect of the joint.

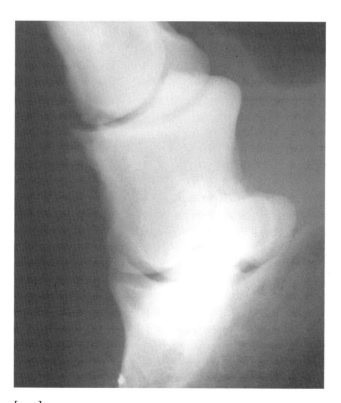

Figure 3.63 Dorsolateral-palmaromedial oblique radiographic view of the proximal interphalangeal joint of the right forelimb of a 12-year-old show jumper. There is extensive periarticular new bone on the dorsomedial aspect of the proximal interphalangeal joint, although no intra-articular abnormalities were seen. Lameness was not alleviated by intra-articular analgesia. There was evidence of chronic desmitis of the oblique sesamoidean ligaments. The current lameness was associated with a complex of soft-tissue injuries within the hoof capsule.

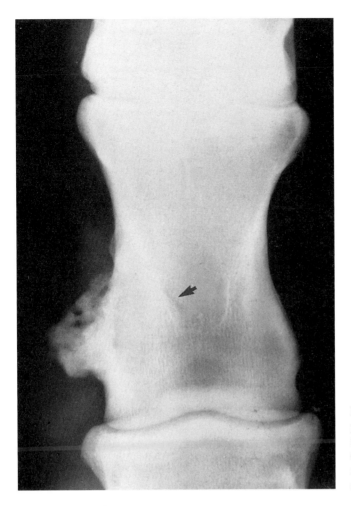

Figure 3.64 Dorsopalmar view of a pastern, showing new bone on the medial aspect of the proximal phalanx caused by repeated trauma (the oblique radiolucent line, arrowed, represents a nutrient vessel).

Irregularly outlined pallisading new bone is sometimes seen on the dorsal diaphysis of the middle phalanx in a lateromedial view (Figure 3.65). This is generally associated with lameness relieved by intra-articular analgesia of the distal interphalangeal joint. The aetiology is unknown, although such new bone has been recognized in association with degenerative joint disease in some horses. The bone lies within the dorsoproximal out-pouching of the distal interphalangeal joint capsule and surgical debridement of this new bone may result in resolution of lameness. Occasionally smoothly outlined new bone is seen at the same site unassociated with clinical signs.

New bone unassociated with the interphalangeal joints may develop, encircling the phalanges. The aetiology is unknown. It is usually associated with chronic lameness.

New bone on the dorsoproximal aspect of the proximal phalanx must be differentiated from that associated with a partial or complete sagittal fracture of the proximal phalanx (see page 144 and Figure 3.68, page 147).

There may be fairly extensive new bone on the dorsal aspect of the proximal phalanx and/or the proximal aspect of the middle phalanx, which

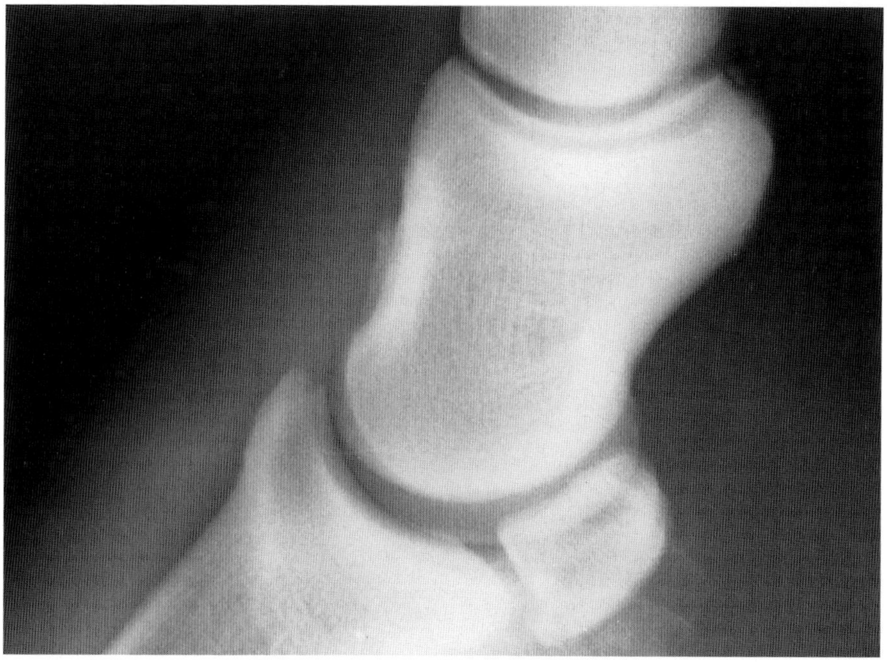

Figure 3.65 Lateromedial view of the proximal and distal interphalangeal joints of an 8-year-old horse, with lameness alleviated by intra-articular analgesia of the distal interphalangeal joint. There is pallisading new bone on the dorsal cortex of the diaphyseal region of the middle phalanx, within the distal interphalangeal joint capsule.

does not extend to the joint margins. If there are no periarticular changes, this new bone is not synonymous with degenerative joint disease (see page 141), although it may be associated with lameness.

New bone (entheseophytes) is often seen at the region of insertion of the oblique distal sesamoidean ligaments on the palmar aspect of the proximal phalanx. This is probably due to chronic or acute stress on the ligaments (see Figure 3.60, page 140). It may cause lameness initially while actively forming, but is not of long-term significance. It should alert the clinician to the possibility of soft-tissue injury. Ultrasonography may be used to assess the ligaments. New bone may be seen at the attachment of the proximal digital annular ligament to the proximal palmar aspect of the proximal phalanx medially and/or laterally, reflecting enthesopathy (see Figure 3.58b, page 135 and Figure 3.66).

Fractures

Fractures of the proximal and middle phalanges are relatively common (see Figure 3.89, page 177). Small chip fractures of the proximal aspect of the proximal phalanx are described elsewhere (see page 167) and are of varying significance.

Midline sagittal fractures occur in both bones, but are more common in the proximal phalanx. They frequently follow a spiral course and are generally visualized as a double radiolucent line extending through the diaphysis of the bone. Each line represents cortical discontinuity (Figure 3.67). There are three principal types of midline sagittal fracture:

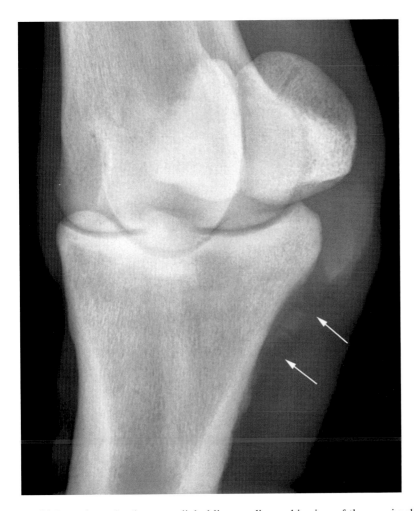

Figure 3.66 Dorsolateral-palmaromedial oblique radiographic view of the proximal aspect of a pastern of a 6-year-old dressage horse. There is irregular new bone on the proximopalmar lateral aspect of the proximal phalanx (arrows), at the site of insertion of the proximal digital annular ligament. The horse resented digital pressure applied to this area. The soft tissue opacity distal to the lateral proximal sesamoid bone is the ergot. Note the concave depression in the skin contour palmar to the ergot.

1   A fracture extending from the proximal to the distal joint, and entering both joints.

2   A fracture extending from either joint and exiting through the cortex.

3   An incomplete sagittal fracture extending from one of the two joints into the diaphysis of the bone (Figures 3.68a and 3.68b). These may only involve the dorsal cortex and most commonly affect the proximal phalanx.

Initially there may be little or no displacement and surprisingly limited clinical signs. The fracture may also be difficult to visualize initially. For this reason a series of oblique views should be obtained if there is any suspicion that such a fracture may be present. A series of oblique views may also be needed to determine the exact configuration of a fracture. Non-displaced sagittal fractures may be accompanied by remarkably little lameness, and this has led to such cases being returned to work undiagnosed, sometimes with disastrous results.

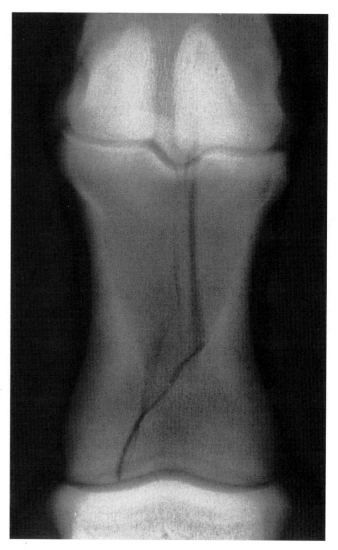

Figure 3.67 Dorsopalmar view of a pastern, showing a complete sagittal fracture of the proximal phalanx (note the double lucent line which represents the fracture through the dorsal and palmar cortices).

Incomplete fractures of the proximal aspect of the proximal phalanx can be very difficult to detect in the acute stage. If the horse is exercised however, such fractures can propagate into catastrophic comminuted fractures. If a fracture is suspected on clinical grounds the horse should be rested and re-radiographed after 10 days, when rarefaction along the fracture line may be more obvious. Nuclear scintigraphy may be useful. Some horses never develop any associated radiographic abnormality. In others an incomplete fracture may not be detected radiographically until callus forms as part of the normal healing process. This is seen as new bone on the dorsoproximal aspect of the proximal phalanx (Figures 3.68a and 3.68b) and may be detected on lateromedial radiographs. Reduced exposures are needed to demonstrate this poorly mineralized new bone. In some cases there is only increased opacity in the midline of the proximal aspect of the proximal phalanx seen in a dorsoproximal-palmarodistal oblique view. Incomplete

[146]

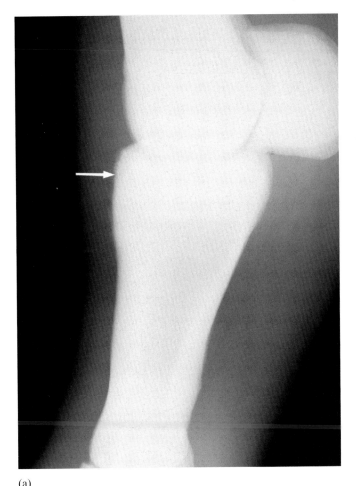

(a)

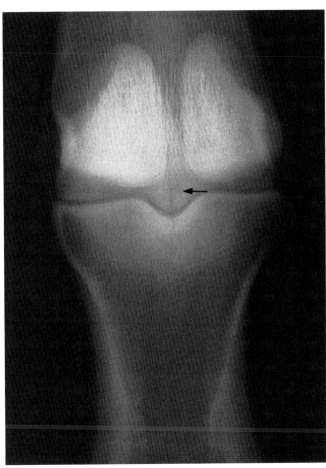

(b)

Figure 3.68(a) Lateromedial view of the pastern, showing new bone on the dorsoproximal aspect of the proximal phalanx (arrow) secondary to an incomplete sagittal fracture of approximately 6 weeks' duration.

Figure 3.68(b) Dorsopalmar view of a pastern, showing an incomplete sagittal fracture of the proximal phalanx (arrow) of approximately 6 weeks' duration. Note that much of the fracture line is superimposed over the distal end of the third metacarpal bone. There is some sclerosis around the fracture in the proximal phalanx.

fractures have a good prognosis with conservative treatment, but repeat radiographs should be obtained to ensure healing does take place. Although most incomplete fractures of the proximal aspect of the proximal phalanx involve the dorsal cortex, less commonly they occur as sagittal fissures midway between the dorsal and palmar cortices, and may be seen as an ill defined lucent area in the most proximal aspect of the proximal phalanx in a dorsoproximal-palmarodistal oblique view.

Simple fractures of the proximal or middle phalanx respond well to internal fixation, but comminuted fractures are common and may be so extensive that any treatment is hopeless. Casting severely comminuted fractures or internal fixation and arthrodesis occasionally save an animal for breeding purposes.

Fractures of the dorsal and palmar/plantar aspects of the proximal end of the proximal phalanx occasionally occur. Dorsal 30° proximal 70° lateral-palmarodistomedial oblique and dorsal 30° proximal 70°

[147]

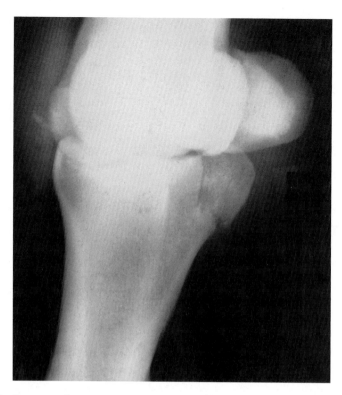

Figure 3.69 Dorsomedial-palmarolateral oblique view of a metacarpophalangeal joint, showing a slightly displaced articular fracture of the medial palmar process of the proximal phalanx. There are some ill defined opacities in the dorsal aspect of the joint.

medial-palmarodistolateral oblique views are helpful for visualization of such fractures (see page 151). These may occur as simple fractures or in combination with sagittal fractures.

Palmar or, more commonly, plantar fractures frequently involve either the medial or lateral tuberosity of the proximal phalanx (Figure 3.69). It is possible for both tuberosities to fracture separately or for a complete fracture of the palmar/plantar aspect of the bone to occur. Fractures of the tuberosity usually involve only a proximal fragment, but occasionally extend down the diaphysis. They may be articular or non-articular, and may require surgical fixation.

Small fractures of the palmar or plantar articular margin (Figure 3.70) occur on the axial aspect of the medial or lateral tuberosity, near the insertion of the cruciate sesamoidean ligaments. These are also more common in hindlimbs and have been referred to as Birkeland fractures. However, some workers suggest that these fragments are associated with osteochondrosis. Surgical removal of these fragments may be indicated.

Dorsal frontal fractures also occur predominantly in hindlimbs. They are often incomplete. Incomplete fractures have a good prognosis with conservative treatment, but complete fractures usually require surgical treatment. Articular fractures of the distal medial or distal lateral aspect of the middle phalanx, close to the site of insertion of the collateral ligament of the distal interphalangeal joint, sometimes occur. Multiple flexed oblique views may be required to identify the fracture (Figure 3.71). Surgical removal usually results in a satisfactory outcome.

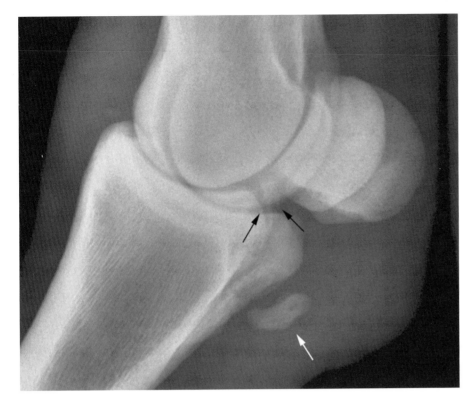

Figure 3.70 Oblique lateromedial radiographic view of the left hind fetlock of an 8-year-old Thoroughbred purchased 1 week previously. There was soft-tissue swelling on the dorsal aspect of the fetlock and mild lameness, which was not altered by distal limb flexion. There is a small articular fragment displaced from the medial plantar tuberosity of the proximal phalanx (black arrows). There is a large smoothly outlined osseous opacity (white arrow) plantar to the lateral plantar tuberosity of the proximal phalanx. There is a small mineralized opacity on the dorsal aspect of the metatarsophalangeal joint.

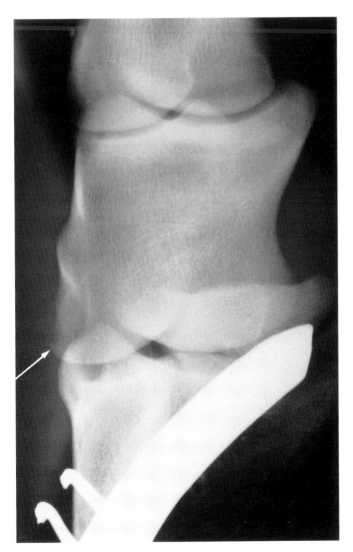

Figure 3.71 Dorsal 45° medial-plantarolateral (flexed) oblique view of the foot and pastern of a horse with acute onset, severe lameness. There is an articular fracture (arrow) of the distal aspect of the lateral condyle of the middle phalanx. The shoe had not been removed for clinical reasons.

Dystrophic mineralization

Dystrophic mineralization occasionally occurs in the distal sesamoidean ligaments. Its significance is equivocal. Ultrasonography may be useful.

Metacarpophalangeal (fetlock) joint

RADIOGRAPHIC TECHNIQUE

Although this section refers to the metacarpophalangeal joint, it applies equally well to the metatarsophalangeal joint.

Equipment

Radiographs of the metacarpophalangeal joint are readily obtained with portable equipment and do not require the use of a grid. High-definition screens and compatible film are recommended when available.

Positioning

Dorsopalmar, lateromedial, dorsolateral-palmaromedial oblique and dorsomedial-palmarolateral oblique views

Standard views of the metacarpophalangeal joint are obtained with the horse weight bearing, using a horizontal x-ray beam. The views should include a minimum of dorsopalmar (dorsoplantar), lateromedial and two 45° oblique views (D45°L-PaMO, D45°M-PaLO). Initial exposures should give good visualization of the trabecular pattern of the distal aspect of the third metacarpal bone, but may be reduced for evaluation of soft tissues, chip fractures or new bone. Although only four standard views need be obtained during a routine examination, dorsal 60° lateral-palmaromedial oblique and dorsal 60° medial-palmarolateral oblique views may be necessary for better visualization of lesions on the dorsal joint margins. Superimposition of the proximal sesamoid bones over the metacarpophalangeal joint space can be avoided by angling the x-ray beam proximodistally at least 10° for a dorsopalmar view and 15° for a dorsoplantar view. The precise angle depends on both the pastern foot axis and the position of the limb. The position of the limb (forelimb or hindlimb) markedly influences the position of the proximal sesamoid bones relative to the third metacarpal or metatarsal bones and the proximal phalanx for all views. Ideally the fetlock should be extended, with the limb as far back as possible while weight bearing, in order to 'lift' the proximal sesamoid bones.

If there is some rotation of the distal limb, it can be difficult to achieve a true lateromedial projection. The position of the metacarpophalangeal joint relative to the foot should be assessed. Usually aligning the x-ray beam 5° palmar to a line tangential to the bulbs of the heel (i.e. L5°Pa-MDO) will result in a true lateromedial view. It may help to palpate the relative positions of the medial and lateral epicondyles of the third metacarpal bone.

This is particularly important in hindlimbs, since many horses stand with the limb rotated toe outwards. A true lateromedial projection is required for proper assessment of the sagittal ridge of the third metacarpal bone, but slightly oblique views may sometimes be helpful for assessment of suspect lesions elsewhere in the joint.

Visualization of the proximal sesamoid bones is only partially achieved on the standard views described above. A dorsopalmar view taken at higher kilovoltage is required to visualize the axial surface of the bones. Further oblique views may also be required (see below).

Flexed lateromedial view

A flexed lateromedial view of the metacarpophalangeal joint gives better visualization of the articular surfaces of the proximal sesamoid bones and of the sagittal ridge of the third metacarpal bone. If slightly oblique, this view may aid in determining the extent of chip fractures of the proximal sesamoid bones. These radiographs may be enhanced by reducing the mAs slightly from that normally required for the third metacarpal bone. The flexed lateromedial view is obtained by resting the horse's toe on a block, preferably 20–25 cm high, with the metacarpophalangeal joint flexed (or positioning the joint similarly, holding the limb at the toe). The x-ray beam is centred on the centre of the radius of curvature of the distal articular surface of the third metacarpal bone. The alignment of the beam may be difficult, as slight abnormalities in conformation result in oblique views. It is most practical to take one view and realign the beam if necessary.

Special oblique views

Standard D45°L-PaMO and D45°M-PaLO views highlight the lateral and medial proximal sesamoid bones respectively, allowing assessment of their shape, internal architecture and the apex, dorsal, palmar and distal borders. Additional information can also be obtained from a lateral 45° proximal-medial distal oblique view (L45°Pr-MDiO) (Figure 3.72a), to highlight the abaxial surface of the medial proximal sesamoid bone (Figure 3.72b) and a medial 45° proximal-lateral distal oblique view (M45°Pr-LDiO) to highlight the abaxial surface of the lateral proximal sesamoid bone.

Evaluation of the proximal palmar (plantar) articular margins of the palmar (plantar) process of the proximal phalanx is sometimes best achieved using a dorsal 30° proximal 70° lateral-palmar distal medial oblique view (D30°Pr70°L-PaDiMO) (Figure 3.73a) or a dorsal 30° proximal 70° medial-palmar distal lateral oblique view (D30°Pr70°M-PaDiLO). This view is particularly useful for identification of palmar (plantar) fragments, and determining their source (see page 169). The D30°Pr70°L-PaDiMO view projects the lateral proximal sesamoid bone distal to the medial proximal sesamoid bone, and highlights the lateral plantar process of the proximal phalanx (Figure 3.73b).

[151]

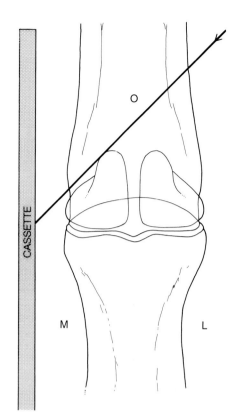

Figure 3.72(a) Technique to obtain lateral 45° proximal-medial distal oblique views to skyline the abaxial surface of the medial proximal sesamoid bone.

Assessment of the lateral and medial palmar (plantar) condyles of the third metacarpal (metatarsal) bone may be facilitated by using a dorsal 45° proximal 45° lateral-palmar distal medial oblique view (D45°Pr45°L-PaDiMO), to project the lateral condyle distal to the medial condyle (Figure 3.74). This view is particularly useful for identification of stress reactions (radiolucency or sclerosis) in the lateral condyle of the third metatarsal bone (see page 175).

Tangential dorsopalmar views

The articular surface of the distal aspect of the third metacarpal bone curves through 180°. On dorsopalmar views, only a limited part of the bone and joint tangential to the beam is clearly visualized. This means that when third metacarpal condylar fractures or osteochondral lesions are suspected, several dorsoproximal-palmarodistal or dorsodistal-palmaroproximal tangential views can be useful for determining the extent of such fractures and confirming possible comminution (Figure 3.75). Improved visualization may be achieved by flexing the metacarpophalangeal joint. The toe of the foot is placed in the standard navicular block (see pages 104 and 156), with the metacarpal region vertical. With the metacarpal region vertical it makes the technique easy to repeat for follow-up examinations, keeping the same angle of the x-ray beam relative to the third metacarpal bone. A horizontal x-ray beam is centred on the joint. The cassette is positioned as closely perpendicular to the x-ray beam as possible. This view moves the proximal sesamoid bones further proximally (see Figure 4.1c, page 191), and

[152]

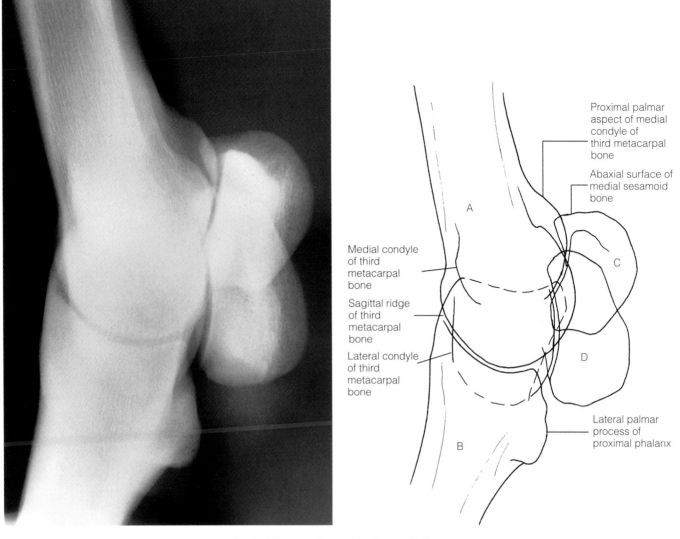

Figure 3.72(b) Lateral 45° proximal-medial distal oblique radiographic view and diagram of the metacarpophalangeal joint of a normal adult horse. A = third metacarpal bone, B = proximal phalanx, C = medial proximal sesamoid bone, D = lateral proximal sesamoid bone.

is particularly useful when evaluating their axial margins. With the limb in the same position the x-ray beam can also be directed distoproximally to assess a more palmar aspect of the articular surface of the metacarpal condyles.

The palmar articular surface may be assessed better with the limb partially extended, with the foot on a flat block (see Figure 4.2, page 192). This technique has the disadvantage of resulting in magnification and geometric distortion. The cassette is positioned approximately vertically. The x-ray beam is directed distoproximally, in the plane of rotation of the metacarpophalangeal joint, at approximately 125° to the metacarpal region. If the limb and x-ray beam are correctly aligned, between one-quarter and one-third of the proximal sesamoid bones are projected below the joint space (see Figure 4.1d, page 191). This view is particularly important when evaluating a vertical condylar fracture; comminution of the palmar articular surface of

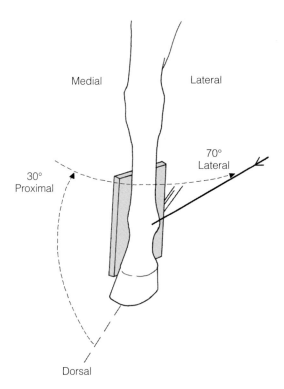

Figure 3.73(a) Positioning to obtain a dorsal 30° proximal 70° lateral-palmarodistal medial oblique view of the metacarpophalangeal joint, to highlight the lateral palmar process of the proximal phalanx.

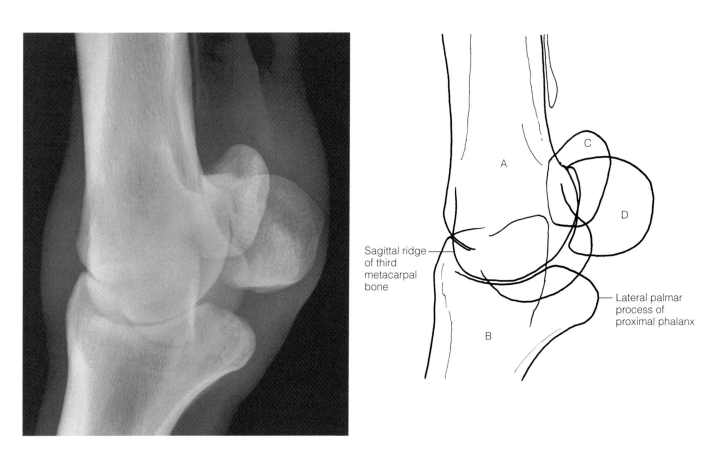

Figure 3.73(b) Dorsal 30° proximal 70° lateral-palmarodistal medial oblique radiographic view and diagram of the metacarpophalangeal joint of a normal adult horse. A = third metacarpal bone, B = proximal phalanx, C = medial proximal sesamoid bone, D = lateral proximal sesamoid bone.

[154]

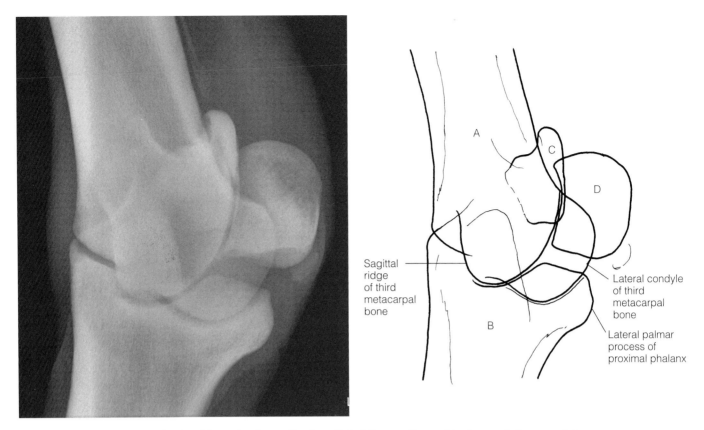

Sagittal ridge of third metacarpal bone

Lateral condyle of third metacarpal bone

Lateral palmar process of proximal phalanx

Figure 3.74 Dorsal 45° proximal 45° lateral-palmarodistal medial oblique radiographic view and diagram of the metacarpophalangeal joint of a normal adult horse. A = third metacarpal bone, B = proximal phalanx, C = medial proximal sesamoid bone, D = lateral proximal sesamoid bone.

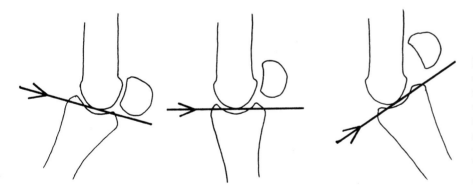

Figure 3.75 Technique to obtain flexed dorsoproximal-palmarodistal oblique and dorsodistal-palmaroproximal oblique views of the metacarpophalangeal joint. Note the different angles made by the x-ray beam to the long axis of the third metacarpal bone, in order to skyline different areas of the third metacarpal bone.

the third metacarpal bone is usually only identifiable in this projection. It is also useful for detecting lucent lesions in the palmar aspect of the condyles of the third metacarpal bone (page 169).

Dorsoproximal-dorsodistal (flexed) view

A dorsoproximal-dorsodistal view of the metacarpophalangeal joint may be a useful view to visualize subtle lesions of the dorsal half of the distal articular surface of the third metacarpal bone. The horse is positioned with the

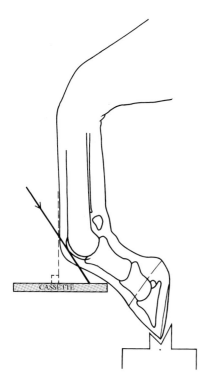

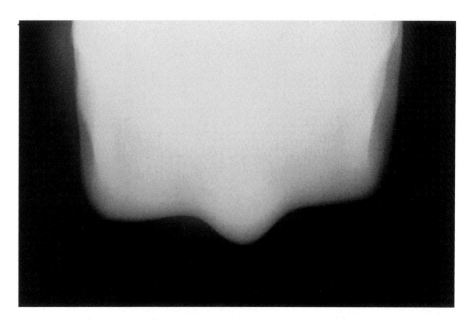

Figure 3.76(b) Dorsoproximal-dorsodistal (flexed) oblique view of a metacarpophalangeal joint, to highlight the sagittal ridge and condyles of the third metacarpal bone.

Figure 3.76(a) Positioning to obtain a dorsoproximal-dorsodistal (flexed) oblique view of the metacarpophalangeal joint, to highlight the dorsal aspect of the sagittal ridge of the third metacarpal bone.

metacarpophalangeal joint flexed and the metacarpal region vertical. The cassette is placed distal to the joint and parallel to the floor. The x-ray tube is positioned dorsal to the limb, with the x-ray beam centred on the meta-carpophalangeal joint, angled dorsal 45–70° proximal-dorsodistal. A series of radiographs may be obtained at slightly different angles to visualize different areas of the joint (Figure 3.76).

Palmaroproximal-palmarodistal oblique view of the proximal sesamoid bones

A palmaroproximal-palmarodistal oblique view of the proximal sesamoid bones is most useful for evaluation of their axial and abaxial margins and for defining the presence of an abaxial fragment and whether or not it is articular. The horse is positioned with the fetlock extended with the limb to be examined palmar to the contralateral limb. The horse stands on a cassette tunnel. The x-ray machine is placed almost vertically above the proximal sesamoid bones. Palmar 85° proximal 15° lateral-palmarodistal medial oblique and palmar 85° proximal 15° medial-palmarodistal lateral oblique views highlight the abaxial aspects of the medial and lateral proximal sesamoid bones respectively (Figure 3.77).

[156]

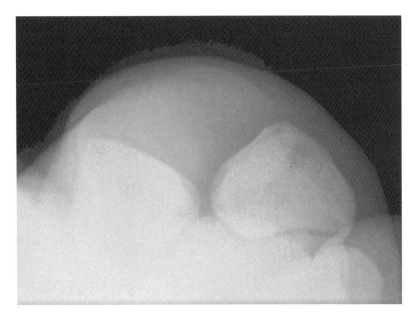

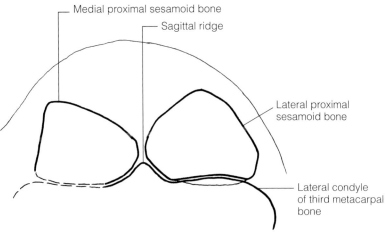

Medial proximal sesamoid bone

Sagittal ridge

Lateral proximal
sesamoid bone

Lateral condyle
of third metacarpal
bone

Figure 3.77 Palmar 85° proximal lateral-palmarodistal medial oblique view of a normal metacarpophalangeal joint. Lateral is to the right. The palmar, axial and abaxial aspects of the proximal sesamoid bones and the palmar aspect of the sagittal ridge of the third metacarpal bone are highlighted.

NORMAL ANATOMY

Immature horse

Prior to fusion of the distal physis of the third metacarpal/metatarsal bone at about 6–8 months of age, the distal metaphysis usually appears irregular (Figures 3.78a and 3.78b). The proximal physis of the proximal phalanx fuses at about 12 months of age.

Each proximal sesamoid bone usually ossifies from a single centre, which in the very young animal may have a slightly irregular margin. In a small percentage of foals there are two ossification centres, one for the proximal one-third and one for the distal two-thirds of the bone. This may occur in one or several proximal sesamoid bones of the same foal. Fusion usually occurs by approximately 60 days of age. This should not be confused with a fracture of the sesamoid bone (see page 178). The cartilage precursor is fully ossified by about 3–4 months, although the bones may continue to enlarge until 18 months of age.

[157]

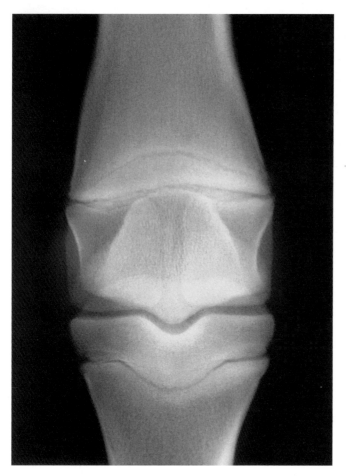

Figure 3.78(a) Dorsopalmar view of a metacarpophalangeal joint of a normal foal 6 weeks of age.

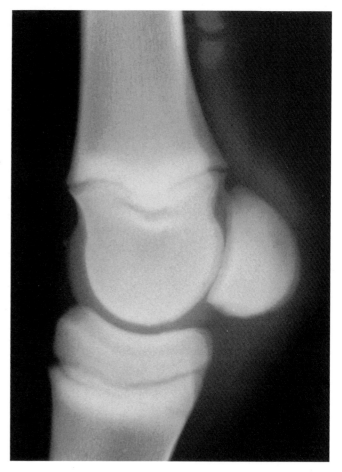

Figure 3.78(b) Lateromedial view of a metacarpophalangeal joint of a normal foal 8 weeks of age. Note also the separate centre of ossification of the distal aspect of the fourth metacarpal bone.

Skeletally mature horse

On a lateromedial view, the joint surface of the distal end of the third metacarpal bone describes a smooth curve, which flattens slightly on the palmarodistal aspect (Figure 3.78c). The third metacarpal bone articulates with the proximal phalanx and the proximal sesamoid bones. The distal metaphysis of the third metacarpal bone may show some irregularity at the level of the fused physis (physeal scar).

On dorsopalmar radiographs, the metacarpophalangeal joint is approximately symmetrical about the prominent sagittal ridge of the distal aspect of the third metacarpal bone, although the medial condyle is slightly wider than the lateral. The sagittal ridge articulates with a groove in the proximal phalanx. The joint space is approximately at right angles to the long axis of the third metacarpal bone (Figure 3.78d). Immediately proximal to the joint, the medial and lateral aspects of the third metacarpal bone have a smooth depression, above which the cortex appears slightly sclerotic.

[158]

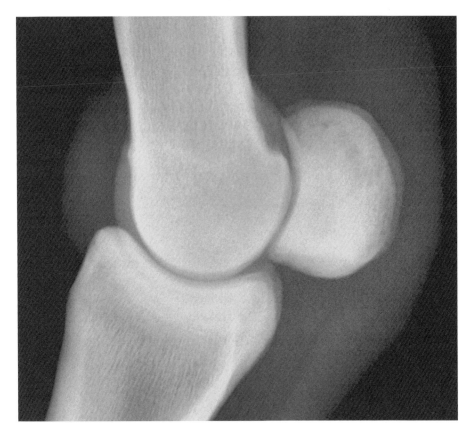

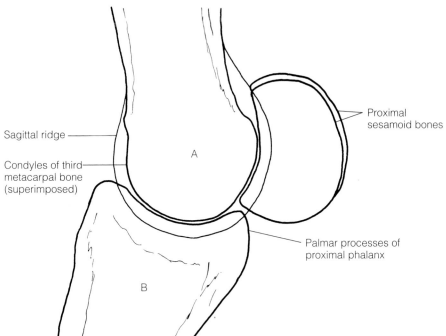

Sagittal ridge

Condyles of third
metacarpal bone
(superimposed)

Proximal
sesamoid bones

Palmar processes of
proximal phalanx

A

B

Figure 3.78(c) Radiograph and diagram of a lateromedial view of a normal adult metacarpophalangeal joint. A = third metacarpal bone, B = proximal phalanx.

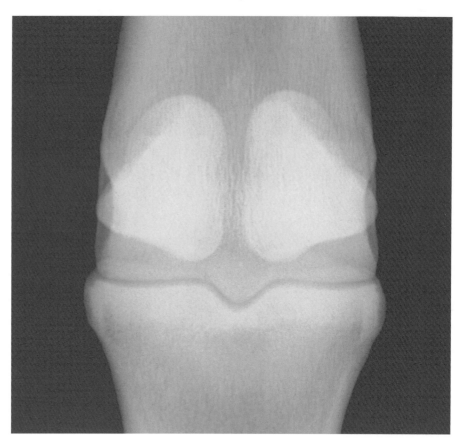

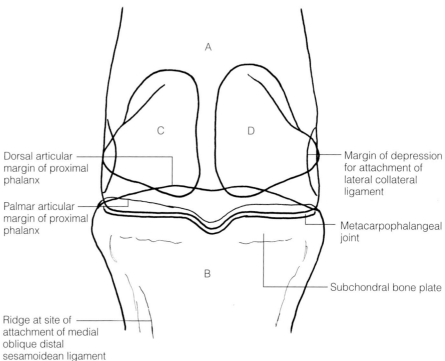

Dorsal articular margin of proximal phalanx

Palmar articular margin of proximal phalanx

Ridge at site of attachment of medial oblique distal sesamoidean ligament

Margin of depression for attachment of lateral collateral ligament

Metacarpophalangeal joint

Subchondral bone plate

Figure 3.78(d) Dorsal 10° proximal-palmarodistal oblique radiographic view and diagram of a normal adult fetlock. A = third metacarpal bone, B = proximal phalanx, C = medial proximal sesamoid bone, D = lateral proximal sesamoid bone.

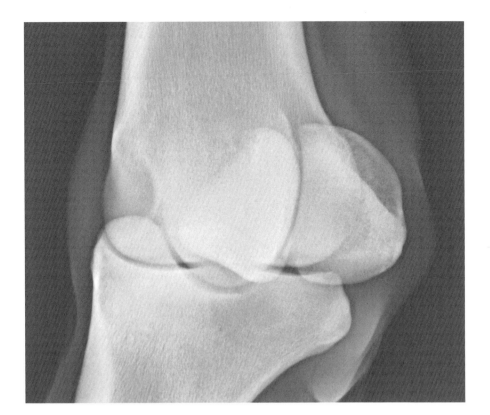

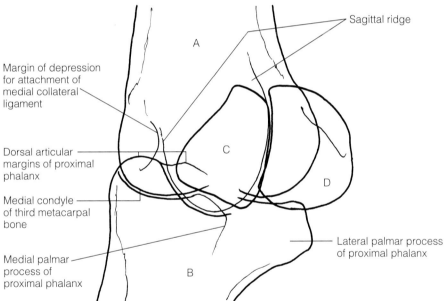

Figure 3.78(e) Radiograph and diagram of a dorsolateral-palmaromedial oblique view of a normal adult metacarpophalangeal joint. A = third metacarpal bone, B = proximal phalanx, C = medial proximal sesamoid, D = lateral proximal sesamoid.

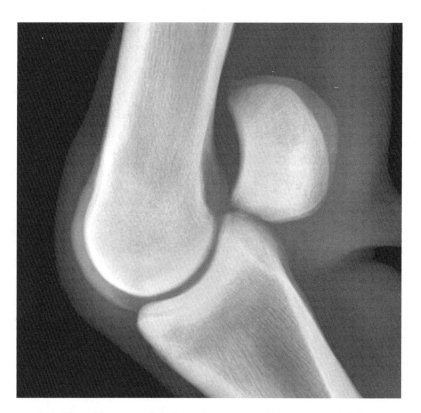

Figure 3.78(f) Flexed lateromedial view of a normal adult metacarpophalangeal joint. Note how the proximal sesamoid bones lift away from the articular surface of the third metacarpal bone.

The proximal subchondral bone plate of the proximal phalanx is best evaluated in a dorsopalmar projection. There is usually a clear demarcation between the subchondral bone plate and the underlying cancellous bone. The subchondral bone plate is of fairly uniform thickness, sometimes slightly thicker laterally than medially. The ergot superimposed over the proximal phalanx may result in an approximately circular region of increased opacity.

The proximal sesamoid bones are difficult to visualize clearly, as on most views they are superimposed over other bones. They are most clearly visualized on the dorsolateral-palmaromedial and dorsomedial-palmarolateral oblique views (Figure 3.78e). They normally have a smooth outline, rounded over their palmar aspects. The axial and abaxial surfaces may show some unevenness, being areas of ligament insertion, but should not have marked roughening. There are faint radiating lucent lines within the bones. On flexed lateromedial views, the proximal sesamoid bones are lifted away from the articular surface of the distal end of the third metacarpal bone (Figure 3.78f).

NORMAL VARIATIONS AND INCIDENTAL FINDINGS

Slight modelling of the dorsoproximal articular margins of the proximal phalanx is a common incidental finding in older horses and is often unassoci-

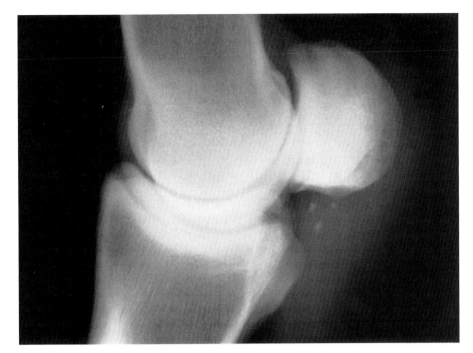

Figure 3.79 Lateromedial view of a metacarpophalangeal joint of an adult horse. There are several small, smoothly rounded mineralized opacities distal to the proximal sesamoid bones, which are unlikely to be of clinical significance. Note that this is not a true lateromedial projection. The condyles of the third metacarpal bone are not superimposed, because the horse was not standing squarely on the limb.

ated with detectable clinical signs, although it may reflect degenerative joint disease (see page 166). A small, smoothly rounded osseous opacity on the midline, on the dorsoproximal aspect of the proximal phalanx sometimes occurs in one or more fetlocks (see page 167). Small palmar or plantar osteochondral fragments and an ununited palmar or plantar process (see page 169) are frequently not associated with clinical signs, although they may affect performance or longevity of career in racehorses. Smoothly rounded osseous opacities are sometimes seen distal to one or both proximal sesamoid bones (Figure 3.79), presumably within the distal sesamoidean ligaments. They are usually asymptomatic and their aetiology is unknown.

An unusually long proximal sesamoid bone indicates previous fracture of the bone in the neonatal period (see page 178).

In maximally flexed lateromedial views, especially of hind fetlocks, a focal radiolucent area may be seen superimposed over the distal aspect of the sagittal ridge of the third metacarpal/metatarsal bone. This is a gas artefact caused by the vacuum effect resulting from maximal flexion, and disappears with reduced flexion.

Intra-articular analgesia of the fetlock joint is often associated with air being introduced into the joint. If radiography is performed within a few hours, radiolucent areas may be seen in the proximal recesses of the joint capsule, and in some views these are superimposed over the third metacarpal bone and mimic lesions (see Figure 1.4, page 14). Such artefacts disappear within 24–48 hours.

[163]

SIGNIFICANT FINDINGS

Soft-tissue swelling

Soft-tissue swelling in the fetlock region can be due to many causes and may be detected radiographically, either alone or with other radiographic abnormalities. The cause of swelling cannot usually be determined radiographically and ultrasonographic evaluation may be indicated. The metacarpophalangeal joint is prone to soft-tissue injury, and although initial radiographs may show only soft-tissue swelling, radiographs obtained 3–6 weeks later may demonstrate new bone at the articular margins, at the points of attachment of the joint capsule and/or collateral ligaments. Entheseophytes and periarticular osteophytes may also develop on the proximal sesamoid bones. Accurate knowledge of the anatomy of soft-tissue attachments is essential for determination of the likely cause of entheseophyte formation. It is important to recognize how far proximal is the location of the origin of the proximal portions of the collateral ligaments of the metacarpophalangeal joint (Figures 3.58 and 3.59, pages 135–139).

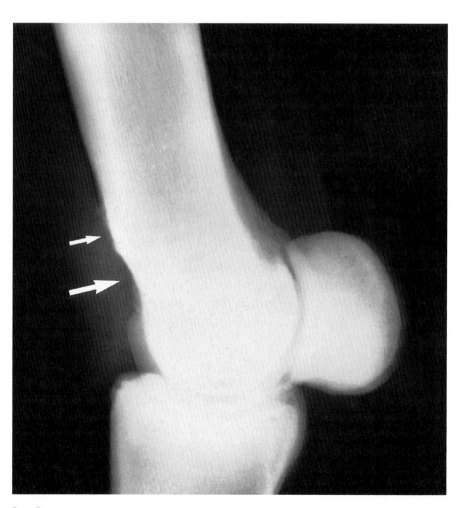

Figure 3.80(a) Chronic proliferative synovitis. Lateromedial view of a metacarpophalangeal joint, showing radiographic changes associated with chronic proliferative synovitis. There is a depression proximal to the sagittal ridge of the third metacarpal bone (large arrow). Proximal to this is periosteal new bone at the site of the capsular attachment (small arrow). This modelling of the dorsal distal aspect of the third metacarpal bone usually relates to chronic proliferative synovitis. The radiograph is deliberately underexposed to demonstrate these abnormalities.

Synovitis is a common problem, visualized radiographically as a distension of the metacarpophalangeal joint capsule. This is most easily seen on the dorsal aspect of the joint on a lateromedial view. Chronic proliferative synovitis (villonodular hypertrophic synovitis) may be suspected if on lateromedial radiographs there is modelling of the dorsal distal aspect of the third metacarpal bone, associated with soft-tissue swelling. In the early stages a depression may be noted just proximal to the sagittal ridge. There may be new bone just proximal to the depression, as entheseophytes form at the capsular attachment (Figure 3.80a). In advanced cases an increased opacity may be evident dorsal to the depression, due to dystrophic mineralization or osseous metaplasia. These changes are most easily identified on a flexed lateromedial view. It may be necessary to introduce positive contrast agent into the joint to outline the soft-tissue mass (Figure 3.80b), however the lesion may also be confirmed ultrasonographically. Clinically there is enlargement of the dorsal pouch of the metacarpophalangeal joint. Treatment is by surgical removal of the mass and adequate rest to allow the joint inflammation to resolve.

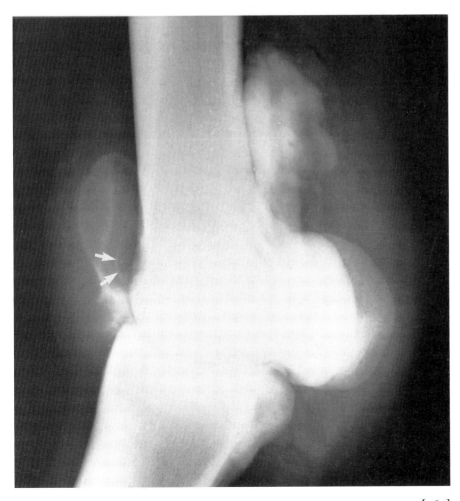

Figure 3.80(b) Chronic proliferative synovitis. Lateromedial view of a metacarpophalangeal joint, with contrast medium in the joint (slightly oblique view). Note the filling defect (arrows) in the dorsal pouch of the joint.

Soft-tissue swelling medially or laterally may reflect injury of a collateral ligament. With severe lameness and marked swelling, stressed dorsopalmar radiographs should be obtained to determine the stability of the joint (see Luxation, page 175). Occasionally there may be an avulsion fracture from the origin of the collateral ligament, which may be substantially displaced distally. Collateral desmitis can occur without obvious swelling and should be considered if lameness is localized to the fetlock region, but there is no response to intra-articular analgesia. In the acute stage radiographs may appear normal, although entheseophyte formation may develop subsequently. Ultrasonography helps diagnosis.

Soft-tissue swelling on the palmar proximal aspect of the metacarpophalangeal joint may be due to distension of the digital flexor tendon sheath. On lateromedial views a depression in the palmar contour of this swelling may indicate functional constriction by the palmar annular ligament. Occasionally mineralization in the sheath or the digital flexor tendon, or abnormalities of the proximal sesamoid bones are seen. Distension of the digital flexor tendon sheath and the metacarpophalangeal joint capsule may be seen in association with infectious or traumatic osteitis of a proximal sesamoid bone (see page 174). Swelling may arise after trauma to the region and results in lameness, which may resolve with prolonged rest, or may require surgical treatment. The prognosis depends on the underlying pathology. Ultrasonographic examination may give additional information about the associated soft-tissue structures.

Degenerative joint disease

On lateromedial and/or oblique views, modelling of the proximodorsal aspect of the proximal phalanx may involve the articular margins, and may indicate early degenerative joint disease (Figure 3.81a). Periarticular osteophytes are best seen in oblique projections and vary from thin, sharply angled periarticular margins to large protuberances of bone. As disease progresses there may be sclerosis of the subchondral bone and loss of normal trabecular architecture. The distal dorsal aspect of the third metacarpal bone may also change in shape. The proximal dorsal attachments of the joint capsule are close to the proximal end of the sagittal ridge, and entheseophyte formation at this point may result from joint trauma or chronic joint capsule distension. This is not synonymous with degenerative joint disease, but may be seen in association with it.

On dorsopalmar views, osteophytes may be seen at the articular margins on the medial or lateral aspects of the proximal phalanx and indicate degenerative joint disease. Entheseophytes at the insertion of the joint capsule develop slightly distal to a periarticular osteophyte, and indicate strain or tension of the capsular attachment. It is often difficult to differentiate between these two types of new bone formation at this location, and careful clinical assessment of their significance is required.

In advanced degenerative joint disease, periarticular osteophytes on the proximal and distal margins of the proximal sesamoid bones may be seen. Associated with this there may be a depression in the distal palmar aspect of the third metacarpal bone, proximal to the condyles. This so-called 'supra-condylar lysis' is associated with fibrous proliferation of the synovial membrane in this region (Figure 3.81b). Positive contrast studies may demonstrate a filling defect in this area.

The joint space is best assessed on a dorsopalmar view. Narrowing of the joint space, particularly unilateral narrowing (usually of the medial side), may be significant and reflects advanced articular cartilage pathology. It is important, however, that this is assessed on weight-bearing views, with the horse standing evenly on all four feet, since the joint can open on either side if unevenly loaded. Narrowing of one side of the joint space may be the only radiographic abnormality detectable in any view in some horses with advanced degenerative joint disease (Figure 3.82). The relatively opaque subchondral bone should be of even thickness. Change in thickness or opacity of the subchondral bone of the third metacarpal bone or the proximal phalanx has been associated with degenerative joint disease. There may also be decreased demarcation between the subchondral bone and the underlying cancellous bone.

Osteochondrosis and osteochondral fragments

The aetiology of some changes in the metacarpophalangeal and metatarsophalangeal joints still remains open to debate, although recent publications are helping to clarify the findings. Some abnormalities formerly thought to be due to osteochondrosis may be traumatic in origin. There appear to be breed differences in the incidence of these abnormalities and their clinical significance is not always easy to determine. Included in this group are fragments arising from the dorsal aspect of the sagittal ridge of the third metacarpal (metatarsal) bone, fragments on the dorsoproximal aspect of the proximal phalanx, palmar or plantar osteochondral fragments, an ununited palmar or plantar eminence of the proximal phalanx and flattening of the palmar or plantar condyle of the third metacarpal or metatarsal bone.

Osteochondrosis of the sagittal ridge may be seen anywhere on the ridge, but is most often seen dorsally on the proximal or middle third (Figure 3.83). A mild lesion is seen as flattening or concavity of the ridge. Such lesions may resolve spontaneously. More severe lesions may result in marked irregularity of the dorsal contour of the sagittal ridge and the presence of osteochondral fragments. These lesions are best seen on a flexed lateromedial view (Figure 3.83b) and may involve all four fetlocks. The prognosis is favourable with surgical management.

Small, well rounded fragments on the midline on the dorsoproximal aspect of the proximal phalanx (Figure 3.90, page 178), readily identifiable on a lateromedial projection, are a common radiographic finding, frequently not associated with clinical signs. They may be present in one or several fetlocks. Their aetiology is unknown but they may result from separate centres of ossification or possibly be a manifestation of osteochondrosis. Occasionally they are associated with synovial effusion and lameness, in which case surgical removal is indicated. A good prognosis is usually warranted.

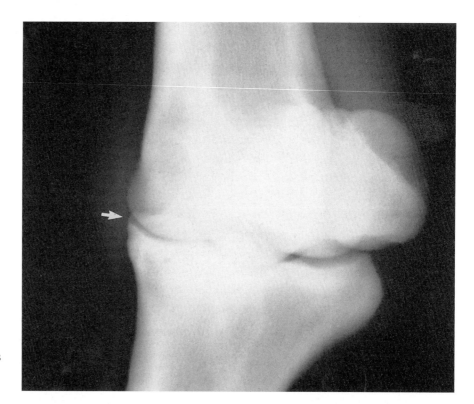

Figure 3.81(a) Degenerative joint disease. Dorsolateral-palmaromedial oblique view of a metacarpophalangeal joint, showing early changes associated with degenerative joint disease. There is modelling of the dorsomedial aspect of the proximal phalanx (arrow).

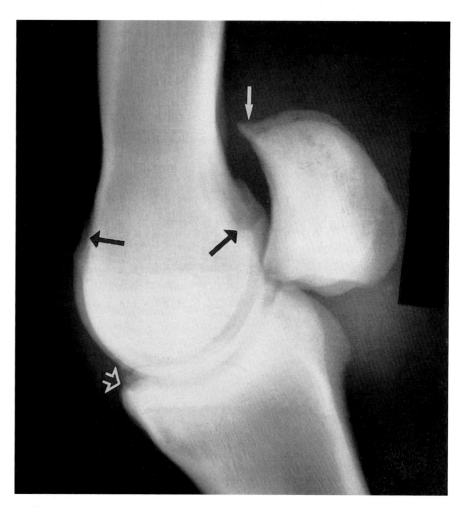

Figure 3.81(b) Degenerative joint disease. Flexed lateromedial view of a metacarpophalangeal joint, showing advanced changes associated with degenerative joint disease. There is modelling of the articular margins of the proximal sesamoid bones (white arrow), the dorsal aspect of the proximal phalanx (open white arrow) and the dorsal and palmar distal aspects of the third metacarpal bone proximal to the sagittal ridge (black arrows).

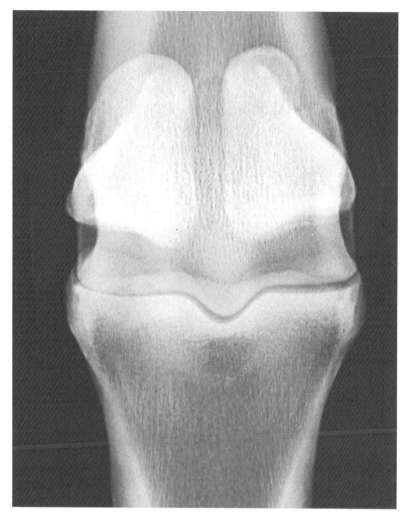

Figure 3.82 Dorsal 15° proximal-palmarodistal oblique radiographic view of a metacarpophalangeal joint of a 12-year-old showjumper. There is marked narrowing of the medial aspect of the metacarpophalangeal joint, reflecting substantial loss of the articular cartilage. Note also the lack of congruity between the sagittal ridge of the third metacarpal bone and the sagittal groove of the proximal phalanx. There was no periarticular modelling, but such joint space narrowing reflects advanced degenerative joint disease.

So-called osteochondrosis involving the palmar (plantar) aspect of the condyles of the third metacarpal (metatarsal) bones usually occurs slightly palmar (plantar) to the transverse ridge. Initially the radiographic changes are flattening and sclerosis of the subchondral bone in the affected area. This may be followed by resorptive changes, resulting in focal radiolucent areas of variable shape. Although this lesion has formerly been classified as osteochondrosis, it now seems probable that it is a traumatic lesion and only seen in athletic horses (see Stress-related bone injury, page 175). Palmar or plantar osteochondral fragments (Figure 3.84a) are usually seen medially or laterally (or both together) at the site of attachment of the short distal sesamoidean ligaments, and occur most commonly in hindlimbs. They have also been referred to as Birkeland fractures. They are best identified in D30°Pr70°L-PaDiMO or D30°Pr70°M-PaDiLO views. Medial fragments are most common. These are believed to represent avulsion fractures, sustained as a foal, and are frequently asymptomatic, although they may compromise performance at high speed.

An ununited palmar or plantar process of the proximal phalanx (Figure 3.84b) usually occurs laterally, either alone or in association with a palmar

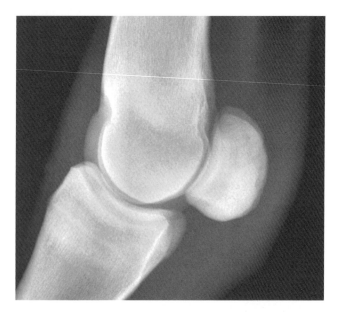

Figure 3.83(a) Lateromedial radiographic view of a metacarpophalangeal joint of a yearling Thoroughbred, obtained as part of a routine screening. There is slightly heterogeneous opacity where the sagittal ridge of the third metacarpal bone is superimposed over the proximal aspect of the proximal phalanx dorsally. Compare with Figure 3.83(b).

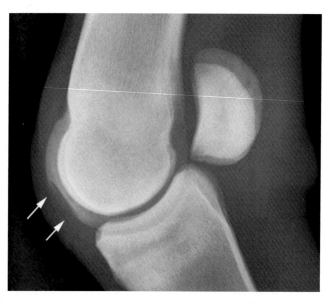

Figure 3.83(b) Flexed lateromedial view of the same fetlock as Figure 3.83(a). There is a large defect in the dorsal aspect of the sagittal ridge of the third metacarpal bone (arrows). This is osteochondrosis.

or plantar osteochondral fragment. It occurs most commonly in hindlimbs and may be articular or non-articular. In some horses it may represent an avulsion fracture of the cruciate distal sesamoidean ligament, sustained as a foal, however in many horses the fragments are located abaxial to the insertion of this ligament. They are frequently asymptomatic.

Physitis

Physitis (epiphysitis) of the distal physis of the third metacarpal bone occurs predominantly in rapidly growing foals. Radiographically the physis is widened and irregular in thickness, frequently with new bone (lipping) at its margins. On dorsopalmar views an angular limb deformity may be evident. The usual clinical history is of a limb deviation developing distal to the metacarpophalangeal joint. Treatment of this condition must be radical and rapid, because of the early closure of the distal physis. Usually restriction of diet and exercise, coupled with corrective trimming of the foot, will be sufficient. In some cases, periosteal elevation, physeal stimulation or transphyseal bridging will be needed.

Osseous cyst-like lesions

Osseous cyst-like lesions occur near the metacarpophalangeal joint, most commonly in the third metacarpal bone, but also in the proximal phalanx. Visualization of these may require a dorsoproximal-palmarodistal angula-

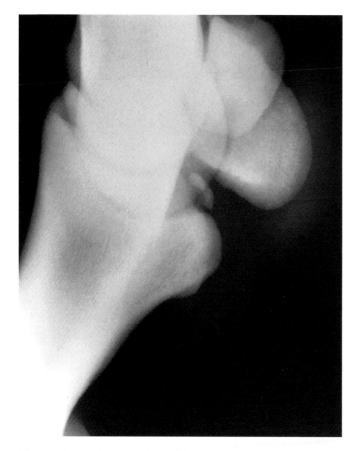

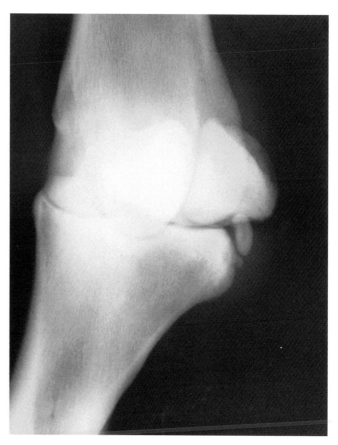

Figure 3.84(a) Dorsal 30° proximal 70° medial-plantarodistal oblique view of a metatarsophalangeal joint of an 8-year-old Danish Warmblood. There is a non-articular osteochondral fragment from the proximoplantar aspect of the medial plantar process of the proximal phalanx.

Figure 3.84(b) Dorsolateral-plantaromedial oblique view of a metatarsophalangeal joint of a 7-year-old Thoroughbred. There are two smoothly rounded osseous opacities in close apposition to the plantar aspect of the lateral plantar process of the proximal phalanx. Each has a trabecular pattern. This is an ununited lateral plantar process of the proximal phalanx.

tion of the x-ray beam. Lesions often start as focal flattening of the subchondral bone and develop through an elliptical lucent area to an oval-shaped lucency, with progressive development of surrounding sclerosis. Conservative treatments warrant a guarded prognosis, but surgical treatment has shown favourable results in the third metacarpal bone.

Ill defined radiolucent areas in the medial or lateral condyles of the third metacarpal bone may also develop as a sequel to trauma (e.g. a fall in a jump) (Figure 3.85). Lameness is usually persistent with conservative management. The success of surgical debridement depends on the location of the lesion relative to the major weight-bearing surface of the bone.

Sesamoiditis

Sesamoiditis is a widely used term that encompasses lucent areas within the bones and new bone production. Radiographic abnormalities are best assessed in D45°M-PaLO and D45°L-PaMO views. The radiographic appearance is variable, ranging from a number of radiolucent areas along the palmar aspect of the bones, with minimal new bone formation, to extensive

Figure 3.85 Dorsal 15° proximal-palmarodistal oblique radiographic view of the right metacarpophalangeal joint of a 7-year-old event horse. Medial is to the left. There is an ill defined radiolucent area in the distal medial aspect of the third metacarpal bone (arrows). There was moderate lameness associated with distension of the joint capsule and exacerbation of lameness by flexion. Arthroscopic examination revealed a large full-thickness cartilage defect extending into a crater in the subchondral bone on the weight-bearing surface of the third metacarpal bone and extensive cartilage fibrillation of the medial condyle of both the third metacarpal bone and the proximal phalanx.

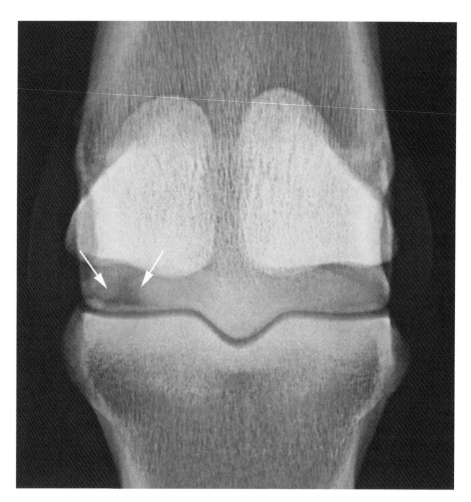

new bone on the axial and abaxial surfaces, with an apparently normal internal structure to the bone. There is often poor correlation between radiological abnormalities and clinical signs.

The lucent areas are sometimes referred to as vascular channels. The number of sharply demarcated vascular channels in a normal horse may vary according to breed and work history. Wide or abnormally shaped lucent areas are likely to be associated with lameness (Figure 3.86a). In racing Thoroughbreds the presence of two or more vascular canals of irregular width as yearlings has been associated with decreased performance when compared with horses with normal vascular canals. The greater the number of vascular channels, the more likely there is to be associated lameness. The new bone on the abaxial and distal surfaces of the bone is often associated with strain of the suspensory ligament and distal sesamoidean ligaments (Figure 3.86b). The lucent zones adjacent to the vascular channels, but outside the normal bone, are areas of fibrous tissue around nutrient vessels. The fibrous tissue resists encroachment of entheseophytes and gives a radiographic appearance of enlarged vascular channels.

In a young horse (less than 3 years) where lucent lesions are the predominant radiographic abnormality, a fair prognosis can be given if the horse receives adequate rest (although the radiographic lesions will persist). The prognosis may be more guarded when these lesions develop in older

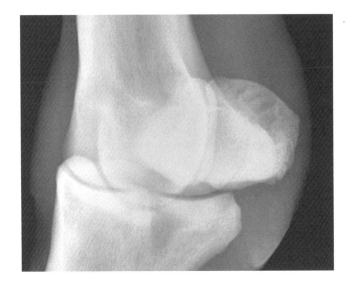

Figure 3.86(a) Dorsolateral-palmaromedial oblique radiographic view of the left metacarpophalangeal joint of a 12-year-old hunter with severe desmitis of the lateral branch of the suspensory ligament. The lateral proximal sesamoid bone has multiple broad radiating lucent lines representing enlarged vascular channels in the proximal one half of the bone. There is mild modelling of the palmar aspect of the bone.

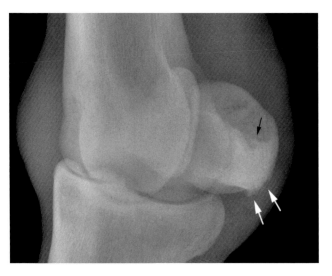

Figure 3.86(b) Dorsomedial-palmarolateral oblique radiographic view of the right metacarpophalangeal joint of an 8-year-old Thoroughbred steeplechaser. There is extensive soft-tissue swelling of the dorsal aspect of the joint. There is irregular new bone on the abaxial (black arrow) and palmarodistal (white arrows) aspects of the medial proximal sesamoid bone. There are ill defined lucent areas in the proximal half of the medial proximal sesamoid bone. There was a large core lesion in the medial branch of the suspensory ligament.

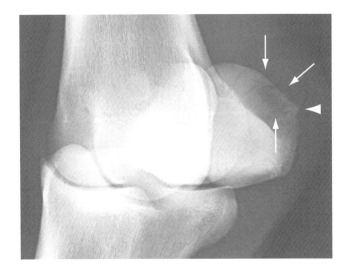

Figure 3.86(c) Dorsolateral-palmaromedial oblique radiographic view of the left metacarpophalangeal joint of a 7-year-old Thoroughbred steeplechaser. There is a large ill defined radiolucent area in the proximal palmar aspect of the lateral proximal sesamoid bone (arrows), with irregular new bone on the palmar aspect of the proximal sesamoid bone distal to it (arrowhead). There are also several narrow radiating radiolucent lines in the bone, normal vascular channels. The horse had sustained an apparently innocuous puncture wound on the palmar aspect of the fetlock 8 weeks previously, but had recently developed a deteriorating lameness. There was marked pain on focal pressure applied to the palmar aspect of the lateral proximal sesamoid bone. Surgical exploration revealed necrotic bone, which was debrided. Note also mild modelling of the dorsoproximal-medial aspect of the proximal phalanx.

[173]

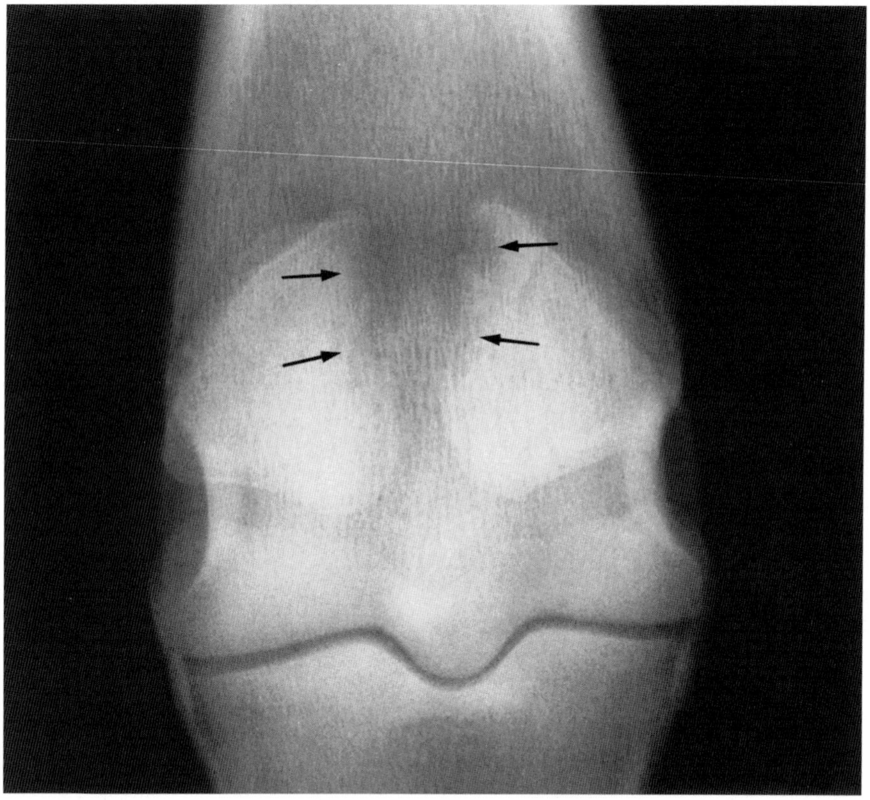

Figure 3.87 Dorsoplantar (flexed) view of a metatarsophalangeal joint of a 3-year-old Thoroughbred with sudden onset of severe lameness 6 weeks previously, associated with diffuse swelling on the plantar aspects of the fetlock and pastern. There is an indistinct axial margin with underlying ill defined lucent zones, involving the proximal half of the medial and lateral proximal sesamoid bones (arrows). This is the result of infection.

horses. Radiating lucent zones may also be seen in association with desmitis of a suspensory ligament branch.

In horses where new bone formation is the predominant radiological finding, there has probably been an associated soft-tissue injury. Ultrasonographic examination of the suspensory apparatus and palmar (plantar) annular ligament in these cases may be useful. The prognosis depends on the amount of new bone formed and the extent of the accompanying soft-tissue injuries.

Periarticular osteophytes seen on the articular margins of the sesamoid bones are an indication of degenerative joint disease. This may be best visualized on a flexed lateromedial view (Figure 3.81b) (see 'Degenerative joint disease', page 166). A discrete lucent zone in the palmar aspect of a proximal sesamoid bone may reflect enthesopathy of the palmar annular ligament (Figure 3.86c). The ligament should also be evaluated ultrasonographically.

Lucent zones restricted to the axial aspect of the proximal sesamoid bones are easily overlooked, unless a dorsopalmar radiographic view is overexposed. For accurate evaluation of the axial margins of the proximal sesamoid bones a flexed dorsopalmar view is extremely useful. Lucent lesions on the axial aspect of the proximal sesamoid bones (Figure 3.87) have been associated with infectious osteitis in horses that have presented with severe lameness, often with distension of the digital flexor tendon sheath. The prognosis is guarded. An irregular axial margin of the proximal sesamoid bones has also been seen with or without desmitis of the inter-sesamoidean ligament and is assumed to be of traumatic origin. Ultrasonographic examination is indicated. The prognosis is guarded with conservative management, but surgical debridement may be indicated in selected cases.

Abnormal position of the proximal sesamoid bones

The position of the proximal sesamoid bones relative to the metacarpophalangeal (metatarsophalangeal) joint should be carefully assessed. Failure of the suspensory apparatus in the metacarpal or, more commonly, metatarsal regions results in an abnormally low position of the proximal sesamoid bones and is a poor prognostic indicator. Severe injury of the superficial digital flexor tendon results in hyperextension of the entire fetlock joint, thus the proximal sesamoid bones will be lower. Complete disruption of the distal sesamoidean ligaments results in proximal displacement of the proximal sesamoid bones. Ultrasonographic evaluation is indicated.

Luxation

Luxation of the metacarpophalangeal joint can occur in lateromedial or dorsopalmar directions. The injury may be obvious radiographically, but it may be necessary to obtain radiographs with the distal limb under stress (see Figures 1.15a and 1.15b, page 31). The radiographs must be carefully examined for concurrent fractures. The prognosis for return to athletic function is very grave, but a guarded prognosis may be given for breeding after casting the limb.

Stress-related bone injury

Stress-related bone injury occurs commonly in the condyles of the third metacarpal and third metatarsal bones in Thoroughbred and Standardbred racehorses. Hindlimbs are more commonly affected. Although the palmar (plantar) aspect of the lateral condyle is most frequently affected, experience with magnetic resonance imaging reveals that evidence of bone trauma may be more widespread. Care must be taken with interpretation, as the subchondral bone in this area is normally slightly flatter than the remainder of the condyle. Flattening of the condyle, or a triangular-shaped sclerotic area in the subchondral bone (Figure 3.88), are best visualized on a lateromedial or flexed lateromedial view, or the dorsal 45° proximal 45° lateral-palmar distal medial oblique view. Nuclear scintigraphy is more sensitive for detection of early and less severe reactions. These lesions may occur bilaterally, especially in the hindlimbs, causing a variable degree of lameness or loss of performance. It is usually difficult to keep affected horses that have radiographic abnormalities sound enough to withstand training.

Fractures

The common fracture sites of the phalanges and metacarpophalangeal joint are shown in Figure 3.89. Small radiopaque bodies at the joint margins may be an incidental finding (Figure 3.90 and page 163).

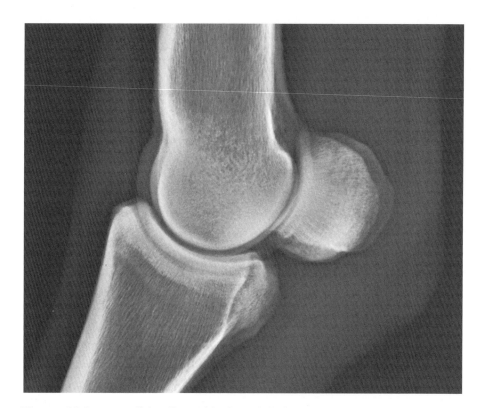

Figure 3.88 Lateromedial radiographic view of the left metatarsophalangeal joint of a 4-year-old Thoroughbred flat racehorse with bilateral hindlimb lameness. There is sclerosis of the plantar aspect of the condyles of the third metatarsal bone. There were no localizing clinical signs. Lameness was abolished by a low four-point block at the plantar and plantar metatarsal nerves, but only slightly improved by intra-articular analgesia, a response typical of subchondral bone pain.

Chip fractures of the proximodorsal and proximopalmar aspects of the proximal phalanx, involving the joint surface, are relatively common and, if only 2–3 mm in diameter, lameness frequently resolves with rest, although it may be recurrent. Larger chips, chips associated with recurrent lameness, or fragments of bone with a roughened appearance or irregular and lucent base usually need surgical removal. Other fractures of the proximal phalanx are referred to under 'Proximal phalanx' on pages 144–148. See also 'Osteochondral fragments', page 167.

Fractures of the proximal sesamoid bones occur frequently, and their significance depends on their position and the degree of associated soft-tissue injury. They may occur in association with fractures of the third metacarpal bone and phalanges, and should not be overlooked.

Fractures of the abaxial surface of the bone are best seen on oblique tangential views (see Figure 3.72a, page 152). Prognosis depends on the degree of suspensory ligament pathology, but is often guarded.

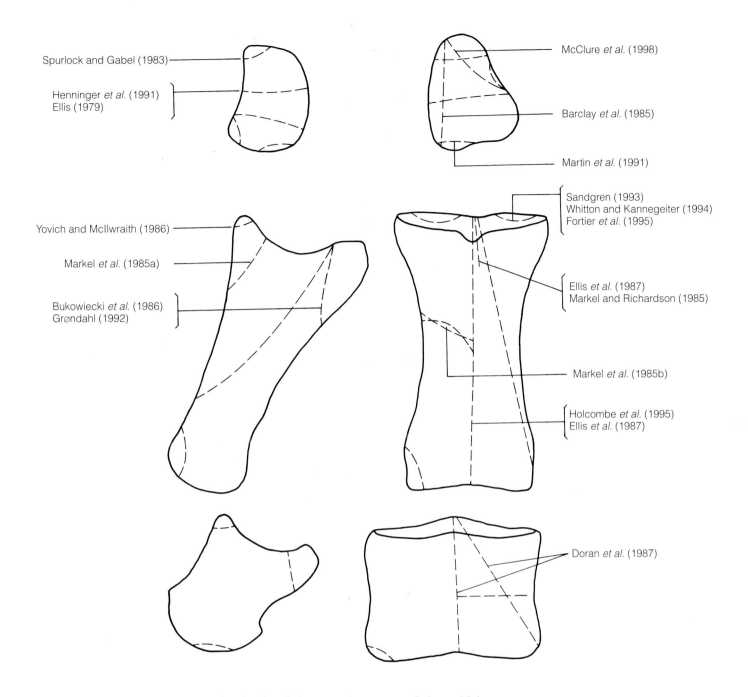

Spurlock and Gabel (1983)

Henninger *et al.* (1991)
Ellis (1979)

Yovich and McIlwraith (1986)

Markel *et al.* (1985a)

Bukowiecki *et al.* (1986)
Grøndahl (1992)

McClure *et al.* (1998)

Barclay *et al.* (1985)

Martin *et al.* (1991)

Sandgren (1993)
Whitton and Kannegeiter (1994)
Fortier *et al.* (1995)

Ellis *et al.* (1987)
Markel and Richardson (1985)

Markel *et al.* (1985b)

Holcombe *et al.* (1995)
Ellis *et al.* (1987)

Doran *et al.* (1987)

Figure 3.89 The common fracture sites for the phalanges and metacarpophalangeal joint.

Fractures of the apical region involving less than one-third of the bone generally respond well to surgical removal of the fragment. Larger fragments should normally be treated by internal fixation or bone grafting, preferably within 10 days of fracture. Even with prompt treatment the prognosis for these fractures is poor. Basilar fragments of bone may be removed surgically, but even with improved arthroscopic technique, some disruption

[177]

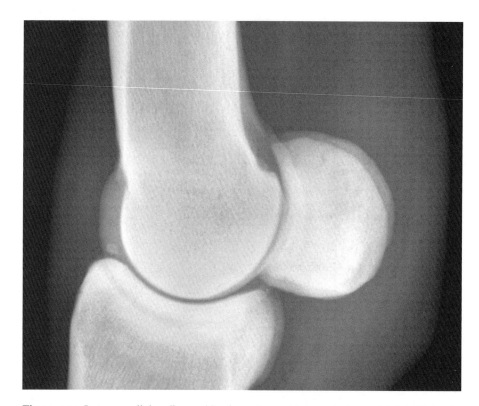

Figure 3.90 Lateromedial radiographic view of a metacarpophalangeal joint. There is a small well rounded mineralized opacity on the dorsoproximal aspect of the proximal phalanx. This was an incidental finding at a pre-purchase examination of this 7-year-old intermediate event horse.

of the distal sesamoidean ligaments is inevitable, resulting in a guarded prognosis.

Sagittal fractures of the proximal sesamoid bones also occur, usually concurrent with other fractures. They warrant a guarded prognosis.

Occasionally an avulsion fracture at the attachment of the palmar annular ligament occurs. These have a favourable outcome with either conservative management or surgical removal.

Care should be taken when interpreting radiographs of foals. The sesamoid bones are not fully mineralized until 3 months of age and the cartilage precursors may tear. This may not be seen radiographically until the sesamoid bones are more completely ossified, when the bones may appear elongated or be visualized as two separated fragments (Figure 3.91). This is a common injury in foals under 1 month of age and may involve all four limbs. It is often seen in even slightly premature foals that have exercised excessively and is associated with mild, transient lameness. With confinement to stall rest, bony union usually develops. The resulting sesamoid bone is usually larger than normal but the prognosis is good if treated promptly.

Fractures of the distal aspect of the third metacarpal bone are described in Chapter 4, page 216.

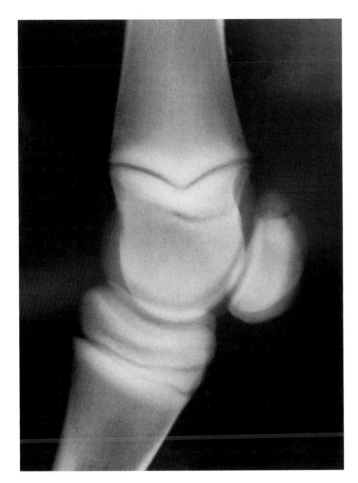

Figure 3.91 Lateromedial view of a metacarpophalangeal joint of a foal 5 weeks of age. There is a non-displaced apical fracture of the lateral proximal sesamoid bone.

FURTHER READING

Foot

Aanes, W.A. (1984) Congenital phalangeal hypoplasia in Equidae. *J. Am. Vet. Med. Ass.*, **185**, 554–556

Ackerman, N., Johnson, J.H. and Dorn, C.R. (1977) Navicular disease in the horse. *J. Am. Vet. Med. Ass.*, **170**, 183–187

Attenburrow, D. and Heyse-Moore, G. (1982) Non-ossifying fibroma in a phalanx of a Thoroughbred yearling. *Equine vet. J.*, **14**, 59–61

Baird, A., Seahorn, T. and Morris, E. (1990) Equine digital sequestration *Vet. Radiol.*, **31**, 210–213

Bathe, A. and Joyner, S. (2003) Limitations and improvements in the quality of navicular flexor view radiographs. *Proc. Am. Ass. Equine Pract.*, **49**, 317–319

Berry, C., O'Brien, T. and Pool, R. (1991) Squamous cell carcinoma of the hoof wall in a stallion. *J. Am. Vet. Med. Ass.*, **199**, 90–92

Berry, C., Pool, R., Stover, S. *et al.* (1992) Radiographic/morphologic investigation of a radiolucent crescent within the flexor central eminence of the navicular bone in Thoroughbreds. *Am. J. Vet. Res.*, **53**, 1604–1611

Bertone, A. and Aanes, W. (1984) Congenital phalangeal hypoplasia in Equidae. *J. Am. Vet. Med. Ass.*, **185**, 554–556

Blunden, T., Dyson, S., Murray, R. and Schramme, M. (2006) Histopathological findings in horses with chronic palmar foot pain and age-matched control horses Part 1: the navicular bone & related structures. *Equine vet. J.*, **38**, 15–22

Boado, A., Kristoffersen, M., Dyson, S. and Murray, R. (2005) Use of nuclear scintigraphy and magnetic resonance imaging to diagnose chronic penetrating wounds in the equine foot. *Equine vet. Educ.*, **17**, 62–68

Boys-Smith, S., Clegg, P., Hughes, I. and Singer, E. (2006) Complete and partial hoof wall resection for keratoma removal: post operative complications and final outcome in 26 horses (1994–2004) *Equine vet. J.*, **38**, 127–133

Busoni, V. and Denoix, J.-M. (2001) Ultrasonography of the podotrochlear apparatus in the horse using a transcuneal approach: technique and reference images. *Vet. Radiol. and Ultrasound*, **42**, 534–540

Cauvin, E. and Munroe, G. (1998) Septic osteitis of the distal phalanx: findings and surgical treatment in 18 cases. *Equine vet. J.*, **30**, 512–519

Colles, C.M. (1979) Ischaemic necrosis of the navicular bone (distal sesamoid bone) of the horse and its treatment. *Vet. Rec.*, **104**, 133–137

Colles, C.M. (1982) The pathogenesis and treatment of navicular disease in the horse. *PhD Thesis*, University of London

Colles, C.M. (2001) How to repair navicular bone fractures in the horse *Proc. Am. Assoc. Equine Pract.*, **47**, 270–277

Colles, C.M. and Hickman, J. (1977) The arterial supply of the navicular bone and its variations in navicular disease. *Equine vet. J.*, **9**, 150–154

Cripps, P. and Eustace, R. (1999a) Radiological measurements from the feet of normal horses with relevance to laminitis. *Equine vet. J.*, **31**, 427–432

Cripps, P. and Eustace, R. (1999b) Factors involved in the prognosis of equine laminitis in the UK. *Equine vet. J.*, **31**, 433–442

Dakin, S., Robson, K. and Dyson, S. (2006) Fracture of the ossified cartilage of the foot: 10 cases. *Equine vet. Educ.*, **18**, 130–136

Dechant, J., Trotter, G., Stashak, T. and Hendrickson, D. (2000) Removal of large extensor process fractures of the distal phalanx via arthrotomy in horses: 14 cases (1992–1998). *J. Am. Vet. Med. Ass.*, **217**, 1351–1355

De Clerq, T., Verschooten, F. and Ysebaert, M. (2000) A comparison of the palmaroproximal-palmarodistal oblique view of the isolated navicular bone to other views. *Vet. Radiol. and Ultrasound*, **41**, 525–533

Dik, K. and Broeck, J. van den (1995) Role of navicular bone shape in the pathogenesis of navicular disease: a radiological study. *Equine vet. J.*, **27**, 390–393

Dik. K., van den Belt, A., Enzerink, E. and van Weeren, R. (2001a) The radiographic development of the distal and proximal double contours of the equine navicular bone on dorsoproximal-palmarodistal oblique (upright pedal) radiographs, from age 1 to 11 months. *Equine vet. J.*, **33**, 70–74

Dik. K., van den Belt, A. and van den Broek, J. (2001b) Relationships of age and shape of the navicular bone to the development of navicular disease: a radiological study. *Equine vet. J.*, **33**, 172–175

Down, S., Dyson, S. and Murray, R. (2007) Ossification of the cartilages of the foot. *Equine vet. Educ.*, **19**, 51–56

Dyson, S. (1991) Lameness due to pain associated with the distal interphalangeal joint: 45 cases. *Equine vet. J.*, **23**, 128–135

Dyson, S. (1998) The puzzle of distal interphalangeal joint pain. *Equine vet. Educ.*, **10**, 119–125

Dyson, S. and Murray, R. (2004) Collateral desmitis of the distal interphalangeal joint in 62 horses (January 2001–December 2003). *Proc. Am. Ass. Equine Pract.*, **50**, 248–256

Dyson, S. and Murray, R. (2007) Magnetic resonance imaging of the equine foot. *Clin. Techniques in Equine Pract.*, **6**, 46–61

Dyson, S., Murray, R., Schramme, M. and Branch, M. (2003) Lameness in 46 horses associated with deep digital flexor tendonitis in the horse: diagnosis confirmed with magnetic resonance imaging. *Equine vet. J.*, **35**, 681–690

Dyson, S., Murray, R., Schramme, M. and Branch, M. (2004) Collateral desmitis of the distal interphalangeal joint in 18 horses (2001–2002). *Equine vet. J.*, **36**, 160–166

Dyson, S., Murray, R. and Schramme, M. (2005) Lameness associated with foot pain and results of magnetic resonance imaging in 199 horses (January 2001–December 2003). *Equine vet. J.*, **37**, 113–121

Dyson, S., Murray, R., Blunden, T. and Schramme, M. (2006) Current concepts of navicular disease. *Equine vet. Educ.*, **18**, 45–56

Fraser, B., Else, R. and Jones, E. (2006) Intraosseous epidermoid cyst of the third phalanx in a Thoroughbred gelding. *Vet. Rec.*, **159**, 360–362

Frecklington, P. and Rose, R. (1981) An unusual case of fracture of the navicular bone in the hindlimb of a horse. *Austr. Vet. Pract.*, **11**, 57–59

Gelatt, K.L., Neuwirth, L., Hawkins, D.L. and Woodard, J.C. (1996) Hemangioma of the distal phalanx in a colt. *Vet. Radiol. and Ultrasound*, **37**, 275–280

Giraldo, L. and Redding, R. (2005) Radiographic diagnosis: Foreign body in the distal interphalangeal joint. *Vet. Radiol. and Ultrasound*, **46**, 304–305

Heitzmann, A. and Denoix, J.-M. (2007) Rupture of the distal sesamoidean impar ligament with proximal displacement of the distal sesamoid bone in a steeplechaser. *Equine vet. Educ.*, **19**, 117–120

Hoegaerts, M., Pille, F., De Clerq, T., Fulton, I. and Saunders, J. (2005) Comminuted fracture of the distal sesamoid bone and distal rupture of the deep digital flexor tendon. *Vet. Radiol. and Ultrasound*, **46**, 234–237

Honnas, C., O'Brien, T. and Linford, R. (1988) Distal phalanx fractures in horses: a survey of 274 horses with radiographic assessment of healing in 36 horses. *Vet. Radiol.*, **29**, 98–107

Honnas, C., Liskey, C., Meagher, D., Brown, D. and Luck, E. (1990) Malignant melanoma in the foot of a horse. *J. Am. Vet. Med. Ass.*, **197**, 756–758

Hunt, R. (1993) A retrospective evaluation of laminitis in horses. *Equine vet. J.*, **25**, 61–64

Jones, V.B. (1938) Veterinary radiology – navicular disease. *Vet. Rec.*, **50**, 676–677

Kaneps, A.J., O'Brien, T.R., Redden, R.F., Stover, S.M. and Pool, R.R. (1993) Characterisation of osseous bodies of the distal phalanx of foals. *Equine vet. J.*, **25**, 285–292

Keegan, K., Twardock, R., Losonsky, J. and Baker, G. (1993) Scintigraphic evaluation of fractures of the distal phalanx in 27 cases (1979–1988). *J. Am. Vet. Med. Assoc.*, **202**, 1993–1997

Kristiansen, K. and Kold, S. (2007) Multivariable analysis of factors influencing outcome of 2 treatment protocols in 128 cases of horses responding positively to intra-articular analgesia of the distal interphalangeal joint. *Equine vet. J.*, **39**, 150–156

Lillich, J., Ruggles, A., Gabel, A., Bramlage, L. and Schneider, R. (1995) Fracture of the distal sesamoid bone in horses: 17 cases (1982–1992). *J. Am. Vet. Med. Ass.*, **207**, 924–927

Linford, R.L., O'Brien, T.R. and Trout, D.R. (1993) Qualitative and morphometric radiographic findings in the distal phalanx and distal soft tissues of sound Thoroughbred racehorses. *Am. J. Vet. Res.*, **54**, 38–51

McDiarmid, A.M. (1998) Distal interphalangeal joint lameness in a horse associated with damage to the insertion of the lateral collateral ligament. *Equine vet. Educ.*, **10**, 114–118

MacGregor, C.M. (1986) Radiographic assessment of navicular bones based on change in the distal nutrient foramina. *Equine vet. J.*, **18**, 203–206

Murray, R., Schramme, M., Dyson, S. and Blunden, A. (2006) MRI characteristics of the foot in horses with palmar foot pain and control horses. *Vet. Radiol. and Ultrasound*, **47**, 1–16

Murray, R., Blunden, A., Schramme, M. and Dyson, S. (2006) How does magnetic resonance imaging represent histological findings in the equine digit? *Vet. Radiol. and Ultrasound*, **47**, 17–31

Murray, R., Dyson, S., Schramme, M. and Branch, M. (2003) Magnetic resonance imaging of the equine digit with chronic laminitis. *Vet. Radiol. and Ultrasound*, **44**, 609–617

Nagy, A., Dyson, S. and Murray, R. (2007) Scintigraphic examination of the cartilages of the foot. *Equine vet. J.*, **39**, 250–256

Nagy, A., Dyson, S. and Murray, R. (2007) A comparison of radiography, nuclear scintigraphy and magnetic resonance imaging of the palmar processes of the distal phalanx. *Equine vet. J.*, **40**, 57–63.

O'Brien, T.R., Millman, T.M., Pool, R.R. and Suter, P.F. (1975) Navicular disease in the Thoroughbred horse: a morphologic investigation relative to a new radiographic projection. *J. Am. Vet. Rad. Soc.*, **16**, 39–50

Ohlsson, J. and Jansson, N. (2005) Conservative treatment of intra-articular distal phalanx fractures in horses not used for racing. *Aust. Vet. J.*, **83**, 221–223

O'Sullivan, C.B., Dart, A.J., Malikides, N., Rawlinson, R.J., Hutchins, D.R., and Hodgson, D.R. (1999) Nonsurgical management of type II fractures of the distal phalanx in 48 Standardbred horses. *Aust. Vet. J.*, **77**, 501–503

Oxspring, G.E. (1935) The radiology of navicular disease, with observations on its pathology. *Vet. Rec.*, **48**, 1445–1454

Petterson, H. (1976) Fractures of the pedal bone in the horse. *Equine vet. J.*, **8**, 104–109

Pickersgill, C. (2000) Recurrent white line abscessation associated with a keratoma in a pony. *Equine vet. Educ.*, **12**, 286–291

Poulos, P. (1983) Correlation of radiographic signs and histological changes in the navicular bone. *Proc. Am. Ass. Equine Pract.*, **29**, 241–255

Poulos, P. (1988) The nature of enlarged 'vascular channels' in the navicular bone of the horse. *Vet. Radiol.*, **29**, 60–64

Puchalski, S., Snyder, J., Hornof, W., Macdonald, M. and Galuppo, L. (2005) Contrast-enhanced computed tomography of the equine distal extremity. *Proc. Am. Assoc. Equine Pract.*, **51**, 389–394

Rabuffo, T. and Ross, M. (2002) Fractures of the distal phalanx in 72 racehorses: 1990–2001. *Proc. Amer. Assoc. Equine Pract.*, **48**, 375–377

Redden, R. (2001) A technique for performing digital venography in the standing horse. *Equine vet. Educ.*, **5**, 172–178

Rendano, V. and Grant, B. (1978) The equine third phalanx: its radiographic appearance. *Vet. Radiol.*, **19**, 125–135

Richardson, G. and O'Brien, T. (1985) Puncture wounds into the navicular bursa of the horse: their radiological evaluation. *Vet. Radiol.*, **26**, 203–207

Robson, K., Kristoffersen, M. and Dyson, S. (2007) Palmar or plantar process fractures of the distal phalanx in riding horses: 22 cases (1994–2003). *Equine vet. Educ.*, **20**, 40–46

Rose, J.R., Taylor, B.J. and Steel, J.D. (1978) Navicular disease in the horse: an analysis of 70 cases and assessment of a special radiographic view. *J. Equine Med. Surg.*, **2**, 492–497

Rucker, A., Redden, R., Arthur, E. et al. (2006) How to perform the digital venogram. *Proc. Am. Ass. Equine Pract.*, **52**, 526–530

Ruohoniemi, M., Tulamo, R-M. and Hackzell, M. (1993) Radiographic evaluation of ossification of the collateral cartilages of the third phalanx in Finnhorses. *Equine vet. J.*, **25**, 453–455

Ruohoniemi, M., Karkkainen, M. and Tervahartiala, P. (1997) Evaluation of the variably ossified collateral cartilages of the distal phalanx and adjacent anatomic structures in the Finnhorse with computed tomography and magnetic resonance imaging. *Vet. Radiol. and Ultrasound*, **38**, 344–351

Ruohoniemi, M. and Tervahartiala, P. (1999) Computed tomographic evaluation of Finnhorse cadaver forefeet with radiographically problematic findings on the flexor aspect of the navicular bone. *Vet. Radiol. and Ultrasound*, **40**, 275–281

Ruohoniemi, M., Makela, M. and Eskonen, T. (2004) Clinical significance of ossification of the cartilages of the front feet based on nuclear scintigraphy, radiography and lameness examinations in 21 Finnhorses. *Equine vet. J.*, **36**, 143–148

Scott, E., McDole, M. and Shires, M. (1979) A review of third phalanx fractures in the horse: sixty-five cases. *J. Am. Vet. Med. Assoc.*, **174**, 1337–1343

Scott, E., Snyder, S., Schmotzer, W. and Pool, R. (1991) Subchondral bone cysts with fractures of the extensor processes in a horse. *J. Am. Vet. Med. Ass.*, **199**, 595–597

Silva, S. and Vulcano, L. (2002) Collateral cartilage ossification of the distal phalanx in the Brazilian jumper horse. *Vet. Radiol. and Ultrasound*, **43**, 461–463

Smallwood, J.E., Albright, S.M., Metcalf, M.R., Thrall, D.E. and Harrington, B.D. (1989) A xeroradiographic study of the developing equine foredigit and metacarpophalangeal region from birth to six months of age. *Vet. Radiol.*, **30**, 98–110

Smith, M., Crowe, O., Ellson, C., Turner, S., Patterson-Kane, J., Schramme, M. and Smith, R. (2005) Surgical treatment of osseous cyst-like lesions in the distal phalanx arising from collateral ligament insertion injury. *Equine vet. Educ.*, **17**, 195–200

Smith, S., Dyson, S. and Murray, R. (2004) Is there an association between distal phalanx angles and deep digital flexor tendon lesions? *Proc. Am. Assoc. Equine Pract.*, **50**, 328–331

Stock, K. and Distl, O. (2006) Genetic analysis of the radiographic appearance of the distal sesamoid bone in Hanoverian Warmblood horses. *Am. J. Vet. Res.*, **67**, 1013–1019

Story, M. and Bramlage, L. (2004) Arthroscopic debridement of subchondral bone cysts in the distal phalanx of 11 horses (1994–2000). *Equine vet. J.*, **36**, 356–361

Ter Braake, F. (2005) Arthroscopic removal of large fragments of the extensor process of the distal phalanx in 4 horses. *Equine vet. Educ.*, **17**, 101–104

Van Hoogmoed, L., Snyder, J., Thomas, H. and Harmon, F. (2003) Retrospective evaluation of equine prepurchase examinations performed between 1991–2000. *Equine vet. J.*, **35**, 375–381

Vaughan, L.C. (1961) Fracture of the navicular bone in the horse. *Vet. Rec.*, **73**, 895–897

Verschooten, F. and deMoor, A. (1982) Subchondral cystic and related lesions affecting the equine pedal bone and stifle. *Equine vet. J.*, **14**, 47–54

Verschooten, F., Wearable, B. Van and Verbeeck, J. (1996) The ossification of cartilages of the distal phalanx in the horse – an anatomical, experimental, radiographic and clinical study. *J. Equine Vet. Sci.*, **16**, 291–305

Verschooten, F., Roels, J., Lampo, P., DeMoor, A. and Picavet, T. (1989) Radiographic measurements from the lateromedial projection of the equine foot with navicular disease. *Res. Vet. Sci.*, **46**, 15–21

Wagner, I. and Hood, D. (1997) Cause of air lines associated with acute and chronic laminitis. *Proc. Am. Ass. Equine Pract.*, **43**, 363–366

Wagner, P. and Balch-Burnett, O. (1982) Surgical management of subchondral bone cysts of the third phalanx. *Equine Pract.*, **4**, 8–14

Watering, C.C. van de and Morgan, J.P. (1975) Chip fractures as a radiological finding in navicular disease of the horse. *J. Am. Vet. Rad. Soc.*, **16**, 206–210

Widmer, W., Buckwalter, K., Fessler, J., Hill, M., Van Sickle, D. and Ivancevich, S. (2000) Use of radiography, computed tomography and magnetic resonance imaging for evaluation of navicular syndrome in the horse. *Vet. Radiol. and Ultrasound*, **41**, 108–117

Wong, D., Scaratt, W., Maxwell, V. and Moon, M. (2003) Incomplete ossification of the carpal, tarsal and navicular bones in a dysmature foal. *Equine vet. Educ.*, **15**, 72–81

Wright, I. (1993) A study of 118 cases of navicular disease: radiological features. *Equine vet. J.*, **25**, 493–500

Wurfel, C. and Hertsch, B. (2005) Study on the diagnostic values of contrast radiography of the navicular bone. *Pferheilkunde*, **21**, 4–12

Yovich, J., Stashak, T., DeBowes, R. and Ducharme, N. (1986) Fractures of the distal phalanx of the forelimb in eight foals. *J. Am. Vet. Med. Ass.*, **189**, 550–554

Pastern

Brasche, S., Rick, M. and Herthel, D. (2004) Treatment of a horse with osteomyelitis following repair of a middle phalangeal fracture via pastern arthrodesis. *Equine vet. Educ.*, **16**, 262–266

Doran, R., White, N. and Allen, D. (1987) Use of a bone plate for treatment of middle phalangeal fractures in horses: 7 cases (1979–1984). *J. Am. Vet. Med. Ass.*, **191**, 575–578

Ellis, D., Simpson, D., Greenwood, R. and Crowhurst, J. (1987) Observations and management of fractures of the proximal phalanx in young Thoroughbreds. *Equine vet. J.*, **19** 43–49

Ellis, D. and Greenwood, R. (1985) Six cases of degenerative joint disease of the proximal interphalangeal joint of young thoroughbreds. *Equine vet. J.*, **17**, 66–68

Holcombe, S.J., Schneider, R.K., Bramlage, L.R., Gabel, A.A., Bertone A.L. and Beard, W.L. (1995) Lag screw fixation of non-comminuted sagittal fractures of the proximal phalanx in racehorses: 59 cases (1973–1991). *J. Am. Vet. Med. Ass.*, **206**, 1195–1199

Kraus, B., Richardson, D., Nunamaker, D. and Ross, M. (2004) Management of comminuted fractures of the proximal phalanx in horses: 64 cases (1983–2001). *J. Am. Vet. Med. Ass.*, **224**, 254–263

Knox, P. and Watkins, J. (2006) Proximal interphalangeal joint arthrodesis using a combination plate–screw technique in 53 horses (1994–2003). *Equine vet. J.*, **38**, 538–542

Kold, S. and Killingbeck, J. (1998) The use of autogenous cancellous bone graft for the treatment of subchondral bone cysts in the distal phalanges; three cases. *Equine vet. Educ.*, **10**, 307–312

Markel, M. and Richardson, D. (1985) Non comminuted fractures of the proximal phalanx in 69 horses. *J. Am. Vet. Med. Ass.*, **186**, 573–579

Markel, M., Martin, B. and Richardson, D. (1985a) Dorsal frontal fractures of the first phalanx in the horse. *Vet. Surg.*, **14**, 36–40

Markel, M., Richardson, D. and Nunamaker, D. (1985b) Comminuted first phalanx fractures in 30 horses. Surgical versus non-surgical treatments. *Vet. Surg.*, **14**, 135–140

Schaer, T., Bramlage, L., Embertson, R. and Hance, S. (2001) Proximal interphalangeal arthrodesis in 22 horses. *Equine vet. J.*, **33**, 360–365

Shiroma, J., Engel, H. and Watrous, B. (1989) Dorsal subluxation of the proximal interphalangeal joint in the pelvic limb of three horses. *J. Am. Vet. Med. Ass.*, **195**, 777–780

Trotter, G., McIlwraith, C., Nordin, R. and Turner, A. (1982) Degenerative joint disease with osteochondrosis of the proximal interphalangeal joint in young horses. *J. Am. Vet. Med. Ass.*, **180**, 1312–1318

Weaver, J., Stover, S. and O'Brien, T. (1992) Radiographic anatomy of soft tissue attachments in the equine metacarpophalangeal and proximal phalangeal region. *Equine vet. J.*, **24**, 310–315

Fetlock

Anthenill, L., Stover, S., Gardner, I., Hill, A. *et al.* (2006) Association between findings on palmarodorsal radiographic images and detection of a fracture in the proximal sesamoid bones of forelimbs obtained from cadavers of racing Thoroughbreds *Am. J. Vet. Res.*, **67**, 858–868

Barbee, D., Allen, J., Grant, B., Crawley, G. and Sande. R. (1987) Detection by computerized tomography of occult osteochondral defects in the fetlock of a horse. *Equine vet. J.*, **19**, 556–558

Barclay, W., Foerner, J. and Phillips, T. (1985) Axial sesamoid fractures associated with lateral condylar fractures. *J. Am. Vet. Med. Ass.*, **186**, 278–279

Barclay, W., Foerner, J. and Phillips, T. (1987) Lameness attributable to osteochondral fragmentation of the plantar aspect of the proximal phalanx: 19 cases. *J. Am. Vet. Med. Ass.*, **191**, 855–857

Barr, E., Clegg, P., Senior, M. and Singer, E. (2005) Destructive lesions of the proximal sesamoid bones as a complication of dorsal metatarsal artery catherisation in three horses. *Vet. Surg.*, **34**, 159–166

Birkeland, R. (1972) Chip fractures of the first phalanx in the metacarpophalangeal joint. *Acta Radiol. Suppl.*, **39**, 73–77

Bukowiecki, C., Bramlage, L. and Gabel, A. (1986) Palmar/plantar process fractures of the proximal phalanx in 15 horses. *Vet. Surg.*, **15**, 383–388

Carlsten, J., Sandgren, B. and Dalin, J. (1993) Development of osteochondrosis in the tarsocrural joints and osteochondral fragments in the fetlock joint in Standardbred trotters. I. A radiological survey. *Equine vet. J. Suppl.*, **16**, 42–47

Cohen, N., Carter, G., Watkins, J. and O'Conor, M. (2006) Association of racing performance with specific abnormal radiographic findings in Thoroughbred yearlings sold in Texas. *J. Equine Vet. Sci.*, **26**, 462–474

Colon, J., Bramlage, L., Hance, S. and Embertson, R. (2000) Qualitative and quantitative documentation of the racing performance of 461 Thoroughbred racehorses after arthroscopic removal of dorsoproximal first phalanx osteochondral fractures (1986–1995). *Equine vet. J.*, **32**, 475–481

Courouce-Malblanc, A., Leleu, C., Bouchilloux, M. and Geffroy, O. (2006) Abnormal radiographic findings in 865 French Standardbred trotters and their relationship to racing performance. *Equine vet. J. Suppl.*, **36**, 417–422

Dabareiner, R., Watkins, J., Carter, G., Honnas, C. and Eastman, T. (2001) Osteitis of the axial border of the proximal sesamoid bones in horses: 8 cases (1993–1999). *J. Am. Vet. Med. Ass.*, **219**, 82–86

Dabareiner, R., White, N. and Sullins, K. (1996) Metacarpophalangeal joint synovial pad fibrotic proliferation in 63 horses. *Vet. Surg.*, **25**, 199–206

Dalin, G., Sandgren, B. and Carlsten, J. (1993) Plantar osteochondral fragments in the metatarsophalangeal joints in Standardbred trotters: result of osteochondrosis or trauma? *Equine vet. J. Suppl.*, **16**, 62–65

Dik, K.J. (1985) Special radiographic projections for the equine proximal sesamoid bones and the caudoproximal extremity of the first phalanx. *Equine vet. J.*, **17**, 244–247

Dyson, S. and Murray, R. (2006) Osseous trauma in the fetlock region of mature sports horses. *Proc. Am. Ass. Equine Pract.*, **52**, 443–456

Dyson, S. and Murray, R. (2007) Magnetic resonance imaging of the equine fetlock. *Clin. Techniques in Equine Pract.*, **6**, 62–77

Ellis, D. (1979) Fractures of the proximal sesamoid bones in Thoroughbred foals. *Equine vet. J.*, **11**, 48–52

Enzerink, E. and Dik, K. (2001) Palmar/plantar ligament insertion injury: a report of 4 cases. *Equine vet. Educ.*, **13**, 75–80

Fortier, L., Foerner, J. and Nixon, A. (1995) Arthroscopic removal of axial osteochondral fragments of the plantar/palmar proximal aspect of the proximal phalanx in horses: 119 cases (1988–1992). *J. Am. Vet. Med. Ass.*, **206**, 71–74

Grøndahl, A. (1992) Incidence and development of ununited proximoplantar tuberosity of the proximal phalanx in Standardbred trotters. *Vet. Radiol. Ultrasound*, **33**, 18–21

Grøndahl, A., Gaustad, G. and Engeland, A. (1994) Progression and association with lameness and racing performance of radiographic changes in the proximal sesamoid bones of young Standardbred trotters. *Equine vet. J.*, **26**, 152–155

Hardy, J., Marcoux, M. and Breton, L. (1991) Clinical relevance of radiographic findings in proximal sesamoid bones of two-year-old Standardbreds in their first year of race training. *J. Am. Vet. Med. Ass.*, **198**, 2089–2094

Haynes, P., Root, C., Clabough, Q. and Roberts, E. (1981) Palmar supracondylar lysis of the third metacarpal bone. *Proc. Am. Ass. Equine Pract.*, **27**, 185–193

Henninger, R., Bramlage, L., Schneider, R. and Gabel, A. (1991) Lag screw and cancellous bone graft fixation of transverse proximal sesamoid fractures in horses: 25 cases (1983–1989). *J. Am. Vet. Med. Ass.*, **199**, 606–612

Hogan, P., McIlwraith, C., Honnas, C. *et al.* (1997) Surgical treatment of subchondral cystic lesions of the third metacarpal bone: results in 15 horses (1986–1994). *Equine vet. J.*, **29**, 477–482

Hornhof, W.J. and O'Brien, T.R. (1980) Radiographic evaluation of the palmar aspect of the equine metacarpal condyles: a new projection. *Vet. Radiol.*, **21**, 161–167

Kane, A., Park, R., McIlwraith, C., Rantanen, N., Morehead, J. and Bramlage, L. (2003a) Radiographic changes in Thoroughbred yearlings. Part 1: Prevalence at the time of sales. *Equine vet. J.*, **35**, 354–365

Kane, A., McIlwraith, C., Park, R., Rantanen, N., Morehead, J. and Bramlage, L. (2003b) Radiographic changes in Thoroughbred yearlings. Part 2: Association with racing performance. *Equine vet. J.*, **35**, 366–374

Kawcak, C., Bramlage, L. and Embertson, D. (1995) Diagnosis and management of incomplete fracture of the distal palmar aspect of the third metacarpal bone in five horses. *J. Am. Vet. Med. Ass.*, **206**, 335–338

McCall, D.J.M. and Kneller, S.K. (1989) Proximodorsal-distodorsal view of the equine metacarpophalangeal joint. *Vet. Technician*, **10**, 617–621

McClure, S., Watkins, J., Glickman, N. *et al.* (1998) Complete fracture of the third metacarpal or metatarsal bone in horses: 25 cases (1980–1986). *J. Am. Vet. Med. Ass.*, **213**, 847–850

Mair, T. and Tucker, R. (2004) Hypertrophic osteopathy (Marie's disease) in horses. *Equine vet. Educ.*, **16**, 308–311

Martin, B., Nunamaker, D., Evans, L., Orsini, J. and Palmer, S. (1991) Circumferential wiring of mid-body and large basilar fractures of the proximal sesamoid bones in 15 horses. *Vet. Surg.*, **20**, 9–14

Medina, L., Wheat, J., Morgan, J. and Pool, R. (1950) Treatment of basal fractures of the sesamoid bones using autogenous bone grafts. *Proc. Am. Ass. Equine Pract.*, **26**, 345–380

Morgan, J., Santschi, E., Zekas, L., Scollay-Ward, M., Radtke, C., Sample, S., Keuler, N. and Muir, P. (2006) Comparison of radiography and computer tomography to evaluate metacarpo/metatarsophalangeal joint pathology of paired limbs of Thoroughbred racehorses with severe condylar fractures. *Vet. Surg.*, **35**, 611–617

Nickels, J.F., Grant, B.D. and Lincoln, S.C. (1975) Villonodular synovitis of the equine metacarpophalangeal joint. *J. Am. Vet. Med. Ass.*, **168**, 1043–1046

Nixon, A. and Pool, R. (1995) Histologic appearance of axial osteochondral fragments from the proximoplantar/proximopalmar aspect of the proximal phalanx. *J. Am. Vet. Med. Ass.*, **207**, 1076–1080

O'Brien, T.R. (1977) Disease of the thoroughbred fetlock joint – a comparison of radiographic signs with gross pathological lesions. *Proc. Am. Ass. Equine Pract.*, **23**, 367–380

O'Brien, T.R., Morgan, J.P., Wheat, J.D. and Suter, P.F. (1971) Sesamoiditis in the thoroughbred: a radiographic study. *J. Am. Vet. Res.*, **12**, 75–87

O'Brien, T.R., Hornhof, W. and Meagher, D. (1981) Radiographic detection and characterisation of palmar lesions in the fetlock joint. *J. Am. Vet. Med. Ass.*, **178**, 231–237

O'Grady, S. (2001) White line disease – an update. *Equine vet. Educ.*, **3**, 66–72

Palmar, S.E. (1982) Radiography of the abaxial surface of the proximal sesamoid bones of the horse. *J. Am. Vet. Ass.*, **181**, 264–265

Poulos, P. (1988) Radiographic and histologic assessment of proximal sesamoid bone changes in young and working horses. *Prox. Am. Ass. Equine Pract.*, **34**, 347–358

Rick, M., O'Brien, T., Pool, R. and Meagher, D. (1983) Condylar fractures of the third metacarpal bone and third metatarsal bone in 75 horses: radiographic features, treatment and outcome. *J. Am. Vet. Med. Ass.*, **183**, 287–296

Riggs, C. (1999) Aetiopathogenesis of parasagittal fractures of the distal condyles of the third metacarpal and third metatarsal bones – review of the literature. *Equine vet. J.*, **31**, 116–121

Riggs, C., Whitehouse, G. and Boyde, A. (1999a) Structural variation of the distal condyles of the third metacarpal bone and third metatarsal bone in the horse. *Equine vet. J.*, **31**, 130–139

Riggs, C., Whitehouse, G. and Boyde, A. (1999b) Pathology of the distal condyles of the third metacarpal bone and third metatarsal bone in the horse. *Equine vet. J.*, **31**, 140–149

Ross, M., Nolan, P., Palmer, J. *et al.* (1991) The importance of the metatarsophalangeal joint in Standardbred lameness. *Proc. Am. Ass. Equine Pract.*, **37**, 741–756

Ross, M. (1998) Scintigraphic and clinical findings in the Standardbred metatarsophalangeal joint: 114 cases (1993–1995). *Equine vet. J.*, **30**, 131–138

Sandgren, B. (1993) Osteochondrosis in the tarsocrural joint and osteochondral fragments in the metacarpo/metatarsophalangeal joints in young Standardbreds. *PhD Thesis*, University of Uppsala, Sweden

Schnabel, L., Bramlage, L., Mohammed, H., Embertson, R., Ruggles, A. and Hopper, S. (2006) Racing performance after arthroscopic removal of apical sesamoid fractures in Thoroughbred horses age ≥2 years: 84 cases (1998–2002). *Equine vet. J.*, **38**, 446–453

Schnabel, L., Bramlage, L., Mohammed, H., Embertson, R., Ruggles, A. and Hopper, S. (2007) Racing performance after arthroscopic removal of apical sesamoid fractures in Thoroughbred horses age <2 years: 151 cases (1998–2002). *Equine vet. J.*, **39**, 64–68

Schleining, J. and Voss, E. (2004) Hypertrophic osteopathy secondary to gastric squamous cell carcinoma in a horse. *Equine vet. Educ.*, **16**, 304–307

Shepherd, M. and Pilsworth, R. (1997) Stress reactions in the plantarolateral condyles of MT III in UK Thoroughbreds: 26 cases. *Proc. Am. Ass. Equine Pract.*, **43**, 128–131

Southwood, L., Trotter, G. & McIlwraith, C. (1998) Arthroscopic removal of abaxial fracture fragments of the proximal sesamoid bone in horses: 47 cases (1989–1997). *J. Am. Vet. Med. Ass.*, **213**, 1016–1021

[186]

Southwood, L. and McIlwraith, C. (2000) Arthroscopic removal of fracture fragments involving a portion of the base of the proximal sesamoid bone in horses: 26 cases (1984–1997). *J. Am. Vet. Med. Ass.*, **217**, 236–240

Spike, D., Bramlage, L., Howard, B. *et al.* (1997) Radiographic proximal sesamoiditis in Thoroughbred sales yearlings. *Proc. Am. Ass. Equine Pract.*, **43**, 132–137

Spike-Pierce, D. and Bramlage, L. (2003) Correlation of racing performance with radiographic changes in the proximal sesamoid bones of 487 Thoroughbred yearlings. *Equine vet. J.*, **35**, 350–353

Spurlock, G. and Gabel, A. (1983) Apical sesamoid fractures in the proximal sesamoid bones in 109 Standardbred horses. *J. Am. Vet. Med. Ass.*, **183**, 76–79

Storgaard, J., Jorgensen, H., Proschowsky, H., Falke-Ronne, J., Willeberg, P. and Hesselholt, M. (1997) The significance of routine radiographic findings with respect to racing performance and longevity in Standardbred trotters. *Equine vet. J.*, **29**, 55–59

Tetens, J., Ross, M. and Lloyd, J. (1997) Comparison of racing performance before and after treatment of incomplete mid-sagittal fractures of the proximal phalanx in Standardbreds. *J. Am. Vet. Med. Ass.*, **210**, 82–86

Thompson, K. and Rooney, J. (1994) Bipartite proximal sesamoid bones in young Thoroughbred horses. *Vet. Radiol. Ultrasound*, **35**, 368–370

Whitton, C. and Kannegeiter, N. (1994) Osteochondral fragmentation of the plantar/palmar proximal aspect of the proximal phalanx in racing horses. *Austr. Vet. J.*, **71**, 318–321

Winberg, F. and Petterson, H. (1994) Diagnosis and treatment of lesions of the intersesamoidean ligament and its adjoining structures. *Vet. Surg.*, **23**, 215

Woodie, J., Ruggles, A., Bertone, A., Hardy, J. and Schneider, R. (1999) Apical fractures of the proximal sesamoid bone in Standardbred horses: 43 cases (1990–1996). *J. Am. Vet. Med. Ass.*, **214**, 1653–1656

Yovich, J., McIlwraith, C. and Stashak, T. (1985) Osteochondrosis dissecans of the sagittal ridge of the third metacarpal and metatarsal bones in horses. *J. Am. Vet. Med. Ass.*, **186**, 1186–1191

Yovich, J. and McIlwraith, C. (1986) Arthroscopic surgery for osteochondral fractures of the proximal phalanx of the metacarpophalangeal and metatarsophalangeal (fetlock) joints in horses. *J. Am. Vet. Med. Ass.*, **188**, 273–279

Zekas, L., Bramlage, L., Embertson, R. and Hance, S. (1999a) Characterisation of the type and location of fractures of the third metacarpal/metatarsal condyles in 135 horses in central Kentucky (1986–1994). *Equine vet. J.*, **31**, 304–308

Zekas, L., Bramlage, L., Embertson, R. and Hance, S. (1999b) Results of treatment of 145 fractures of the third metacarpal/metatarsal condyles in 135 horses in central Kentucky (1986–1994). *Equine vet. J.*, **31**, 309–313

Zubrod, C., Schneider, R., Tucker, R. *et al.* (2004) Use of magnetic resonance imaging for identifying subchondral bone damage in horses: 11 cases (1999–2003). *J. Am. Vet. Med. Ass.*, **224**, 411–418

Chapter 4
The metacarpal and metatarsal regions

Throughout this chapter, although reference is made to the metacarpal region it also applies to the metatarsal region. Significant differences of the metatarsal region are highlighted.

A standard radiographic examination of the metacarpal region comprises lateromedial, dorsopalmar, dorsolateral-palmaromedial oblique and dorsomedial-palmarolateral oblique views. In selected cases dorsoproximal-palmarodistal oblique views may yield valuable additional information about the distal end of the third metacarpal bone (see Chapter 3, page 152). Occasionally a flexed lateromedial view of the proximal metacarpal region is helpful for identifying avulsion fractures at the origin of the suspensory ligament. Special projections for evaluating the proximal sesamoid bones are discussed in Chapter 3 (pages 153–156).

In many instances the clinical examination will suggest which views are necessary and at which level the x-ray beam should be centred. In some cases a complete examination is not required, although many views with only slight differences in angle of projection may be needed (e.g. for evaluation of a dorsal cortical fatigue fracture of the third metacarpal bone). It is difficult to evaluate the entire length of the metacarpal region properly using small (30 cm) cassettes.

RADIOGRAPHIC TECHNIQUE

Lateromedial, dorsopalmar and oblique views

The metacarpal region may be radiographed using a portable x-ray machine and either high-definition or rare earth screens and compatible film. A grid is unnecessary. All the standard projections are ideally obtained with the horse bearing full weight on the limb, with the metacarpal region vertical. The second and fourth metacarpal bones are best evaluated using dorsomedial-palmarolateral oblique and dorsolateral-palmaromedial oblique views, respectively. The x-ray beam is centred on the area of principal interest. In some cases it may be helpful to use a long (43 cm) cassette so that the entire length of the metacarpal region can be seen on a single radiograph, but in an adult horse some obliquity of projection at the extremities of the bones is inevitable (see Figure 4.3, pages 194–195). Therefore it is usually preferable to use more than one projection and create a 'jigsaw' of the length of the bone.

Many of the radiographic abnormalities in this region are subtle and are only visible with correct angulation of the x-ray beam and appropriate

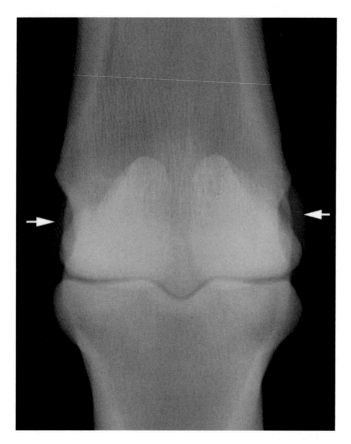

Figure 4.1(a) Horizontal dorsopalmar view of the distal metacarpal region of a normal adult horse. The proximal sesamoid bones are superimposed over the condyles of the third metacarpal bone. Note the curved outline of the medial and lateral aspects of the distal end of the third metacarpal bone (arrows) and the variable opacity in these areas. This may be exaggerated in a slightly oblique projection.

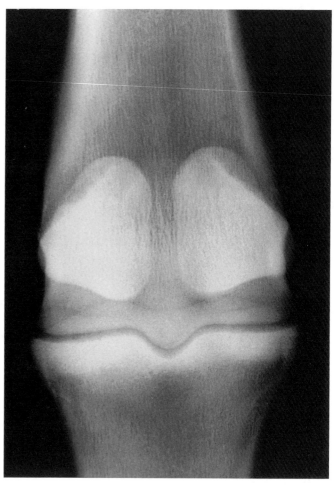

Figure 4.1(b) Dorsal 10° proximal-palmarodistal oblique view of the distal metacarpal region of a normal adult horse. The proximal sesamoid bones are projected proximally giving excellent visualization of the metacarpal condyles.

exposure factors. Fatigue fractures of the dorsal cortex of the third metacarpal bone are readily missed unless multiple oblique views are obtained. Early periosteal proliferative reactions, less opaque than the parent bone (e.g. a 'splint') are easily overexposed. Thus reduced exposure factors should be used. The timing of the radiographic examination is also critical, since many radiographic abnormalities will not be present until at least 7–21 days after the onset of clinical signs. Sequential radiographic examinations may therefore be helpful.

Dorsoproximal-palmarodistal oblique views

In a dorsopalmar view of the distal aspect of the metacarpal region, the proximal sesamoid bones are projected over the distal aspect of the third metacarpal bone (Figure 4.1a) and lesions involving the condyles may easily be missed (e.g. an incomplete vertical condylar fracture). The proximal sesamoid bones are projected further proximally if the x-ray beam is angled proximodistally at least 10°, i.e. a dorsal 10° proximal-palmarodistal oblique

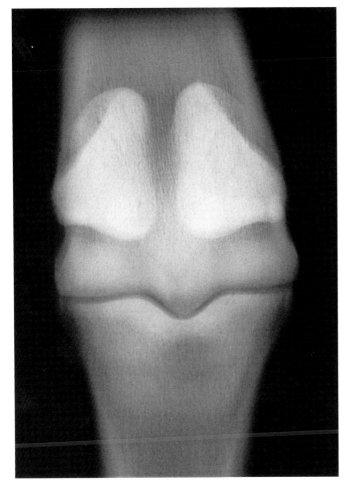

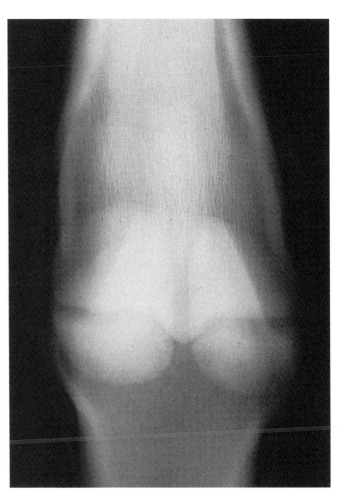

Figure 4.1(c) Dorsopalmar (flexed) view of the distal metacarpal region of a normal adult horse. The proximal sesamoid bones are projected more proximally than in Figure 4.1(b). This view highlights a more distal articular margin of the condyles of the third metacarpal bone.

Figure 4.1(d) Dorsodistal-palmaroproximal oblique view of the distal metacarpal region of a normal adult horse. The proximal sesamoid bones are superimposed over the metacarpophalangeal joint, but this view gives visualization of the palmar aspect of the metacarpal condyles.

(D10°Pr-PaDiO) view (Figure 4.1b). This view is particularly important for the identification of incomplete, vertical articular condylar fractures, although these lesions may still be difficult to detect. Improved visualization may be achieved by flexing the metacarpophalangeal joint. The toe of the foot is placed in the standard navicular block (see page 104), with the metacarpal region vertical. A horizontal x-ray beam is centred on the joint. The cassette is positioned as near perpendicular to the x-ray beam as possible. This view moves the sesamoid bones further proximally (Figure 4.1c). If the x-ray beam is directed dorsodistal-palmaroproximal a more palmar region of the articular surface can be examined.

The palmar articular surface may be assessed better with the limb partially extended with the foot on a flat block (Figure 4.2). The cassette is held approximately parallel to the metacarpal region. The x-ray beam is directed dorsodistal-palmaroproximally in the plane of rotation of the metacarpophalangeal joint, at approximately 125° to the third metacarpal bone. If the limb and the x-ray beam are correctly aligned, between one-quarter and

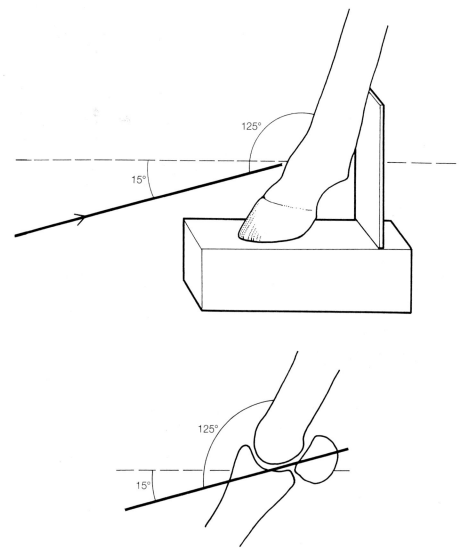

Figure 4.2 Position of the limb, x-ray machine and cassette to obtain a dorsodistal-palmaroproximal oblique view of the distal metacarpal region (see Figure 4.1d).

one-third of the proximal sesamoid bones are projected below the joint space (Figure 4.1d). This view is especially important when evaluating a vertical condylar fracture; comminution of the palmar articular surface of the third metacarpal bone is usually only identifiable in this projection. It is also useful for detecting lucent lesions in the palmar aspect of the third metacarpal bone condyles (see Chapter 3, page 169). Other oblique views of the condyles of the third metacarpal bone and the proximal sesamoid bones are described in detail on pages 151–156.

Other imaging techniques

Nuclear scintigraphy offers a more sensitive method for detection of acute fatigue fractures. Ultrasonography provides a means of evaluating the metacarpal soft-tissue structures. It must be remembered that bony and soft-tissue lesions may occur concurrently and this may have an important bearing on the prognosis (e.g. fractures of the distal one-third of the second or fourth metacarpal bones often occur together with suspensory desmitis).

NORMAL RADIOGRAPHIC ANATOMY: ITS VARIATIONS AND INCIDENTAL FINDINGS

Lateromedial view

The dorsal cortical contour of the third metacarpal bone is usually straight, but that of the third metatarsal bone is relatively convex (Figures 4.3a and 4.3b). The dorsal cortex is thicker than the palmar (plantar) cortex especially on the dorsomedial aspect of the forelimb. The smoothness of the dorsal cortex should always be evaluated carefully under high-intensity illumination or by using the windowing of a digital system. The dorsal cortices of the third metacarpal or metatarsal bones may be unusually convex and thicker than normal as a result of previous trauma, or adaptation to previous work. Small, uniformly opaque, clinically silent osteophytes or entheseophytes are sometimes seen on the dorsoproximal aspect of the third metatarsal bone (see Chapter 7, page 325). The principal nutrient canal is frequently seen in the palmar cortex, at approximately the distal margin of the proximal third of the bone. It may course horizontally, or curve proximally.

Dorsopalmar view

The proximal articular surface of the third metacarpal bone is concave; therefore part of the carpometacarpal joint is superimposed over the third carpal bone (Figure 4.4b, page 197). The subchondral bone plate is a relatively opaque band of uniform thickness. A series of small, circular lucent zones, nutrient foramina, may be seen in the subchondral bone of the proximal aspect of the third metacarpal bone depending on the angle of projection (Figure 4.4b). The proximal and distal quarters of the third metacarpal bone have a relatively coarse, but uniformly opaque trabecular pattern (see Figures 4.1a–c; 4.4b; and 4.17c, page 213). The trabeculae are orientated approximately parallel to the long axis of the bone. In some horses there is a narrow, vertical, more opaque line in the middle of the proximal quarter of the third metacarpal bone, representing a ridge between the heads of the suspensory ligament. This is seen more commonly in hindlimbs. Increased opacity of the proximolateral aspect of the third metatarsal bone may be a response to normal biomechanical loading. The principal nutrient foramen is usually seen as an oval-shaped lucent area superimposed on the medullary cavity, at the junction between the proximal and middle thirds of the bone (Figure 4.4a). Occasionally it may be linear in appearance, or there may be more than one nutrient foramen.

In this view and some oblique projections the second and fourth metacarpal bones are partially superimposed over the third metacarpal bone, and this may result in some confusing lucent lines. These lucent lines (Mach

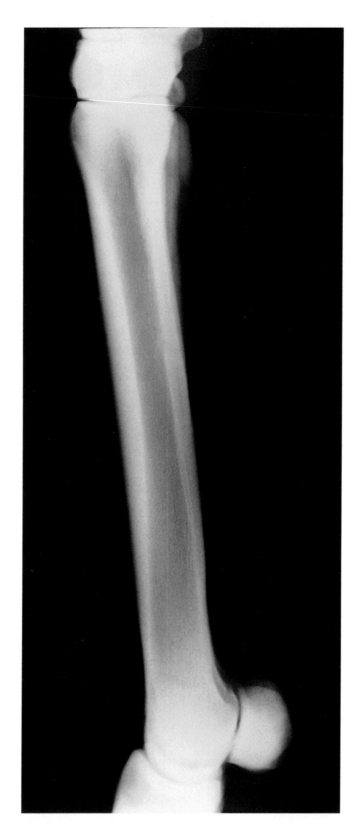

Figure 4.3(a) Lateromedial view of a
normal adult metacarpal region. Note
the obliquity of projection at the distal
end of the bone. To evaluate this area
better, a view centred on this region is
required.

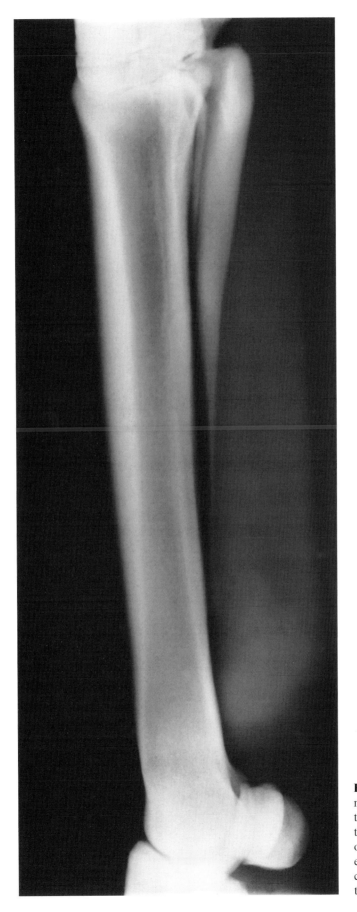

Figure 4.3(b) Lateromedial view of a
normal adult metatarsal region. Due to
the increased length of the bone relative
to the metacarpal region there is greater
obliquity at the proximal and distal
extremities of the bone. Note the slightly
convex contour of the dorsal cortex of
the third metatarsal bone.

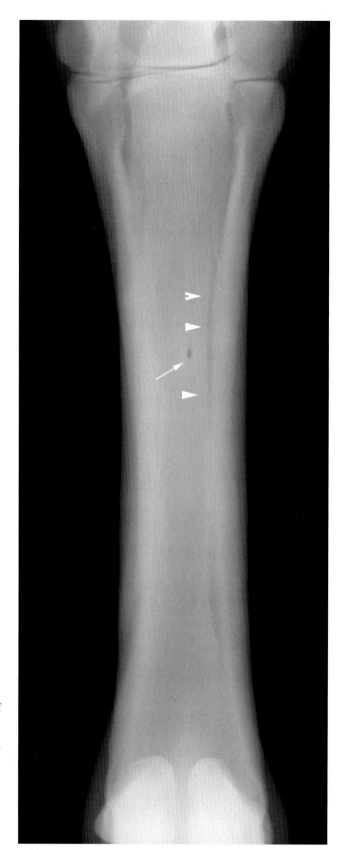

Figure 4.4(a) Dorsopalmar projection of
the metacarpal region of a normal adult
horse. Medial is to the left. Note the
vertical lucent line on the axial aspect of
the fourth metacarpal bone
(arrowheads) created by an edge effect.
The lucent zone in the middle of the
third metacarpal bone (arrow)
represents the principal nutrient
foramen.

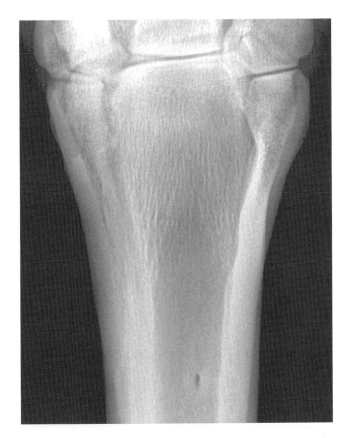

Figure 4.4(b) Dorsopalmar radiographic view of the proximal third of the metacarpal region of a normal adult horse.

lines or bands) are due to edge enhancement, the effect of one bone edge crossing another (Figure 4.5), and should not be confused with fractures. This appearance may be more marked with digital images, where computerized edge enhancement of images may be performed. The second and fourth metacarpal bones are most readily evaluated in the oblique views.

The proximal metacarpal physis is closed at birth. The distal metacarpal physis closes radiographically at approximately 3–6 months of age (Figure 4.6).

The proximal sesamoid bones are superimposed over the distal end of the third metacarpal bone. Their position depends on the angle of projection (see Figures 4.1a–d, pages 190–191). Radiographic features of these bones are discussed in Chapter 3 (page 162).

Dorsolateral-palmaromedial oblique and dorsomedial-palmarolateral oblique views

The dorsolateral-palmaromedial oblique view (Figure 4.7a) highlights the dorsomedial cortex of the third metacarpal bone and the fourth metacarpal bone. The second metacarpal bone is superimposed over the third. The proximal end or base of the fourth metacarpal bone articulates with the fourth carpal bone. The base of the fourth metatarsal bone articulates with the fourth tarsal bone (Figure 4.7b). It may have a prominent plantar

[197]

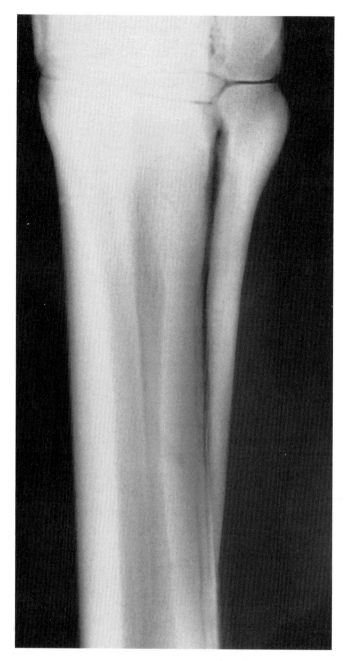

Figure 4.5 Palmarolateral-dorsomedial oblique view of a normal adult metacarpal region. Note the vertical lucent lines on the palmar aspect of the third metacarpal bone which are the result of edge enhancement (Mach lines).

protuberance. Occasionally this protuberance has a small bony spur on its plantar aspect (Figure 4.8) which in the authors' experience is usually of no significance, although it may reflect previous injury.

The dorsomedial-palmarolateral oblique view (Figure 4.9) highlights the dorsolateral cortex of the third metacarpal bone and the second metacarpal bone. The second metacarpal bone articulates with the second and third carpal bones. The second metatarsal bone articulates with the first and second tarsal bones (these are usually fused).

[198]

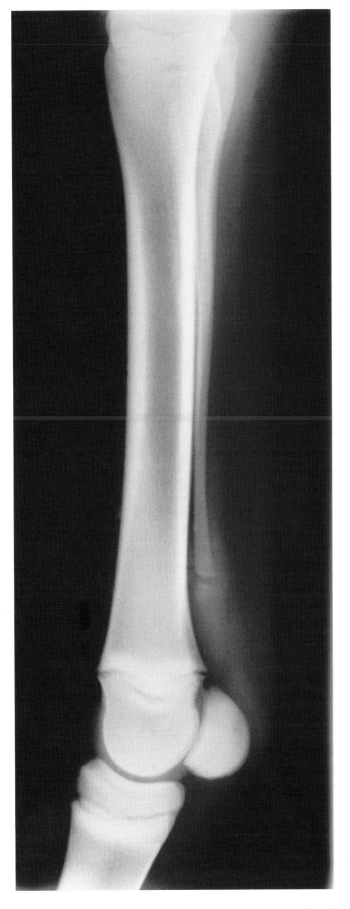

Figure 4.6 Lateromedial view of the
metacarpal region of a normal foal of 8
weeks of age.

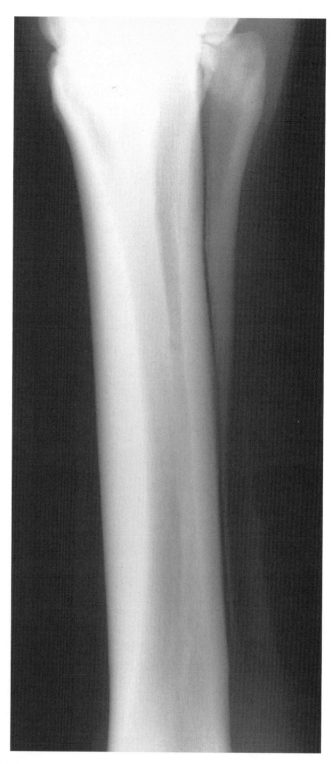

Figure 4.7(a) Dorsolateral-palmaromedial oblique view of a normal adult metacarpal region. The fourth metacarpal bone is highlighted.

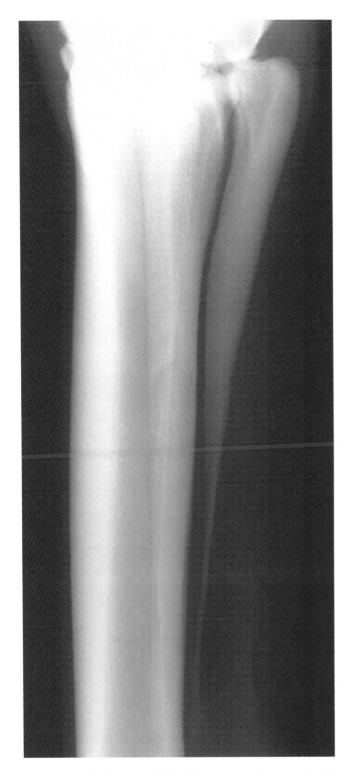

Figure 4.7(b) Dorsolateral-plantaromedial oblique view of a normal adult metatarsal region. The fourth metatarsal bone is highlighted.

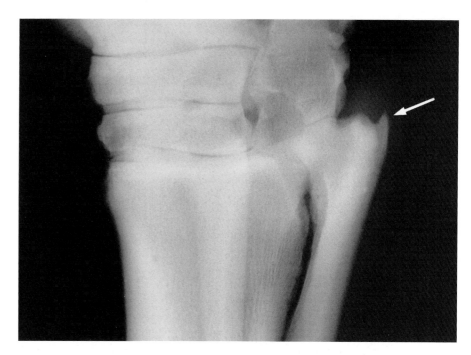

Figure 4.8 Dorsolateral-plantaromedial oblique view of the proximal metatarsal region of a clinically normal adult horse. There is a smoothly outlined bony spur (arrow) on the proximal plantar aspect of the fourth metatarsal bone, of no clinical significance.

The principal nutrient foramen of the third metacarpal bone may be projected as a lucent line across the second or fourth metacarpal bones and should not be confused with a fracture (Figure 4.10). The second and fourth metacarpal bones are relatively straight, but may curve away from the third metacarpal bone distally. There is considerable variation in their length and shape. There is a variably sized and shaped enlargement on the distal ends of the second and fourth metacarpal bones (this is particularly marked, but clinically insignificant, in certain breed lines of the Irish Draught horse); the distal epiphyses are cartilaginous at birth and gradually ossify (Figure 4.6, page 199), but are separate from the body of the bone until approximately 1–9 months of age.

The contour of the second and fourth metacarpal bones is clearly defined, but many horses have smoothly outlined exostoses reflecting previous trauma to the bone (Figure 4.11a). Sometimes there is irregular periosteal new bone with distinct margins; this must not be misinterpreted as an active periosteal reaction (compare Figures 4.11b, page 205 and 4.15, page 208).

In some horses there is a large exostosis on the proximolateral aspect of the third and fourth metatarsal bones (Figure 4.12). This is usually smoothly demarcated and of no clinical significance, despite usually being associated with intense focal increased radiopharmaceutical uptake.

With the correct obliquity of the x-ray beam, and provided that there is no mineralization or ossification of the interosseous ligaments, a lucent space may be seen between the second and third, and fourth and third metacarpal bones. In some horses it may be necessary to obtain several views at slightly different angles in order to evaluate the entire interosseous space. Many horses have some mineralization or ossification of the interosseous ligaments (Figure 4.13). Occasionally ossification is complete. There may be an ill defined lucent zone in the base (head) of the second metacarpal bone. This is usually seen in association with the presence of a first carpal bone (see Figure 5.12b, page 250).

In some horses there is a lucent line in the proximal one-third of either or both of the second and fourth metacarpal bones. This extends distally from the medullary cavity and ends on the dorsal aspect of the bone (Figure 4.14); it represents a nutrient foramen and should not be misinterpreted as a fracture.

SIGNIFICANT RADIOLOGICAL ABNORMALITIES

Periostitis

Periostitis resulting from direct trauma to bone

Direct trauma to any of the metacarpal bones may result in inflammation of the periosteum and/or a subperiosteal haematoma and subsequent periosteal new bone. The smoothness of the margin and the opacity of the new bone help to determine the activity and age of the lesion. New bone is usually not detectable for at least 14 days and appears first as a slightly opaque area in the soft tissues adjacent to the metacarpal bone, with an irregular margin (Figures 4.15a and 4.15b). The new bone becomes progressively more opaque and smoother in outline as it is modelled (see Figures 4.11a and 4.11b, page 205). Trauma to the bone may alternatively be detected ultrasonographically as early as 5 days.

The second and fourth metacarpal bones seem particularly susceptible to production of very irregular new bone. Pillars of relatively opaque bone may be separated by more lucent bone. This palisade-like appearance, which may be due to invasion of the proliferative new bone by some fibrous tissue, may persist when the lesion has become inactive (Figure 4.11b, page 205). The pattern of mineralization can result in a lucent line, or lines, which traverse the periosteal reaction and may mimic a fracture (Figure 4.15b), although a fracture line may indeed be present.

Provided that there is no further trauma to the bone, an active periosteal reaction usually becomes quiescent within 6–12 weeks. A horse with an active periosteal reaction usually resents pressure applied to the lesion but may not be lame; nevertheless, it is likely that the reaction will heal more quickly if the horse is confined to box rest.

Periostitis produced in response to microfractures

Sore shins or 'bucked shins' is a relatively common syndrome in racing Thoroughbreds and Quarter Horses, resulting in localized heat, pain and swelling and a variable degree of lameness.

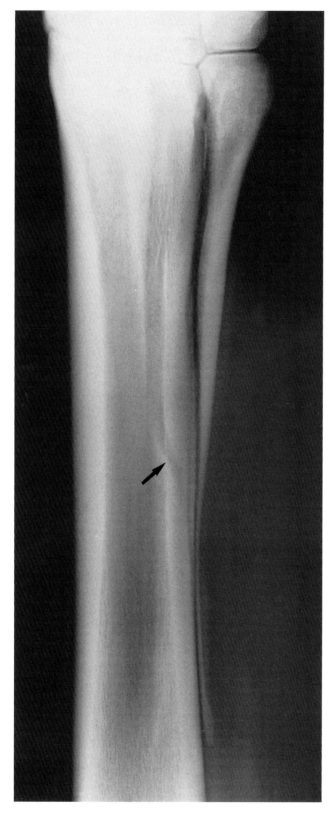

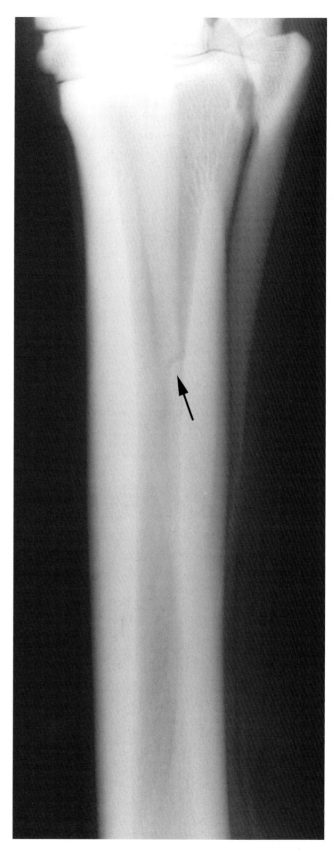

Figure 4.9 Dorsomedial-palmarolateral oblique view of a normal adult metacarpal region. Note the oblique lucent line in the middle of the third metacarpal bone (arrow): this represents the nutrient foramen.

Figure 4.10 Dorsolateral-plantaromedial oblique view of a normal adult metatarsal region. Note the oblique lucent line crossing the second metatarsal bone (arrow). This is the nutrient foramen and should not be confused with a fracture.

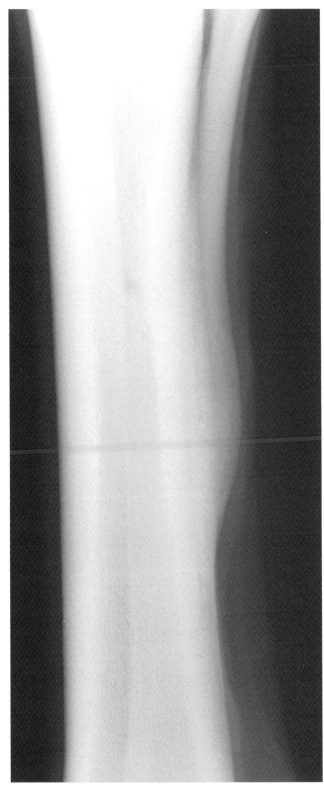

Figure 4.11(a) Dorsomedial-palmarolateral oblique view of an adult metacarpal region. There is a smoothly outlined exostosis on the second metacarpal bone and some mineralization in the interosseous space, of no clinical significance.

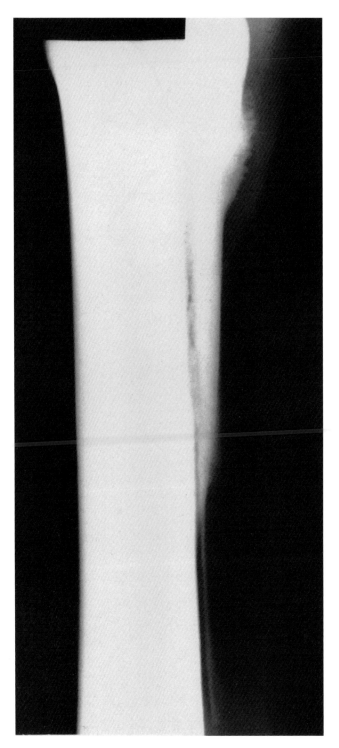

Figure 4.11(b) Dorsomedial-palmarolateral oblique view of an adult metacarpal region. There is irregular periosteal new bone with distinct margins on the proximal aspect of the second metacarpal bone (compare with Figures 4.15a and 4.15b, page 208). Despite the irregularity the margin is distinct, which makes it likely that this change is inactive. There is also smoothly outlined new bone involving the diaphysis and mineralization in the interosseous space. This is inactive and not of current clinical significance.

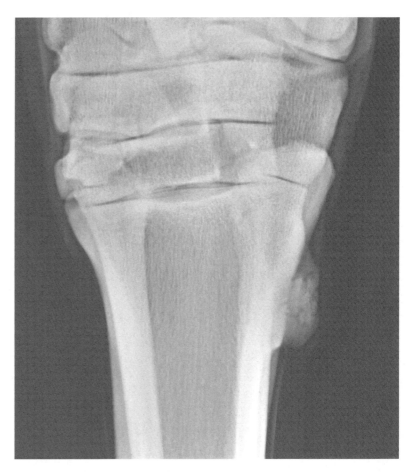

Figure 4.12 Dorsoplantar radiographic view of the proximal metatarsal region of a 9-year-old event horse. There is a smoothly marginated exostosis on the proximolateral aspect of the third metatarsal bone. The interior of the exostosis has a heterogeneous opacity. There is an ill defined oblique radiolucent line in the cortex of the third metatarsal bone. This exostosis was cool and non-painful and not associated with lameness.

Cortical modelling is an adaptive response to increased loading during normal exercise. During training of 2- and 3-year-old horses, cortical modelling is particularly intense and often creates focal areas of porosity in the cortex. Cyclic loading of the immature third metacarpal bone may ultimately result in fatigue microfractures in the middle or distal one-thirds of the dorsal cortex which are not detectable radiographically. They may also be seen occasionally in older horses that have not previously undergone training. Microfractures may result only in periosteal and endosteal reactions, and if the training programme is moderated a fracture may never be detected radiographically. If early clinical signs are overlooked and the horse is kept in training, an overt, radiographically detectable fracture may result. Alternatively acute fractures do occur without any preceding periosteal reaction.

When clinical signs are first recognized, high-quality radiographs are essential to identify radiographic abnormalities. Nuclear scintigraphy dem-

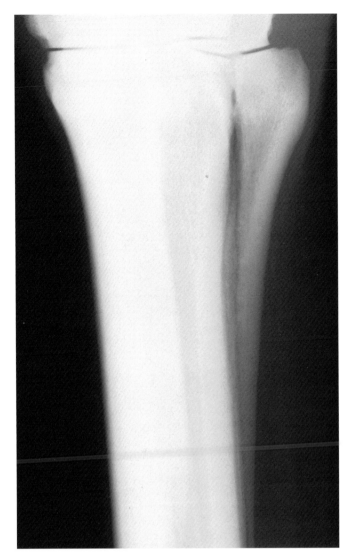

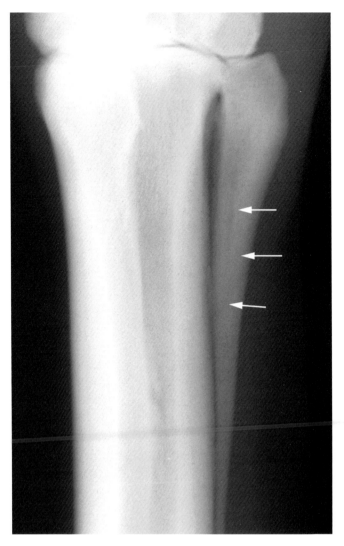

Figure 4.13 Dorsolateral-palmaromedial oblique view of an adult metacarpal region. There is mineralization between the third and fourth metacarpal bones of no clinical significance.

Figure 4.14 Dorsolateral-palmaromedial oblique view of a normal adult metacarpal region. There is a lucent line (arrows) in the proximal one-third of the fourth metacarpal bone which represents a nutrient foramen.

onstrates focal increased uptake of technetium-99m (^{99m}Tc). Intracortical fissures or indistinct lucent areas in the dorsal cortex are sometimes demonstrable, with or without localized periostitis and an endosteal reaction. Periostitis is not detectable using plain radiography until at least 2 weeks after the onset of the clinical signs.

Using high-quality radiographic technique and multiple oblique views it may be possible to detect small fractures in the dorsal cortex of the bone. Most fractures traverse distoproximally at an angle of approximately 30° to the long axis of the bone and end at the junction of the middle and inner one-thirds of the cortex (Figures 4.16a and 4.16b). Some fractures extend to form a complete semi-circle or 'saucer'; occasionally only the proximal half of the saucer can be seen. Multiple fractures sometimes occur.

[207]

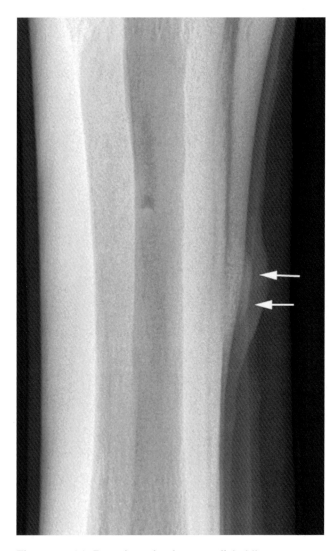

Figure 4.15(a) Dorsolateral-palmaromedial oblique radiographic view of the mid metacarpal region of a 6-year-old event horse. There is soft tissue swelling overlying an ill defined exostosis (arrows) on the abaxial aspect of the fourth metacarpal bone. There was focal pain on pressure over this area and mild lameness.

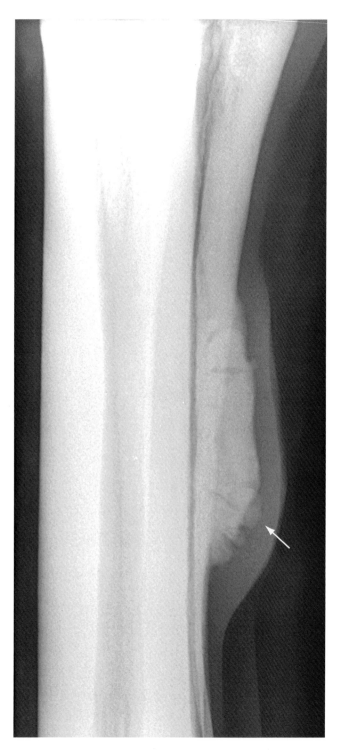

Figure 4.15(b) Dorsomedial-palmarolateral oblique radiographic view of the metacarpal region of an 8-year-old Warmblood with mild lameness evident only on a circle. There is soft-tissue swelling overlying a large generally well defined old exostosis involving the diaphysis of the second metacarpal bone. Within the exostosis are relatively lucent lines. These are the result of new bone formation and should not be confused with fractures. On the distal palmar aspect of the exostosis there is less well defined active periosteal new bone (arrow).

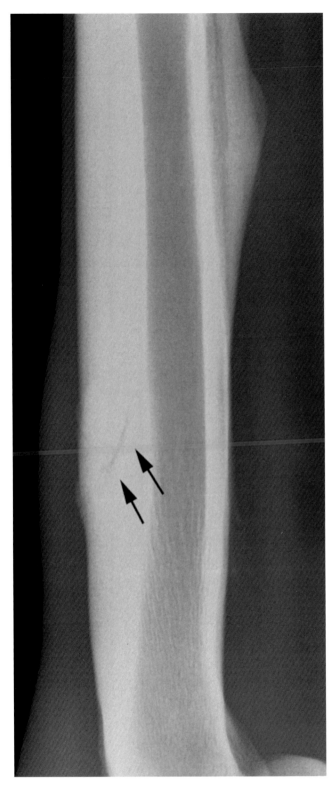

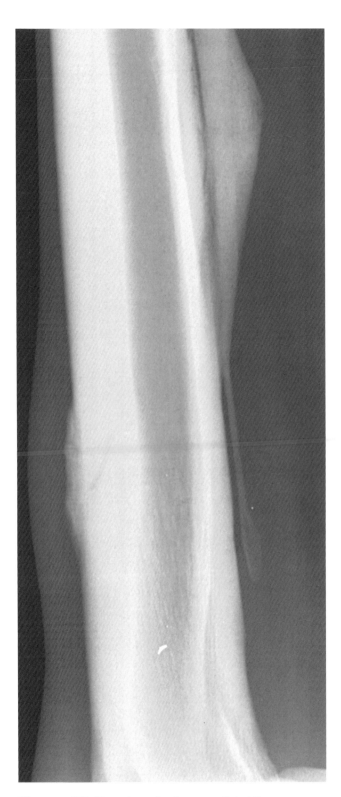

Figure 4.16(a) Lateromedial radiographic view of the metacarpal region of a 3-year-old Thoroughbred flat racehorse. There is an oblique radiolucent line in the dorsal cortex of the third metacarpal bone (arrows), a dorsal cortical stress fracture. There is subtle periosteal and endosteal new bone at the same level and overlying soft tissue swelling. Note also the smoothly marginated exostosis involving the diaphyseal region of the fourth metacarpal bone. See also Figure 4.16(b).

Figure 4.16(b) Dorsolateral-palmaromedial oblique radiographic view of the metacarpal region of the same limb as in Figure 4.16(a). In this view much more extensive periosteal new bone can be seen in the region of the incomplete dorsal cortical fracture of the third metacarpal bone.

Rest results in resolution of clinical signs, but follow-up radiography or nuclear scintigraphy is important to monitor bone healing. Some fractures heal satisfactorily within 8–12 weeks and training can be resumed, but in some horses there appears to be minimal change in the radiographic appearance of the fracture and, in selected cases, surgical intervention may be necessary. In order to monitor healing it is very important to obtain identical radiographic views to those that initially demonstrated the lesion best.

Periostitis between the second and third or fourth and third metacarpal bones (splints)

Periostitis between the second and third or fourth and third metacarpal bones develops secondary to damage of the interosseous ligament. The reaction, which is of variable size, usually involves the proximal half of the second or fourth metacarpal bones. Splints develop most frequently between the second and third metacarpal bones in the forelimb and the fourth and third metatarsal bones in the hindlimb. Several oblique views may be necessary in order to evaluate the interosseous space properly.

The condition occurs most commonly in young horses when regular work commences, but is also seen in older horses. There may be associated lameness, deteriorating with work. Careful palpation reveals a localized area of pain. If the metacarpal region is set lateral relative to the central axis of the antebrachium and carpus, or there is an angular limb deformity, the horse is particularly prone to the development of both ossification between the second and third metacarpal bones, and new bone on the medial aspect of the second metacarpal bone, as the bones model according to Wolff's law. This often develops without associated lameness. New bone formation may also occur suddenly in older horses without lameness.

In an early lesion there is some slightly opaque bone between the two metacarpal bones and cortical bone remodelling may be detectable. With time the periosteal new bone becomes more opaque and will eventually look solid. The amount of periosteal new bone produced is extremely variable and sometimes an active bony reaction may mimic a fracture with associated callus. It is not possible to differentiate radiographically between this condition and periostitis developing secondary to direct trauma. With rest the active bone reaction usually settles within 6 weeks, but can take several months. The new bone may model once it is no longer active. Lameness will recur if work is resumed when the periosteal reaction is still active.

Occasionally, if extensive new bone develops on the axial surface of the second or fourth metacarpal bones, this may result in associated suspensory ligament desmitis and adhesion formation. The significance of the new bone must be assessed in the light of clinical signs and ultrasonographic examination. Surgical treatment is usually necessary. Occasionally magnetic resonance imaging may also be helpful if the results of ultrasonography are equivocal.

Syndesmopathy, inflammation of the interosseous ligament between the third and second or fourth metacarpal/metatarsal bones, occasionally occurs but magnetic resonance imaging is usually required to confirm diagnosis.

Endosteal reaction and entheseophyte formation in the area of attachment of the suspensory ligament

The suspensory ligament originates from the proximal palmar aspect of the third metacarpal bone. Tearing of the attachment may result in entheseophyte formation (periostitis), due to subperiosteal haematoma formation, or endosteal new bone formation. Radiographic examination may reveal a localized area of increased opacity in the proximal aspect of the bone with or without small patchy lucent zones. In the early stages this is seen only in high-quality dorsopalmar views (Figures 4.17a–d), and comparison with the contralateral limb is often helpful. Endosteal new bone is seen as a region of increased opacity of the palmar subcortical bone in a true lateromedial view (see below). The presence of radiographic abnormalities associated with proximal suspensory desmitis is seen more commonly in hindlimbs than forelimbs and is usually a sign of chronicity. However, increased opacity of the proximal third metatarsal bone may be seen as an incidental finding in dorsoplantar projections and is not necessarily synonymous with active desmitis. In the forelimb the lesions predominantly involve the medial half of the third metacarpal bone, whereas in the hindlimb the lateral half of the third metatarsal bone is more frequently involved. In dorsopalmar views it is difficult to differentiate between endosteal and periosteal new bone; ultrasonography can be a more sensitive way of detecting entheseous new bone.

If entheseophyte formation is extensive it may also be seen in a lateromedial view as an area of increased opacity superimposed over the second or fourth metacarpal bones.

Fatigue (stress) fractures of the palmar cortex of the third metacarpal bone can result in increased opacity of the proximomedial aspect of the third metacarpal bone and a lucent vertical or oblique line or lines may be detectable (Figure 4.26, page 225). The opaque region may extend further distally compared with that associated with proximal suspensory desmitis and abnormalities are usually not detectable on a lateromedial projection.

Increased opacity seen in a dorsopalmar view may also be due to sclerosis of the trabeculae, which may be seen in the subcortical bone in a lateromedial view, i.e. endosteal new bone (Figure 4.17b). The trabeculae may be orientated more obliquely than usual. The suspensory ligament *per se* should be evaluated ultrasonographically. Nuclear scintigraphy may also be helpful to determine the degree of bony activity. In some horses injury appears to be principally entheseous, with little or no detectable abnormality of the suspensory ligament itself. There may be focal increased radiopharmaceutical uptake, or signal alterations in the third metacarpal bone at its insertion seen on magnetic resonance images, but no detectable radiographic abnormality. Severe trauma may result in an avulsion fracture of

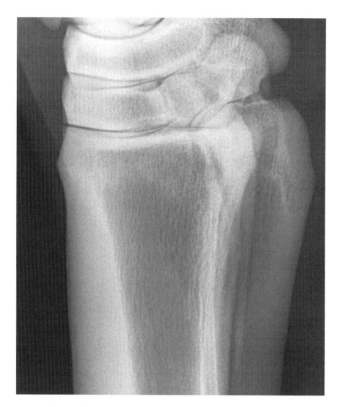

Figure 4.17(a) Lateromedial radiographic view of the proximal metatarsal region of a normal adult horse. Note the regular, linear orientation of the trabeculae and the definition between the cortical and medullary bone.

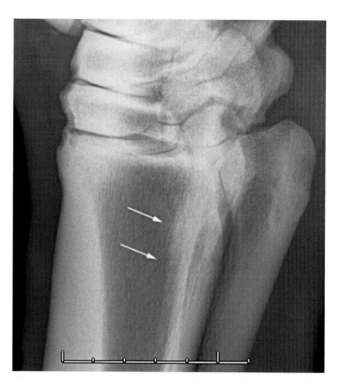

Figure 4.17(b) Lateromedial radiographic view of the proximal metatarsal region of a 6-year-old Thoroughbred event horse with chronic proximal suspensory desmitis. There is endosteal new bone on the proximoplantar aspect of the third metatarsal bone (arrows). Note also the small osteophyte on the dorsoproximal aspect of the third metatarsal bone.

the origin of the suspensory ligament from the third metacarpal bone (see page 221).

Periosteal new bone on the proximal third of the second or fourth metacarpal bones

Extensive palisading periosteal new bone involving the base and proximal metaphyseal region of the second or fourth metacarpal bones can be seen in association with localized narrowing of the carpometacarpal joint (Figure 4.18). It is usually associated with chronic lameness.

Infectious osteitis and osteomyelitis

The third metacarpal bone is only protected by a thin layer of soft tissues and is therefore susceptible to infection following severe skin wounds and trauma to the bone. An open fracture of any of the metacarpal bones may also result in infection. The thick dorsal cortex of the diaphysis of the third metacarpal bone may predispose it to sequestrum formation in its outer one-third, since trauma to the bone may deprive it of its periosteal

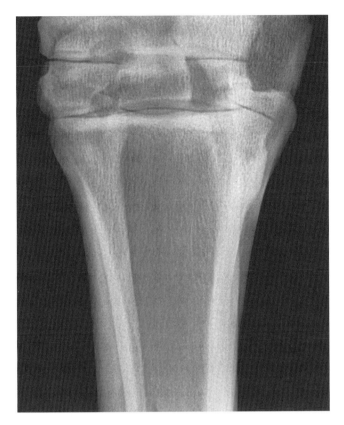

Figure 4.17(c) Dorsoplantar radiographic view of the proximal metatarsal region of a normal adult horse. Note the regular linear orientation of the trabeculae and the clear definition between the proximal subchondral bone plate and the medulla.

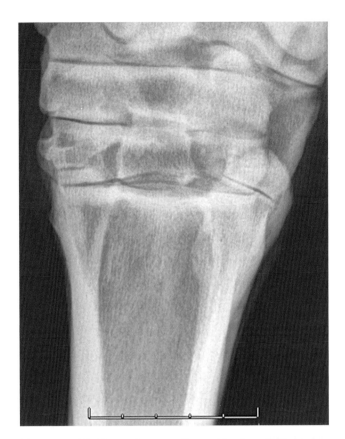

Figure 4.17(d) Dorsoplantar radiographic view of the proximal metatarsal region of a 6-year-old Thoroughbred event horse with chronic proximal suspensory desmitis. There are generalized patchy areas of increased opacity over the proximal aspect of the third metatarsal bone. The apparent narrowing of the lateral aspect of the centrodistal joint space is an artefact.

blood supply and leave it dependent on medullary vessels traversing the cortex.

Radiographic signs of osteitis are not detectable until at least 7–14 days after the injury when subtle lucent areas may be seen in the cortex. These may be restricted to lucent lines parallel to the margin of the bone, in the outer one-third of the cortex, followed by the development of periosteal reaction and more diffuse areas of reduced opacity in the cortex (Figure 4.19a). Earlier diagnosis of infectious osteitis is possible using ultrasonography. In most cases this progresses to sequestrum formation; a central opaque piece of bone (the sequestrum) is surrounded by a lucent zone (purulent material or granulation tissue) which in turn is bordered by more sclerotic bone (the involucrum) (Figures 4.19b and 4.19c). Periostitis may develop proximal and distal to the sequestrum but does not involve the sequestrum itself. Although antibiotic therapy may control clinical signs, removal of the sequestrum is usually required for complete recovery.

[213]

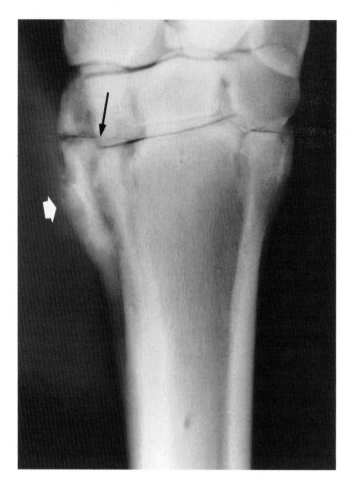

Figure 4.18 Dorsopalmar view of the proximal metacarpal region of an aged pleasure horse, with lameness associated with pain in this area. There is narrowing of the carpometacarpal joint medially (black arrow) with ill defined lucent areas in the adjacent subchondral bone. There is irregularly outlined new bone (white arrow) on the abaxial aspect of the second metacarpal bone.

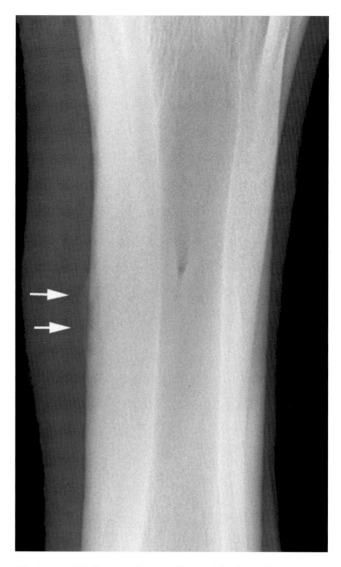

Figure 4.19(a) Dorsopalmar radiographic view of a metacarpal region of an 11-year-old Draught cross which had been kicked 1 month previously. There was a discharging wound on the medial aspect of the mid metacarpal region. Medial is to the left. There is ill defined periosteal new bone on the medial aspect of the diaphysis of the third metacarpal bone (arrows); a lucent line can be seen between this new bone and the third metacarpal bone and there are ill defined lucent areas in the cortex of the third metacarpal bones. This is early infectious osteitis.

Angular limb deformities originating in the diaphysis of the third metacarpal or metatarsal bone

This is a rare condition, which may be congenital. The abnormal limb angulation is noted clinically, but the site of deformity is confirmed radiographically. The limb deviation usually originates in the proximal one-third of the third metacarpal or metatarsal bone. There may be cortical thickening on the concave side of the bone. To correct the condition wedge osteotomy

[214]

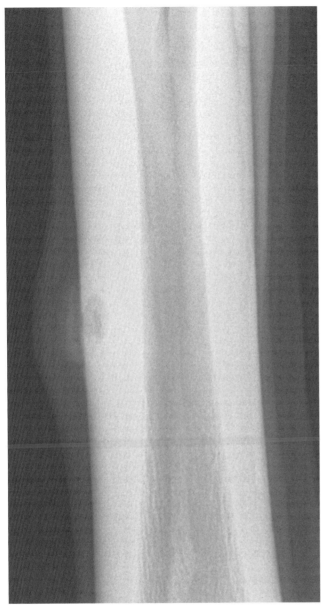

Figure 4.19(b) Dorsolateral-palmaromedial oblique radiographic view of a metacarpal region of a 5-year-old crossbred horse which had been kicked 2 months previously. There is soft-tissue swelling overlying ill defined periosteal new bone. In the cortex of the third metacarpal bone there is an oval-shaped radiolucent area with a central area of further reduced opacity. This is a sequestrum.

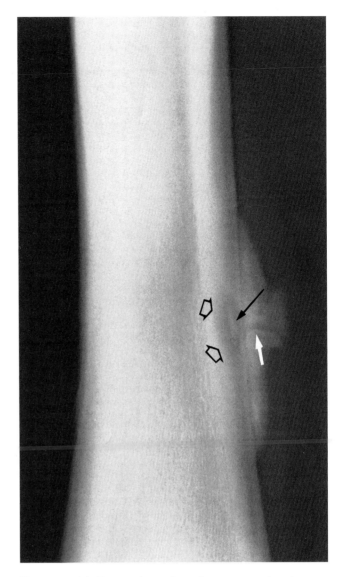

Figure 4.19(c) Dorsopalmar view of a metacarpal region. There is a sequestrum (filled black arrow) and involucrum (open arrows), and extensive periosteal new bone formation with a lucent cloaca (white arrow) and overlying soft-tissue swelling.

may be considered. A deformity of the distal aspect of the third metatarsal bone occurs occasionally, in which the bone describes a smooth 'bend', either laterally or medially. Treatment must be instituted as early as possible, using corrective trimming and shoe extensions. The limb may remodel adequately as it grows if sufficiently aggressive treatment is started early enough in life.

[215]

Physitis of the third metacarpal bone

Physitis (physeal dysplasia) of the distal physis of the third metacarpal bone may result in enlargement of the bone and an angular limb deformity of the metacarpophalangeal joint. Radiographically the metaphysis of the bone is broadened and asymmetrical. There is sclerosis of the metaphysis adjacent to the physis, which may be more irregular in appearance than normal, with narrow vertical radiolucent lines or conical areas representing retained cartilage cones. The cortices of the bone may be abnormally thick. The epiphysis may appear wedge shaped. Surgical correction of the deviation may be needed, and should be performed before 8 weeks of age, despite the 'open' radiographic appearance of the physis.

Mineralization in the soft tissues

Dystrophic mineralization may occur in the soft tissues, particularly in the suspensory ligament or the digital flexor tendons, as the result of trauma or injection of a medicament. This may or may not be of clinical significance. A thorough clinical appraisal of the structure involved and ultrasonographic examination are indicated.

Hypertrophic osteopathy

Shifting limb lameness associated with variable oedematous swelling of a limb or limbs is the most common clinical feature of hypertrophic osteopathy (Marie's disease) (see Chapter 1, page 22). Careful palpation of the metaphyses and diaphyses of the bones may reveal unusual heat and tenderness. Radiographically the disease is typified by periosteal new bone, which often appears active and extends along the metaphyses and diaphyses (Figure 4.20). The third metacarpal and metatarsal bones are frequently involved. The periosteal reaction must be differentiated from other causes of periostitis and osteitis. Thoracic or abdominal opacities may or may not be detectable.

Fractures

Third metacarpal bone

FRACTURES OF THE DISTAL PHYSIS

Fractures of the distal physes of the third metacarpal and metatarsal bones in foal are not uncommon and usually have a Salter-Harris type II configuration (see Chapter 1, page 25). Internal fixation is probably the treatment of choice and, provided that the foal is not less than 8 weeks of age, the longitudinal growth of the bone should not be compromised. Immobilization of the limb in a full-limb cast has been successful in some cases.

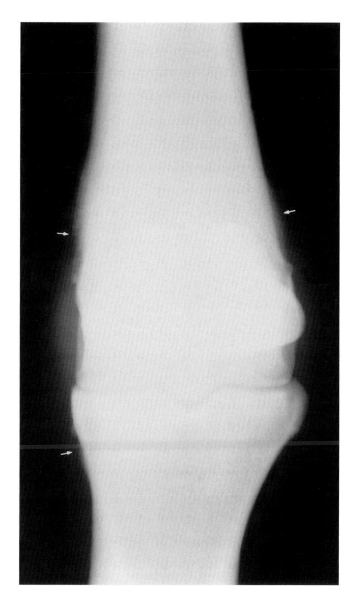

Figure 4.20 Slightly oblique dorsopalmar view of the metacarpal region and proximal phalanx of a 3-year-old Thoroughbred colt with hypertrophic osteopathy. There is extensive ill defined, active periosteal new bone along the distal diaphysis and metaphysis of the third metacarpal bone and the proximal metaphysis of the proximal phalanx (arrows). The primary lesion was an aortic aneurysm (identified *post mortem*). The radiograph was deliberately underexposed to demonstrate this new bone formation.

FATIGUE FRACTURES OF THE DORSAL CORTEX ('SAUCER' FRACTURES)

Fatigue fractures of the dorsal cortex have been discussed previously (pages 203–208).

CONDYLAR FRACTURES

Fracture of either the medial or, more commonly, the lateral condyle is a common injury in racehorses (Thoroughbreds, Standardbreds and Quarter

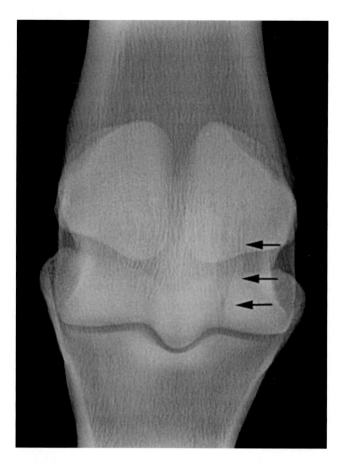

Figure 4.21 Flexed dorsopalmar radiographic view of the metacarpophalangeal joint of a 3-year-old Thoroughbred flat racehorse. Medial is to the left. There is an incomplete lateral condylar fracture of the third metacarpal bone (arrows). The fracture could not be seen in other views. Ideally a dorsodistal-palmaroproximal oblique view is also required to evaluate better the articular surface to establish whether or not there is comminution.

Horses). There is usually distension of the metacarpophalangeal joint capsule, pain on flexion of the joint, and moderate to severe lameness. If the fracture is incomplete the lameness may resolve temporarily following rest. The fractures either occur adjacent to the sagittal ridge (Figure 4.21) or in the mid-condyles (see Figure 4.23, page 220) and may be incomplete with minimal displacement. Some of these fractures extend longitudinally through the diaphysis. Many fractures are complete and 'break out' through the cortex approximately 5–8 cm proximal to the articular surface. Any fracture extending longer than 7.5 cm is likely to be complete. In both the forelimbs and the hindlimbs the lateral condyle is most commonly involved (Figure 4.21). Medial condylar fractures are more often incomplete and extend into the diaphysis, especially in hindlimbs (Figures 4.22a and 4.22b).

If the fracture is incomplete it is very important to examine the entire metacarpal region. All the standard views should be used, and extra oblique views at 5° increments may be necessary to establish whether the fracture

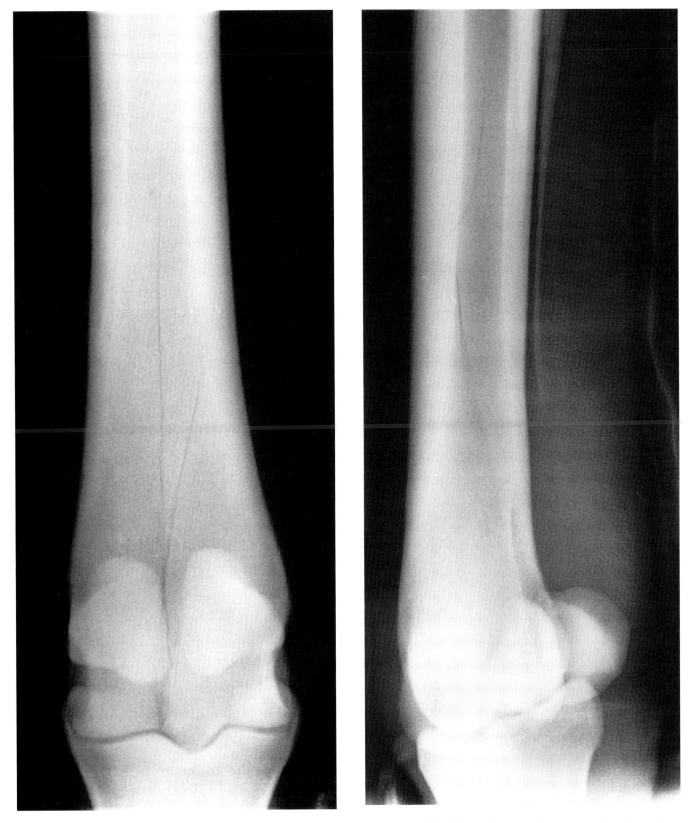

Figure 4.22 Dorsoplantar (lateral to the right) (a) and plantarolateral-dorsomedial oblique (b) views of a metatarsal region of a 4-year-old Thoroughbred. There is an incomplete medial condylar fracture which spirals proximally in the diaphysis. The limb is in a cast incorporating the foot, extending to the hock.

extends into the diaphysis. Even with radiographs of excellent quality it may not be possible to identify all the components of the fracture. A dorsodistal-palmaroproximal oblique view to examine the palmar articular surface is important to identify comminution, which cannot be detected in standard views. The proximal sesamoid bones should also be inspected carefully since occasionally they suffer concurrent fractures. Computed tomography may give more information than radiography. Some incomplete, non-displaced fractures are extremely difficult to detect radiographically in the acute stage, and nuclear scintigraphy may be useful to confirm the results of trauma to bone. Follow-up radiographs obtained after 7–10 days may demonstrate the fracture. Simple, non-displaced fractures may be successfully treated by lag screw fixation or, in selected cases, immobilization in a cast and box rest. Displaced fractures require reduction and internal fixation. The presence

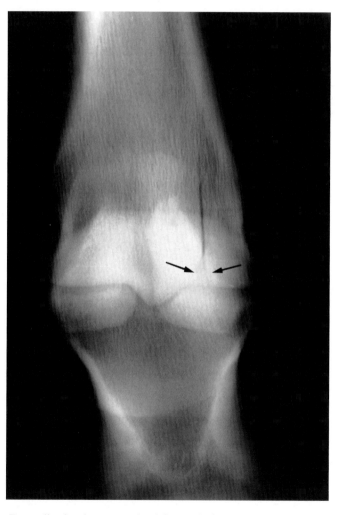

Figure 4.23 Dorsodistal-palmaroproximal (extended) oblique view of the metacarpophalangeal joint of a 5-year-old Thoroughbred racehorse with acute onset forelimb lameness of 2 weeks' duration. Lateral is to the right. There is a fracture of the lateral condyle of the third metacarpal bone. Note the Y-shaped comminution (arrows) at the articular surface. This is not visible in standard projections.

of Y-shaped fragments at the articular surface (Figure 4.23) is associated with a poorer prognosis. Long-term persistence of a radiographically detectable lucent fracture line is associated with reduced performance, compared with horses in which the fracture line disappears.

METAPHYSEAL AND DIAPHYSEAL FRACTURES

Incomplete transverse fractures through the palmar or dorsal aspect of the distal diaphysis or metaphysis occur occasionally and may be bilateral (Figure 4.24a–d). They are associated with moderate to severe lameness and pain can be induced by applying pressure on the palmar or dorsal cortex. These fractures, which are usually incomplete, are best seen in lateromedial and oblique projections. A lucent line traverses the bone horizontally from either the palmar or the dorsal cortex. Within 7–10 days some callus may be identified at the site where the fracture passes through the cortex. These fractures heal satisfactorily with rest.

Fractures of the diaphysis of the third metacarpal bone usually occur in transverse, spiral or comminuted configurations and are often compound. Clinical signs include severe lameness, readily detectable crepitus and possibly swelling of the fetlock joint, but in some cases non-displaced fractures may be very difficult to detect clinically. Radiography is used to confirm the orientation of the fractures. Many oblique views may be needed to follow the complete course of the fracture(s). The radiographs should be inspected carefully to establish whether involvement of the nutrient foramen has occurred, as this will adversely influence the prognosis. Internal fixation using dynamic compression plates and lag screws may result in complete recovery.

Incomplete oblique sagittal dorsal cortical fractures occur occasionally in young Thoroughbred racehorses. These fractures are orientated in a proximolateral-distomedial direction, within the dorsal cortex, at an angle of 20–30° to the long axis of the bone. They are best identified in palmar-odorsal views.

Avulsion fractures of the origin of the suspensory ligament cause a variable degree of lameness that may be relieved by subcarpal local analgesia. Similar fractures may occur slightly distal to the site of attachment of the suspensory ligament; the aetiology of these is unknown. Radiographically these fractures are identified as lucent crescent-shaped lesions in the metaphysis seen in a dorsopalmar view, or as a 'punched-out' radiopacity (Figure 4.25) or separate bone fragments on the palmar aspect, in a lateromedial or a flexed lateromedial projection. They occur in both the forelimb and the hindlimb. Ultrasonography may be more sensitive in identifying some small avulsed fragments and is helpful to determine the presence of concurrent suspensory desmitis. Lameness usually resolves satisfactorily with rest, although in racing trotters the prognosis with rest alone is less favourable and surgery may be required.

Similar clinical signs may be associated with fatigue fractures of the palmar cortex of the proximal one-third of the third metacarpal bone. In a

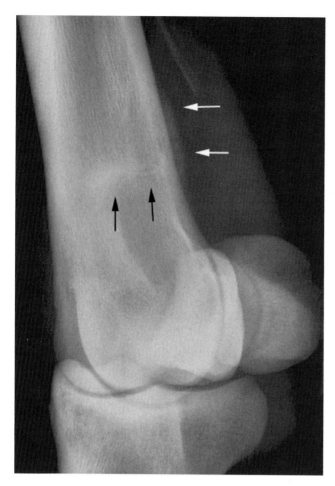

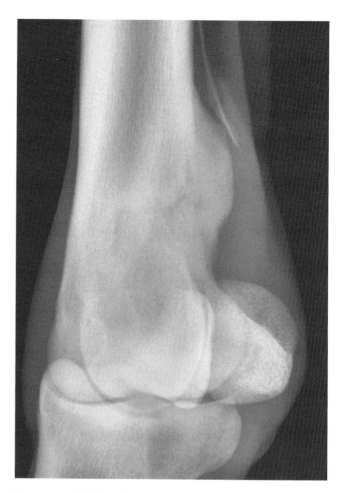

Figure 4.24(a) Dorsolateral-palmaromedial oblique radiographic view of the distal metacarpal region of a 4-year-old polo pony with acute onset of moderate lameness of 2 weeks' duration and considerable swelling in the distal metacarpal and fetlock regions, but no joint effusion. There is extensive periosteal new bone on the palmarolateral-distal diaphyseal and proximal metaphyseal regions of the third metacarpal bone (white arrows). Note also the horizontal line of increased opacity traversing the third metacarpal bone (black arrows). This was an incomplete horizontal fracture of the palmar aspect of the third metacarpal bone. The distal aspect of the fourth metacarpal bone is distorted because of the soft-tissue swelling. Compare with Figures 4.24(b) to 4.24(d).

Figure 4.24(b) Dorsolateral-palmaromedial oblique radiographic views of the same limb as in Figure 4.24(a), obtained 5 weeks later. There is very well consolidated callus and a more obvious radiolucent line traversing the metaphyseal region of the third metacarpal bone. There is slight modelling of the distorted distal aspect of the fourth metacarpal bone.

dorsopalmar view these are evident radiographically as subtle vertical lucent lines (the fracture seen 'end-on') in the metaphyseal region, sometimes extending distally into the diaphysis, usually with surrounding sclerosis of the trabecular bone (Figure 4.26). Fatigue fractures occur most often in the medial half of the third metacarpal bone. Sometimes no fracture line is detectable, only medullary sclerosis. This is particularly so in the less lame limb of a bilaterally lame horse. Development of sclerosis, the result of micro-fractures, may precede the onset of lameness. Less commonly the

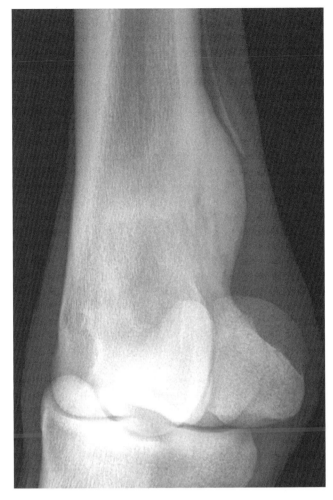

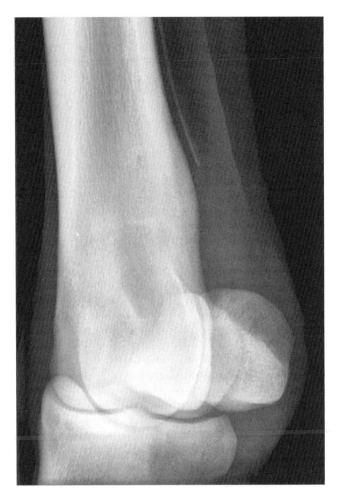

Figure 4.24(c) Dorsolateral-palmaromedial oblique radiographic view of the same limbs as Figures 4.24(a and b), obtained 4½ months after the onset of lameness. There has been further modelling of the callus. An ill defined horizontal radiopaque line is seen in the metaphyseal region of the third metacarpal bone.

Figure 4.24(d) Dorsolateral-palmaromedial oblique radiographic view of the same limb as Figures 4.24a, b and c, 13 months after initial injury. There has been remarkable modelling of the callus and the distal aspect of the fourth metacarpal bone. A faint linear horizontal radiopaque line persists in the third metacarpal bone at the fracture site.

fracture is seen only in an oblique view, although increased opacity is seen on a dorsopalmar projection. Increased opacity should be differentiated from that associated with chronic proximal suspensory desmitis (see page 211). Nuclear scintigraphy enables earlier detection of these fractures and may also aid interpretation of subtle alterations in the trabecular pattern of the bone. It also permits detection of some fractures that never become radiographically apparent. Scintigraphy may also provide a more accurate indicator of healing than radiography. Lameness usually resolves satisfactorily with rest (3 months).

Articular fractures of the dorsoproximal medial aspect of the third meta-carpal bone have been identified in Standardbred racehorses (pacers). These fractures are best identified in a dorsolateral-palmaromedial

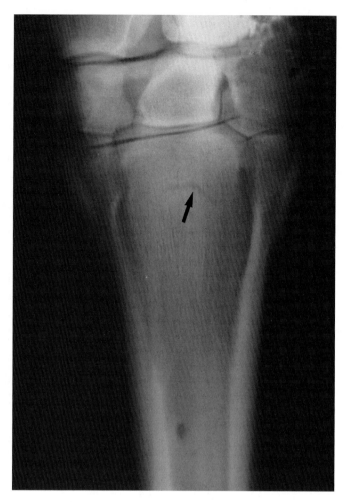

Figure 4.25 Dorsopalmar view of a metacarpal region of a 6-year-old steeplechaser with sudden onset of lameness 12 days previously. Lameness was alleviated by subcarpal analgesia. There is a curved lucent line in the third metacarpal bone (arrow) which probably represents an incomplete avulsion fracture of the origin of the suspensory ligament. The horse was treated conservatively and made a complete recovery.

oblique projection. Satisfactory healing usually occurs with conservative management.

Third metatarsal bone

Incomplete articular fractures of the dorsoproximal aspect of the third metatarsal bone have been seen in association with osteophyte formation on the dorsal aspect of the tarsometatarsal joint in young Thoroughbred racehorses and occasionally in older performance horses. These fractures are difficult to identify radiographically unless the x-ray beam passes through the fracture plane. They are usually best seen in a projection that superimposes the lateral and medial trochlea tali. Similar complete fractures have

[224]

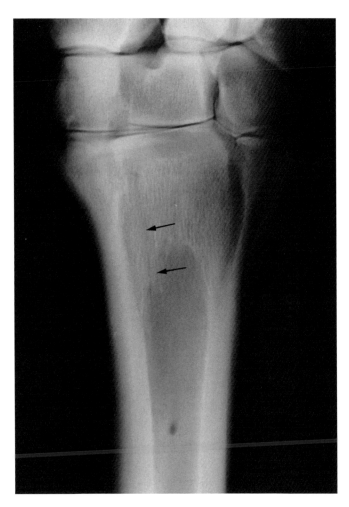

Figure 4.26 Dorsopalmar view of a
metacarpal region of a 5-year-old
hurdler with recurrent lameness of
several weeks' duration. Lameness was
alleviated by subcarpal analgesia. There
is an ill defined approximately vertical
lucent line (arrows) in the medial half of
the third metacarpal bone with
surrounding sclerosis of the trabecular
bone. This is a palmar cortical fatigue
fracture. The horse was treated
conservatively and made a complete
recovery.

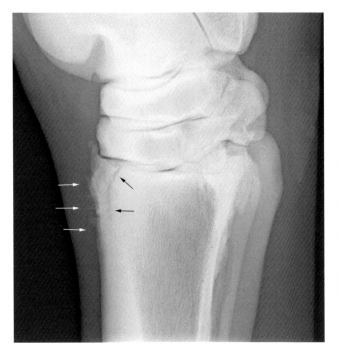

Figure 4.27 Lateral 10° plantar-
dorsomedial oblique radiographic view
of the hock and proximal metatarsal
region of a 2-year-old Thoroughbred
flat racehorse. There is an incomplete
articular stress fracture of the
dorsoproximal aspect of the third
metatarsal bone (black arrows). There
is extensive active-appearing periosteal
new bone on the dorsoproximal aspect
of the third metatarsal bone (white
arrows) and a large periarticular
osteophyte.

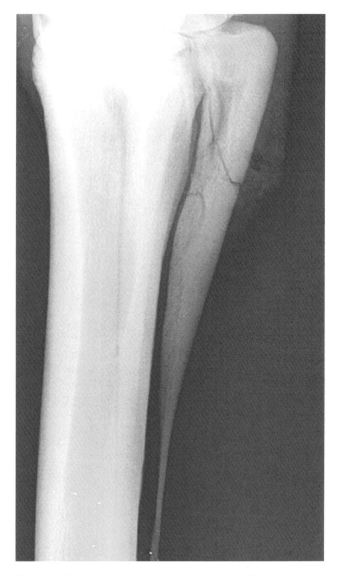

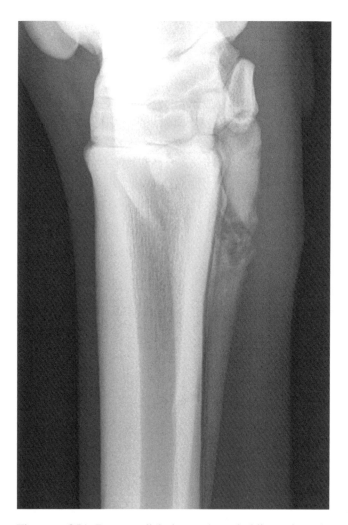

Figure 4.28(a) Dorsolateral-plantaromedial oblique view of the proximal metatarsal region of a 7-year-old showjumper that had been kicked 8 hours previously. There is a comminuted non-displaced fracture of the fourth metatarsal bone. There is overlying soft-tissue swelling and a radiolucent line extends from the skin surface to the bone representing gas in an open wound. The horse was treated conservatively and made an excellent recovery.

Figure 4.28(b) Dorsomedial-plantarolateral oblique view of the proximal metatarsal region of a Thoroughbred gelding, kicked 5 weeks previously. There was mild lameness and localized soft-tissue swelling over the second metatarsal bone. There is a healing fracture of the proximal aspect of the second metatarsal bone.

been identified in Standardbred racehorses. Lameness is moderate but acute in onset, and is alleviated either by intra-articular analgesia of the tarsometatarsal joint or by perineural analgesia of the fibular and tibial nerves. Nuclear scintigraphy may be useful to focus attention on the proximal metatarsal region. In both Thoroughbreds and Standardbreds there is frequently pre-existing periarticular new bone formation on the dorsoproximal aspect of the third metatarsal bone (Figure 4.27). Abnormal bone may predispose to fracture. The prognosis for return to full athletic function without recurrent lameness is guarded. Although the fracture may heal, there is often further development of periarticular new bone or degenerative changes within the tarsometatarsal joint.

Second and fourth metacarpal/metatarsal bones

Fractures involving the proximal half of the second and fourth metacarpal bones are usually the result of external trauma and may be comminuted. There is a high risk of secondary infection, especially if the fracture is open. Ultrasonography may be useful for assessment. Surgical stabilization may be required, since weight is transmitted through the second and fourth metacarpal bones. Surgical stabilization may also be needed if there is tearing of the collateral ligaments of the carpometacarpal joint. Fractures of the proximal third of the second or fourth metatarsal bones, however, can usually be treated conservatively, with complete success (Figure 4.28a and 4.28b). The carpal bones should be inspected for evidence of a concurrent fracture, which will adversely influence the prognosis (see also page 267).

A fracture at the junction between the middle and distal one-thirds of the second or fourth metacarpal bones is often seen in association with suspensory desmitis, but may be the result of external trauma. The fracture may not be detectable clinically without radiographic examination, especially if there is widespread swelling. The suspensory ligament should be carefully assessed ultrasonographically and the proximal sesamoid bones radiographed if indicated. If the fracture is displaced distally (Figure 4.29a), a non-union may result. The fracture fragment often does not cause a problem if left *in situ*, but may be removed surgically. The majority of fractures that are treated conservatively do heal within 2 months (Figure 4.29b), although there may be considerable callus formation (Figure 4.29c) and small lucent defects may persist. The callus models and often reduces in size, but some enlargement of the bone persists. Simple fractures of the second and fourth metacarpal (metatarsal) bones have a good prognosis, but associated suspensory ligament desmitis warrants a more guarded prognosis. Surgical removal of the distal aspect of the affected bone from a site proximal to the fracture may be indicated if there is a malunion or adhesion to the suspensory ligament.

Figure 4.30 summarizes common fracture sites in the metacarpal and the metatarsal regions.

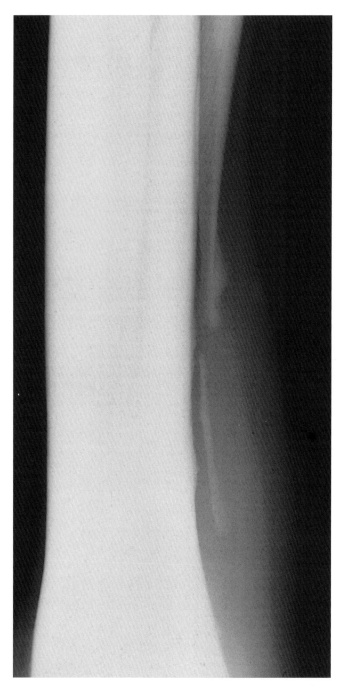

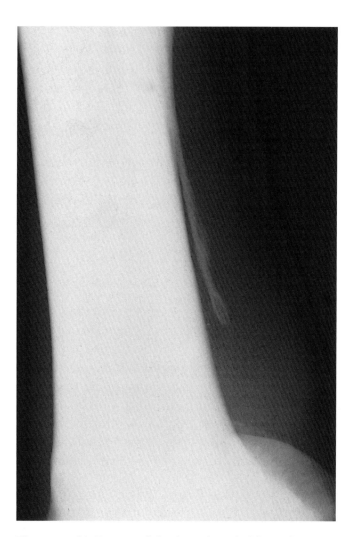

Figure 4.29(b) Dorsomedial-palmarolateral oblique view of a metacarpal region. There is a healed fracture of the distal aspect of the second metacarpal bone. Note also the rather curved configuration of the bone, suggestive of possible adhesions with adjacent soft tissues.

Figure 4.29(a) Dorsomedial-plantarolateral oblique view of a metatarsal region. There is soft-tissue swelling and an old displaced non-union fracture of the second metatarsal bone. Note also the irregular contour of the plantar cortex of the third metatarsal bone. Soft-tissue swelling is due to concurrent suspensory desmitis.

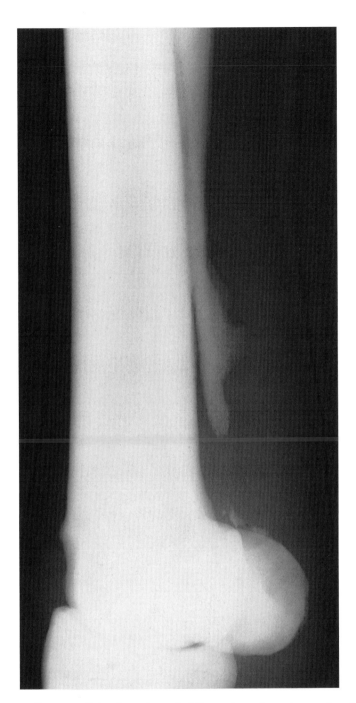

Figure 4.29(c) Dorsomedial-palmarolateral oblique view of a metacarpal region. There is considerable modelling of the distal end of the second metacarpal bone, the result of a previous fracture and excessive callus formation. Note also the mineralization proximal to the proximal sesamoid bones reflecting associated suspensory desmitis.

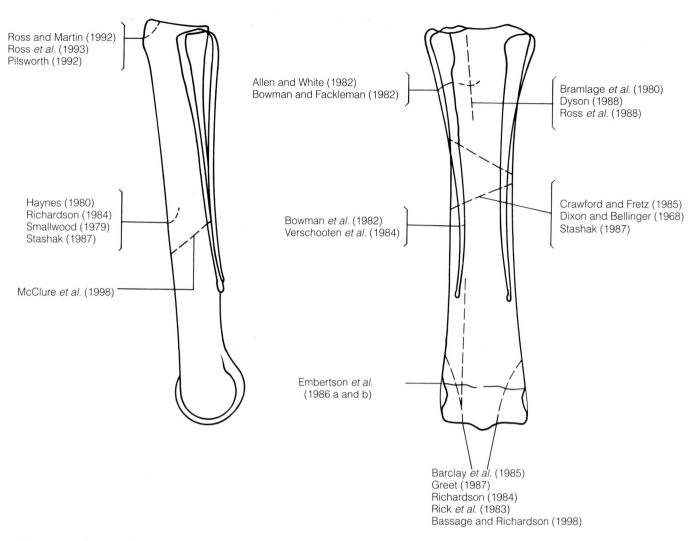

Ross and Martin (1992)
Ross et al. (1993)
Pilsworth (1992)

Allen and White (1982)
Bowman and Fackleman (1982)

Bramlage et al. (1980)
Dyson (1988)
Ross et al. (1988)

Haynes (1980)
Richardson (1984)
Smallwood (1979)
Stashak (1987)

Bowman et al. (1982)
Verschooten et al. (1984)

Crawford and Fretz (1985)
Dixon and Bellinger (1968)
Stashak (1987)

McClure et al. (1998)

Embertson et al.
(1986 a and b)

Barclay et al. (1985)
Greet (1987)
Richardson (1984)
Rick et al. (1983)
Bassage and Richardson (1998)

Figure 4.30 Common fracture sites in the metacarpal and metatarsal regions, and recommended references (see 'Further reading').

FURTHER READING

Allen, D. and White, N. (1982) Management of proximal splint fractures and exostoses in the horse. *Proc. Am. Ass. Equine Pract.*, **28**, 89–95

Barclay, W., Foerner, J. and Phillips, T. (1985) Axial sesamoid injuries associated with lateral condylar fractures in horses. *J. Am. Vet. Med. Ass.*, **186**, 278–279

Bassage, L. and Richardson, D. (1998) Longitudinal fractures of the condyles of the third metacarpal and metatarsal bones in racehorses: 224 cases (1986–1995). *J. Am. Vet. Med. Ass.*, **212**, 1757–1764

Baxter, G., Doron, R. and Allen, D. (1992) Complete excision of a fractured fourth metacarpal bone in eight horses. *Vet. Surg.*, **21**, 273–278

Booth, L. (1998) Superficial septic osteitis and sequestrum formation in the horse. *Equine vet. Educ.*, **10**, 233–237

Bowman, K. and Fackleman, G. (1982) Surgical treatment of complicated fractures of the splint bones in horses. *Vet. Surg.*, **11**, 121–124

Bowman, K., Evans, L. and Herring, M. (1982) Evaluation of surgical removal of fractured distal splint bones in the horse. *Vet. Surg.*, **11**, 116–120

Bowman, K., Sweeney, C. and Tate, L. (1987) Compression plating of a medial condylar fracture of the third metatarsal bone in a Thoroughbred filly. *J. Am. Vet. Med. Ass.*, **190**, 305–307

Bramlage, L., Gabel, A. and Hackett, R. (1980) Avulsion fractures of the origin of the suspensory ligament in the horse. *J. Am. Vet. Med. Ass.*, **176**, 1004–1010

Caron, J., Barber, S., Doige, C. and Pharr, J. (1987) The radiographic and histologic appearance of controlled surgical manipulation of the equine periosteum. *Vet. Surg.*, **16**, 13–20

Crawford, W. and Fretz, P. (1985) Long bone fractures in large animals: a retrospective study. *Vet. Surg.*, **14**, 259–302

Dixon, R. and Bellinger, C. (1968) Fissure fractures of the equine metacarpus and metatarsus. *J. Am. Vet. Med. Ass.*, **153**, 1289–1291

Dyson, S. (1988) Some observations on lameness associated with the proximal metacarpal region in the horse. *Equine vet. J.*, Suppl. **6**, 43–52

Dyson, S. (1991) Proximal suspensory desmitis: clinical, radiographic and ultrasonographic features in 42 horses. *Equine vet. J.*, **23**, 25–31

Dyson, S. (1994) Proximal desmitis in the hindlimb: 42 cases. *Br. Vet. J.*, **150**, 279–291

Dyson, S. (2003) Proximal metacarpal and metatarsal pain: a diagnostic challenge. *Equine vet. Educ.*, **15**, 134–138

Embertson, R., Bramlage, L. and Gabel, A. (1986a) Physeal fractures in the horse: Management and outcome. *Vet. Surg.*, **15**, 230–236

Embertson, R., Bramlage, L., Herring, D. and Gabel, A. (1986b) Physeal fractures in the horse: classification and incidence. *Vet. Surg.*, **15**, 223–229

Greet, T. (1987) Condylar fractures of the cannon bone with axial sesamoid fracture in 3 horses. *Vet. Rec.*, **120**, 223–225

Haynes, P. (1980) Disease of the metacarpophalangeal joint and the metacarpus. *Vet. Clin. N. Am.: Large Anim. Pract.*, **2**(1), 33–59

Hornhof, W. and O'Brien, T. (1980) Radiographic evaluation of the palmar aspect of the equine metacarpal condyles: a new projection. *Vet. Radiol.*, **21**, 161–167

Huskamp, B. and Nowak, M. (1988) Insertion desmopathies in the horse. *Pferdheilkunde*, **4**, 3–12

Jackson, N., Furst, A., Hassig, M. and Auer, J. (2007) Splint bone fractures in the horse: a retrospective study 1992–2001. *Equine vet. Educ.*, **19**, 324–335

Jensen, P., Gaughan, E., Lillich, J. and Bryant, J. (2004) Segmental ostectomy of the second and fourth metacarpal and metatarsal bones in horses: 17 cases (1993–2002). *J. Am. Vet. Med. Ass.*, **224**, 271–274

Kawcak, C., Bramlage, L. and Embertson, D. (1995) Diagnosis and management of incomplete fracture of the distal palmar aspect of the third metacarpal bone in five horses. *J. Am. Vet. Med. Ass.*, **206**, 335–337

Launois, T., Desbrosse, F. and Perrin, R. (2003) Percutaneous osteostixis as treatment of the palmar/plantar third metacarpal/metatarsal cortex at the origin of the suspensory ligament in 29 horses. *Equine vet. Educ.*, **15**, 126–138

Lloyd, K., Koblik, P., Ragle, C., Wheat, J. and Lakritz, J. (1988) Incomplete palmar fractures of the proximal extremity of the third metacarpal bone in the horse: ten cases (1981–1986). *J. Am. Vet. Med. Ass.*, **192**(6), 798–803

Mair, T. and Tucker, R. (2004) Hypertrophic osteopathy (Marie's disease) in horses. *Equine vet. Educ.*, **16**, 308–311

McClure, S., Watkins, J., Glickman, N. *et al.* (1998) Complete fracture of the third metacarpal or metatarsal bone in horses: 25 cases (1980–1986). *J. Am. Vet. Med. Ass.*, **213**, 847–850

Moens, Y., Verschooten, F., De Moor, A. and Wouters, L. (1980) Bone sequestration as a consequence of limb wounds in the horse. *Vet. Radiol.*, **21**, 40–44

Momiya, N., Tagami, M., Tsunoda, N. and Taniyama, H. (1999) Aneurysmal bone cyst in a colt. *Equine vet. Educ.*, **11**, 243–246

O'Sullivan, C. and Lumsden, J. (2002) Distal third metacarpal bone palmar cortical stress fractures in four Thoroughbred racehorses. *Equine vet. Educ.*, **14**, 70–73

Pilsworth, R. (1992) Incomplete fracture of the dorsal aspect of the proximal cortex of the third metatarsal bone as a cause of hindlimb lameness in the racing Thoroughbred: a review of 3 cases. *Equine vet. J.*, **24**, 147–150

Pilsworth, R., Hopes, R. and Greet, T. (1988) Use of a flexed dorsopalmar (plantar) projection of the fetlock joint to demonstrate lesions of the distal third metacarpal (tarsal) bone in the horse. *Vet. Rec.*, **122**, 332–333

Pinchbeck, G. and Kriz, N. (2001) Two cases of incomplete longitudinal fracture of the proximopalmar aspect of the third metacarpal bone. *Equine vet. Educ.*, **13**, 187–194

Ramzan, P. (2002) Enostosis-like lesions: 12 cases. *Equine vet. Educ.*, **14**, 143–148

Richardson, D. (1984) Dorsal cortical fractures of the equine metacarpus. *Comp. Cont. Educ.*, **6**, S248–254

Richardson, D. (1984) Medial condylar fractures of the third metatarsal bone in horses. *J. Am. Vet. Med. Ass.*, **185**, 761–765

Rick, M., O'Brien, T., Pool, R. and Meagher, D. (1983) Condylar fractures of the third metacarpal bone and third metatarsal bone in 75 horses: radiographic features, treatments and outcome. *J. Am. Vet. Med. Ass.*, **183**, 287–296

Rose, R. (1978) Surgical treatment of osteomyelitis in the metacarpal and metatarsal bones of the horse. *Vet. Rec.*, **102**, 498–500

Ross, M. and Martin, B. (1992) Dorsomedial articular fracture of the proximal aspect of the third metacarpal bone in Standardbred racehorses: seven cases (1978–1990). *J. Am. Vet. Med. Ass.*, **201**, 332–335

Ross, M., Ford, T. and Orsini, P. (1988) Incomplete longitudinal fracture of the proximal palmar cortex of the third metacarpal bone in horses. *Vet. Surg.*, **17**, 82–86

Ross, M., Sponseller, M., Gill, H. and Moyer, W. (1993) Articular fracture of the dorsoproximolateral aspect of the third metatarsal bone in five Standardbred racehorses. *J. Am. Vet. Med. Ass.*, **203**, 698–700

Russell, T. and Maclean, A. (2006) Standing surgical repair of propagating metacarpal and metatarsal condylar fractures in racehorses. *Equine vet. J.*, **38**, 423–427

Sampson, S. and Tucker, R. (2007) Magnetic resonance imaging of the proximal metacarpal and metatarsal regions. *Clin. Techniques in Equine Pract.*, **6**, 78–85

Smallwood, J. (1979) Evaluation of the 'bucked shin syndrome' using xeroradiography. *Equine Pract.*, **1**(2), 28–35

Stashak, T. (1987) The metacarpus and metatarsus. In: *Adams' Lameness In Horses*, 4th edn, Lea and Febiger, Philadelphia, pp. 596–624

Verschooten, F., Gasthuys, F. and De Moor, A. (1984) Distal splint bone fractures in the horse: an experimental and clinical study. *Equine vet. J.*, **16**, 532–536

Watt, B., Foerner, J. and Haines, G. (1998) Incomplete oblique sagittal fracture of the dorsal cortex of the third metacarpal bone in six horses. *Vet. Surg.*, **27**, 337–341

White, K. (1983) Diaphyseal angular limb deformities in 3 foals. *J. Am. Vet. Med. Ass.*, **182**, 272–279

Zubrod, C., Schneider, R. and Tucker, R. (2004) Use of magnetic resonance imaging to identify suspensory desmitis and adhesions between exostoses of the second metacarpal bone and the suspensory ligament in four horses. *J. Am. Vet. Med. Ass.*, **224**, 1815–1819

Chapter 5
The carpus and antebrachium

RADIOGRAPHIC TECHNIQUE

The carpus consists of three principal joints: antebrachiocarpal (radiocarpal), middle carpal (intercarpal) and carpometacarpal. Articulations also exist between adjacent bones in each row of carpal bones. This causes overlying images that may confuse interpretation. Therefore it is necessary to obtain at least five standard views.

The distal aspect of the radius is included in standard views of the carpus, but to evaluate the majority of the radius four standard views centred on the area of interest are required.

Equipment

Portable x-ray machines are adequate for radiography of the carpus and antebrachial regions and a grid is not required. Using conventional radiography, high-definition screens and films are preferable, although rare earth screens and compatible films can be used. The faster screen and film combinations tend to lack contrast and definition. A grid may be useful if the carpal region is very swollen.

Positioning for the carpus

Examinations are best carried out with the horse standing. Sedation may be required in fractious animals.

All examinations should include lateromedial, dorsopalmar, dorsal 45° lateral-palmaromedial oblique and dorsal 45° medial-palmarolateral oblique views. Flexed lateromedial views are very helpful in many cases, to separate the dorsodistal margin of the radial and intermediate carpal bones, where bone fragmentation frequently occurs in racehorses. If degenerative joint disease is suspected it may also be helpful to obtain dorsal 75° lateral-palmaromedial oblique and dorsal 75° medial-palmarolateral oblique views to evaluate the entire joint margins better. For suspected fractures, it is often necessary to take further oblique views at different angles, as well as dorsoproximal-dorsodistal oblique ('skyline') views. Consistency of the angle of the views will greatly aid film reading.

Lateromedial, dorsopalmar and oblique views

Lateromedial, dorsopalmar and oblique views are all obtained with the horse standing bearing weight evenly on all four limbs, with the limb to be radiographed vertical. Dorsopalmar and most oblique views are obtained with the x-ray beam aligned horizontally and the cassette held vertically, at right angles to the beam. The joints slope distally to a varying degree towards their lateral or medial aspects. For this reason the x-ray beam may need to be angled slightly up or down in order to give good visualization of the joints on lateromedial views. The x-ray beam should be centred on the middle carpal joint or on a site of particular interest. In order to obtain true lateromedial and dorsopalmar views of the joints the x-ray beam should be orientated relative to the limb, rather than the trunk of the horse.

Flexed lateromedial views

The flexed lateromedial view is of great assistance to separate some of the overlying bone images. Chip fractures are often most easily seen on this view.

The horse should stand squarely on all four limbs. The limb to be radiographed is then lifted by an assistant who stands against, or just behind, the shoulder of the horse, facing in the same direction as the horse. The toe of the foot is rested on the assistant's leg to help keep the limb steady and also to enable the limb to be repositioned accurately if subsequent films are needed. It is important not to rotate the limb and the foot should be supported vertically below the elbow (Figure 5.1). The x-ray beam is initially maintained horizontal, at right angles to the long axis of the limb. Slight changes in alignment of the x-ray beam may need to be made subsequently to allow better visualization of specific lesions.

Flexed dorsoproximal-dorsodistal oblique (skyline) views

Flexed dorsoproximal-dorsodistal oblique views of the carpus are essential to visualize some slab fractures, to establish their extent and to detect

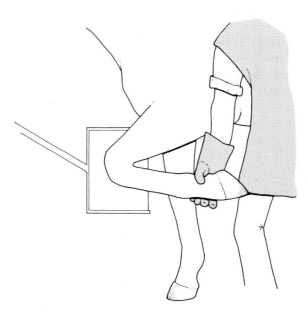

Figure 5.1 Positioning to obtain a flexed lateromedial view of the carpus.

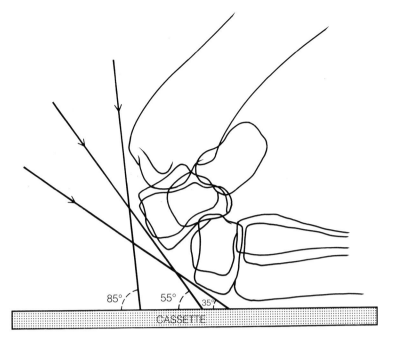

Figure 5.2 Positioning to obtain dorsoproximal-dorsodistal oblique views of the carpus. The three different angles of the x-ray beam allow visualization of the distal radius, proximal row of carpal bones, or distal row of carpal bones.

pathology not apparent in the standard views (see also 'Degenerative joint disease', page 252, 'Sclerosis of the third carpal bone', page 258 and 'Sagittal fracture of the third carpal bone', page 266).

An assistant holds the limb to be examined with the carpus flexed and slightly in front of the carpus of the contralateral limb, trying to keep the metacarpal region horizontal (Figure 5.2). The cassette is placed against the dorsal aspect of the third metacarpal bone, with its centre level with the carpus. Alternatively the flexed limb and cassette may be placed on a block of sufficient height, with restraint of the limb at the toe. This can help to reduce movement. The degree of flexion of the carpus that can be achieved depends on the amount of pain induced by flexion. The angle of the x-ray beam required to visualize the distal radius and proximal and distal rows of carpal bones is therefore variable. The radiographer must try to visualize the positions of the radius and the carpal bones in relation to the degree of flexion. In a fully flexed carpus the following guide can be given (Figure 5.2):

● To project an image of the distal radius, the x-ray beam is aligned at approximately 85° to the cassette, pointing obliquely downward through the flexed carpus. This is often most easily achieved if the carpus is allowed to drop towards the ground.

● To project an image of the proximal row of carpal bones, the beam is aligned at approximately 55° to the cassette.

● To project an image of the distal row of bones, the beam is aligned at approximately 35° to the cassette.

Positioning for the antebrachium (radius)

The horse should stand bearing full weight with the antebrachium positioned vertically. The most common reason to be examining this region is

[235]

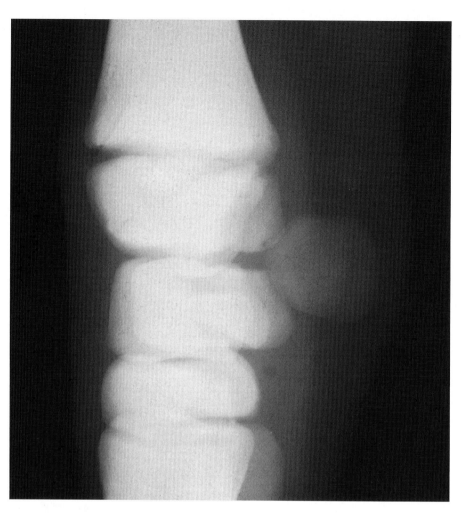

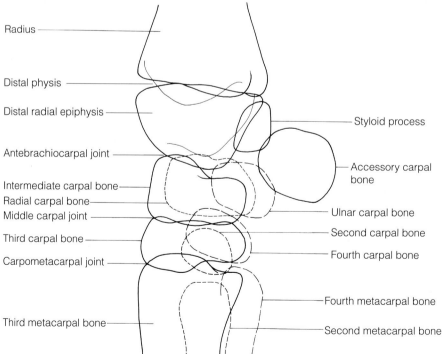

Radius

Distal physis

Distal radial epiphysis

Antebrachiocarpal joint

Intermediate carpal bone
Radial carpal bone
Middle carpal joint

Third carpal bone

Carpometacarpal joint

Third metacarpal bone

Styloid process

Accessory carpal bone

Ulnar carpal bone

Second carpal bone

Fourth carpal bone

Fourth metacarpal bone

Second metacarpal bone

Figure 5.3(a) Lateromedial view and diagram of a carpus of a normal 5-day-old foal (see text on page 239).

[236]

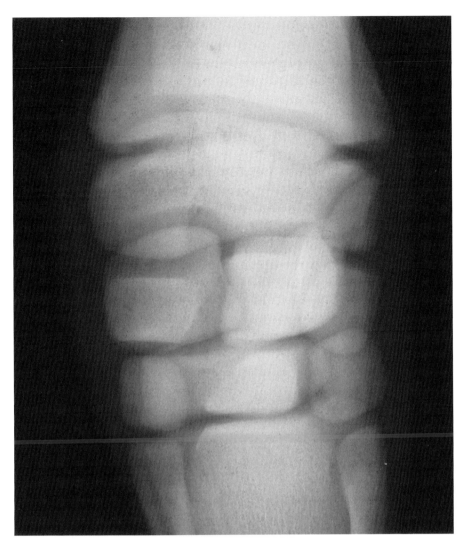

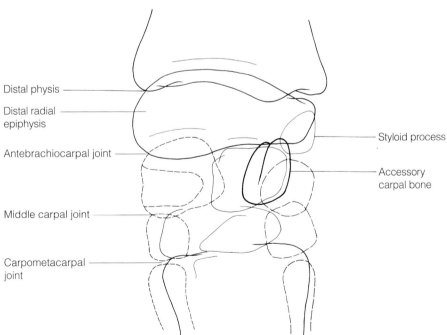

Distal physis

Distal radial
epiphysis

Antebrachiocarpal joint

Middle carpal joint

Carpometacarpal
joint

Styloid process

Accessory
carpal bone

Figure 5.3(b) Dorsopalmar view and
diagram of a carpus of a normal 5-day-
old foal. Lateral is to the right (see text
on page 239).

[237]

to determine the presence of an incomplete fracture of the radius following a kick injury. The x-ray beam should initially be centred at the site of suspected trauma, but if a fracture line is identified, additional more proximal views may be required to determine the full extent of the fracture. Craniocaudal, lateromedial and several oblique views are normally required.

NORMAL ANATOMY

Immature horse

The distal radius has two ossification centres. The lateral styloid process (morphologically the distal end of the ulna) is separate at birth and fuses with the epiphysis in the first year of life. Oblique views of the carpus in a skeletally mature horse may demonstrate a radiolucent line between the styloid process and the distal radius. This line is more pronounced in young

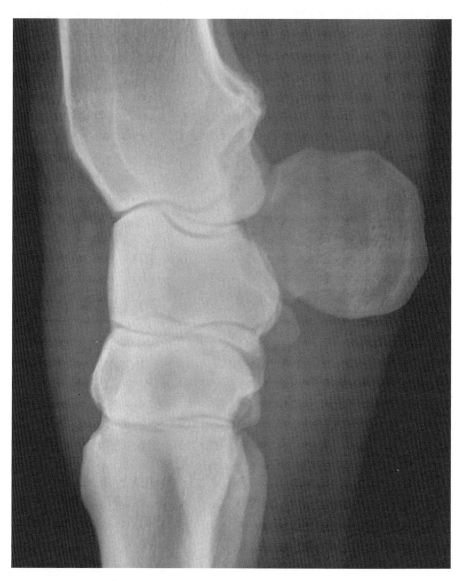

Figure 5.4 Lateromedial view and diagram of a normal adult carpus (see text on page 240).

horses, but may persist to varying degrees throughout life. The distal radial physis closes at about 20 months of age.

At birth the joint spaces appear wider than in the mature horse, since endochondral ossification is incomplete and therefore the cartilage is thicker (Figures 5.3a, page 236, and 5.3b, page 237). The carpal bones should be approximately cuboidal. Rounded margins to the bones indicate that they are incompletely ossified (see 'Incomplete carpal ossification', page 261).

Each of the carpal bones ossifies from a single centre and is fully developed by 18 months of age.

The third metacarpal bone has a proximal epiphysis, which is fused with the metaphysis at birth.

Skeletally mature horse

The carpus is complex and it may be necessary to compare images from several different views to ensure that suspected lesions are not due to overlying images.

Lateromedial view

The distal aspect of the radius has a prominent transverse ridge caudally, to which, medially and laterally, the medial and lateral collateral ligaments of the carpus attach. Immediately distal to the ridge are depressions for

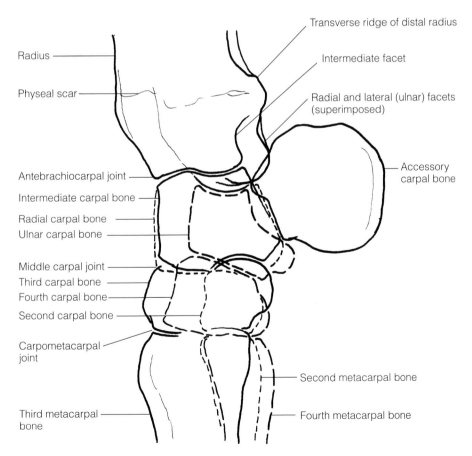

Figure 5.4 *Cont'd*

[239]

attachment of carpal ligaments. This transverse ridge is not the origin of the accessory ligament of the superficial digital flexor tendon, which arises from a longitudinal ridge approximately 10–15 cm proximal to the antebrachio-carpal joint.

The lateromedial view (Figure 5.4, page 238) demonstrates the two rows of carpal bones clearly delineated by the antebrachiocarpal, middle carpal and carpometacarpal joints. These joints are represented by double lucent lines, as they undulate, rather than forming flat parallel planes. It is possible to eliminate the double line in local areas by altering the angle of the beam and/or the point at which it is centred.

On a true lateromedial view, the bone projected most dorsally in the proximal row is the intermediate carpal. This bone has a relatively

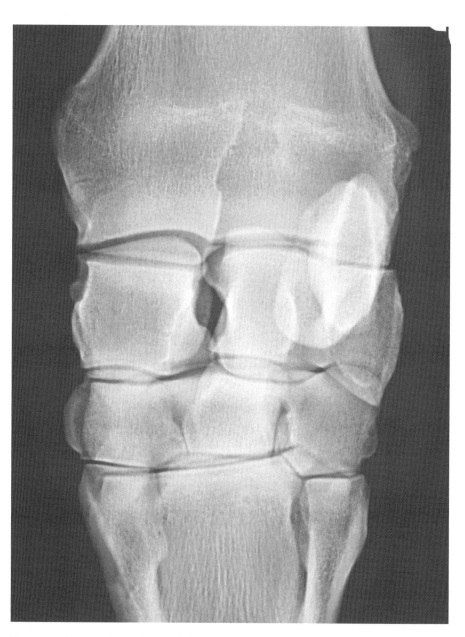

Figure 5.5 Dorsopalmar view and diagram of a normal adult carpus. Lateral is to the right.

straight dorsal border, well defined proximally and distally where it meets the articular surfaces at approximately a right angle. Very slight dorsolateral-palmaromedial obliquity will make the radial carpal bone most prominent.

The most dorsal of the distal row of carpal bones is the third carpal. The middle third of this bone often protrudes dorsally. The dorsal surface meets the articular surfaces at approximately a right angle.

The accessory carpal bone is relatively thin, but thickens at its palmar aspect where there are tendon and ligament insertions. There is a vertical radiolucent line close to the palmar surface caused by edge enhancement.

One or two focal radiolucencies may be seen in the soft tissues on the dorsal aspect of the antebrachiocarpal joint. These represent fat in the joint capsule and lie palmar to the synovial sheath of the extensor carpi radialis tendon. Distension of the joint capsule may obscure these lucent areas.

Dorsopalmar views

There is a large approximately circular lucent zone in the centre of the distal end of the radius, which is caused by a depression (between the medial and lateral styloid processes) in the caudal surface of the bone.

Figure 5.5 shows the individual carpal bones seen on the dorsopalmar radiograph and the reader is referred to this figure for their identification. A radiolucent canal is normally seen between the radial and intermediate carpal bones on this projection.

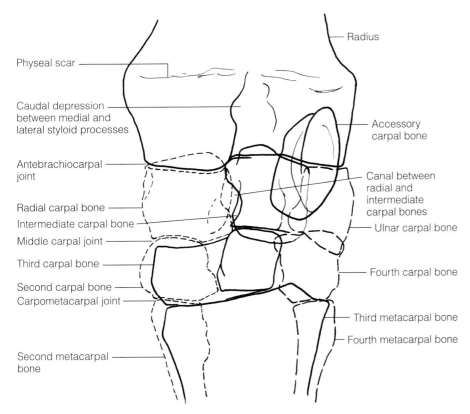

Figure 5.5 *Cont'd*

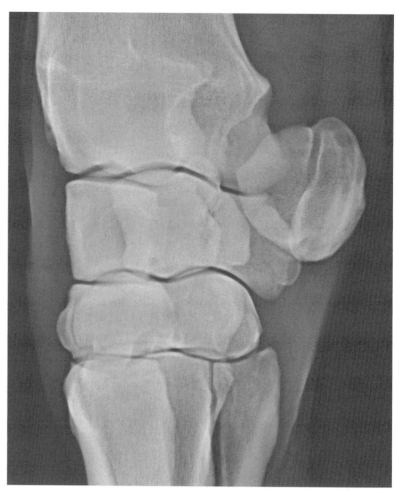

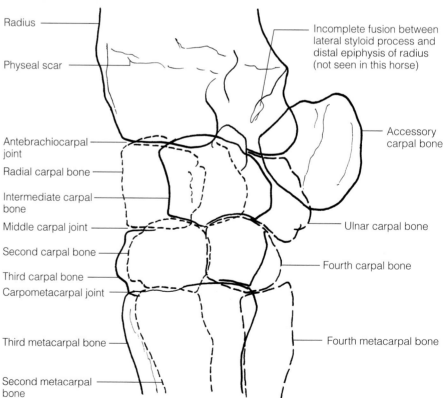

Radius

Physeal scar

Incomplete fusion between
lateral styloid process and
distal epiphysis of radius
(not seen in this horse)

Antebrachiocarpal
joint

Radial carpal bone

Intermediate carpal
bone

Middle carpal joint

Second carpal bone

Third carpal bone

Carpometacarpal joint

Accessory
carpal bone

Ulnar carpal bone

Fourth carpal bone

Third metacarpal bone

Fourth metacarpal bone

Second metacarpal
bone

Figure 5.6 Dorsal 45° lateral-
palmaromedial oblique view and
diagram of a normal adult carpus (see
text on page 244).

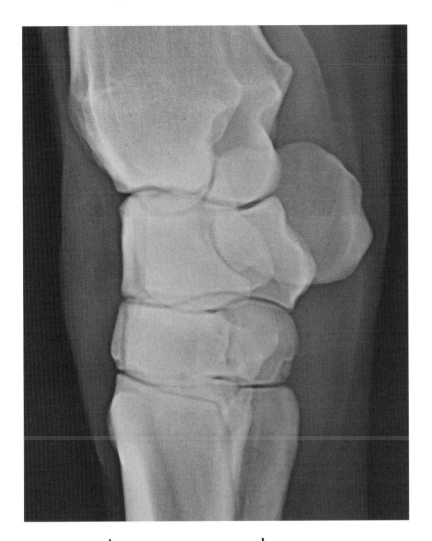

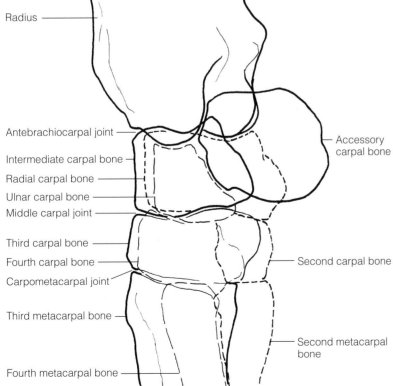

Radius

Antebrachiocarpal joint

Intermediate carpal bone

Radial carpal bone

Ulnar carpal bone

Middle carpal joint

Third carpal bone

Fourth carpal bone

Carpometacarpal joint

Third metacarpal bone

Fourth metacarpal bone

Accessory carpal bone

Second carpal bone

Second metacarpal bone

Figure 5.7 Dorsal 45° medial-palmarolateral oblique view and diagram of a normal adult carpus.

Oblique views

Standard oblique views are shown in Figures 5.6 (page 242) and 5.7 (page 243), but their appearance is greatly affected by the degree of obliquity. Interpretation of oblique radiographs is therefore facilitated by comparison with an anatomical specimen.

Flexed lateromedial view

In the flexed lateromedial view (Figure 5.8) the distal end of the radius will normally be projected as three distinct articular surfaces, that with the largest radius of curvature being the radial facet, the smallest the intermediate facet, and the lateral or ulnar facet having an intermediate radius of curvature.

As the carpus is flexed, the accessory carpal bone gradually rotates around a horizontal axis, and so appears slightly shorter in a proximal to distal direction than on a standing lateral view.

The majority of carpal flexion occurs at the antebrachiocarpal joint, with some flexion at the middle carpal joint. As the carpus flexes, the intermediate carpal bone moves proximally relative to the radial carpal bone. The proximal border of the fourth carpal bone is seen proximal to the third, and the dorsal surface of the third is dorsal to the fourth. The carpometacarpal joint does not open appreciably during flexion. The first and/or the fifth carpal bones, if present, are easily seen.

Dorsoproximal-dorsodistal oblique views

It is necessary to obtain separate views to evaluate the distal radius and the proximal and distal rows of carpal bones.

The distal radius has a continuous outline, with two distinct grooves on the dorsal aspect (Figure 5.9a). The outline of the proximal row of carpal bones may be seen superimposed on the image of the radius on overexposed radiographs.

In the proximal row of carpal bones (Figure 5.9b) the dorsal borders of the radial and intermediate carpal bones are clearly outlined, with their articulation near the midline. The ulnar carpal bone can be seen laterally.

In the distal row of carpal bones (Figure 5.9c) the third carpal bone is central, with the second and fourth carpal bones at the medial and lateral aspects respectively.

Each carpal bone should have a smooth outline, with an even trabecular pattern and sharply defined corticomedullary border.

NORMAL VARIATIONS AND INCIDENTAL FINDINGS

In a lateromedial or slightly oblique lateromedial view there is a smoothly outlined prominence on the caudolateral and caudomedial aspects of the radius at the level of the fused physis. The distal caudal aspect of the radius proximal to the physis may have a rather irregular outline (Figure 5.10). The

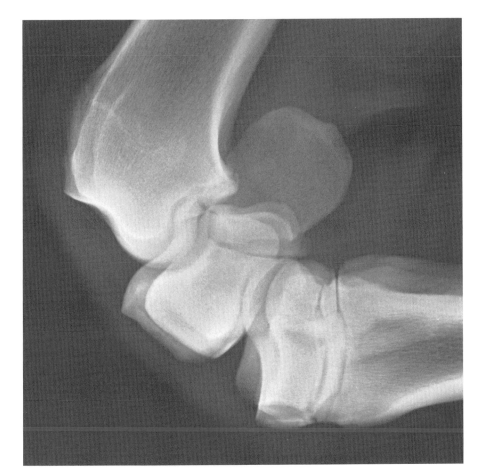

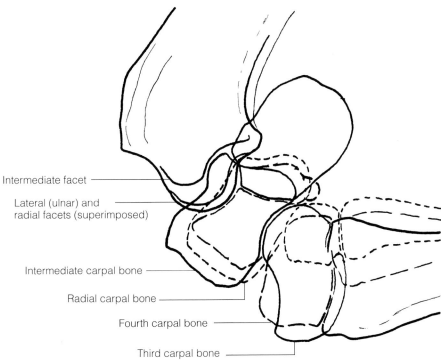

Intermediate facet

Lateral (ulnar) and
radial facets (superimposed)

Intermediate carpal bone

Radial carpal bone

Fourth carpal bone

Third carpal bone

Figure 5.8 Flexed lateromedial view and diagram of a normal adult carpus.

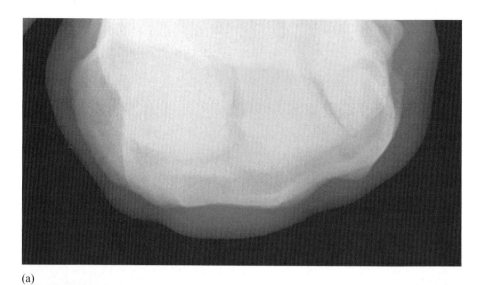

(a)

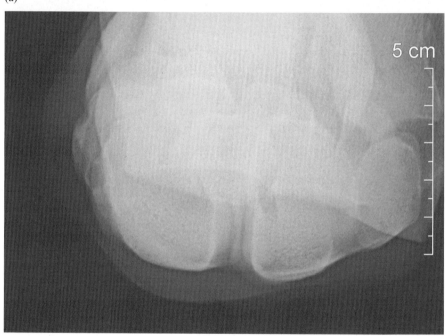

(b)

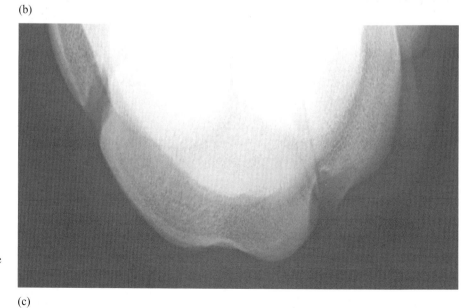

Figure 5.9 Dorsoproximal-dorsodistal oblique views and diagrams of a carpus of a normal adult horse, showing: (a) the distal radius; (b) the proximal row of carpal bones; (c) the distal row of carpal bones. Lateral is to the right.

(c)

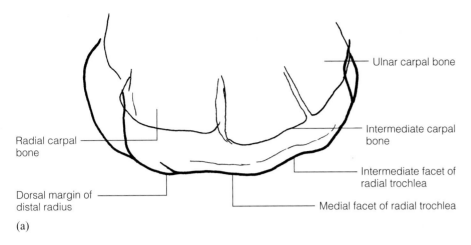

Ulnar carpal bone

Intermediate carpal bone

Intermediate facet of radial trochlea

Medial facet of radial trochlea

Radial carpal bone

Dorsal margin of distal radius

(a)

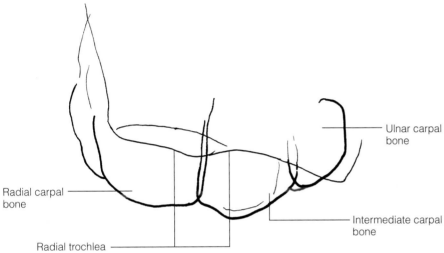

Ulnar carpal bone

Radial carpal bone

Intermediate carpal bone

Radial trochlea

(b)

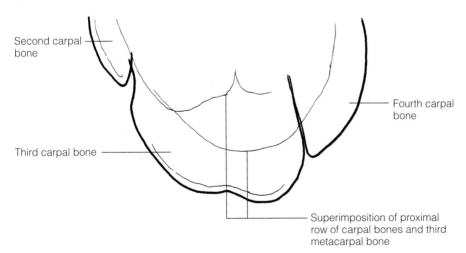

Second carpal bone

Fourth carpal bone

Third carpal bone

Superimposition of proximal row of carpal bones and third metacarpal bone

(c)

Figure 5.9 *Cont'd*

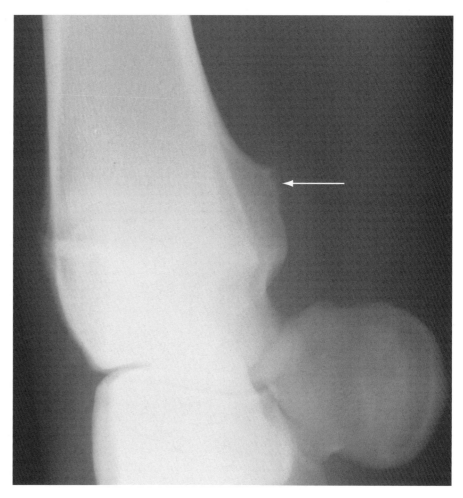

Figure 5.10 Lateromedial view of a carpus from a normal adult horse, showing marked irregularity of the caudal aspect of the radius (arrow) proximal to the level of the fused distal radial physis.

transverse ridge on the distal caudal aspect of the radius often appears slightly roughened and does not reflect previous tearing of the accessory ligament of the superficial digital flexor tendon (superior check ligament), which arises further proximally from a longitudinal ridge approximately 10–15 cm proximal to the antebrachiocarpal joint. Oblique views may demonstrate an incomplete lucent line in the distal lateral aspect of the radius (see page 238).

Although the distal end of the ulna is vestigial in the horse, it may continue to the distal tuberosity of the radius as a fibrous cord. In some cases this is partially ossified, when it can be seen on radiographs. It is variable in size and appearance (Figures 5.11a and 5.11b). In some small pony breeds, e.g. the Shetland, a complete ulna may be present.

The palmar aspect of the ulnar carpal bone is variable in shape, but is usually bilaterally symmetrical. A lucent zone is sometimes seen in the ulnar carpal bone, with or without an adjacent osseous opacity (Figure 5.11a). In a dorsopalmar projection they may appear to be on the axial border of the bone. They may possibly be associated with previous intercarpal ligament avulsion. They are not generally associated with lameness in sports horses; however, such lesions have been associated with lameness in racehorses (see page 259) and arthroscopic assessment may be indicated. Osseous cyst-like lesions are also occasionally seen in conjunction with an extra small bone on the palmarolateral aspect of the proximal row of carpal bones.

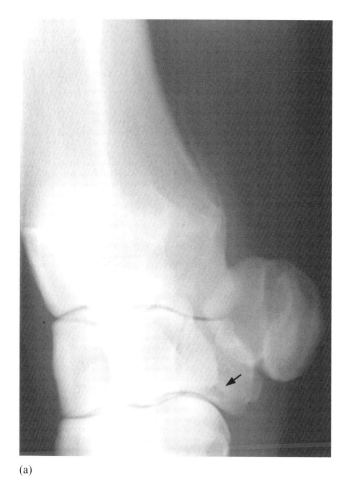

(a)

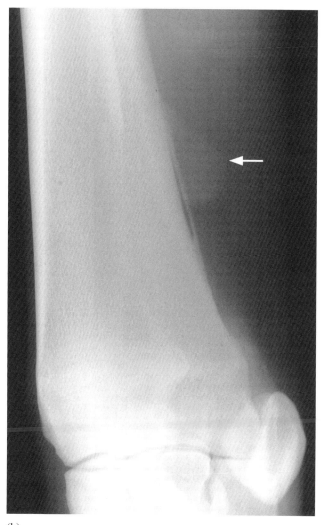

(b)

Figure 5.11 Dorsolateral-palmaromedial oblique views of a distal radius and carpus of normal adult horses showing:
(a) a vestigial distal ulna – there is also a radiolucent zone (arrow) with surrounding sclerosis in the ulnar carpal bone, which is an incidental finding;
(b) a vestigial distal ulna – there is also a clearly demarcated opacity (arrow) caused by the torus carpeus (chestnut).

The first carpal bone is seen in approximately one-third of horses, in one or both limbs. It is variable in size, ranging from pinpoint to 12–15 mm in diameter. It may, but need not, articulate with the second carpal bone (Figure 5.12a–c), and occasionally also articulates with the second metacarpal bone. If it is separated from the second carpal bone, it usually has a uniformly opaque appearance. If it is in close proximity to the second carpal or metacarpal bones, these bones may have focal lucent areas within them.

Occasionally a fifth carpal bone is present on the palmarolateral aspect of the distal row of carpal bones. Very occasionally there is a separate ossification centre in the proximal row of carpal bones. The size, shape and articulations of these bones are variable, but they are usually uniformly opaque. These separate ossification centres should not be confused with fractures.

Some degree of sclerosis of the radial facet of the third carpal bone may be seen in dorsoproximal-dorsodistal oblique views of horses in full work, but this is generally mild and bilaterally symmetrical.

[249]

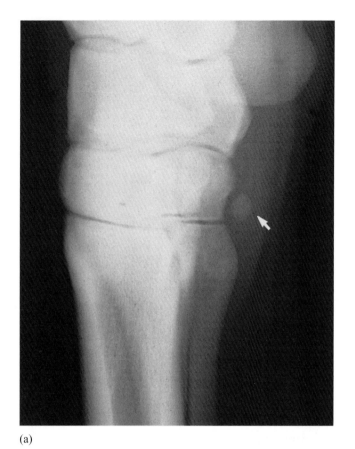
(a)

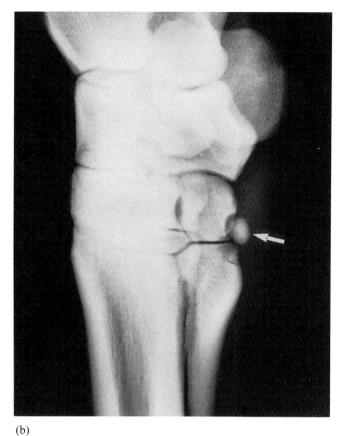
(b)

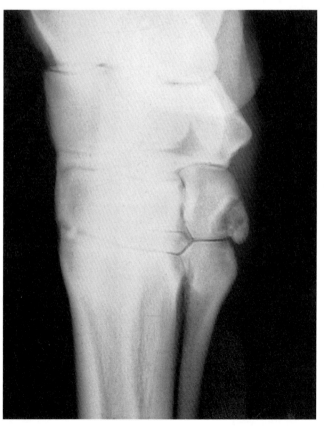
(c)

Figure 5.12 Dorsomedial-palmarolateral oblique view of the carpus of normal horses, showing variations of the first carpal bone.

(a) The first carpal bone (arrow) is well separated from the second carpal bone.

(b) The first carpal bone (arrow) appears to articulate with the second carpal bone. Note that the distal palmar aspect of the second carpal bone appears relatively lucent.

(c) The first carpal bone appears to articulate with the second carpal bone. The distal palmar aspect of the second carpal bone is relatively lucent. There are ill defined lucent areas within the first carpal bone.

Marginal osteophyte formation may be seen, particularly on the medial aspect of the antebrachiocarpal and middle carpal joints in older horses with marked conformational abnormalities of the distal limb. This is most common if the metacarpal region is set on lateral to the central axis of the antebrachium. It is not necessarily associated with lameness, but this may depend on the athletic demands placed on the horse.

SIGNIFICANT FINDINGS

Soft-tissue swelling

Soft-tissue injury and swelling of the carpus is common. It can generally be appreciated radiographically but it is frequently not possible to determine its cause. The site of maximum swelling may be located near the site of the injury, but frequently the swelling is too extensive for this to be of diagnostic assistance. Gravity will also change the appearance of the swelling. Swelling may be restricted to, or by, periarticular structures or involve the carpal joint capsules. It may indicate the presence of synovitis and/or infection, or result from contusion or ligament strains.

The antebrachiocarpal (radiocarpal) joint usually does not communicate with the middle carpal joint. Synovitis of these joints may therefore occur separately. Distension of the antebrachiocarpal joint capsule may obscure the focal radiolucencies, which represent fat, on the dorsal aspect of the joint. If there is swelling of the middle carpal joint capsule, a dorsoproximal-dorsodistal oblique view of the distal row of carpal bones should be obtained (see 'Sclerosis of the third carpal bone', page 258). Diffuse soft-tissue swelling on the dorsal aspect of the carpus may be due to a hygroma, an acquired bursa. Usually there are no associated radiographic abnormalities other than the soft-tissue swelling. Occasionally herniation of a joint capsule may occur, to cause a synoviocoele, usually on the dorsolateral aspect of the carpus. Distension of the tendon sheath of the extensor carpi radialis, common digital extensor or lateral digital extensor may result in a chronic longitudinal swelling on the dorsal aspect of the carpus. Occasionally communication develops between two of the above structures. Positive and double contrast radiographic techniques are useful to aid differentiation of these swellings, and to identify filling defects due to synovial proliferation or adhesion formation. Ultrasonography may yield additional information. Chronic distension of the tendon sheath of the extensor carpi radialis is often seen in association with irregular periosteal new bone formation on the distal cranial radius; however, this new bone is not necessarily of clinical significance.

Intercarpal ligament desmitis

Each of the carpal bones is connected to the adjacent bone by horizontally orientated intercarpal ligaments, within the joint. In addition there are medial and lateral palmar intercarpal ligaments connecting the proximal and distal row of carpal bones. There are also dorsal intercarpal ligaments connecting the dorsal aspect of adjacent carpal bones. Palmar intercarpal

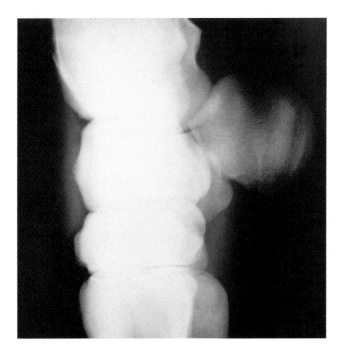

Figure 5.13(a) Dorsolateral-palmaromedial oblique view of a carpus. There is new bone on the dorsal aspect of the radial carpal bone at the site of the intercarpal ligament attachment. This is often not of long-term clinical significance.

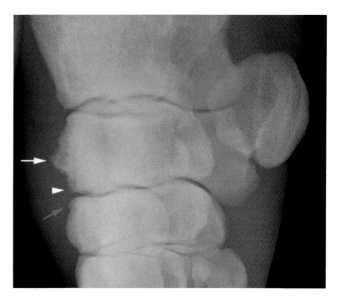

Figure 5.13(b) Dorsolateral-palmaromedial oblique radiographic view of a carpus of a 3-year-old Thoroughbred flat racehorse, with lameness which was improved by intra-articular analgesia of the middle carpal joint. There is extensive irregular entheseophyte formation on the dorsal aspect of the radial carpal bone (white arrow), at the attachment of the dorsal intercarpal ligament. There is reduced opacity of the distal dorsal aspect of the radial carpal bone (arrow head) and mild modelling of the proximodorsal aspect of the third carpal bone (grey arrow). Diagnostic arthroscopy of the middle carpal joint revealed extensive cartilage degeneration on the radial facet of the third carpal bone.

ligament desmitis or rupture has been recognized arthroscopically un-associated with detectable radiographic abnormality, although resultant instability may predispose to osteophyte formation on the dorsal margin of the joint. Dorsal intercarpal ligament injury is associated with the development of entheseous new bone on the dorsal aspect of affected bones (Figures 5.13a and 5.13b), often the radial and intermediate carpal bones in racehorses. Desmitis of the horizontal intra-articular intercarpal ligaments has not been well recognized; this may be associated with subtle new bone on the axial aspect of the affected carpal bone and some entheseous reaction. It may be associated with the development of an osseous cyst-like lesion on the axial aspect of the ulnar carpal bone (see Osseous cyst-like lesions, page 259). There may be no detectable radiographic abnormality and diagnosis may be dependent on magnetic resonance imaging.

Degenerative joint disease

The radiographic changes associated with degenerative joint disease are described elsewhere (see Chapter 1, page 34). The most frequent abnormalities identified in the carpus are periarticular osteophytes, rounding of the normally right-angled shape of the articular margins of the carpal

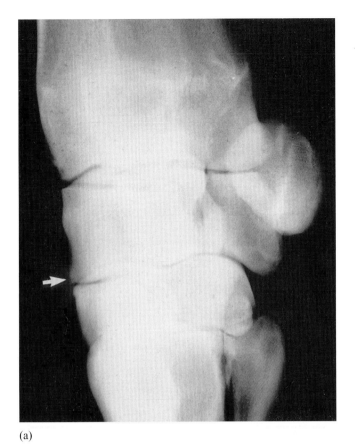

(a)

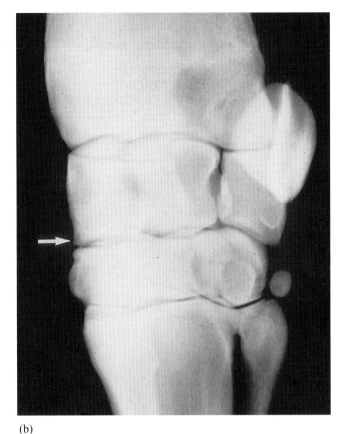

(b)

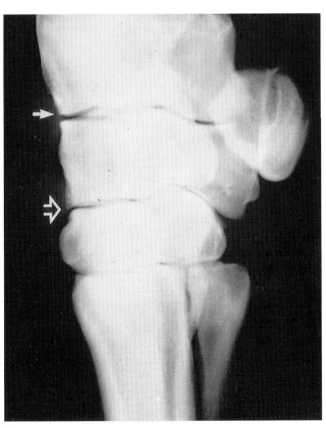

(c)

Figure 5.14 Radiographs of the carpus of adult horses, showing changes associated with early degenerative joint disease (the significance of these radiographic abnormalities must be determined in the light of the clinical examination).

(a) Dorsolateral-palmaromedial oblique view of a carpus of an 8-year-old Thoroughbred cross. There is slight osteophyte formation on the distal aspect of the radial carpal bone (arrow) and slight loss of trabecular pattern in the proximal aspect of the third carpal bone.

(b) Dorsolateral-palmaromedial oblique view of a carpus of a 3-year-old Thoroughbred. There is modelling of the distal aspect of the radial carpal bone, with alteration of the trabecular pattern (arrow) and rounding of the proximal aspect of the third carpal bone. Note also the large fifth carpal bone.

(c) Dorsolateral-palmaromedial oblique view of a carpus of a 5-year-old crossbred. There is slight osteophyte formation (solid arrow) on the medial aspect of the antebrachiocarpal joint, with more extensive modelling of the distal aspect of the radiocarpal bone (open arrow). Note the small radiolucent zone in the distal aspect of the ulnar carpal bone.

[253]

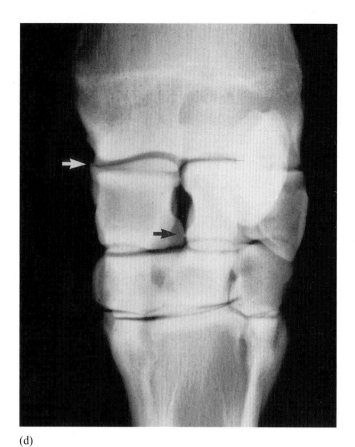
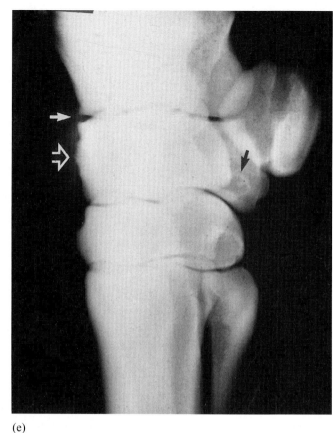

(d)   (e)

Figure 5.14 (d) Dorsopalmar view of a carpus of a 14-year-old Thoroughbred. Lateral is to the right. There is osteophyte formation on the distal medial aspect of the radius and the proximal aspect of the radial carpal bone (white arrow). There is a small clearly outlined spur on the distal medial aspect of the intermediate carpal bone (black arrow), the clinical significance of which is unknown.

(e) Dorsolateral-palmaromedial oblique view of a carpus of a 3-year-old Thoroughbred. There is osteophyte formation on the dorsomedial aspect of the antebrachiocarpal joint, involving the distal radius and the radial carpal bone (solid white arrow). The dorsal aspect of the radial carpal bone is modelled at the site of the intercarpal ligament attachments (open white arrow). There is rounding of the distal aspect of the radial carpal bone. Note the apparent lucent zone in the distal aspect of the ulnar carpal bone, surrounded by a rim of sclerosis (black arrow). This is an incidental finding.

bones and sclerosis or lucent zones in the subchondral trabecular bone (Figure 5.14a–e). The antebrachiocarpal and middle carpal joints are most commonly affected, especially the antebrachiocarpal joint in sports horses and the middle carpal joint in racehorses.

Periarticular osteophytes are most commonly seen at the proximal and distal dorsal aspects of the radial carpal bone, the proximodorsal aspect of the third carpal bone and, less commonly, the proximodorsal aspect of the intermediate carpal bone. Because of this positioning, examinations for degenerative joint disease of the carpus should always include dorsal 45° lateral-palmaromedial and dorsal 75° lateral-palmaromedial oblique views. Care should also be taken to evaluate the palmar margins of the joints, since periarticular osteophyte formation may also develop here, especially in more advanced cases of degenerative joint disease. Small bone spurs or modelling of the joint margins may be found in apparently sound horses in work, and their significance must be assessed in relation to the age of the

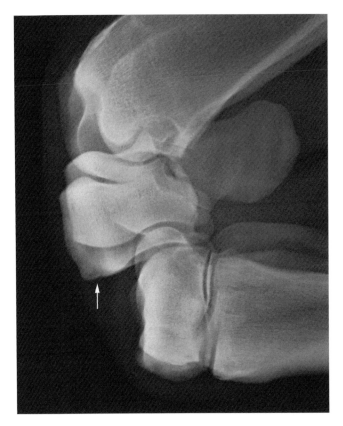

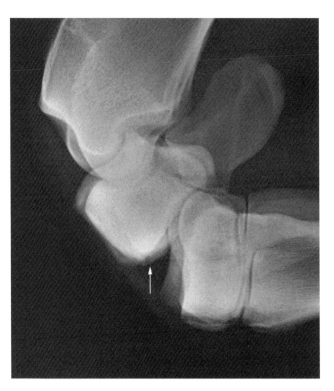

Figure 5.15(a) Flexed lateromedial radiographic view of a carpus of a 4-year-old Thoroughbred flat racing horse. Dorsal is to the left. The horse had shown intermittent lameness for many months but had been kept in training and had raced successfully. There is an ill defined small radiolucent area in the distal dorsal aspect of the radial carpal bone (arrow).

Figure 5.15(b) Flexed lateromedial radiographic view of a carpus of a 2-year-old Thoroughbred flat racing horse, with bilateral forelimb lameness. Dorsal is to the left. There is an ill defined small radiolucent area in the distal dorsal aspect of the radial carpal bone (arrow). See also Figure 5.17a.

horse, conformation, the work previously carried out, current lameness and future work required. Thus these would be of more significance if found at a purchase examination of a young top-grade performance horse, than if seen as an incidental finding in an old pleasure horse. Quite extensive abnormalities of the antebrachiocarpal joint in sports and pleasure horses can be present without lameness, although there is often restricted flexion of the joint and pain induced by flexion. Radiographic abnormalities of either the antebrachiocarpal or middle carpal joint are more likely to be associated with lameness in racehorses.

In the young Thoroughbred in training, subtle remodelling changes of the radial and third carpal bones may have important consequences. Initially there may be slight loss of opacity on the dorsal distal aspect of the radial carpal bone (Figure 5.15a); the distal articular margin becomes more rounded and 'cut back' (Figure 5.15b). This effectively moves the articulation with the third carpal bone in a slightly palmar direction. Subsequently the dorsoproximal aspect of the third carpal bone becomes less opaque. This modelling may predispose to fracture of the third carpal bone. Subtle lucent areas on the distal dorsal aspect of the radial carpal

[255]

bone are usually associated with significant cartilage pathology and may lead to fragmentation.

Narrowing of a joint space or ankylosis are rarely seen except in the carpometacarpal joint.

Degenerative changes are sometimes seen involving only part of the carpometacarpal joint, either the articulation between the second carpal and second metacarpal bone, or the fourth carpal and fourth metacarpal bone. There is narrowing of the joint space and subchondral lucent zones or sclerosis, often in association with irregular periosteal new bone on the metaphysis and proximal diaphysis of the second or fourth metacarpal bone (Figure 4.18, page 214). This is associated with mild but chronic lameness.

New bone formation

New bone formation is seen in several locations:
• New bone formed at the margins of the joints (periarticular osteophytes) is associated with degenerative joint disease (see above).
• New bone formed on the dorsal aspect of one or more carpal bones, not involving the joint margins, may be associated with tearing or strain of the intercarpal ligaments (entheseophyte formation), or direct trauma to the periosteum (periosteal osteophytes) (Figure 5.13a and 5.13b). Its significance will depend to some extent on its activity at the time of examination, as well as on the amount of bone formed. The new bone will gradually remodel, but may remain irregular. If it has well defined smooth opaque margins it is unlikely to be of long-term significance. Entheseophyte formation on the dorsal aspects of the carpal bones is sometimes seen in association with degenerative joint disease, but may also be seen as an incidental observation in young Thoroughbreds in training. Entheseophyte formation reflects ligamentous damage, resulting in slight instability of the joints. This may cause secondary degenerative joint disease, but need not do so.
• New bone formation is quite often seen on the transverse ridge of the distal caudal aspect of the radius, unassociated with clinical signs.
• Mineralization or new bone beginning to bridge the antebrachiocarpal, middle carpal and/or carpometacarpal joints, as well as new bone between the carpal bones in either row, is rare but usually the result of infection or repeated intra-articular administration of corticosteroids (so-called steroid arthropathy). Both steroid arthropathy and infection result in destruction of bone and thus irregular lucent areas in the bones. Infection is usually associated with sclerosis, and either condition may result in ankylosis of joints and extensive new bone formation. In either case, a poor or hopeless prognosis must be given.
• New bone formation occasionally occurs at the origin of the accessory ligament of the superficial flexor tendon (superior check ligament) at the caudal aspect of the radius. Its significance should be assessed in the light of clinical signs. Lameness, if present, will usually resolve with rest. Ultrasonographic evaluation is important to assess the integrity of the ligament.
• A small spur on the caudal aspect of the radius at the level of the distal physis may be subtle and difficult to detect radiographically but can cause

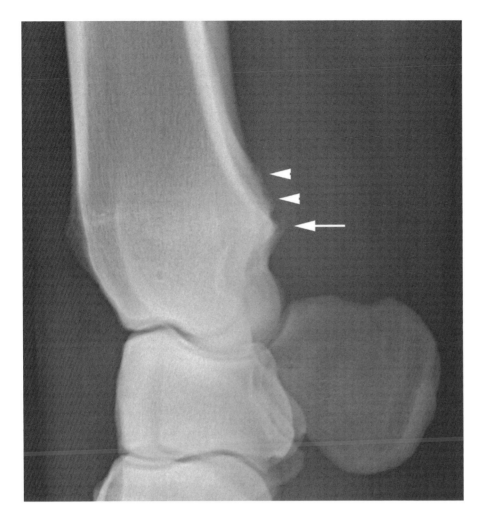

Figure 5.16 Lateromedial radiographic view of a distal radius and carpus of an 8-year-old Warmblood dressage horse with sporadic lameness. When present the lameness was accentuated by carpal flexion, in association with mild distension of the carpal sheath. Dorsal is to the left. There is an exostosis on the caudal aspect of the radius at the level of the distal radial physis (arrow). Ultrasonographic examination confirmed that this spike was impinging on the deep digital flexor tendon. Note also the slightly irregular periosteal new bone on the caudal aspect of the radius proximal to the physis (arrow heads).

an impingement lesion on the deep digital flexor tendon and cause episodic lameness with or without distension of the carpal sheath (Figure 5.16). Ultrasonography may be necessary to confirm the diagnosis. Surgical removal usually has a successful outcome.

● Distension of the carpal sheath, lameness and resentment of pressure applied to the distal caudal aspect of the radius may be associated with an osteochondroma on the distal diaphysis or metaphysis of the radius. Radiographically this appears as a variably shaped bony protuberance on the distocaudal aspect of the radius (see Figure 5.22, page 264). This mass has a thin cortex that appears to be continuous with the cortex of the radius. Sequential radiographs may demonstrate progressive enlargement of the mass. Treatment by surgical removal of the osteochondroma is usually successful in resolving both the lameness and carpal sheath swelling.

[257]

Figure 5.17(a) Dorsoproximal-dorsodistal oblique radiographic view of the distal row of carpal bones of a 2-year-old Thoroughbred flat racing horse. Medial is to the left. There is extensive sclerosis of the radial facet of the third carpal bone. There are several ill defined lucent lines within the sclerotic bone. The dorsal margin of the bone is slightly irregular medially. Lameness was improved by intra-articular analgesia of the middle carpal joint. Compare with the trabecular structure of the fourth carpal bone. See also Figure 5.15b.

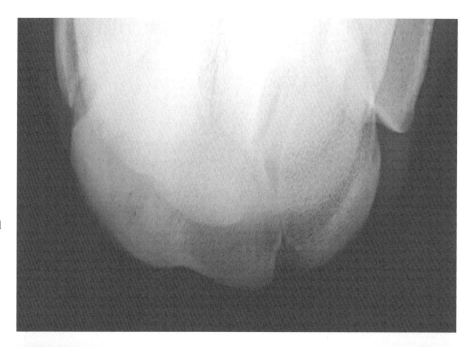

Figure 5.17(b) Dorsoproximal-dorsodistal oblique radiographic view of the distal row of carpal bones of a 3-year-old Thoroughbred racehorse. Medial is to the left. There is extensive sclerosis of the radial facet of the third carpal bone and multiple lucent zones on the dorsal aspect of the bone. Lameness was partially improved by intra-articular analgesia of the middle carpal joint and abolished by perineural analgesia of the median and ulnar nerves.

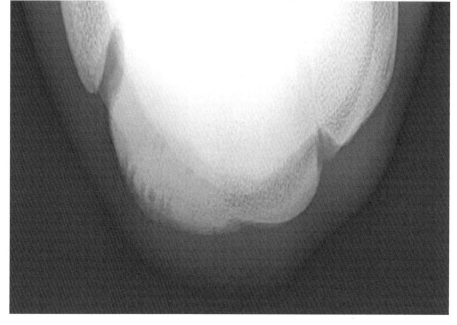

● New bone formation may occur on the distal cranial radius, often in conjunction with distension of the tendon sheath of the extensor carpi radialis. This is usually the result of repeated trauma, but is rarely of long-term significance. Occasionally surgical debridement is indicated.

Sclerosis of the third carpal bone

A mild degree of sclerosis of the third carpal bone is believed to be a normal modelling feature in young Thoroughbreds and Standardbreds in training and usually involves the radial facet. These changes can only be appreciated radiographically in dorsoproximal-dorsodistal oblique views, which highlight the third carpal bone. Marked sclerosis of either the radial (Figure 5.17a) and/or intermediate facet is abnormal. This change is appreciated radiographically as a loss of both the trabecular structure and the definition between the cortex and medulla. Often there is associated joint capsule distension of the middle carpal joint, a finding that should lead to further evaluation of the third carpal bone. Small poorly circumscribed lucent zones are abnormal (Figure 5.17b) and may be a precursor to fracture. The third carpal bone may be compared carefully with the fourth carpal bone since the trabecular pattern of the latter is generally normal. If the fourth carpal bone appears sclerotic the radiograph is probably underexposed and should be repeated. The radial facet can also be compared with the remainder of the third carpal bone. Sclerosis of the third carpal bone can be seen in conjunction with lameness improved or alleviated by intra-articular analgesia of the middle carpal joint, with no other identifiable abnormality.

Lameness usually resolves with rest and the sclerotic bone may slowly remodel, although lameness may be recurrent when full work is resumed. Magnetic resonance imaging and computed tomography have demonstrated that lesions may be more extensive than appreciated radiographically, involving bones more proximal and distal in the same sagittal plane, e.g. the distal aspect of the radius, the radial carpal bone and the third metacarpal bone. Excessive sclerosis in the radial facet has been shown to predispose to subsequent fracture. Sometimes intra-articular analgesia does not alleviate the lameness associated with third carpal bone sclerosis, but nuclear scintigraphic examination reveals increased modelling activity in the third carpal bone.

Sclerosis of the radial facet of the third carpal bone has occasionally been identified as the cause of lameness in sports horses.

Osseous cyst-like lesions

Osseous cyst-like lesions have been described in all the carpal bones, as well as at the proximal end of all three metacarpal bones and the distal radius. They are frequently, but not always incidental findings unassociated with lameness. However, in young foals osseous cyst-like lesions may represent E-type osteomyelitis (see page 32) and should lead to further diagnostic tests for 'joint ill' (Figures 5.18a and 5.18b). Aggressive broad-spectrum antimicrobial therapy may be required. Very large osseous cyst-like lesions close to a joint margin are probably more likely to be associated with lameness (see Chapter 1, page 33). Significant lesions may become clinically silent with conservative treatment or may require surgery.

Osseous cyst-like lesions in the axial aspect of the ulnar carpal bone, with avulsion fragments at the insertion of the interosseous ligament, have been seen as a cause of lameness in racehorses. However similar lesions have been seen in sports horses as incidental abnormalities unassociated with lameness. Occasionally osseous cyst-like lesions are seen in any of the

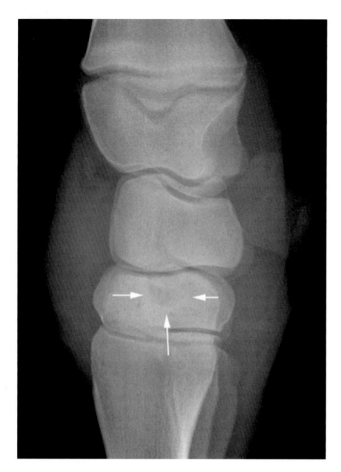

Figure 5.18(a) Lateromedial radiographic view of a carpus of a 2.5-month-old crossbred foal. Dorsal is to the left. There is massive soft-tissue swelling on the dorsal and palmar aspects of the carpus centred around the middle carpal joint. There is a large radiolucent area in the third carpal bone (arrows), consistent with type E osteomyelitis. Synovial fluid from the middle carpal joint contained 97% neutrophils.

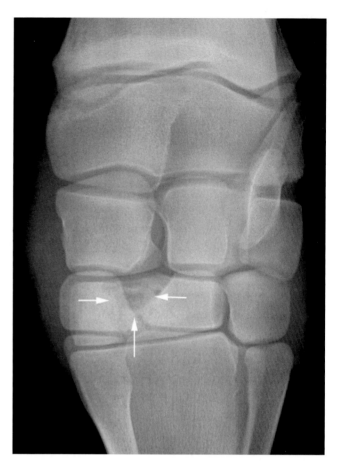

Figure 5.18(b) Dorsopalmar radiographic view of a carpus of the same foal as Fig. 5.18a. Medial is to the left. There is an ill defined radiolucent lesion in the third carpal bone (arrows).

carpal bones associated with interosseous desmitis, a diagnosis that can be confirmed using magnetic resonance imaging.

Polydactyly

Polydactyly has been recorded in the horse, arising from the carpus or distally and often represents a non-rudimentary second or fourth metacarpal bone. The extra appendage tends to cause limb deviation and therefore requires surgical removal at an early age.

Physitis (epiphysitis)

The radiographic appearance of physitis is described fully in Chapter 1 (page 21). It is relatively common in the distal radius of rapidly growing yearlings and in young racehorses as they commence work.

[260]

Physitis is characterized radiographically by an irregular widening of the physis. There may be 'lipping' medially and laterally (Figure 5.19). Frequently limb deviation will also result. Clinically the limb may be swollen immediately proximal to the carpus, and may be hot and painful to palpation. Treatment is by restricting feed and exercise until an adequate clinical response is seen.

Carpal angular limb deformities

Many limb deviations arise from the carpus and may be congenital or acquired. If a deviation is severe, or a moderate deviation fails to respond to conservative treatment, radiographic examination is indicated. For valgus and varus deviations, dorsopalmar views on long (43 cm) cassettes are most useful. The extent of the deviation can be measured and monitored by drawing the lines that bisect the radius and third metacarpal bones. These will intersect at or near the point at which the deviation arises, and the angle at the point of intersection indicates the degree of deviation (Figure 5.20). Subsequent films to evaluate change in angle must be identical in position to the first set.

Radiographic abnormalities may include one or more of the following:
- Irregularity in width of the distal radial physis
- A wedge-shaped distal radial epiphysis
- Incomplete ossification of one or more carpal bones (see below)
- Malformation of one or more carpal bones. This probably results from weight bearing on incompletely ossified bones
- Delayed development of the lateral styloid process

If the limb deformity is related to changes in the distal physis or epiphysis, treatment carries a reasonable prognosis if carried out well before closure of the physis. Malformation of the carpal bones warrants a poor prognosis. Incomplete ossification requires early identification and treatment for a successful outcome (see below). An angular limb deformity may be coexistent with rotation (usually outwards) of the limb, which should be assessed clinically. Radiographs can give limited information about rotation and the direction of the x-ray beam must be governed by this clinical assessment. In general terms, if a limb is outwardly rotated and a radiograph is obtained perpendicular to the antebrachium, the carpal bones will appear slightly superimposed upon one another. However, if the x-ray beam is perpendicular to the carpus the bones will be separated normally.

Incomplete carpal ossification

This condition is seen in very young foals (often dysmature or twins) with a carpal angular limb deformity. On radiographs the distal radial physis usually appears normal, but one or more of the carpal bones will be small and rounded, lacking the normal cuboidal shape (Figure 5.21).

Successful treatment requires prompt action in the first days of life to straighten the limb and support it in a cast, until ossification of the affected bones is normal.

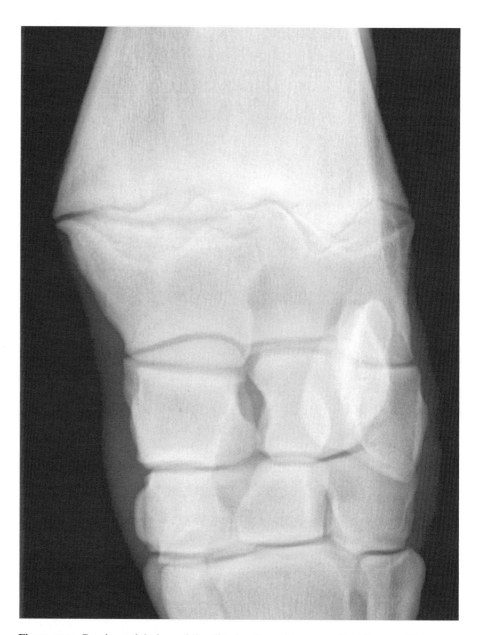

Figure 5.19 Craniocaudal view of the distal radius of a 14-month-old potential event horse. Medial is to the left. The medial aspect of the distal radial physis is broader than laterally. The distal metaphyseal region is flared medially. The central axes of the radius and the metacarpal regions are not in alignment.

Osteochondroma

The caudodistal aspect of the radius is the site where osteochondromas are most frequently identified radiographically. They are variable in size and shape, and may have an irregular outline (Figure 5.22). It may be possible to identify a communication with the marrow cavity of the radius. Although they may be benign and not associated with clinical signs, they may result in lameness often with distension of the carpal sheath. These lesions are usually solitary, but may be associated with lesions elsewhere. They can be removed surgically and this treatment carries a good prognosis for return to work.

[262]

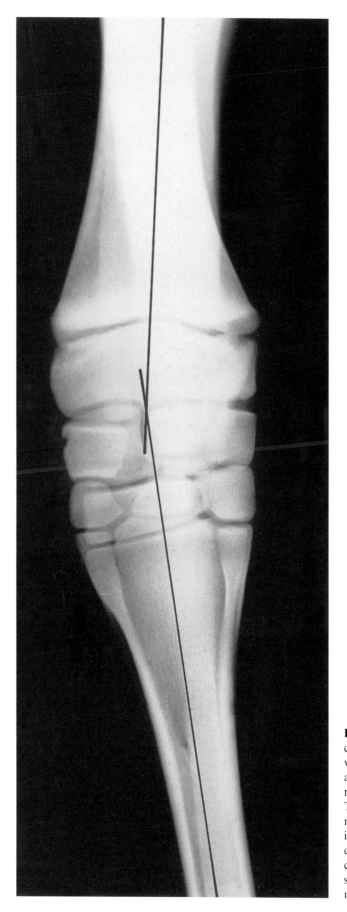

Figure 5.20 Dorsopalmar view of a carpus of a 3-week-old foal with a carpal valgus deformity, centred close to the antebrachiocarpal joint. Lateral is to the right. Deviation is approximately 12°. The lateral styloid process of the distal radius is incompletely ossified and there is a discrete fragment distal to it. The distal radial epiphysis and the third carpal bone are wedge shaped, being shorter on their lateral aspects than medially.

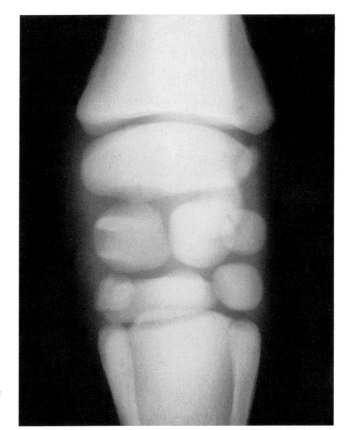

Figure 5.21 Dorsopalmar view of a carpus of a Quarterhorse foal, born at 323 days of gestation, obtained 6 days after birth. Lateral is to the right. The carpal bones are incompletely ossified; note their rounded contour. Note also the incompletely ossified separate centre of ossification of the lateral styloid process of the ulna.

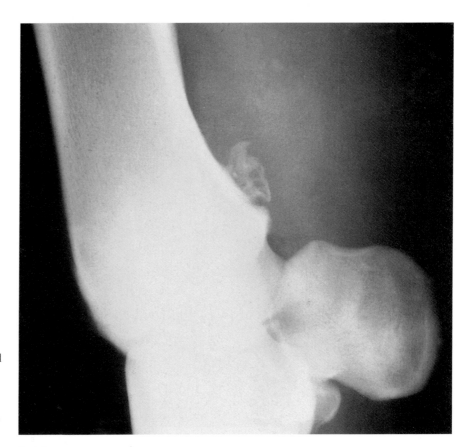

Figure 5.22 Lateromedial view of a distal radius of a mature horse. There is a solitary osteochondroma on the caudal aspect of the distal radius, which was associated with distension of the carpal sheath and severe lameness. After surgical removal of the osteochondroma the clinical signs resolved.

Carpal subluxation

Carpal subluxation is rare and may occur at the antebrachiocarpal, middle carpal or carpometacarpal joint. The latter site is most common. There may be concurrent fractures. Occasionally stressed radiographic views are required to confirm the diagnosis. The prognosis for athletic function is poor.

Carpal fractures

Chip fractures of the carpal bones

These fractures occur frequently, especially in racehorses (Figure 5.23). They may be defined as fractures that involve only one joint surface of the

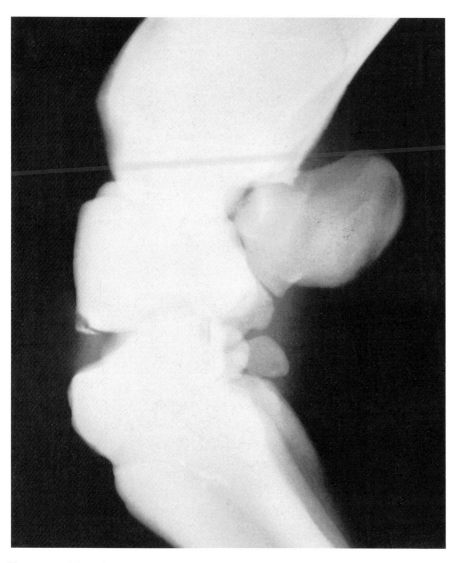

Figure 5.23 Flexed lateromedial view of a carpus, showing a chip fracture of the distal border of the radial carpal bone. The fracture was poorly demonstrated on other views. Note the large first carpal bone. (The radiograph was taken with reduced exposure to highlight the fracture.)

bone. Their visualization may require several oblique views, although they are often most readily observed on the flexed lateromedial view. The most common sites for chip fractures are the distal border of the dorsal aspect of the radius, the radial carpal bone (slightly to the medial side of the midline) and the opposing radial facet of the third carpal bone; also, the distal dorsal aspect of the intermediate carpal bone. Less commonly fractures occur in the proximal aspect of the radial and intermediate carpal bones. Lameness due to small fracture fragments may resolve with rest. Surgical removal should always be considered in cases in which horses are required to return to athletic performance, and in cases with larger fragments. A good prognosis can generally be given, provided that no other lesions are present. A degree of cartilage damage will have occurred and degenerative joint disease may subsequently develop.

Chip fractures can also involve the lateral, medial and palmar aspects of the carpal bones. These are less common and carry a more guarded prognosis. Fractures on the palmar aspect of the carpal joints alone are usually the result of trauma, for example poor recovery from general anaesthesia. They may initially be minimally distracted and are easily missed. Osteochondral fragments on the palmar aspect of the joint may be seen in conjunction with dorsal fragments in racehorses. They may also arise dorsally and migrate palmad. Multiple small fragments warrant a more guarded prognosis for return to racing.

Degenerative joint disease (see page 252) may be pre-existing and may have predisposed to a fracture. The radiographs should be carefully scrutinized to evaluate the entire carpus, both for evidence of degenerative joint disease and for the presence of more than one fracture. Since fractures frequently occur bilaterally, both carpi should be examined radiographically.

Slab fractures

Slab fractures (involving both proximal and distal articular surfaces) occur most commonly at the dorsal aspect of the third, fourth or radial carpal bones (Figure 5.24). These fractures can usually be detected on lateromedial radiographs, but dorsoproximal-dorsodistal oblique views should also be obtained to ascertain the extent and degree of comminution of the fracture. This view will also show fractures that are not easily recognized on lateromedial views, and may show sclerosis of the third carpal bone (see page 258). Slab fractures have also been recorded at the palmar aspect of the third carpal bone.

Dorsal or oblique slab fractures of the radial and third carpal bones are usually repaired by lag screw fixation, but if the fracture fragment is very thin it may be removed.

Sagittal fractures of the third carpal bone are generally only detectable on dorsoproximal-dorsodistal oblique views (Figures 5.25a and 5.25b). Internal fixation is possible, but a fair prognosis can be given for conservative treatment provided that there is minimal displacement and no degenerative joint disease.

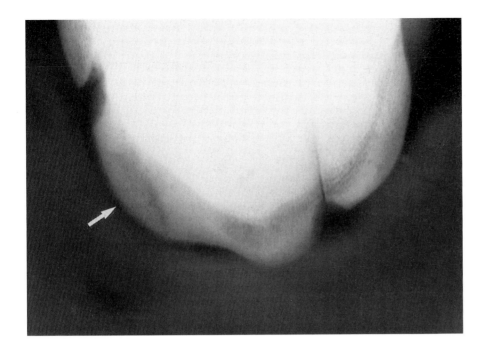

Figure 5.24 Dorsoproximal-dorsodistal oblique view of a carpus of a 2-year-old Thoroughbred. Lateral is to the right. There is a frontal (slab) fracture of the third carpal bone (arrow), which probably occurred secondarily to the marked sclerosis of the radial facet. Compare the trabecular pattern of the medial aspect of the third carpal bone with that of the fourth (see also Figure 5.17).

Fractures of the accessory carpal bone

These fractures most frequently occur in a vertical plane approximately through the middle of the bone. The fractures may be simple or comminuted and can occur in any plane. The pull of the flexor tendons that insert on the palmar aspect of the bone may result in the palmar fragment being pulled proximally and medially. With prolonged rest (6–8 months) and restricted exercise, approximately 80% of cases will return to work. Healing is by fibrous union and a lucent line persists (Figure 1.14, page 29). Some horses will develop chronic lameness, and internal fixation at the time of fracture should be considered.

Chip fractures may occasionally occur close to the articular surface, often proximodorsally. On a lateromedial view this may be partially superimposed over other carpal bones, and a dorsal 80° lateral-palmaromedial oblique view may give better visualization (Figure 5.26). Surgical removal may be required.

Fractures of the second or fourth carpal bones

Fractures of the second or fourth carpal bones are often comminuted. These fractures are often accompanied by fractures of the proximal aspect of the second or fourth metacarpal bones. This will result in marked lateromedial instability of the carpometacarpal joint. Such fractures require internal

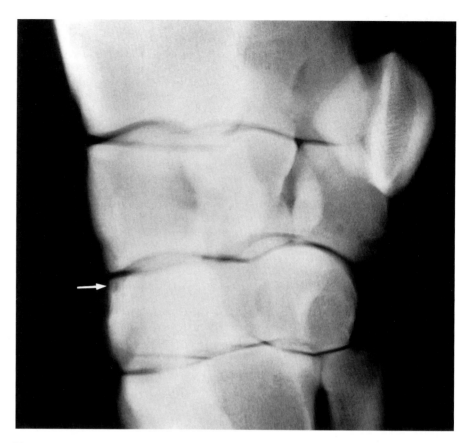

Figure 5.25(a) Dorsolateral-palmaromedial oblique view of a carpus of a 3-year-old Thoroughbred with a sagittal fracture of the third carpal bone. Note the irregular lucency of the dorsoproximal aspect of the third carpal bone (arrow).

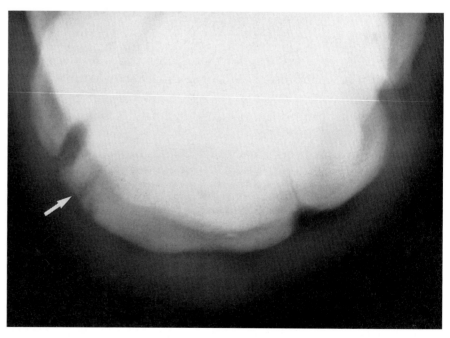

Figure 5.25(b) Dorsoproximal-dorsodistal oblique view of the same carpus to highlight the distal row of carpal bones. Lateral is to the right. Note the sagittal fracture on the medial aspect of the radial facet of the third carpal bone (arrow).

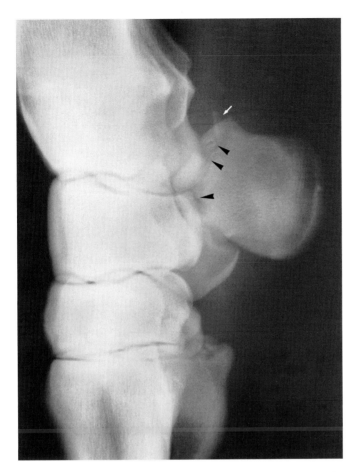

Figure 5.26 Dorsal 80° lateral-palmaromedial oblique view of a carpus of a 3-year-old Thoroughbred with acute onset of lameness of 2 days' duration. There is a comminuted articular fracture (arrow heads) of the accessory carpal bone. One small fragment (white arrow) has been displaced proximally. Note also the osseous opacity in close apposition to the fourth carpal bone, this is a fifth carpal bone.

fixation and carry a guarded prognosis (see also 'Metacarpal fractures', page 227).

FURTHER READING

Auer, J., Smallwood, J., Morris, E., Martens, R. *et al.* (1982) The developing equine carpus from birth to 6 months. A radiographic study. *Equine Pract.*, **4**, 35–55

Auer, J., Watkins, J., White, N. *et al.* (1986) Slab fractures of the fourth and intermediate carpal bones in 5 horses. *J. Am. Vet. Med. Assoc.*, **188**, 595–601

Bailey, J., Barber, S., Fretz, P. and Jacobs, K. (1984) Subluxation of the carpus in thirteen horses. *Can. Vet. J.*, **25**, 311–314

Barr, A., Sinnott, M. and Denny, H. (1990) Fractures of the accessory carpal bone in the horse. *Vet. Rec.*, **127**, 432–434

Beinlich, C. and Nixon, A. (2004) Radiographic and pathologic characterization of lateral palmar intercarpal ligament avulsion fracture in the horse. *Vet. Radiol. and Ultrasound*, **45**, 532–537

Bramlage, L., Schneider, R. and Gabel, A. (1988) A clinical perspective on lameness originating in the carpus. *Equine vet. J.*, Suppl. **6**, 12–18

Burguez, P.N. (1986) Interpreting radiographs 4: the carpus. *Equine vet. J.*, **16**, 159–163

Catcott, E.J. and Smithcors, J.F., Eds (1972) *Equine Medicine and Surgery*, 2nd edn, American Veterinary Publications, Illinois

Dabareiner, R., White, N. and Sullins, K. (1996) Radiographic and arthroscopic findings associated with subchondral lucency of the distal radial carpal bone in 71 horses. *Equine vet. J.*, **28**, 93–97

De Haan, C., O'Brien, T. and Koblick, P. (1987) A radiographic investigation of third carpal bone injury in 42 racing thoroughbreds. *Vet. Radiol.*, **28**, 88–92

Dietze, A. and Rendano, V. (1984) Fat opacities dorsal to the equine antebrachiocarpal joint. *Vet. Radiol.*, **25**, 205–209

Dixon, R.T. (1969) Radiography of the equine carpus. *Aust. Vet. J.*, **45**, 171–174

Dyson, S. (1988) Some observations on lameness associated with pain in the proximal metacarpal region. *Equine vet. J.*, Suppl. **6**, 43–52

Dyson, S. (1990) Fractures of the accessory carpal bone. *Equine vet. Educ.*, **2**(4), 188–190

Ellis, D. (1985) Some observations on bone cysts in the carpal bones of young thoroughbreds. *Equine vet. J.*, **17**, 63–65

Fischer, A. and Stover, S. (1987) Sagittal fractures of the third carpal bone in horses: 12 cases (1977–1985). *J. Am. Vet. Med. Ass.*, **191**, 106–108

Gertson, K.E. and Dawson, H.A. (1976) Sagittal fracture of the third carpal bone in a horse. *J. Am. Vet. Med. Ass.*, **169**, 633–634

Getman, L., Southwood, L. and Richardson, D. (2006) Palmar carpal osteochondral fragments in racehorses: 31 cases (1994–2004). *J. Am. Vet. Med. Ass.*, **228**, 1551–1558

Hopper, B., Steel, C., Richardson, L., Alexander, G. and Robertson, I. (2004) Radiographic evaluation of sclerosis of the third carpal bone associated with exercise and the development of lameness in Standardbred horses. *Equine vet. J.*, **36**, 441–446

Kraus, B., Ross, M. and Boston, R. (2005) Surgical and nonsurgical management of sagittal slab fractures of the third carpal bone in racehorses: 32 cases. *J. Am. Vet. Med. Ass.*, **226**, 945–950

Lucas, J., Ross, M. and Richardson, D. (1999) Post operative performance of racing Standardbreds treated arthroscopically for carpal chip fractures: 176 cases (1986–1993). *Equine vet. J.*, **31**, 48–52

Magnusson, L. and Ekman, S. (2001) Osteoarthritis of the antebrachiocarpal joint of 7 riding horses. *Acta. Vet. Scand.*, **42**, 429–434

Malone, E., Les, C. and Turner, T. (2003) Severe carpometacarpal osteoarthritis in older Arabian horses. *Vet. Surg.*, **32**, 191–195

Manning, J.P. and St. Clair, L.E. (1972) Carpal hyperextension and arthrosis in the horse. *Proc. Am. Ass. Equine Pract.*, **18**, 173–181

Martens, P. (1999) Identification of an ossicle associated with the palmar aspect of the carpus in a horse. *Vet. Radiol. and Ultrasound*, **40**, 342–345

Mason, T.A. and Bourke, J.M. (1973) Closure of the distal radial epiphysis and its relationship to unsoundness in two year old thoroughbreds. *Aust. Vet. J.*, **49**, 221–228

May, K., Holmes, L., Moll, H. and Jones, J. (2001) Computed tomographic imaging of comminuted carpal fractures in a gelding. *Equine vet. Educ.*, **13**, 303–308

Mayrhofer, W., Stanek, C., Lutz, H. and Hiedbrink, U. (2006) Wertigkeit klinischer, radiologischer und computertomographischer Befunde bei der Diagnostik von Karpalgelenkserkrankungen beim Pferd. *Pferdeheilkunde*, **22**, 773–784

Murray, R. (2007) Magnetic resonance imaging of the equine carpus. *Clin. Techniques Equine Pract.*, **6**, 86–95

Myers, V.S. (1965) Confusing radiological variation at the distal end of the radius of the horse. *J. Am. Vet. Med. Ass.*, **147**, 1310–1312

Nixon, A., Schachter, B. and Pool, R. (2004) Exostoses of the caudal perimeter of the radial physis as a cause of carpal synovial sheath tenosynovitis and lameness in horses: 10 cases (1999–2003). *J. Am. Vet. Med. Ass.*, **224**, 264–270

Park, R.D., Morgan, J.P. and O'Brien, T. (1970) Chip fractures in the carpus of the horse; a radiographic study of their incidence and location. *J. Am. Vet. Med. Ass.*, **157**, 1305–1312

Platt, D. and Wright, I. (1997) Chronic tenosynovitis of the carpal extensor tendon sheaths in 15 horses. *Equine vet. J.*, **29**, 11–17

Schneider, R., Bramlage, A., Barone, L. and Kantrowitz, B. (1988) Incidence, location and classification of 371 third carpal bone fractures in 313 horses. *Equine vet. J.*, Suppl. **6**, 33–42

Sisson, S. and Grossman, J.D. (1953) *Anatomy of the Domestic Animals*, 4th edn, W.B. Saunders, Philadelphia

Smallwood, U. and Shiveley, M. (1979) Radiographic and xeroradiographic anatomy of the equine carpus. *Equine Pract.*, **1**, 22–38

Specht, T., Nixon, A. and Colahan, P. (1988) Subchondral cyst-like lesions in the distal portion of the radius in 4 horses. *J. Am. Vet. Med. Assoc.*, **193**, 949–952

Stashak, T.S. (1987) *Adams' Lameness in Horses*, 4th edn, Lea and Febiger, Philadelphia

Stephens, P., Richardson, D. and Spencer, F. (1988) Slab fractures of the third carpal bone in Standardbreds and Thoroughbreds: 155 cases (1977–1984). *J. Am. Vet. Med. Assoc.*, **193**, 353–358

Ter Braake, F. and Rijkenhuizen, A. (2001) Endoscopic removal of osteochondroma at the caudodistal aspect of the radius: and evaluation in 4 cases. *Equine vet. Educ.*, **13**, 90–93

Thrall, D.E., Lebel, J.L. and O'Brien, T.R. (1971) A five-year survey of the incidence and location of equine carpal chip fractures. *J. Am. Vet. Med. Ass.*, **158**, 1366–1368

Uhlorn, H., Ekman, S., Haglund, A. and Carlsten, A. (1998) The accuracy of the dorso-proximal-dorsodistal projection in assessing third carpal bone sclerosis in Standardbred trotters. *Vet. Radiol. and Ultrasound*, **39**, 412–417

Uhlorn, H. and Carlsten, J. (1999) Retrospective study of subchondral sclerosis and lucency in the third carpal bone of Standardbred trotters. *Equine vet. J.*, **31**, 500–505

Waselau, M., Bertone, A. and Green, W. (2006) Computed tomographic documentation of a comminuted fourth carpal bone fracture associated with carpal instability treated by partial carpal arthrodesis in an Arabian filly. *Vet. Surg.*, **35**, 618–625

Whitton, C., Kannegeiter, N. and Rose, R. (1997) The intercarpal ligaments of the equine mid carpal joint. Part 3. Clinical observations in 32 racing horses with mid-carpal joint disease. *Vet. Surg.*, **26**, 374–381

Wilke, M., Nixon, A., Malark, J. *et al.* (2001) Fractures of the palmar aspect of the carpal bones in horses: 10 cases (1984–2000). *J. Am. Vet. Med. Ass.*, **219**, 801–804

Wintzer, H.J. (1986) *Equine Diseases*, Paul Parey, Berlin

Wong, D., Scaratt, W., Maxwell, V. and Moon, M. (2003) Incomplete ossification of the carpal, tarsal and navicular bones in a dysmature foal. *Equine vet. Educ.*, **15**, 72–81

Young, A., O'Brien, T. and Pool, R. (1988) Exercise related sclerosis in the third carpal bone of the racing thoroughbred. *Proc. Am. Ass. Equine Pract.*, **34**, 339–346

Chapter 6
The shoulder, humerus, elbow and radius

Scapulohumeral (shoulder) joint and humerus

RADIOGRAPHIC TECHNIQUE

Equipment

The scapulohumeral joint may be radiographed with the horse standing if a high-output x-ray machine is available. Better-quality radiographs are generally obtained with the horse under general anaesthesia in lateral recumbency. With the horse anaesthetized, positioning is easier and longer exposure times can be used without risk of movement, so a lower output x-ray machine may be used. The radiation hazard to personnel is also reduced. Digital systems, or rare earth screens and appropriate film, are essential due to the high exposures required to penetrate the large muscle mass in this area. A grid is recommended to reduce the effects of scattered radiation, and lead should be placed behind the cassette to limit back scatter. There is less soft tissue to penetrate cranially; therefore it may be necessary to repeat a view with different exposure factors in order to assess both the cranioproximal aspect of the humerus and the more caudally situated scapulohumeral joint properly. Alternatively an aluminium wedge filter can be used to modify the exposure. For mediolateral radiographs obtained with the horse standing, the cassette should be mounted in a holder and not hand held. Both mediolateral and oblique views are required for a complete assessment of the scapulohumeral joint, and in selected cases arthrography yields valuable additional information.

Positioning

Mediolateral view

STANDING

The forelimb to be examined is positioned next to the cassette and the limb is protracted as much as the horse will comfortably allow, to avoid superimposition of the left and right shoulder joints (Figure 6.1). If possible the shoulder joint is superimposed over the trachea, to give the best images. Some horses resist protraction of the limb and this may result in movement blur and partial superimposition of the left and right shoulder joints. Sedation may be helpful, but the horse may relax and lower its neck so that a

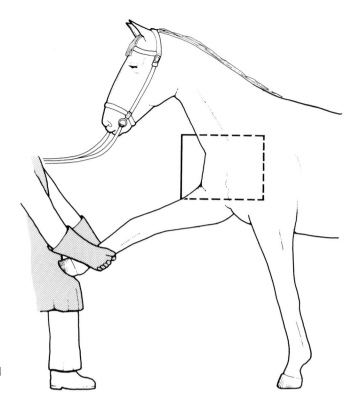

Figure 6.1 Positioning of the horse and cassette to obtain a mediolateral radiographic view of the scapulohumeral joint.

larger proportion of the distal scapula is superimposed over the cervical and thoracic vertebrae. Raising the head and neck can help to minimize this. The use of an analgesic such as butorphanol facilitates the examination of horses suffering severe pain.

LATERAL RECUMBENCY

The anaesthetized horse is placed in lateral recumbency, lying on the limb to be radiographed. This limb is protracted, the contralateral forelimb is retracted and the neck is extended. It may be helpful to restrain the fore-limbs using ropes. The position of the endotracheal tube is adjusted so that its distal end is not superimposed over the scapulohumeral joint. The examination is performed most easily if the horse is lying on a cassette tunnel, to avoid having to lift the horse in order to place the cassette beneath it. With appropriate sedation a foal may be restrained in lateral recumbency without the need for general anaesthesia.

CENTRING THE X-RAY BEAM

The x-ray beam is centred approximately 10 cm cranial to the distal aspect of the scapular spine of the limb contralateral to that being radiographed. This is approximately equivalent to centring at the level of the greater tubercle of the humerus of the protracted limb. It is helpful to mark the point at which the beam is centred (e.g. with sticky tape) so that appropriate corrections can be made for subsequent exposures.

If the scapulohumeral joint is positioned distal to the trachea, up to one-third of the distal scapula can be seen without superimposition of the cervical and thoracic vertebrae and the ribs. Evaluation of the proximal two-thirds

CHAPTER 6
*The shoulder, humerus,
elbow and radius*

of the scapula is difficult because of the superimposed bones and the flatness of the scapula. If either rim of the glenoid cavity of the scapula or the proximal articular surface of the humerus are superimposed over the proximal or distal borders of the trachea, the summation of opacities makes interpretation difficult and additional radiographs may be required. It is sometimes helpful to position the scapulohumeral joint over the trachea. Although this can be achieved in the standing horse, it is most easily done if the horse is anaesthetized.

The distal two-thirds of the humerus is examined using a similar technique, but centring further distally. This examination is usually only indicated when a fracture is suspected and associated pain often makes adequate protraction of the limb very difficult. High exposure factors may therefore be required in order to obtain adequate penetration of the large muscle mass.

Cranial 45° medial-caudolateral oblique view

This view is most easily obtained with the horse standing. The forelimb to be examined is usually protracted and the cassette is held caudal to the shoulder muscle mass in order to position it sufficiently far medially. This inevitably results in some magnification. A grid is unnecessary, which allows lower exposure factors. The x-ray beam is centred at the level of the greater tubercle of the humerus. Alternatively a caudolateral-craniomedial oblique view may be obtained, but this usually results in greater magnification.

These views help to clarify some intra-articular lesions, especially those in the sagittal plane. They also permit identification of some fractures not visible in a mediolateral projection and help to determine the direction of a luxation of the humerus.

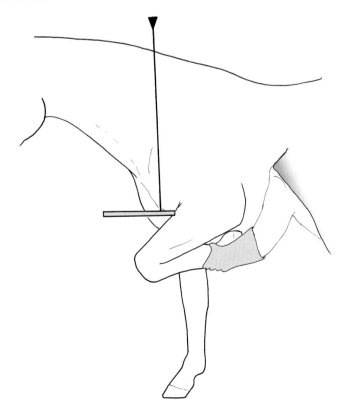

Figure 6.2 Positioning to obtain a cranioproximal-craniodistal oblique view of the proximal aspect of the humerus. The limb is held with the carpus flexed maximally. The imaging plate is held horizontally distal to the shoulder. The horse's head and neck are turned away from the limb to be examined. The x-ray beam is directed ventrally.

[275]

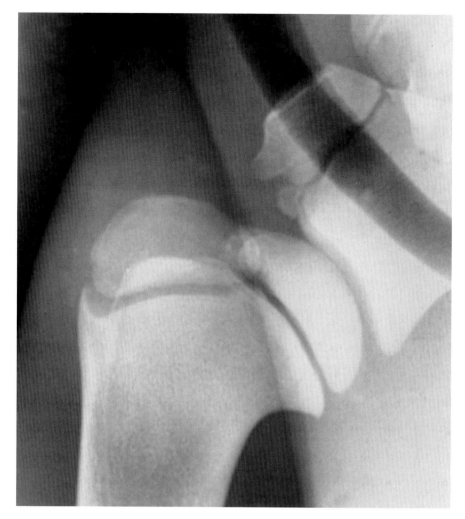

Figure 6.3 Mediolateral view and diagram of a shoulder of a 12-day-old foal. The cranial centre of ossification of the glenoid cavity of the scapula and the lesser tubercle of the humerus are incompletely ossified. The curvature of the glenoid cavity of the scapula is more shallow and the ventral angle is more rounded compared with an adult shoulder.

Cranioproximal-craniodistal oblique 'skyline' view of the proximal aspect of the humerus

This view can be obtained either in the standing horse or with the horse under general anaesthesia. The limb is held with the carpus and elbow flexed (Figure 6.2), with the x-ray cassette positioned horizontally distal to the humeral tubercles. The horse's head and neck are turned away from the limb to be examined. The x-ray machine is positioned proximal to the shoulder and the x-ray beam is directed ventrally, centred on the humeral tubercles. This view helps to identify fractures of the greater, or less commonly lesser, tubercles of the humerus, that may be difficult to identify in other projections.

Caudolateral-craniomedial oblique view

This view is obtained with the horse standing. The x-ray machine is positioned against the thorax, on the ipsilateral side of the shoulder to be examined. A horizontal x-ray beam is used, angled at approximately 40° lateral to the sagittal midline (i.e., caudal 40° lateral-craniomedial oblique view). The x-ray cassette is positioned cranial to the shoulder, perpendicular

[276]

CHAPTER 6
*The shoulder, humerus,
elbow and radius*

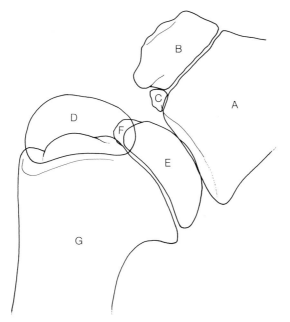

Figure 6.3 *Cont'd* A = body of scapula, B = ossification centre for the supraglenoid tubercle and coracoid process, C = ossification centre for the cranial part of the glenoid of the scapula, D = ossification centre for the greater tubercle of the humerus, E = ossification centre for the humeral head and lesser tubercle, F = incompletely ossified lesser tubercle, G = diaphysis of humerus.

to the x-ray beam. This view may highlight a fracture of the cranial part of the greater tubercle of the humerus.

Arthrography

Arthrography can be performed with the horse standing or in lateral recumbency under general anaesthesia. In the latter position the technique is more complicated because, after injecting the contrast medium with the limb to be examined uppermost, the horse must then be turned over for radiography. A small volume (7–10 ml) of a 60% mixture of sodium and meglumine amidotrizoate (Urografin 60%, Schering AG) is recommended. Dilution of the contrast agent with a balanced polyionic electrolyte solution may help definition of the articular cartilage. The technique can be used to highlight articular cartilage defects and subtle bone lesions and to identify dissecting cartilage flaps in cases of osteochondrosis.

RADIOGRAPHIC ANATOMY, NORMAL VARIATIONS AND INCIDENTAL FINDINGS

Birth to 3 years old

Scapula

The scapula has four centres of ossification: the scapular cartilage, the body of the scapula, the cranial part of the glenoid cavity of the scapula and the supraglenoid tubercle (Figure 6.3). The latter two may be incompletely ossified at birth and have a fuzzy, irregular outline. The cranial part of the glenoid cavity of the scapula fuses with the body by 5 months after birth. The physis of the supraglenoid tubercle closes by 12–24 months after birth.

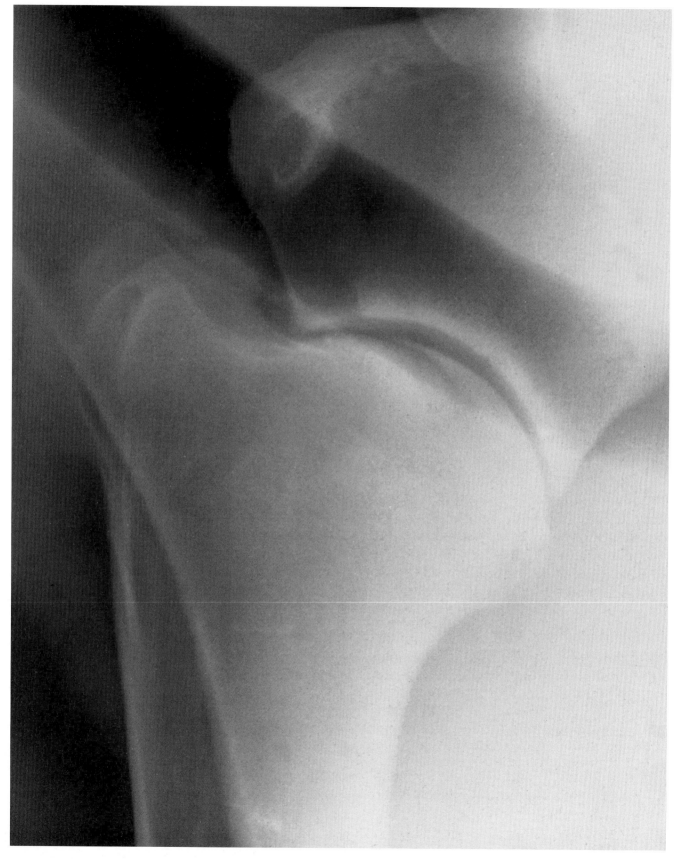

Figure 6.4(a) Mediolateral view and diagram of a normal adult scapulohumeral joint (compare with Figure 6.6). See text regarding Figure 6.4(a) on page 280.

[278]

CHAPTER 6
*The shoulder, humerus,
elbow and radius*

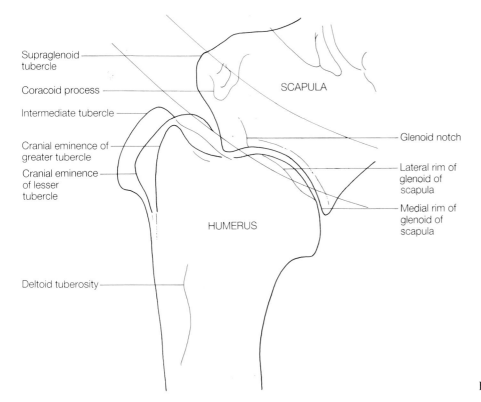

Supraglenoid
tubercle

Coracoid process

Intermediate tubercle

Cranial eminence of
greater tubercle

Cranial eminence
of lesser
tubercle

SCAPULA

Glenoid notch

Lateral rim of
glenoid of
scapula

Medial rim of
glenoid of
scapula

HUMERUS

Deltoid tuberosity

Figure 6.4(a) *Cont'd*

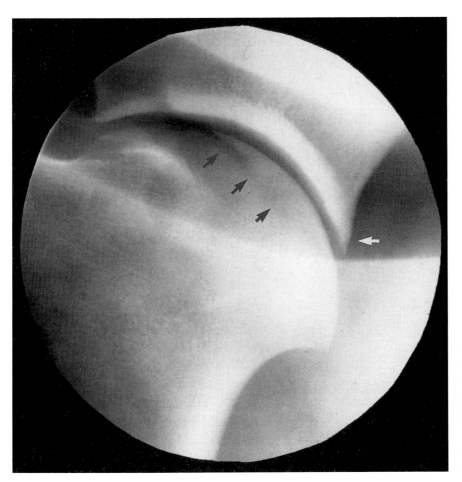

Figure 6.4(b) Coned down mediolateral
view of a normal scapulohumeral joint,
superimposed over the trachea. Note the
congruity of the articulation between the
scapula and the humerus and the sharply
pointed ventral angle of the scapula
(white arrow). The lucent line (black
arrows) traversing the humeral head is
normal, an edge effect created by the
overlying lateral rim of the glenoid
cavity of the scapula.

Humerus

The proximal humerus ossifies from three centres: the diaphysis, the humeral head and the greater tubercle. The lesser tubercle develops from the same ossification centre as the humeral head. It is usually incompletely ossified at birth and has a fuzzy outline and a granular opacity. The centres of ossification of the proximal humeral epiphysis merge by 3–4 months of age and gradually assume a more adult shape; the proximal humeral physis closes by 24–36 months.

Skeletally mature horse

Mediolateral view

There is little variation in the normal radiographic anatomy of the scapulohumeral joint except as a result of positioning. The medial rim of the glenoid cavity of the scapula is projected proximal to the lateral rim and is smoothly curved (Figure 6.4a, pages 278 and 279). Its caudal edge, the ventral angle of the scapula, is sharply pointed. The lateral rim of the glenoid cavity of

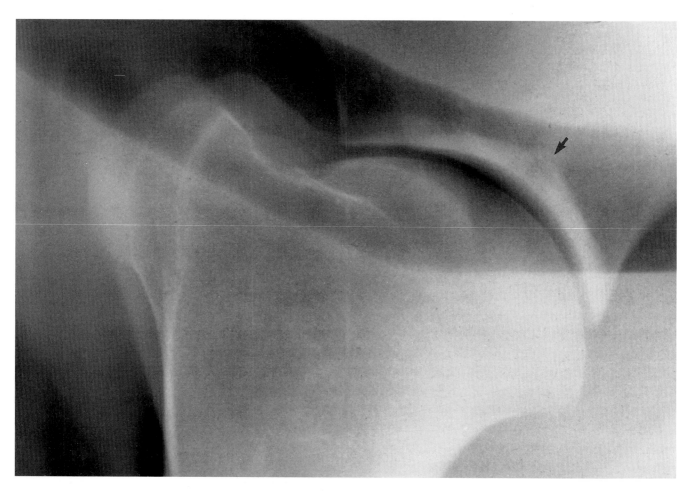

Figure 6.5 Mediolateral view of a normal adult scapulohumeral joint. There is an irregularly shaped radiolucent area (arrow) in the subchondral bone of the middle of the glenoid cavity of the scapula (see text on page 283).

CHAPTER 6
*The shoulder, humerus,
elbow and radius*

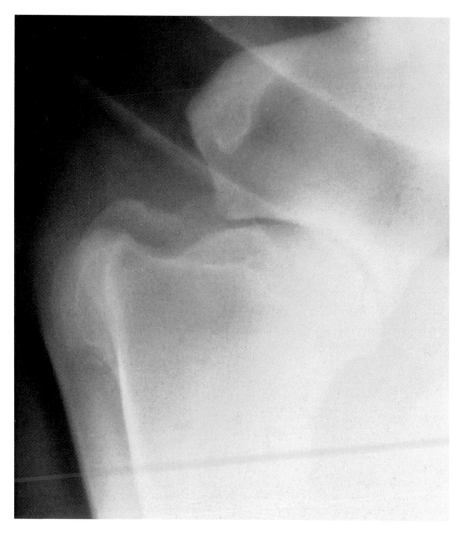

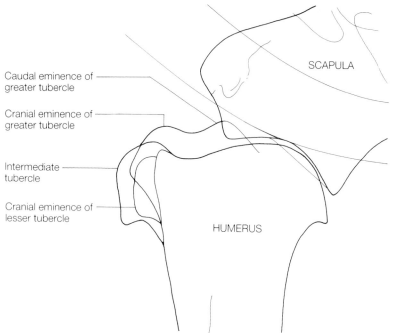

Caudal eminence of
greater tubercle

Cranial eminence of
greater tubercle

Intermediate
tubercle

Cranial eminence of
lesser tubercle

SCAPULA

HUMERUS

Figure 6.6 Mediolateral view and
diagram of a normal adult
scapulohumeral joint (compare with
Figure 6.4a). Due to slight differences
in position of the proximal humerus,
the greater tubercle appears more
prominent. Note also the slightly more
rounded ventral angle of the scapula
compared with Figure 6.4(b). The caudal
aspect of the joint is slightly
underexposed.

[281]

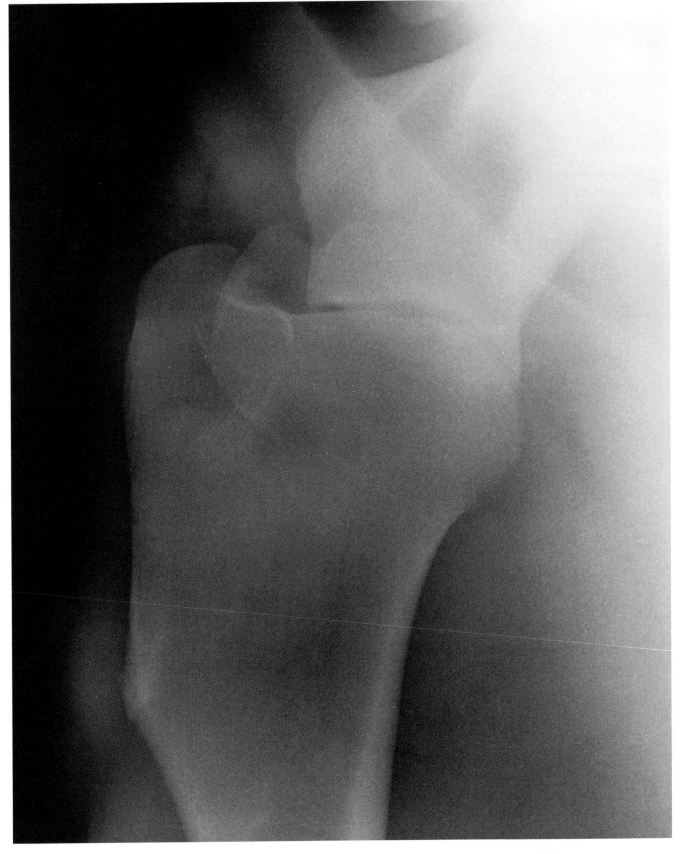

Figure 6.7 Cranial 45° medial-caudolateral oblique view and diagram of a normal adult scapulohumeral joint.

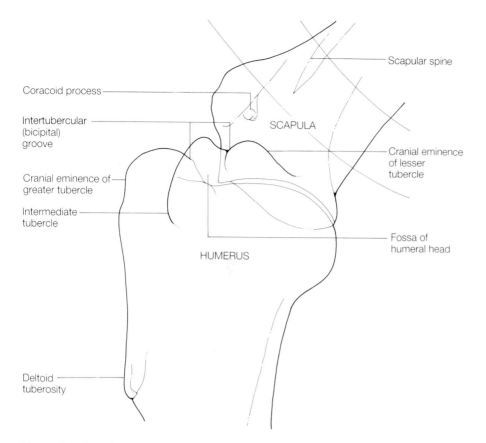

Scapular spine

Coracoid process

Intertubercular
(bicipital)
groove

SCAPULA

Cranial eminence
of lesser
tubercle

Cranial eminence of
greater tubercle

Intermediate
tubercle

HUMERUS

Fossa of
humeral head

Deltoid
tuberosity

Figure 6.7 *Cont'd*

the scapula is seen as a relatively less opaque area immediately distal to the medial rim and may make the latter appear poorly defined. It may be super-imposed over the humeral head, resulting in a relatively lucent area in the cranial part of the humeral head which should not be mistaken for a lucent lesion in the subchondral bone of the humeral head (Figure 6.4b, page 279). The lateral rim of the glenoid cavity forms the proximal border of this lucency.

There is a clearly demarcated band of opaque, sclerotic bone, of uniform width, around the caudal two-thirds of the glenoid cavity of the scapula. In approximately 5% of horses there is a small lucent zone (up to 0.5 cm diameter) in the middle of the glenoid cavity of the scapula within the opaque band (Figure 6.5, page 280). A faint vertical lucent line is sometimes seen at the junction of the cranial and middle thirds of the glenoid cavity. This represents the glenoid notch. Cranial to the glenoid notch the opaque band is usually narrower.

The outline of the humeral head is smoothly curved. The greater, lesser and intermediate tubercles may be slightly separated or superimposed upon each other depending on the positioning of the humerus (Figures 6.3 and 6.6).

There is reasonable congruity between the outlines of the glenoid cavity of the scapula and the humeral head, although in some horses the glenoid cavity of the scapula is more curved, resulting in apparent widening of the joint space in the middle of the joint.

[283]

CHAPTER 6
The shoulder, humerus,
elbow and radius

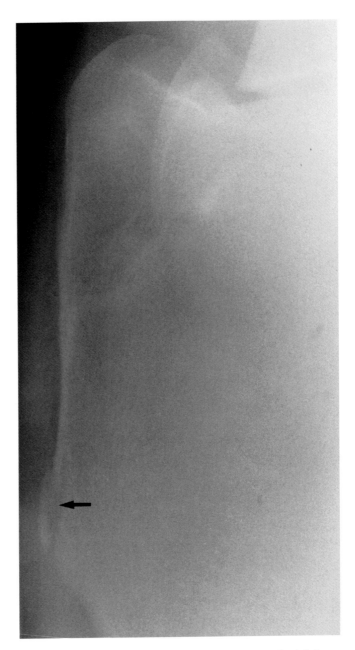

Figure 6.8 Craniomedial-caudolateral oblique view of a normal adult humerus. The 'lip' of the deltoid tuberosity is projected (arrow) and should not be confused with a chip fracture.

Cranial 45° medial-caudolateral oblique

In this projection the width of the scapulohumeral joint space is more variable than in the mediolateral view. The cranial eminence of the lesser tubercle, the intermediate tubercle and the intertubercular groove are highlighted and the deltoid tuberosity is outlined (Figure 6.7). The 'lip' of the deltoid tuberosity, which curves caudolaterally, may be projected in this view and should not be confused with a chip fracture (Figure 6.8).

CHAPTER 6
*The shoulder, humerus,
elbow and radius*

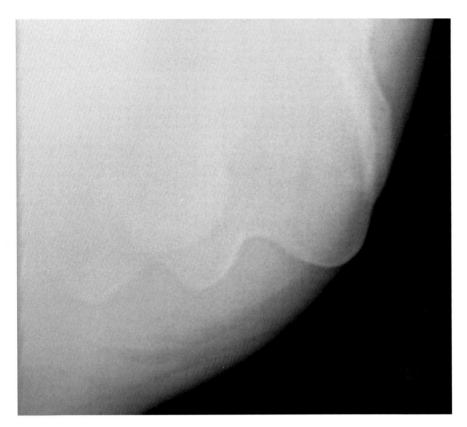

Figure 6.9 Cranioproximal-craniodistal oblique view of the humeral tubercles of a normal adult horse (medial is to the left).

Cranioproximal-craniodistal oblique view of the proximal aspect of the humerus

This view skylines the humeral tubercles, the medial (lesser), intermediate and lateral (greater), which should have a smooth contour (Figure 6.9).

Arthrography

A narrow band of contrast outlines the articular surfaces of the scapula and humerus (Figure 6.10). Some contrast may also be superimposed over the distal scapula and the humeral head. This outlines the proximal cul-de-sac of the scapulohumeral joint capsule and distal aspect of the joint capsule, respectively. In a small proportion of normal horses, arthrography will demonstrate communication between the scapulohumeral joint capsule and the intertubercular bursa.

SIGNIFICANT RADIOLOGICAL ABNORMALITIES

Osteochondrosis

Radiographic abnormalities associated with osteochondrosis are identified in the scapula, the humerus or both. The changes predominantly involve the caudal half of the joint and result in loss of congruity between the

[285]

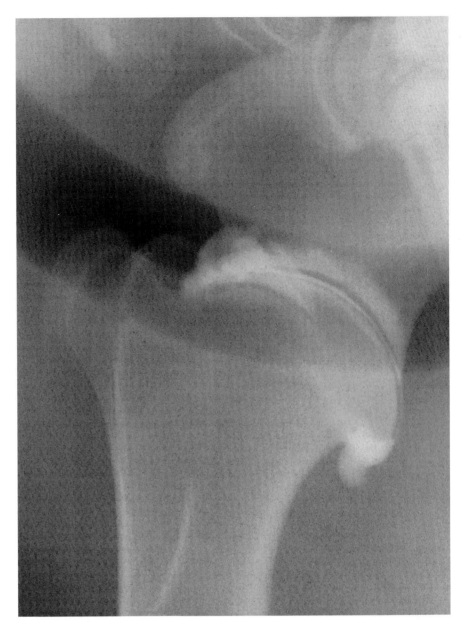

Figure 6.10 Mediolateral arthrogram of a normal adult scapulohumeral joint.

subchondral bone adjacent to the articular surfaces of the scapula and humerus. In some cases there is only subtle variation in contour of the articular surfaces (Figure 6.11a). In other cases there are extensive, irregularly outlined lucent zones in the subchondral bone, which may be surrounded by some sclerosis (Figure 6.11b). There is often flattening of the subchondral bone of the humeral head and/or the glenoid cavity of the scapula (Figure 6.11c). The caudoventral angle of the scapula, which is usually sharply pointed, may be modelled so that it is more bulbous. The rim of the glenoid cavity of the scapula may have a blurred outline. Some of the modelling of the scapula and the humerus is due to secondary degenerative joint disease. Osteochondrosis may occur unilaterally or bilaterally, usually in horses less than 3 years of age. It causes a variable degree of

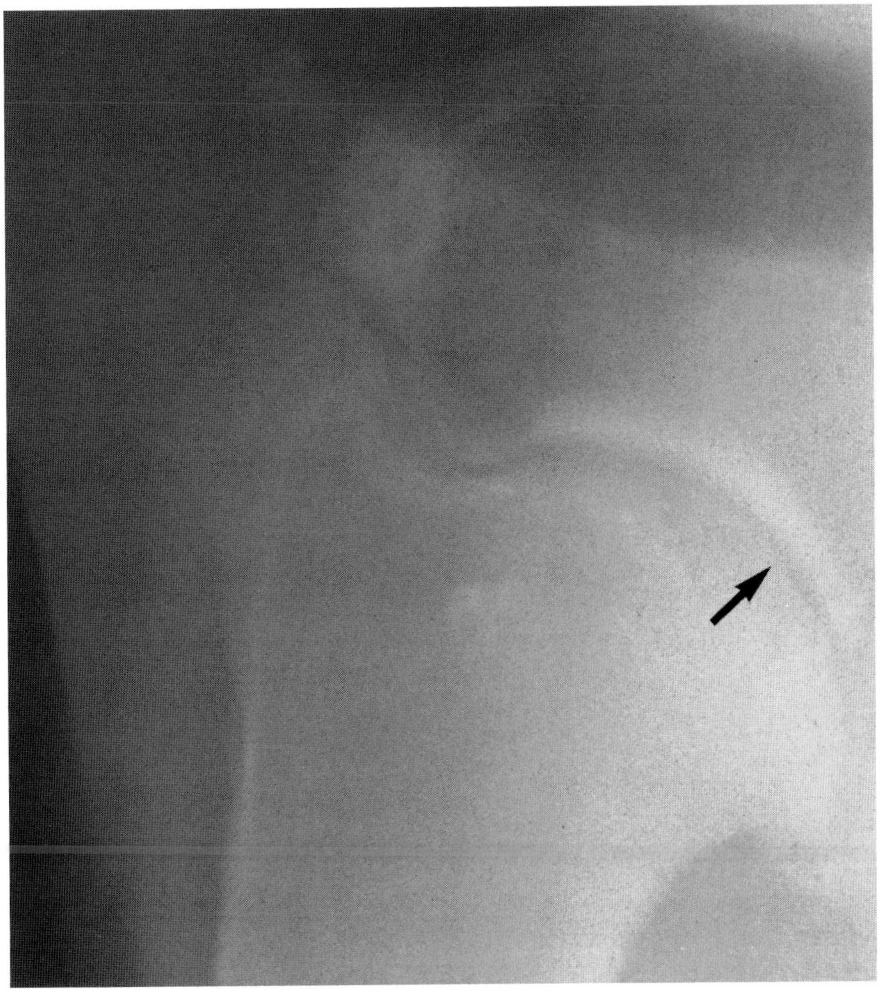

Figure 6.11(a) Mediolateral view of the scapulohumeral joint of a 3-year-old Thoroughbred with osteochondrosis. There is a slight depression in the humeral head (arrow).

lameness. Lameness may or may not be improved by intra-articular anaesthesia.

The majority of horses treated conservatively remain lame; surgical treatment has given encouraging results in immature horses.

In older horses focal osteochondral lesions in the distal aspect of the scapula and the proximal aspect of the humeral head have been associated with lameness. Lesions include focal sclerosis deep to the subchondral bone of the distal aspect of the scapula, small focal radiolucent zones in the distal aspect of the scapula and focal flattening of the humeral head. Arthroscopy invariably reveals associated cartilage defects. The aetiology of these lesions is uncertain; they may be the result of osteochondrosis or trauma. Surgical treatment is recommended.

Osseous cyst-like lesions

Poorly defined lucent zones of irregular shape in the subchondral bone of either the scapula or the humerus are a manifestation of osteochondrosis (Figure 6.11b), but distinct, large circular lucent areas (osseous cyst-like lesions) may be a different clinical condition (or conditions) and are considered separately here.

[287]

CHAPTER 6
*The shoulder, humerus,
elbow and radius*

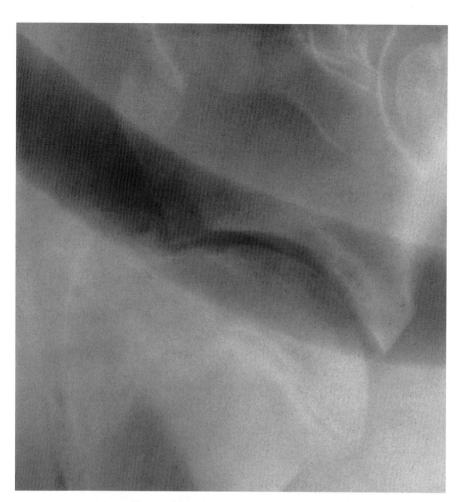

Figure 6.11(b) Mediolateral view of the
scapulohumeral joint of a yearling
Thoroughbred with osteochondrosis.
There are extensive lucent areas in the
subchondral bone of the distal scapula
with surrounding sclerosis. There is
considerable modelling of the caudal
one-third of the glenoid cavity of the
scapula and its ventral angle, resulting in
loss of congruity between the scapula
and humerus. There is an ill defined
lucent area in the subchondral bone of
the middle of the humeral head, but at
post-mortem examination the overlying
cartilage was intact and firmly adherent
to the subchondral bone.

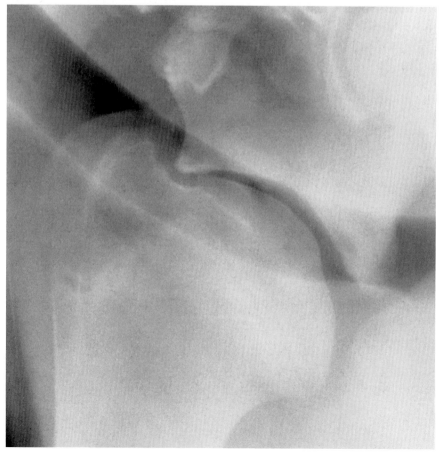

Figure 6.11(c) Mediolateral view of the
scapulohumeral joint of a yearling
Thoroughbred with osteochondrosis.
There is extensive modelling of the
distal scapula and proximal humerus.
The outline of the caudal aspect of the
glenoid cavity and of the ventral angle
of the scapula is rather blurred due to
new bone formation. There are ill
defined lucent zones in the caudal aspect
of the distal scapula.

CHAPTER 6
*The shoulder, humerus,
elbow and radius*

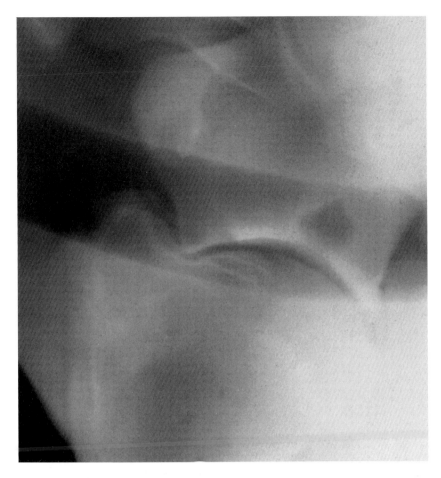

Figure 6.12(a) Mediolateral view of a
scapulohumeral joint of a 2-year-old
Thoroughbred. There is a well defined
single osseous cyst-like lesion in the
distal scapula, surrounded by sclerosis.
When first identified several months
previously, the lesion was smaller, closer
to the articular surface and less well
demarcated without surrounding
sclerosis. There is no detectable
modelling of the scapula (compare with
Figure 6.12b). Post-mortem examination
revealed a true subchondral bone cyst.

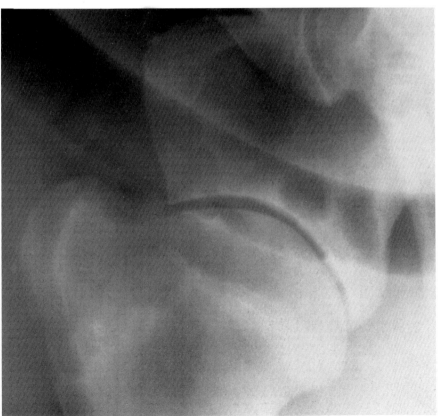

Figure 6.12(b) Mediolateral view of a
scapulohumeral joint of a 2-year-old
Thoroughbred with two large osseous
cyst-like lesions in the distal scapula.
Note the modelling of the ventral angle
of the scapula. The horse ultimately
raced successfully despite radiographic
persistence of the lesions.

CHAPTER 6
*The shoulder, humerus,
elbow and radius*

Figure 6.12(c) Coned mediolateral radiographic view of the left scapulohumeral joint of a 9-year-old Warmblood showjumper with sporadic lameness, which was also variable in severity. There is a large, well defined osseous cyst-like lesion in the centre of the distal aspect of the scapula, caudal to which are two less well defined areas of reduced radiopacity. Lameness was improved by intra-articular analgesia of the scapulohumeral joint.

A small lucent area within the sclerotic subchondral bone of the middle of the glenoid cavity of the scapula has been identified in normal horses (Figure 6.5, page 280) and is of questionable clinical significance. However, horses have been reported which were rendered sound by intra-articular anaesthesia and had this as the only detectable radiographic 'abnormality'; subsequent arthroscopic evaluation revealed focal lesions.

Osseous cyst-like lesions are not common. They may occur singly or there may be more than one (Figures 6.12a and 6.12b). They occur most frequently either in the middle of the distal scapula or the middle of the humeral epiphysis, and are usually surrounded by a rim of sclerotic bone. Associated lameness is usually improved by intra-articular anaesthesia, although it may not be abolished. Lesions in the distal scapula are usually close to the articular surface when first recognized, but appear to move further away with time and become surrounded by a broader rim of sclerotic bone, associated with which there may be improvement in lameness. Osseous cyst-like lesions in the distal scapula occur most commonly in young horses, but are occasionally seen in association with sudden-onset lameness in mature horses. In older horses the cyst-like lesions are often more difficult to detect radiographically and may be easily missed if the radiograph is underexposed (Figure 6.12c). Secondary modelling of the

[290]

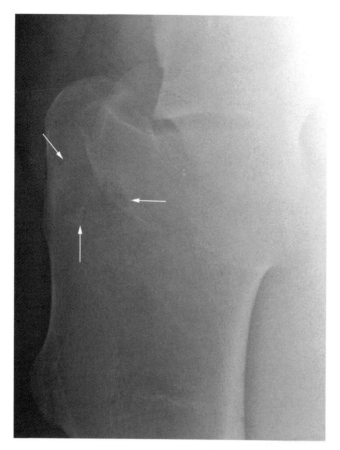

Figure 6.13 Cranial 45° medial-caudolateral oblique radiographic view of a scapulohumeral joint and proximal humerus of an 8-year-old Thoroughbred gelding with moderate lameness, unaltered by any local analgesic technique. There was focal intense increased radiopharmaceutical uptake in the cranioproximal aspect of the humerus. There is an ill defined radiolucent area, an osseous cyst-like lesion, in the cranioproximal aspect of the humerus (arrows), which coincided with the region of increased radiopharmaceutical uptake. No radiographic abnormality was detectable in a mediolateral projection.

ventral angle of the scapula is a variable feature. Not all osseous cyst-like lesions behave similarly and some in the proximal humerus 'fill in' with resolution of lameness. Some young horses with osseous cyst-like lesions in the middle of the distal aspect of the scapula have shown resolution of lameness following intra-articular medication with corticosteroids, but the response in adult horses has been poor. Occasionally modelling of the distal scapula is seen in association with an osseous cyst-like lesion in the proximal humerus.

Poorly defined osseous cyst-like lesions have also been seen to develop in the cranioproximal aspect of the humerus, caudal to the humeral tubercles, following known trauma to the shoulder region (Figure 6.13). Associated lameness has generally resolved with conservative management. Some lesions have not been detectable in a mediolateral projection, but have been seen in a craniomedial-caudolateral oblique view. Such lesions are usually not improved by intra-articular analgesia or intrathecal analgesia of the intertubercular bursa, but are associated with focal increased radiopharmaceutical uptake.

Degenerative joint disease

Degenerative joint disease (DJD) of the scapulohumeral joint occurs rarely compared with the incidence in other joints, except as a sequel to

CHAPTER 6
*The shoulder, humerus,
elbow and radius*

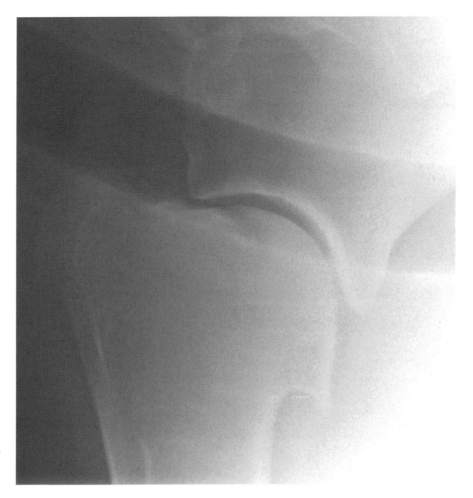

Figure 6.14 Mediolateral radiographic
view of the left scapulohumeral joint of
a 5-year-old Warmblood dressage horse
which had become lame within 3 weeks
of purchase from a dealer. The lameness
was not altered by any local analgesic
technique. There was mild increased
radiopharmaceutical uptake in the distal
caudal aspect of the scapula. There is
extensive modelling of the ventral angle
of the scapula and the proximal caudal
aspect of the humerus. There is loss of
joint surface congruity caudally in the
scapulohumeral joint, due to flattening
of the caudal aspect of the humerus. This
is degenerative joint disease, probably
secondary to osteochondrosis.

osteochondrosis, trauma, infection or an intra-articular fracture in which
cases it inevitably follows rapidly. Some of the modelling of the scapula and
humerus described in conjunction with osteochondrosis is due to secondary
DJD. Radiographic features of DJD include loss of congruity between the
outlines of the distal scapula and the proximal humerus due to flattening of
the humeral head and/or modelling of the ventral angle of the scapula
(Figure 6.14). Subtle abnormalities of the cranial aspects of the joint may
also be seen, including small periarticular osteophytes, especially on the
distal scapula. In addition there may be variations in opacity of the subchondral bone. Narrowing of the joint space may be seen in advanced cases.
The prognosis for return to athletic function is extremely poor.

Mineralization in the tendon of biceps brachii

Mineralization in the tendon of biceps brachii can occur as a sequel to a
fracture of the supraglenoid tubercle (Figure 6.15), but has also been
described as a bilateral condition in association with DJD of the scapulohumeral joints. It can also occur as a sequel to chronic tendonitis of biceps

CHAPTER 6
*The shoulder, humerus,
elbow and radius*

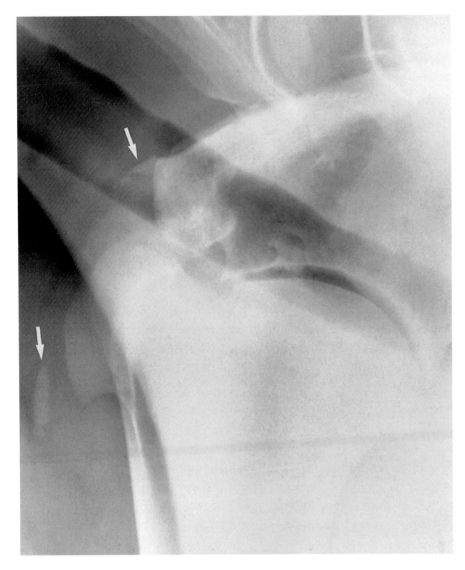

Figure 6.15 Mediolateral view of a scapulohumeral joint of an aged horse. There are discrete mineralized areas (arrows) in the tendon of biceps brachii. Note the modelled supraglenoid tubercle, subsequent to previous fracture, the articular fracture fragment and the abnormally pointed distal cranial aspect of the scapula.

brachii. Mineralization is most easily identified radiographically in a mediolateral view and is seen as a variably sized opacity in the soft tissues cranioproximal to the tubercles of the humerus. The lesion is easily missed if the radiographs are overexposed. Ultrasonography may give additional information. Prognosis for future soundness is guarded.

Lesions of the humeral tubercles

Trauma to the cranial aspect of the shoulder may result in lesions of the humeral tubercles that may be difficult to identify in standard radiographic projections of the shoulder. Nuclear scintigraphy may be necessary to highlight the presence of a potential lesion. A defect in the cortical bone may be detected in some horses using a flexed cranioproximal-craniodistal oblique 'skyline' view. The intermediate tubercle is most commonly affected.

[293]

CHAPTER 6
*The shoulder, humerus,
elbow and radius*

In other horses ultrasonography has been required to identify the lesion. Lameness is usually acute in onset and not responsive to any local analgesic technique. Conservative management usually results in resolution of the lameness.

Congenital abnormalities of the bicipital apparatus

Congenital abnormalities of the tubercles of the humerus have been identified rarely in mature horses with chronic forelimb lameness. These include an abnormal shape (usually narrowed) of the intertubercular sulcus seen in a mediolateral view. Absence of the minor tubercle is best seen in a skyline view of the tubercles. Radiographic evidence of secondary osteoarthritis of the scapulohumeral joint may also be seen. Ultrasonography is useful to assess the intertubercular bursa and tendon of biceps brachii, which is usually luxated medially.

Abnormalities of the scapulohumeral joint in Shetland Ponies and Miniature Horses

Dysplasia of the scapulohumeral joint, with or without subluxation of the scapulohumeral joint or secondary degenerative joint disease, has been seen in both Shetland Ponies and Miniature Horses (Figure 6.16). Unilateral degenerative joint disease, thought to be traumatic in origin, may occur in Shetland Ponies and Miniature Horses associated with sudden-onset, moderate to severe lameness. Radiographic abnormalities may not be present at the time of onset of lameness, and if mild may only be visible in a craniomedial-caudolateral oblique view. This view is also useful for assessment of congruity of the joint surfaces. Radiographic abnormalities include modelling of the articular margins of the glenoid cavity of the scapula and entheseophyte formation at the insertion of the joint capsule (Figures 6.16a–d). Mild subluxation of the joint is occasionally seen. Fragmentation of the ventral angle of the scapula has also been seen in young Shetland Ponies with acute-onset severe lameness (Figure 6.16d). Defective bone, possibly developmental in origin, may predispose to fracture. The response to intra-articular medication is poor and most ponies remain lame.

Infection

Septic arthritis of the scapulohumeral joint occurs most commonly in young foals and may result from osteomyelitis of the distal scapula or proximal humerus (type E) or the humeral physis (type P) (see Chapter 1, page 32). In adult horses septic arthritis is usually iatrogenic. Osteomyelitis of the distal scapula is characterized by lucent zones in the subchondral bone (Figure 6.17) and an irregular outline of the glenoid cavity. There may be periosteal new bone, especially on the caudodistal aspect of the scapula. Similar changes may be seen in the proximal humeral epiphysis. Osteomyelitis of the proximal humeral physis results in areas of lucency and an irregular width of the physis. This may be focal or extend along the entire width of the physis, with or without new bone at the cortices. These changes must be differentiated from those due to osteochondrosis. Septic arthritis may result in apparent widening of the joint space due to excess synovial fluid. The granular opacity and irregular outline of incompletely ossified bones (see Figure 6.3, page 276) should not be confused with the results of infection.

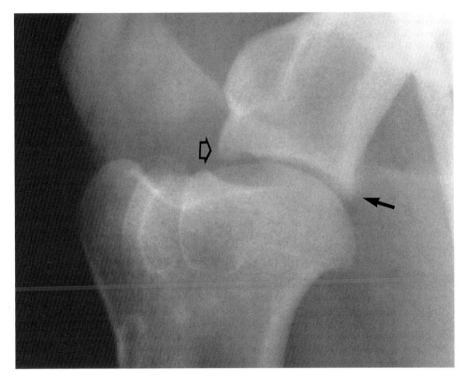

Figure 6.16(a) Craniomedial-caudolateral oblique view of a scapulohumeral joint of a Miniature Horse. No radiological abnormalities were detected in a mediolateral projection. In this oblique view there is poorly defined periosteal new bone on the ventral angle of the scapula (solid arrow). The craniolateral aspect of the scapula is less sharply defined than normal (open arrow).

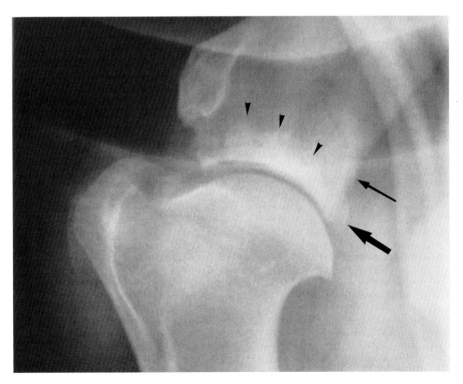

Figure 6.16(b) Mediolateral view of a scapulohumeral joint of a 4-year-old Shetland Pony. There is fairly extensive new bone on the caudal aspect of the ventral angle of the scapula (large arrow), extending proximally along the caudodistal margin of the scapula (small arrow). There is generalized increased opacity of the distal scapula (arrow heads), probably due to the extensive nature of the new bone formation around the distal scapula.

CHAPTER 6
*The shoulder, humerus,
elbow and radius*

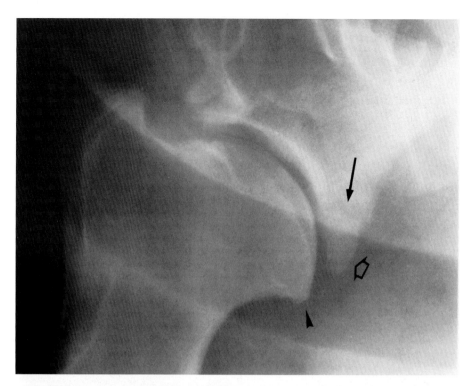

Figure 6.16(c) Mediolateral view of a
scapulohumeral joint of a 4-year-old
Shetland Pony. There is slight modelling
on the articular margin of the
proximocaudal aspect of the humerus
(arrowhead). There is extensive new
bone on the caudoventral aspect of the
scapula, and an abnormal contour of the
ventral angle of the scapula (open
(arrow). There is an ill defined lucent
line (solid arrow) crossing the ventral
angle into the scapulohumeral joint. A
large discrete fragment was identified at
arthroscopic examination.

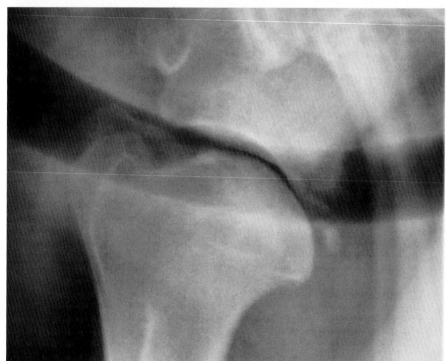

Figure 6.16(d) Mediolateral view of a
scapulohumeral joint of a 5-year-old
Shetland Pony. The joint surfaces of the
scapula and humerus are abnormally flat
and there is subluxation of the joint.
There is extensive new bone on the
caudoventral aspect of the scapula, and a
separate mineralized opacity caudally.

Septic physitis in the proximal humeral physis has also been recognized
in 2-year-old Thoroughbreds in race training with sudden onset of forelimb
lameness. Radiographs are characterized by a large radiolucent zone in the
caudal aspect of the physis, with surrounding sclerosis and periosteal new
bone on the caudal physeal and metaphyseal regions of the proximal aspect
of the humerus. Long-term antimicrobial therapy may be successful in the
treatment of this condition.

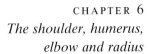

CHAPTER 6
The shoulder, humerus,
elbow and radius

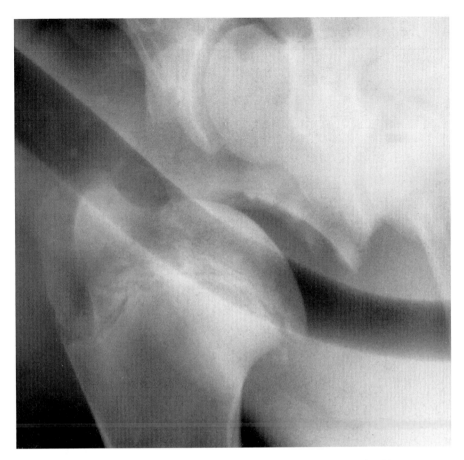

Figure 6.17 Mediolateral view of a scapulohumeral joint of a 7-month-old Thoroughbred with osteomyelitis of the distal scapula and the proximal humerus and septic arthritis. Note the ill defined lucent zones in the distal scapula, the flattened shape of the humeral head due to its partial collapse and the widened joint space. There is periosteal new bone around the ventral angle of the scapula.

Luxation of the scapulohumeral joint

Luxation of the scapulohumeral joint causes firm swelling in the shoulder region and severe lameness. The humerus may be displaced proximally and cranially (Figure 6.18) or proximally and caudally and is readily seen radiographically in a mediolateral projection, the proximal humerus being superimposed over the distal scapula. An oblique view is invaluable for determining whether the luxation is medial or lateral and for identification of any concurrent fracture. A simple luxation must be reduced rapidly, with the horse anaesthetized. Full return to athletic function has been recorded. The presence of a concurrent fracture warrants a guarded prognosis.

Fractures

Fractures of the shoulder region are usually the result of a fall, a kick or a collision with a solid object. They cause moderate to severe lameness with a variable amount of soft-tissue swelling, with or without audible or palpable crepitus.

[297]

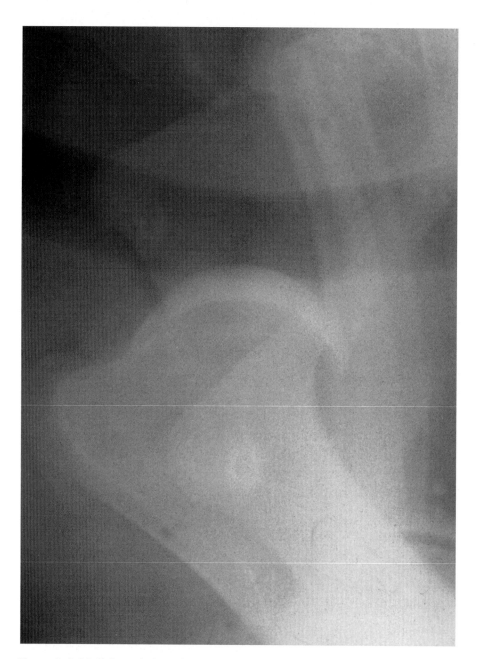

Figure 6.18 Mediolateral view of a scapulohumeral joint of a mature pony with cranioproximal luxation of the humerus. Craniomedial-caudolateral oblique views should also be obtained to ensure that there is no concurrent fracture. This luxation was successfully reduced and the pony ultimately resumed full athletic function.

Fracture of the supraglenoid tubercle

This is the most common fracture in the shoulder region. The fracture may be simple or comminuted and there is often an articular component. There may be a separate fracture through the glenoid notch (this represents the separate centre of ossification of the cranial part of the glenoid cavity of the scapula). The supraglenoid tubercle is usually displaced cranially and distally resulting in a non-union fracture. Lameness may initially improve, but usually persists unless the fracture is treated surgically. Mineralization in the tendon of biceps brachii may be a sequel.

[298]

CHAPTER 6
*The shoulder, humerus,
elbow and radius*

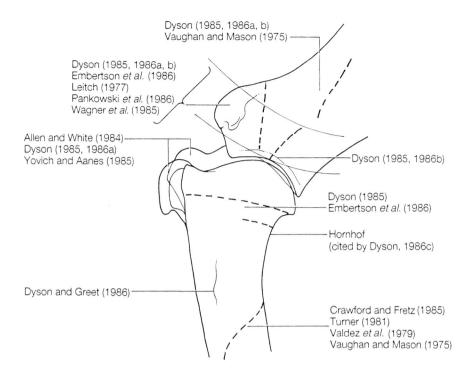

Dyson (1985, 1986a, b)
Vaughan and Mason (1975)

Dyson (1985, 1986a, b)
Embertson *et al.* (1986)
Leitch (1977)
Pankowski *et al.* (1986)
Wagner *et al.* (1985)

Allen and White (1984)
Dyson (1985, 1986a)
Yovich and Aanes (1985)

Dyson (1985, 1986b)

Dyson (1985)
Embertson *et al.* (1986)

Hornhof
(cited by Dyson, 1986c)

Dyson and Greet (1986)

Crawford and Fretz (1985)
Turner (1981)
Valdez *et al.* (1979)
Vaughan and Mason (1975)

Figure 6.19 Location of common fractures of the scapula and humerus, and recommended references (see 'Further reading').

Other fractures

Other common sites of fractures are illustrated in Figure 6.19. Fractures restricted to the glenoid cavity of the scapula may be difficult to identify in a mediolateral view, but may be seen in an oblique projection. Fractures of the body or neck of the scapula are not uncommon and may be articular. Short fractures of the neck and body are easily overlooked due to superimposition of the cervical and thoracic vertebrae and the ribs. A fracture of the scapular spine may be very difficult to identify radiographically except in tangential views. Such fractures are sometimes associated with a chronic draining sinus due to sequestrum formation.

Fractures of the deltoid tuberosity and the greater, lesser and intermediate tubercles of the humerus may only be identifiable in a craniomedial-caudolateral oblique projection (Figure 6.20), cranioproximal-craniodistal oblique view or, for the greater tubercle, a caudolateral-craniomedial oblique view. Fatigue (stress or fissure) fractures of the caudal aspect of the proximal humeral metaphysis or cranial aspect of the distal humeral metaphysis occur occasionally. They can be difficult to identify radiographically in the acute phase, although they may be demonstrable using nuclear scintigraphy. Fractures of the humeral diaphysis are usually oblique or spiral with considerable overriding, with or without comminution. The prognosis for a fracture in the shoulder region depends on its location and configuration, and readers are advised to consult the references listed under 'Further reading'.

[299]

CHAPTER 6
*The shoulder, humerus,
elbow and radius*

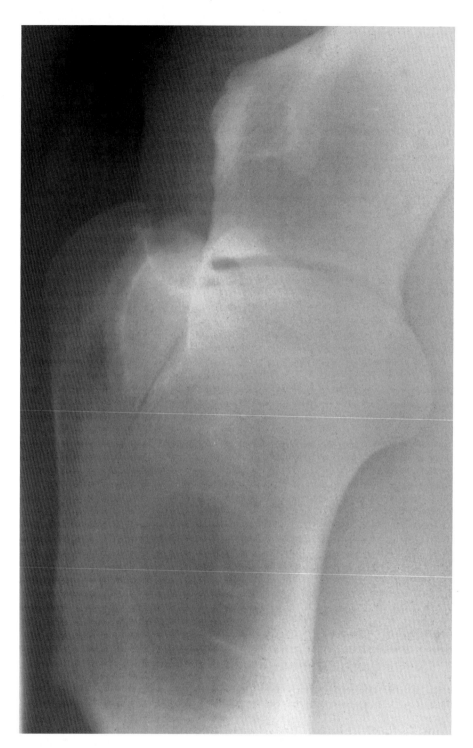

Figure 6.20 Craniomedial-caudolateral oblique view of a proximal humerus of a 3-year-old Thoroughbred. There is a non-displaced fracture of the deltoid tuberosity. No abnormality was detectable in a mediolateral view. The filly was treated conservatively and made a complete recovery.

CHAPTER 6
*The shoulder, humerus,
elbow and radius*

Humeroradial, humeroulnar and radioulnar (elbow) joints and radius

RADIOGRAPHIC TECHNIQUE

Equipment

The elbow joint and the radius are readily examined radiographically using a portable machine, with the horse standing. Sedation and administration of analgesics may facilitate positioning of the limb. Digital systems or fast screens are recommended, but a grid is not essential. An aluminium wedge filter is useful; otherwise it may be necessary to obtain two mediolateral views to obtain correct exposures of the olecranon of the ulna and the humeroradial joint.

Positioning

Mediolateral view

For radiography of the elbow the horse is positioned with the limb to be radiographed next to the cassette. The x-ray machine is placed on the opposite side of the horse. The forelimb to be examined is protracted so that the olecranon of the ulna is cranial to the muscles of the contralateral limb. The x-ray beam is centred approximately at the junction between the cranial two-thirds and caudal one-third of the forearm, at the level of the proximal articular surface of the radius.

The majority of the radius can be examined radiographically with the horse bearing weight on the limb. The x-ray beam is centred at the point of interest and is aligned at right angles to the limb.

Craniocaudal views

Craniocaudal radiographic views of the elbow joint are usually obtained with the horse bearing weight on the limb, and the cassette held caudal to the forearm, beneath the thorax. It is helpful to rotate the cassette so that it can be held as high under the thorax as possible. It may be necessary to direct the x-ray beam approximately 10–15° from cranioproximally to caudodistally, depending on the shape of the rib cage, in order to examine the distal humerus and the humeroradial joint properly. Unfortunately this technique will cause some distortion of the radiographic image.

Alternatively the limb may be protracted, the cassette held parallel with the ulna and the x-ray beam directed perpendicular to it. There is more likely to be movement blur using this technique, and if there is a fracture of the ulna it may be difficult to straighten the limb adequately. Good-quality craniocaudal views, with minimal distortion, are obtained more readily with the horse anaesthetized.

[301]

The radius is radiographed with the horse bearing weight on the limb. The beam is centred at the area of interest.

Oblique views

A craniomedial-caudolateral oblique view is the easiest oblique view to obtain with the horse bearing weight on the limb (see Figure 6.25, page 308). A craniolateral-caudomedial oblique view of the proximal radius is feasible, but due to the relative positions of the sternum and distal humerus, it is impractical to obtain a similar view of the humerus.

RADIOGRAPHIC ANATOMY, NORMAL VARIATIONS AND INCIDENTAL FINDINGS

Birth to 3 years old

The distal humerus develops from three ossification centres: the diaphysis, the distal epiphysis and the epiphysis of the medial epicondyle. The radius has a single proximal epiphysis and the ulna has a single proximal apophysis (Figure 6.21); the ulna may also have a separate centre of ossification for the anconeal process (Figure 6.22). At birth the ossification centres are rounded and may be irregular in outline because they are incompletely ossified. The apophysis of the ulna is small and widely separated from the metaphysis. It gradually enlarges to cover the proximal ulnar metaphysis by 10–12 months. The physis appears very irregular (Figure 6.22) and remains open until 24–36 months after birth. The distal humeral physes and the proximal radial physis close between 11 and 24 months. The distal radial physis closes by between 22 and 42 months of age; there is a separate centre of ossification of the lateral styloid process which fuses with the rest of the distal epiphysis within the first year of life.

Skeletally mature horse

Mediolateral view

There is little variation in the normal radiographic appearance of the adult elbow except as a result of positioning (Figure 6.23). The anconeal process of the ulna may be sharply pointed or rounded. The trochlear notch of the ulna is divided into an articular zone proximally and a synovial fossa distally, separated by a distinct ridge. It is important to differentiate between these two areas when assessing a fracture involving the trochlear notch. The interosseous space between the ulna and radius may be clearly or poorly defined, depending upon the angle of projection. The ulna is incomplete in the majority of horses and fuses distally with the radius. Some horses have a vestigial distal ulna (see Figures 5.11a and 5.11b, page 249) and occasionally the ulna is complete. The cranial margin of the proximal articular surface of the radius has several 'lips' which must not be confused with osteophyte formation.

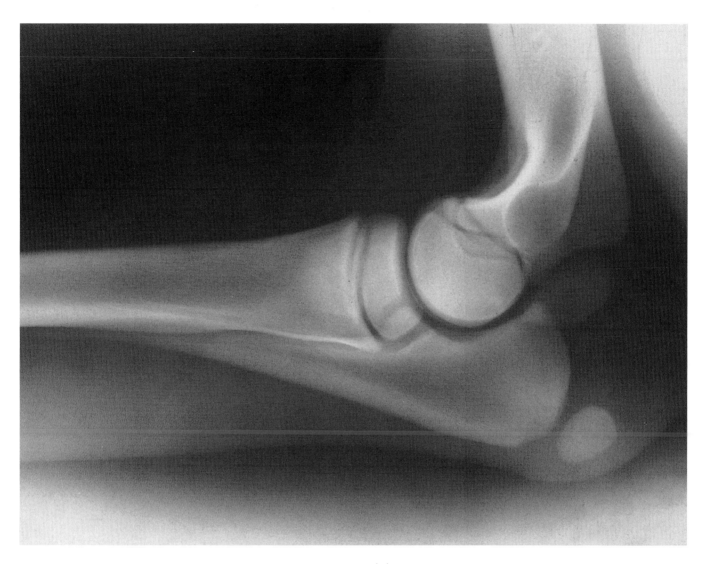

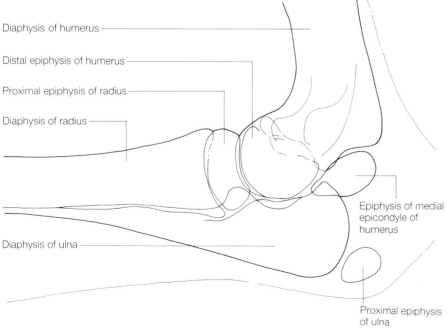

Diaphysis of humerus

Distal epiphysis of humerus

Proximal epiphysis of radius

Diaphysis of radius

Diaphysis of ulna

Epiphysis of medial epicondyle of humerus

Proximal epiphysis of ulna

Figure 6.21 Mediolateral view and diagram of a normal elbow of a 12-day-old foal. Note the position of the incompletely ossified proximal epiphysis of the ulna.

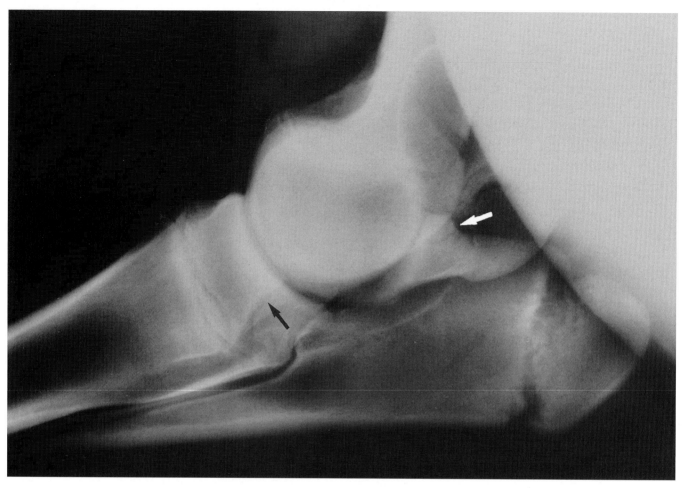

Figure 6.22 Mediolateral view of a normal elbow of an 11-month-old filly. The proximal ulnar epiphysis has enlarged compared with Figure 6.21 and is fusing with the metaphysis, but the physis is extremely irregular. There is a radiolucent line (black arrow) in the caudal aspect of the proximal radial physis which represents part of the radioulnar articulation. Positioning is not ideal, since the opacity of the pectoral muscles is superimposed over the proximal aspect of the ulna. The anconeal process (white arrow) is a separate centre of ossification.

The radial tuberosity is smoothly outlined, but may appear irregular in a slightly oblique mediolateral projection. The medial aspect of the head of the radius is wider craniocaudally than the lateral aspect. Therefore the radioulnar articulation is not in a single plane, and in a mediolateral view the articulation of the lateral aspect of the ulna with the proximal radius is seen as a lucent line through the caudal aspect of the radius (Figure 6.22).

There is an irregularly outlined bony prominence, the transverse crest, on the distocaudal aspect of the radius. Its size depends on the angle of projection, since slight obliquity will enhance it. The mottled opacity of the torus carpeus (chestnut) on the caudal aspect of the radius must not be confused with dystrophic mineralization of soft tissues. Other radiographic characteristics of the distal radius are discussed in Chapter 5 (pages 239–248).

[304]

CHAPTER 6
*The shoulder, humerus,
elbow and radius*

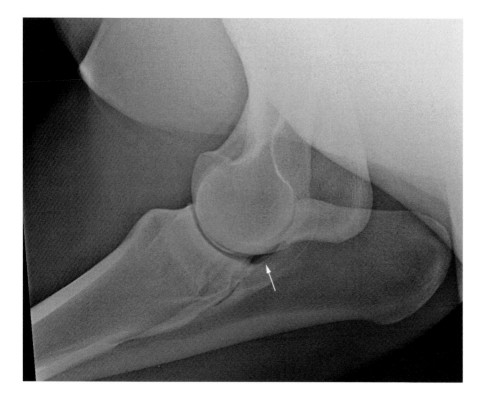

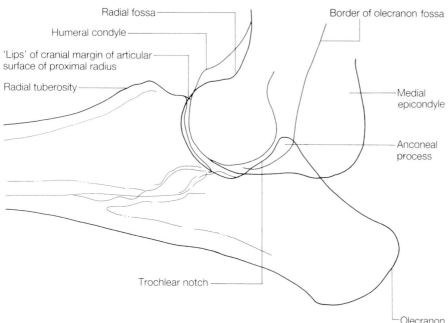

Figure 6.23 Mediolateral view and diagram of a normal adult elbow. The non-articular portion of the trochlear notch of the ulna is arrowed.

CHAPTER 6
*The shoulder, humerus,
elbow and radius*

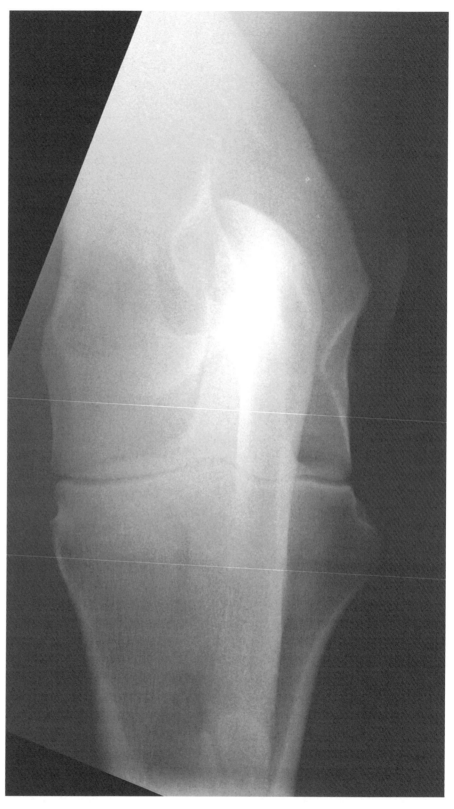

Figure 6.24 Craniocaudal view and diagram of a normal adult elbow. Lateral is to the right.

CHAPTER 6
*The shoulder, humerus,
elbow and radius*

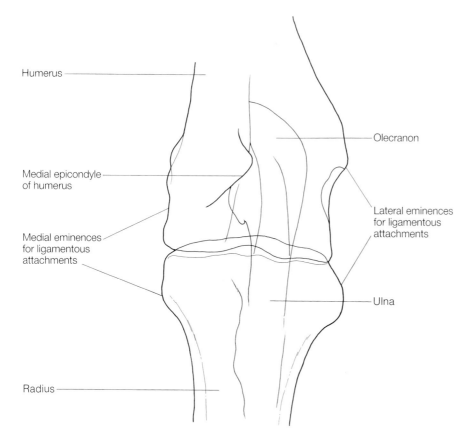

Figure 6.24 *Cont'd*

Craniocaudal views

The humeroradial joint space often appears wider medially than laterally. There are smoothly outlined eminences on the medial and lateral aspects of the distal humerus and proximal radius for attachment of the collateral ligaments (Figure 6.24).

SIGNIFICANT RADIOLOGICAL ABNORMALITIES

Osteochondrosis

Osteochondrosis of the elbow in the horse is rare. It has been documented at post-mortem examination involving the medial condyle of the humerus and the medial proximal aspect of the radius. Lameness associated with a separate bone fragment detached from the anconeal process of the ulna has been described in a 2-year-old Standardbred. The lameness was relieved by intra-articular anaesthesia of the elbow. The anconeal process is best assessed in a mediolateral view, and detachment of its apex may be an osteochondritic lesion. Care must be taken in the assessment of young foals in which the anconeal process may be a separate centre of ossification.

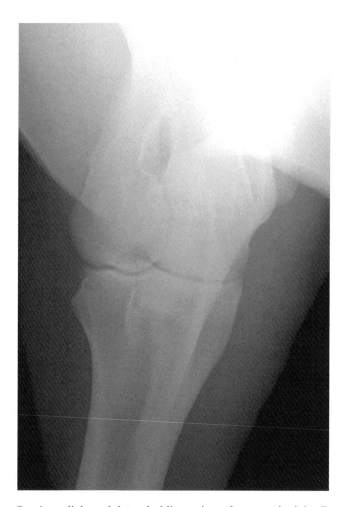

Figure 6.25 Craniomedial-caudolateral oblique view of a normal adult elbow.

Osseous cyst-like lesions

Osseous cyst-like lesions occasionally occur close to the elbow joint and are usually seen in young horses. They occur most commonly in the medial aspect of the proximal radial epiphysis in association with periosteal reactions at the site of insertion of the medial collateral ligament of the humeroradial joint (Figures 6.26a and 6.26b). These cyst-like lesions may ultimately 'fill-in' radiographically, but degenerative joint disease may be a sequel. The response to conservative treatment has been variable; surgical treatment might yield better results. The joint should be inspected carefully for evidence of secondary degenerative joint disease, before contemplating surgery.

Osseous cyst-like lesions occur less commonly in the distal aspect of the radius. Surgical treatment may be successful.

Degenerative joint disease

Degenerative joint disease of the humeroradial, humeroulnar and radioulnar joints is uncommon except as a sequel to an osseous cyst-like lesion,

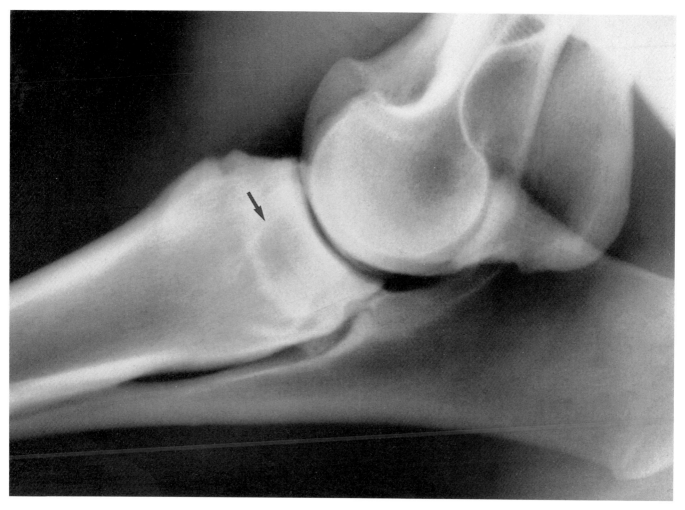

Figure 6.26(a) Mediolateral view of an elbow of a 2-year-old Thoroughbred. There is an irregularly outlined radiolucent area (arrow) in the proximal radial epiphysis and the physis is remodelled. (See also Figure 6.26(b).) The filly was treated conservatively and raced successfully.

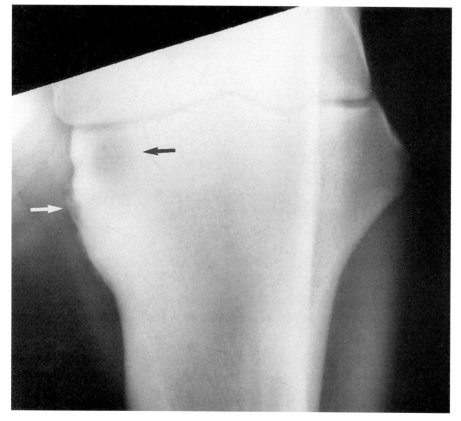

Figure 6.26(b) Craniocaudal view of the same elbow as Figure 6.26(a). Lateral is to the right. The osseous cyst-like lesion (black arrow) is in the medial part of the epiphysis. There is periosteal new bone (white arrow) in the region of insertion of the medial collateral ligament.

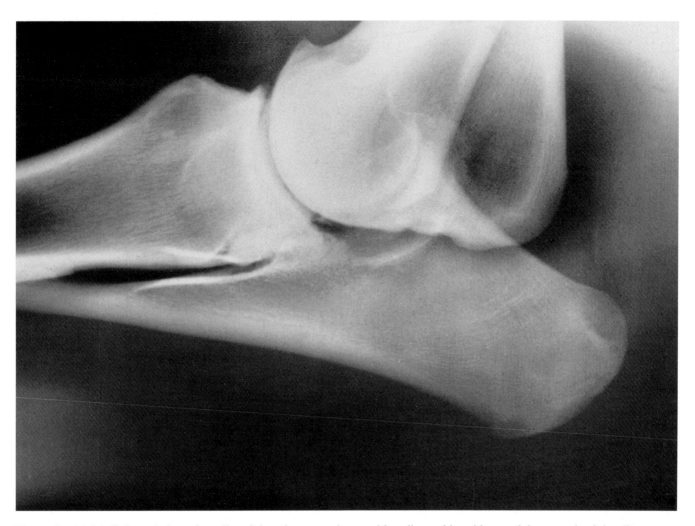

Figure 6.27(a) Mediolateral view of an elbow joint of an event horse with radiographic evidence of degenerative joint disease. There is osteophyte formation on the cranioproximal aspect of the radius (compare with Figure 6.23) and modelling of the anconeal process of the ulna. Lameness was substantially improved by intra-articular analgesia.

collateral ligament damage or an articular fracture. In a mediolateral view the 'lips' of the proximal articular surface of the radius (see page 302) should not be confused with osteophytes. Craniocaudal views are more helpful for the diagnosis of degenerative joint disease. Typically, osteophyte formation is seen on the medial and lateral aspects of the distal humerus and/or the proximal radius (Figures 6.27a and 6.27b). In advanced cases there may be narrowing of the humeroradial joint space with subchondral bone sclerosis. The prognosis for return to athletic function is poor.

Periosteal proliferative reactions (enthesopathy) at the site of insertion of biceps brachii on the radial tuberosity

Entheseous new bone, with or without discrete bony fragments, may develop at the insertion of biceps brachii on the radial tuberosity, and is best seen

CHAPTER 6
*The shoulder, humerus,
elbow and radius*

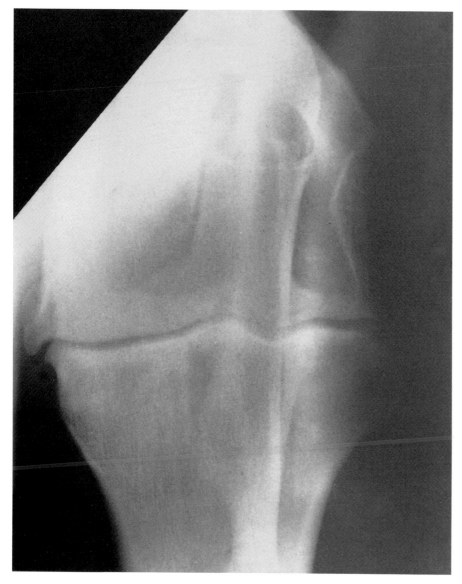

Figure 6.27(b) Craniocaudal view of an elbow (same horse as Figure 6.27a). Lateral is to the right. There is considerable osteophyte formation on the medial aspect of the humeroradial joint and rather irregular opacity of the subchondral bone on the medial aspect of the joint.

on a mediolateral view (Figure 6.28). New bone may not be identifiable until 3–6 weeks after the onset of lameness, so nuclear scintigraphy is more sensitive in the acute phase and may help to interpret the significance of entheseous new bone in a horse with more chronic lameness. In the acute phase there may be some pain on manipulation of the joint, but in more chronic cases there may be no localizing signs. Lameness may resolve with rest, but often persists.

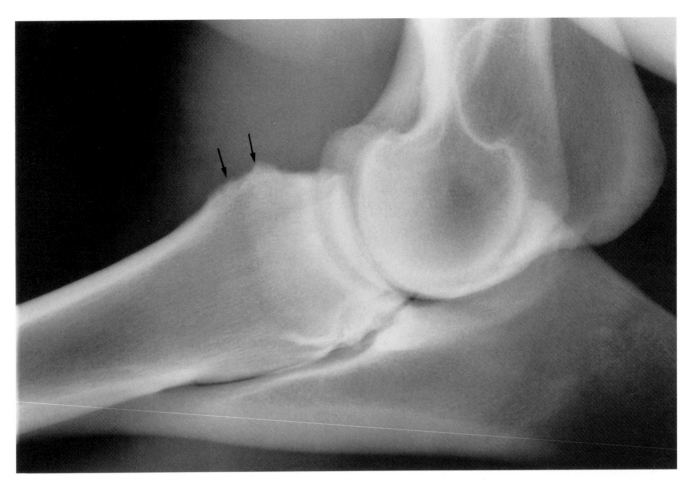

Figure 6.28 Mediolateral view of an elbow of a 7-year-old advanced event horse, with lameness of several months' duration. There is periosteal new bone formation on the cranioproximal aspect of the radius (arrows), which represents entheseophyte formation at the insertion of biceps brachii.

Entheseous new bone at the sites of attachment of the collateral ligaments of the humeroradial joint

Sprain of the lateral collateral (or, less commonly, the medial collateral) ligament of the humeroradial joint may be followed by the development of entheseous new bone on the humeral epicondyle and proximal radius, best seen in a craniocaudal projection (Figure 6.29). Occasionally a fragment may be avulsed, especially from the proximal attachment. Diagnostic ultrasonography is useful to determine the degree of ligamentous damage. Chronic instability of the joint makes degenerative joint disease a likely sequel.

Periosteal reaction at the site of origin of the accessory ligament of the superficial digital flexor tendon

Periostitis may develop proximal to the transverse ridge, on the distal caudomedial aspect of the radius, secondary to tearing of the attachment of the

CHAPTER 6
*The shoulder, humerus,
elbow and radius*

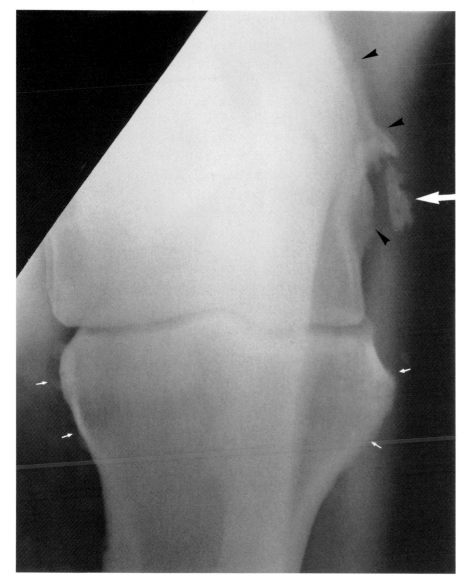

Figure 6.29 Craniocaudal view of an elbow of a 10-year-old riding school pony with chronic lameness. Lateral is to the right. There is extensive new bone on the lateral aspect of the epicondyle of the humerus (arrow heads). There is periosteal roughening and new bone on the lateral and medial aspects of the proximal radius (small white arrows). This is entheseophyte formation at the sites of attachment of the collateral ligaments of the humeroradial joint. There is also mineralization in the soft tissues laterally (large white arrow). There was also slight osteophyte formation on the articular margins of the joint, seen only in a mediolateral view.

accessory ligament of the superficial digital flexor tendon (the superior or radial check ligament). Clinical signs include very subtle lameness, sometimes associated with distension of the carpal sheath in acute cases. This injury may occur concurrently with superficial digital flexor tendonitis and it is therefore prudent to examine the tendon ultrasonographically. Radiographic changes are usually only detectable in chronic cases, and rest (for 2 months) generally results in resolution of clinical signs.

Luxation of the elbow joint

Luxation of the elbow joint is not common and has only been reported concurrent with a fracture of the radius or ulna.

Infection

Infection occurs most commonly in young foals but, since the lateral aspect of the radius is poorly protected by soft tissues, a deep wound in this area may penetrate the elbow joint capsule or cause localized infection. This may spread to the joint or result in osteomyelitis of the radius or ulna in an adult horse. If the degree of lameness associated with a wound in the elbow region is unexpectedly severe, or if there is a discharging sinus, radiographic examination is indicated. Injection of as much radiopaque contrast medium as possible, via a Foley catheter, should establish whether a sinus communicates with the joint capsule or with sequestered bone (Figure 14.9b, page 707). It may also demonstrate a filling defect representing a foreign body. Ultrasonographic evaluation may also be helpful.

Osteochondroma of the distal radius

Distension of the carpal sheath, lameness and resentment of pressure applied to the distal caudal aspect of the radius may be associated with an osteochondroma on the distal diaphysis or the metaphysis of the radius.

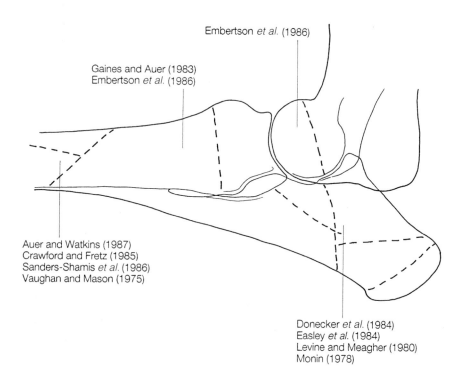

Figure 6.30 Location of common fractures in the elbow region, and recommended references (see 'Further reading').

Radiographically this appears as a variably shaped bony protuberance on the distocaudal aspect of the radius usually proximal to the physeal scar (see Figure 5.22, page 264). This mass has a thin cortex which appears to be continuous with the cortex of the radius. Sequential radiographs may demonstrate progressive enlargement of the mass. Treatment by surgical removal of the abnormal bone is usually successful in resolving both the lameness and carpal sheath swelling.

Hereditary multiple exostosis

Hereditary multiple exostosis is a rare condition characterized by multiple bony projections on growing long bones, the ribs, the pelvic bones and the dorsal spinous processes of the thoracic and lumbar vertebrae. These swellings are present at birth and may enlarge progressively until skeletal maturity. They may be asymptomatic unless impinging upon adjacent soft tissues, but may cause distension of synovial structures. The radiographic appearance is similar to that of solitary osteochondroma. There is no known treatment, but it is a hereditary condition, transmitted by an autosomal dominant gene.

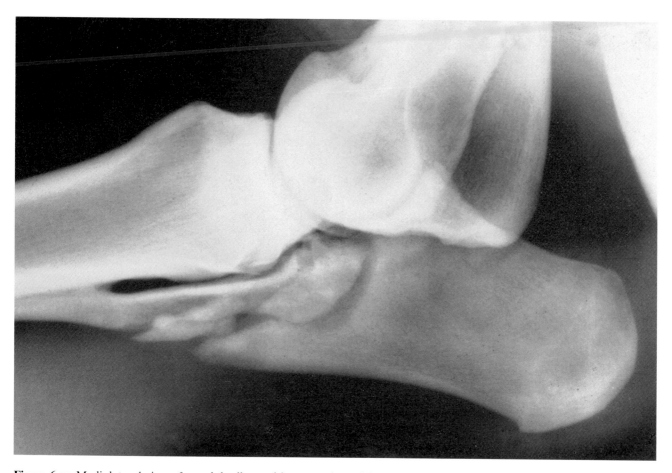

Figure 6.31 Mediolateral view of an adult elbow with a comminuted fracture of the olecranon. Although one of the fracture lines enters the trochlear notch of the ulna, it involves the non-articular area.

CHAPTER 6
*The shoulder, humerus,
elbow and radius*

Hypertrophic osteopathy

This condition is discussed in detail in Chapter 1 (page 22). Periosteal new bone along the diaphysis and the metaphyses of the radius may be due to hypertrophic osteopathy. The multifocal nature of the disease should help to differentiate it from other causes of periostitis.

Fractures (Figure 6.30, page 314)

Physeal fractures

Fractures of the distal physis of the humerus occur occasionally and warrant a poor prognosis. In an immature horse, the open proximal physis of the ulna should not be confused with a fracture. The apophysis may be displaced proximally (Salter-Harris type 1 fracture) (see Chapter 1, page 25) and it is important to compare its position with a horse of similar age. Radiographic examination of the contralateral limb provides an ideal comparison. These fractures and both proximal and physeal fractures of the radius have a fair prognosis.

Ulnar fractures

Fracture of the olecranon of the ulna is a common sequel to trauma in the elbow region. Lameness is usually severe and the horse may stand with the elbow 'dropped'. There may or may not be associated soft-tissue swelling. Radiographic examination of a suspected facture should include both mediolateral and craniocaudal views in order to assess its configuration accurately. A fracture which enters the trochlear notch must be assessed carefully to determine whether or not it involves the articular or non-articular region (Figure 6.31). Provided that ulnar fractures are recognized and treated early, the prognosis depends primarily on whether the fracture is simple or compound, the extent of comminution and the degree of displacement of the fracture fragments. Internal fixation offers the best chance for full return to athletic function.

Radial fractures

Radial fractures are a common result of trauma and occur in many configurations, incomplete parasagittal (see page 317), comminuted, transverse and physeal being the most frequent. Multiple radiographic views may be necessary to assess the full extent of a fracture. Repair may be successful in immature horses, but the prognosis in adult horses for complete fractures is extremely guarded. Incomplete fissure (stress) fractures or incomplete fractures resulting from kick injuries (Figures 6.32a and 6.32b) often heal with conservative treatment (3–6 months' box rest) provided external stability is maximal.

Fatigue or stress fractures of the radial diaphysis occur in young (2- and 3-year-old) Thoroughbreds in training. Although they may not be detectable radiographically in the acute phase, there may be localized increased opacity of the medulla. Nuclear scintigraphy is a more sensitive diagnostic

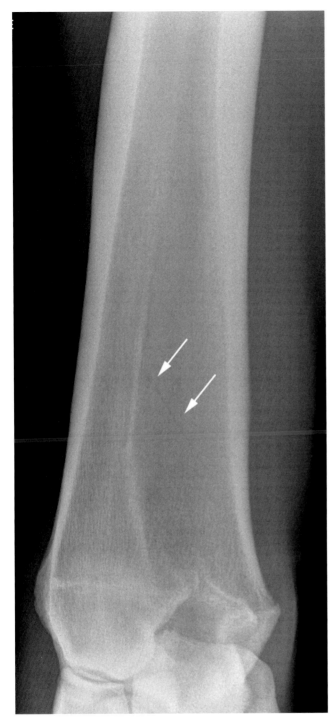

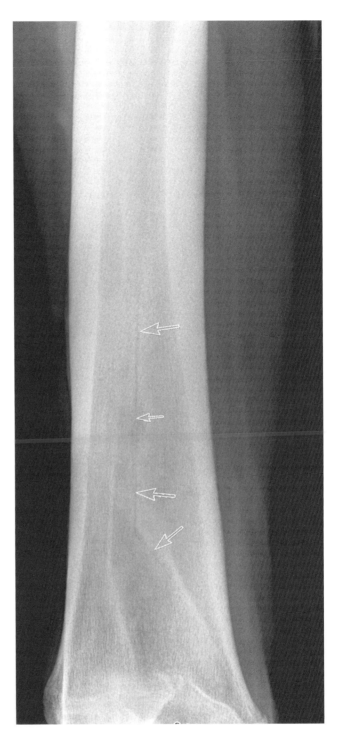

Figure 6.32(a) Craniomedial-caudolateral oblique radiographic view of the radius of a 16-year-old hunter, which had been kicked on the antebrachium 2 weeks previously. There was a discharging wound and the horse was non-weight-bearing on the limb. There is an oblique radiolucent line (arrows), representing an incomplete fissure fracture.

Figure 6.32(b) Craniomedial-caudolateral oblique view of the same horse as in Figure 6.32(a), obtained 10 days later. The fracture line is now much more obvious (arrows), extends much further proximally than was previously apparent and is surrounded by some more opaque bone, representing callus.

CHAPTER 6
*The shoulder, humerus,
elbow and radius*

technique. Medullary sclerosis in the mid-diaphyseal region reflects endosteal callus and should be differentiated from an enostosis-like lesion.

Enostosis-like lesions

The radius is one of the more common sites for enostosis-like lesions, which are seen most commonly in young Thoroughbred racehorses and cause acute, often severe lameness. There are usually no localizing clinical signs and diagnosis is usually dependent on the identification of focal increased radiopharmaceutical uptake in the radial diaphysis, often close to the nutrient foramen. Radiographic examination reveals focal increased opacity. Lameness usually resolves with time, although in some horses it shifts between limbs.

FURTHER READING

Allen, D. and White, N. (1984) Chip fracture of the greater tubercle of a horse. *Comp. Cont. Educ.*, **6**, S39–41

Auer, J. and Watkins, J. (1987) Treatment of radial fractures in adult horses: an analysis of 15 clinical cases. *Equine vet. J.*, **19**, 103–110

Bertone, A., McIlwraith, C., Powers, P., Stashak, T., Aanes, W. and Turner, A. (1986) Subchondral osseous cystic lesions of the elbow of horses: conservative versus surgical treatment. *J. Am. Vet. Med. Ass.*, **189**, 540–546

Bohn, A., Papageorges, M. and Grant, B. (1992) Ultrasonographic evaluation and surgical treatment of humeral osteitis and bicipital tenosynovitis in a horse. *J. Am. Vet. Med. Ass.*, **201**, 305–306

Booth, T. (1999) Lameness associated with the bicipital bursa in an Arab stallion. *Vet. Rec.*, **145**, 194–198

Boswell, J., Schramme, M., Wilson, A. and May, S. (2000) Radiological study to evaluate suspected scapulohumeral joint dysplasia in Shetland ponies. *Equine vet. J.*, **32**, 510–514

Boys Smith, S. and Singer, E. (2007) Mineralisation of the biceps brachii tendon in a 6-year-old Cob mare. *Equine vet. Educ.*, **19**, 74–79

Brown, M. and MacCallum, F. (1974) Anconeal process of ulna: separate centre of ossification in the horse. *Br. Vet. J.*, **130**, 434–438

Chopin, J., Wright, J., Melville, L. and Robinson, W. (1997) Lateral collateral ligament avulsion of the humeroradial joint in a horse. *Vet Radiol. and Ultrasound*, **38**, 50–54

Coudry, V., Allen, K. and Denoix, J.-M. (2005) Congenital abnormalities of the bicipital apparatus in four mature horses. *Equine vet. J.*, **37**, 272–275

Crawford, W. and Fretz, P. (1985) Long bone fractures in large animals: a retrospective study. *Vet. Surg.*, **14**, 295–302

Crawley, G. and Grant, B. (1986) Repair of elbow joint luxation without concomitant fracture in a horse. *Equine Pract.*, **8**(5), 19–26

Davidson, E. and Martin, B. (2004) Stress fracture of the scapula in 2 horses. *Vet. Radiol and Ultrasound*, **45**, 407–410

Derungs, S., Fuerst, A., Haas, C., Geissbuhler, U. and Auer, J. (2001) Fissure fractures of the radius and tibia in 23 horses: a retrospective study. *Equine vet. Educ.*, **13**, 313–318

Donecker, J., Bramlage, L. and Gabel, A. (1984) Retrospective analysis of 29 fractures of the olecranon process of the equine ulna. *J. Am. Vet. Med. Ass.*, **185**, 183–189

Doyle, P. and White, N. (2000) Diagnostic findings and prognosis following arthroscopic treatment of subtle osteochondral lesions in the shoulder joint of horses. *J. Am. Vet. Med. Ass.*, **217**, 1878–1882

Dyson, S. (1985) Sixteen fractures of the shoulder region in the horse. *Equine vet. J.*, **17**, 104–110

CHAPTER 6
*The shoulder, humerus,
elbow and radius*

Dyson, S. (1986a) Shoulder lameness in the horse: an analysis of 58 suspected cases. *Equine vet. J.*, **18**, 29–36

Dyson, S. (1986b) The differential diagnosis of shoulder lameness in the horse. *Thesis*, Fellowship of the Royal College of Veterinary Surgeons

Dyson, S. (1986c) Interpreting radiographs 7: Radiology of the equine shoulder and elbow. *Equine vet. J.*, **18**, 352–361

Dyson, S. and Greet, T. (1986) Repair of a fracture of the deltoid tuberosity of the humerus in a pony. *Equine vet. J.*, **18**, 230–232

Easley, K., Schneider, J., Guffy, M. and Boero, M. (1984) Equine ulnar fractures: a review of 25 clinical cases. *Equine Vet. Sci.*, **3**(1), 5–12

Edwards, G. and Vaughan, L. (1978) Infective arthritis of the elbow joint in the horse. *Vet. Rec.*, **103**, 227–229

Embertson, R., Bramlage, L. and Gabel, A. (1986) Physeal fractures in the horse II: management and outcome. *Vet. Surg.*, **14**, 295–302

Firth, E., Dik, K., Goedegebuure, S., Hagens, F., Verberne, L., Merkens, H. and Kersjes, A. (1980) Polyarthritis and bone infection in foals. *Zbl. Vet. Med.*, **B27**, 102–124

Fitch, G. and Martinelli, M. (1998) Conservative management of a sequestrum involving the radial cortex in 2 horses. *Equine vet. Educ.*, **10**, 228–232

Forresu, D., Lepage, O. and Cauvin, D. (2006) Septic bicipital bursitis, tendonitis and arthritis of the scapulohumeral joint in a mare. *Vet. Rec.*, **159**, 352–354

Fugaro, M. and Adams, S. (2002) Biceps brachii tenotomy or tenectomy for the treatment of bicipital bursitis, tendonitis and humeral osteitis in 3 horses. *J. Am. Vet. Med. Ass.*, **220**, 1508–1511

Gaines, J. and Auer, J. (1983) Treatment of a Salter Harris Type III epiphyseal fracture in a young horse. *Comp. Cont. Educ.*, **5**, S102–106

Hardy, J., Marcoux, M. and Eisenberg, H. (1986) Osteochondrosis-like lesion of the anconeal process in 2 horses. *J. Am. Vet. Med. Ass.*, **189**, 802–803

Kay, A. (2006) An acute subchondral cystic lesion of the equine shoulder causing lameness. *Equine vet. Educ.*, **18**, 316–319

Leitch, M. (1977) A review of treatment of tuber scapulae fractures in the horse. *J. Equine Med. Surg.*, **1**, 234–240

Levine, S. and Meagher, D. (1980) Repair of an ulnar fracture with radial luxation in a horse. *Vet. Surg.*, **9**, 58–60

Mackey, V., Trout, D., Meagher, D. and Hornhof, W. (1987) Stress fractures of the humerus, radius and tibia in horses. *Vet. Radiol.*, **28**, 26–31

Meagher, D., Pool, R. and Brown, M. (1979) Bilateral ossification of the tendon of biceps brachii muscle in the horse. *J. Am. Vet. Med. Ass.*, **174**, 282–285

Meagher, D., Pool, R. and O'Brien, T. (1973) Osteochondrosis of the shoulder joint in the horse. *Proc. Am. Ass. Equine Pract.*, **19**, 247–256

Mez, J., Dabareiner, R., Cole, R. and Watkins, J. (2007) Fracture of the greater tubercle of the humerus in horses: 15 cases (1986–2004). *J. Am. Vet. Med. Assoc.*, **230**, 1350–1355

Monin, T. (1978) Repair of physeal fractures of the tuber olecranon in the horse using a tension band method. *J. Am. Vet. Med. Ass.*, **172**, 287–290

Nixon, A., Stashak, T., McIlwraith, W., Aanes, W. and Martin, G. (1985) A muscle separating approach to the equine shoulder joint for the treatment of osteochondritis dissecans. *Vet. Surg.*, **5**, 247–256

Nyack, B., Morgan, J., Pool, R. and Meagher, D. (1981) Osteochondrosis of the shoulder joint of the horse. *Cornell Vet.*, **71**, 149–163

Oikawa, M. and Narama, I. (1998) Enthesopathy of the radial tuberosity in two Thoroughbred racehorses. *J. Comp. Path.*, **118**, 135–143

Ordidge, R. (2001) Pathological fracture of the radius secondary to an aneurysmal bone cyst. *Equine vet. Educ.* **13**, 239–242

O'Sullivan, C. and Lumsden, J. (2003) Stress fractures of the tibia and humerus in Thoroughbred racehorses: 99 cases (1992–2000). *J. Am. Vet. Med. Ass.*, **222**, 491–498

Pankowski, R., Grant, B., Sande, R. and Nickels, F. (1986) Fracture of the supraglenoid tubercle: treatment and results in 5 horses. *Vet. Surg.*, **15**, 33–39

Parks, A. and Nickels, F. (1986) Scapular sequestrum in a horse: a case report. *Vet. Surg.*, **15**, 389–391

Ramzan, P. and Pilsworth, R. (2001) Suspected septic physitis of the proximal humerus in two cases of Thoroughbred horses age two years. *Equine vet. J.*, **33**, 514–518

[319]

CHAPTER 6
*The shoulder, humerus,
elbow and radius*

Ramzan, P. (2002) Enostosis-like lesions: 12 cases. *Equine vet. Educ.* **14**, 143–148

Ramzan, P. (2004) Osseous cyst-like lesion of the intermediate tubercle of a horse. *Vet. Rec.*, **154**, 534–536

Sanders-Shamis, M., Bramlage, L. and Gabel, A. (1986) Radius fractures in the horse: a retrospective study of 47 cases. *Equine vet. J.*, **18**, 432–437

Semevolos, S., Watkins, J. and Auer, J. (2003) Scapulohumeral arthrodesis in Miniature horses. *Vet. Surg.*, **32**, 416–420

Swineboard, E., Dabareiner, R., Swor, T., Carter, K., Watkins, J. et al. (2003) Osteomyelitis secondary to trauma involving the proximal end of the radius in horses: five cases (1987–2001). *J. Am. Vet. Med. Ass.*, **223**, 486–491

Swor, T., Watkins, J., Bahr, A. and Honnas, C. (2003) Results of plate fixation of type 1b olecranon fractures in 24 horses. *Equine vet. J.*, **35**, 670–675

Swor, T., Watkins, J., Bahr, A., Epstein, K. and Honnas, C. (2006) Results of plate fixation of type 5 olecranon fractures in 20 horses. *Equine vet. J.*, **37**, 30–34

Tudor, R., Crosier, M., Love, N. and Bowman, K. (2001) Radiographic diagnosis: fracture of the caudal aspect of the greater tubercle of the humerus in a horse. *Vet. Radiol. and Ultrasound*, **42**, 244–245

Turner, A.S. (1981) Long bone fractures in horses Part 1. Initial management. *Comp. Cont. Educ.*, **3**, S347–353

Valdez, H., Morris, D. and Auer, J. (1979) Compression plating of long bone fractures in foals. *J. Vet. Orthop.*, **1**, 10–18

Vaughan, L. and Mason, B. (1975) *A Clinicopathological Study of Racing Accidents in Horses*, Adlard and Son, Bartholomew Press, Dorking, Surrey

Wagner, P., Watrous, B., Shires, G. and Riebold, T. (1985) Resection of the supraglenoid tubercle of the scapula in a colt. *Comp. Cont. Educ.*, **7**, S36–40

Wilson, R. and Reynolds, W. (1984) Scapulohumeral joint luxation with treatment by closed reduction in a horse. *Aust. Vet. J.*, **61**, 300–301

Yovich, J. and Aanes, W. (1985) Fracture of the greater tubercle of the humerus in a filly. *J. Am. Vet. Med. Ass.*, **187**, 74–75

Zamos, D. and Parks, A. (1992) Comparison of surgical and non-surgical treatment of humeral fractures in horses: 22 cases (1980–1989). *J. Am. Vet. Med. Ass.*, **201**, 114–116

Chapter 7
The tarsus

RADIOGRAPHIC TECHNIQUE

Equipment

Radiographic examination of the tarsus (hock) is easily performed using a portable x-ray machine and high-definition screens. A grid is unnecessary unless there is considerable periarticular soft-tissue swelling. A minimum of four views, lateromedial, dorsoplantar, dorsolateral-plantaromedial oblique and dorsomedial-plantarolateral oblique (or plantarolateral-dorsomedial oblique), is required. In selected cases, flexed lateromedial and dorsoplantar (flexed) views yield valuable additional information. The first four views are best obtained with the horse bearing full weight on the limb, with the metatarsal region positioned vertically. It is preferable for the horse to bear weight evenly on both hindlimbs. If the horse is reluctant to bear full weight on the limb due to excessive pain, administration of an analgesic such as butorphanol may be helpful. Sedation with detomidine may facilitate examination of a difficult horse, which may otherwise refuse to stand still, or may kick repeatedly.

The hindlimbs should be spread apart sufficiently to allow positioning of the cassette without it touching either limb. The person holding the cassette can position it more accurately if the horse's tail is tied in a knot and the hock is not obscured. A long-handled cassette holder should be used.

Positioning

Lateromedial view

The talocalcaneal-centroquartal (proximal intertarsal), the centrodistal (distal intertarsal) and the tarsometatarsal joints are not horizontal, but slope proximodistally, from laterally to medially. In order to avoid confusing overlap of the joint spaces it is helpful to angle the x-ray beam $10°$ proximodistally (i.e. L$10°$Pr-MDiO view), centring at the approximate level of the centrodistal joint. Alternatively a horizontal x-ray beam is centred at the level of the talus (tibiotarsal bone), thus making use of a divergent x-ray beam through the lower joints of the hock. For a true lateromedial view the x-ray beam is directed parallel to a line joining the medial and lateral malleoli of the tibia, or to a line tangential to the heel of the foot.

A flexed lateromedial view can be useful to evaluate the proximal aspects of the trochlear ridges of the talus, the coracoid process of the calcaneus and the plantar distal aspect of the tibia (see Figure 7.3b, page 327). An assistant stands beside the horse's abdomen facing the tail and holds the distal metatarsus so that the angle between the tibia and the third metatarsal bone is approximately 50°. Care should be taken to hold the limb close to the horse's body, to avoid rotation of the tarsus. The x-ray beam is centred on the talus.

Dorsoplantar view

Many horses stand slightly 'toe-out', which is helpful since it obviates the need to position the x-ray machine beneath the horse's abdomen in order to obtain a dorsoplantar view. A horizontal x-ray beam is used, centred at the centrodistal joint. In some horses it is impossible for all of the centro-distal joint to be assessed simultaneously, due to the slope of the distal joints of the hock: two views may be required. If the x-ray beam is horizontal and centred at the centrodistal joint, the lateral side of the joint may appear normal but the medial side may appear abnormally narrow. If the x-ray beam is angled 5–10° proximodistally, the medial side of the centrodistal joint may then look normal. Abnormalities of the medial and lateral malleoli may be missed in a dorsoplantar projection. A dorsal 15° medial-plantarolateral oblique view is useful to assess the lateral malleolus, and a dorsal 15° lateral-plantaromedial oblique projection is helpful to evaluate the medial malleolus (see Figure 7.6b, page 333).

Oblique views

Due to the complex structure of the equine tarsus, changes in the degree of obliquity of the x-ray beam can result in considerable alteration in the radiographs obtained. It is therefore essential to establish a consistent technique (e.g., dorsal 35° lateral-plantaromedial oblique). The x-ray beam is centred at the site of principal interest (often the centrodistal joint). A horizontal beam is employed. It is often easier and safer to obtain a plantarolateral-dorsomedial oblique, rather than a dorsomedial-plantarolateral oblique view, although either technique can be used.

Dorsoplantar (flexed) view

The hindlimb is held flexed with the hock as far behind the horse as possible (Figure 7.1). Many horses in which this view is required resent flexion of the limb and administration of an analgesic such as butorphanol will facilitate this examination. The cassette is held parallel to the plantar aspect of the tuber calcanei and the x-ray beam is directed as nearly perpendicular to it as possible. It may be easier to obtain a plantarodorsal (flexed) view depending on the degree of flexion of the hock that can be achieved. These

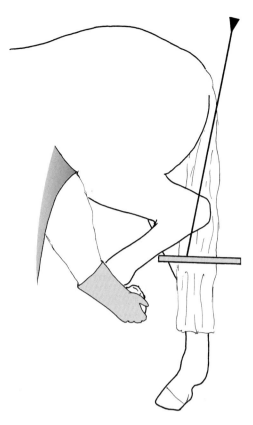

Figure 7.1 Positioning of the limb, cassette and x-ray machine to obtain a dorsoplantar (flexed) view of the calcaneus and sustentaculum tali of the fibular tarsal bone.

projections are particularly useful for evaluation of the tuber calcanei, the sustentaculum tali of the calcaneus and the talocalcaneal joint.

RADIOGRAPHIC ANATOMY: NORMAL VARIATIONS AND INCIDENTAL FINDINGS

It is important to recognize that some of the variations in radiographic appearance discussed below are the result of a previous problem that is now clinically silent. They cannot be regarded as normal, but are unlikely to be of clinical significance.

Immature horse

At birth the malleoli of the tibia and the trochlear ridges may be incompletely ossified and have an irregular, rough contour and a granular opacity (Figures 7.2a and 7.2b). There is a separate ossification centre for the lateral malleolus of the tibia, which represents the distal epiphysis of the fibula. This well circumscribed, oval opacity fuses to the tibia by 3 months of age and should not be misinterpreted as a fracture. Adult features such as the medial proximal and distal tubercles of the talus are undeveloped. There is a separate ossification centre for the tuber calcanei, which may be absent

[323]

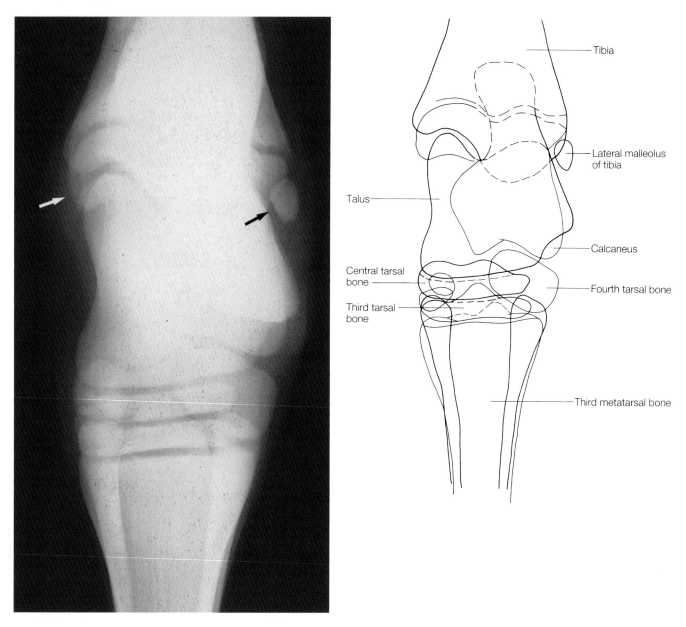

Figure 7.2(a) Dorsoplantar view and diagram of a hock of a 1-day-old foal. The small tarsal bones are rounded and the joint spaces wide compared with those of an adult. The medial malleolus of the tibia (white arrow) is incompletely ossified. There is a separate ossification centre of the lateral malleolus of the tibia (black arrow).

at birth but gradually ossifies and fuses to the calcaneus by 16–24 months of age. The centres of ossification have rounded corners, especially those of the central and third tarsal bones. The joint spaces appear wider than in an adult, because there is proportionally more cartilage present. The first and second tarsal bones may be unfused. The proximal physis of the third metatarsal bone is closed at birth.

Skeletally mature horse

In order to understand the complicated radiographic anatomy of the tarsus it is useful to compare the radiographs with a bone specimen and to visual-

[324]

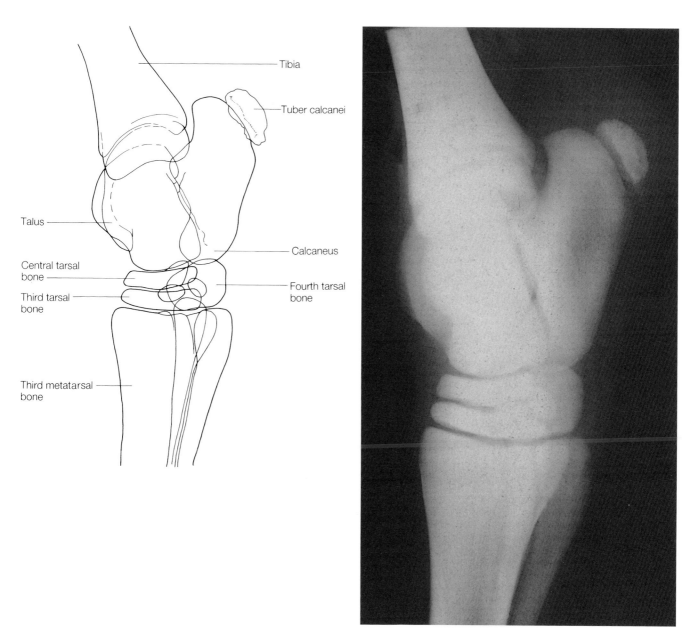

Figure 7.2(b) Lateromedial view and diagram of a hock of a 1-day-old foal. Note the relatively flat contour of the trochlear ridges of the talus compared with those of an adult, the widened joint spaces and the incompletely ossified tuber calcanei.

ize the shapes of the individual, disarticulated bones (see Figures 7.3; 7.6, pages 332 and 333; 7.7, pages 334 and 335; and 7.8, pages 336 and 337).

Lateromedial view

A normal lateromedial view and a flexed lateromedial view are illustrated in Figures 7.3a and 7.3b. In some horses there is a separate bony fragment at the craniodistal aspect of the tibia: its exact location is established from the oblique views, the most common site being the distal intermediate ridge of the tibia (see Figure 7.13, page 343). This may be an accessory ossification centre or a manifestation of osteochondrosis. It is often clinically silent, particularly if small, although its presence may be associated with distension

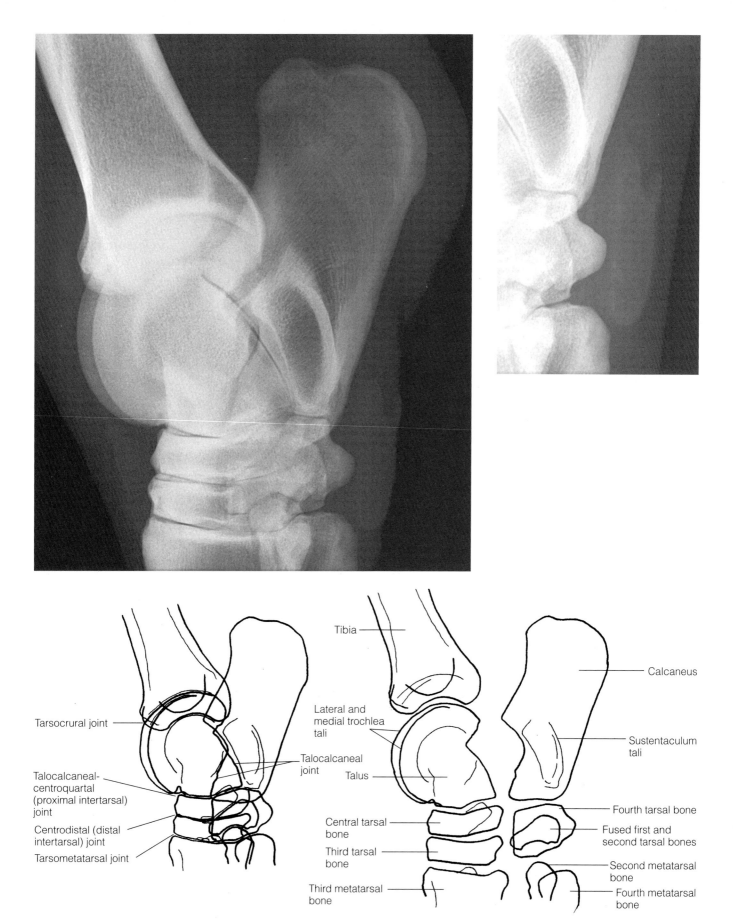

Figure 7.3(a) Lateromedial view and diagram of a normal adult hock. On a soft exposure (inset) the torus tarseus (chestnut) is readily seen.

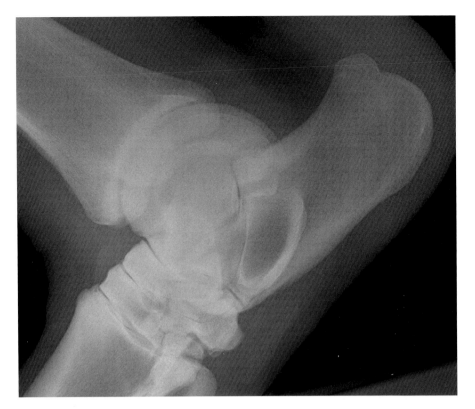

Figure 7.3(b) Flexed lateromedial view of a hock of an adult horse. There is slight modelling of the dorsoproximal aspect of the third metatarsal bone, of no clinical significance in this horse.

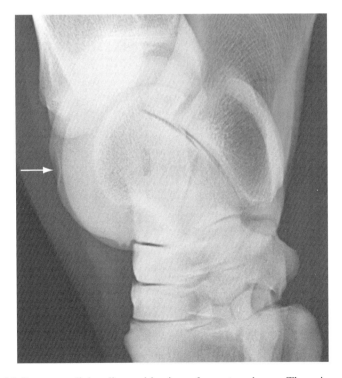

Figure 7.3(c) Lateromedial radiographic view of a mature horse. There is a smoothly outlined concave depression in the lateral trochlea of the talus (arrow), of no clinical significance. Note the bifid protuberance on the distal aspect of the medial trochlea, another normal variant. There is also subtle modelling of the dorsoproximal aspect of the third tarsal bone.

[327]

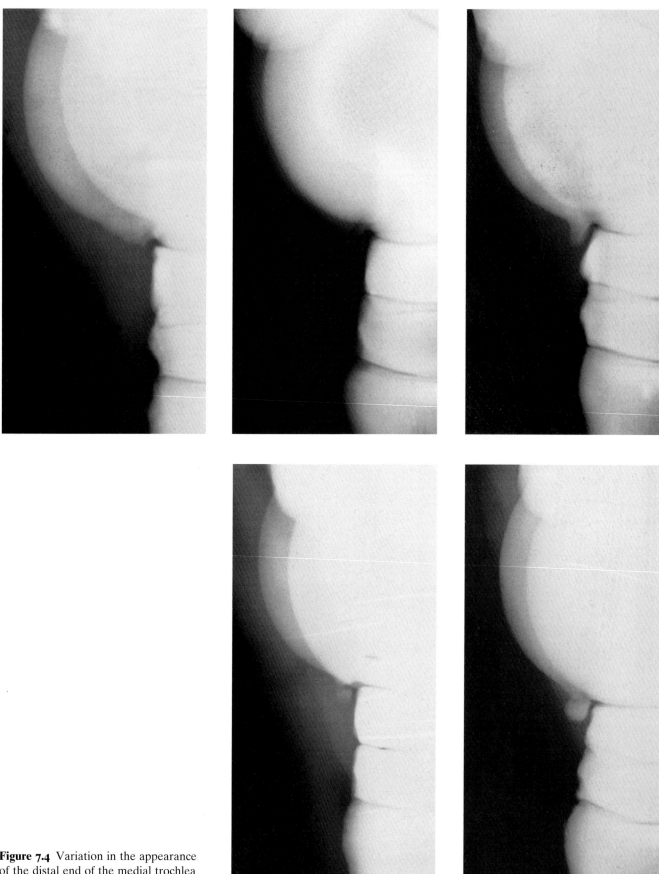

Figure 7.4 Variation in the appearance of the distal end of the medial trochlea tali (trochlear ridge).

of the tarsocrural joint capsule (bog spavin), with or without lameness. The medial and lateral trochlear ridges of the talus are smoothly curved, but may be slightly flattened in the mid-region, especially in Warmblood and heavy horse breeds. There is sometimes a smoothly outlined depression in the middle one-third of the lateral trochlear ridge of the talus, with normal subchondral bone opacity or slight sclerosis seen in either a lateromedial or dorsomedial-plantarolateral oblique view (Figure 7.3c). There is some controversy as to whether these represent a manifestation of osteochondrosis, however they are invariably asymptomatic. There may be an ill defined narrow lucent area in the subchondral bone of the medial trochlea representing the presence of a synovial fossa. The lateral ridge has a distinct large notch at its distal end, whereas the medial ridge has a variably sized protuberance distally. This protuberance may be small, with or without a lucent line (a nutrient vessel) extending through it, or may be large and rounded or pointed. Sometimes there are one or two discrete bony opacities distal to it (Figure 7.4), which should not be confused with fractures. The two trochlear ridges are more widely separated in the oblique views.

Depending on the exposure factors used, a variable number of lucent lines can be identified in the region where the calcaneus and talus are superimposed. These represent the talocalcaneal and tarsocrural articulations and should not be confused with fractures.

The central and third tarsal bones are fairly regular in height (proximodistally) from their dorsal to plantar aspects. The first and second and fourth tarsal bones are projected superimposed upon each other; the smoothly irregular plantar contour of the fourth tarsal bone is highlighted in this view. The plantar surfaces of the calcaneus and fourth tarsal and metatarsal bones are sometimes smoothly modelled, reflecting previous tearing of the attachment of the plantar ligament ('curb').

There is sometimes a small osseous 'spur' on the dorsoproximal aspect of the third metatarsal bone (Figures 7.5a–f). This may be an osteophyte or an entheseophyte at the site of attachment of the dorsal tarsometatarsal ligament, peroneus (fibularis) tertius, or the cranial tibial tendon, reflecting a previous injury. In the absence of other radiographic abnormalities, an osteophyte or an entheseophyte does not necessarily signify degenerative joint disease, although they may be associated with it. An osteophyte of no significance should have a smooth margin and be of uniform opacity (Figures 7.5a and 7.5b). An irregular margin or variable opacity (both of which may only be discernible when the radiograph is viewed over high-intensity illumination) suggest bony activity (Figures 7.5c and 7.5d).

The mottled opacity of the torus tarseus (chestnut) may be seen on the plantar aspect of the fourth tarsal bone (Figure 7.3a, page 326) and must not be confused with pathological mineralization of the soft tissues.

Dorsoplantar view

The medial and lateral malleoli are seen as smoothly rounded protuberances of the distal tibia (Figure 7.6). Smooth irregularity of outline may reflect previous damage to the attachment of the collateral ligaments of the tarsus.

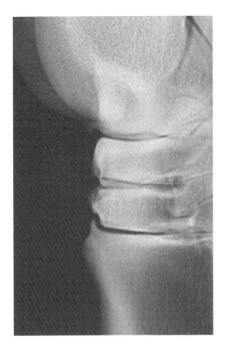

Figure 7.5(a) Lateromedial radiographic view of the left hock of an 11-year-old Warmblood show jumper with a good competition record. There is a uniformly opaque spur on the dorsoproximal aspect of the third metatarsal bone. This radiograph was obtained at a pre-purchase examination. There was no detectable lameness, although mild lameness was induced by flexion. The horse was purchased and has remained sound and in full work.

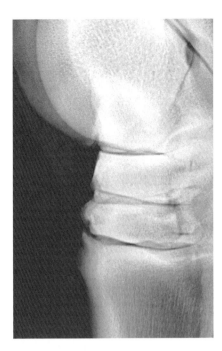

Figure 7.5(b) Slightly oblique lateromedial radiographic view of the right hock of a 7-year-old Thoroughbred cross gelding used for unaffiliated competition. There is a well consolidated periarticular osteophyte on the dorsoproximal aspect of the third metatarsal bone. Lameness was associated with proximal suspensory desmitis. Intra-articular analgesia of the tarsometatarsal joint did not alter the lameness.

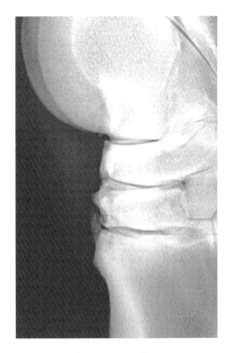

Figure 7.5(c) Lateromedial radiographic view of the left hock of a 13-year-old Thoroughbred used for general purposes. There is a large osteophyte on the dorsoproximal aspect of the third metatarsal bone which is less opaque than the parent bone. This is an active lesion. There is also subtle modelling of the distal dorsal aspect of the third tarsal bone. Lameness was improved by intra-articular analgesia of the tarsometatarsal joint.

The concave proximal articular surface of the central tarsal bone results in its plantar aspect being superimposed over the talus. There are many confusing opacities and lucent lines in the region of the central and third tarsal bones because of superimposition of the first and second and fourth tarsal bones and the bases (proximal ends) of the second and fourth metatarsal bones. The bases of the latter two bones are sloping and their articulations with the fused first and second tarsal bone and the fourth tarsal bone, respectively, are superimposed over the proximal one-third of the third tarsal bone. The resultant lucent lines should not be confused with pathological lesions. There are sometimes well defined oval lucent areas centred on either or both of the talocalcaneal-centroquartal or the centrodistal joints. These represent non-articular depressions and should not be confused with osseous cyst-like lesions.

This is the best view for evaluating the width of the intertarsal articulations, provided that these joints are in the centre of the radiograph and bearing in mind the limitations imposed by the slope of the articular surfaces mentioned previously (page 321). Sometimes one side of the joint space appears narrowed, but this may be an artefact. The view should be

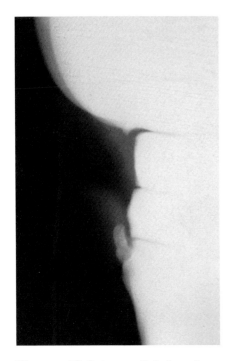 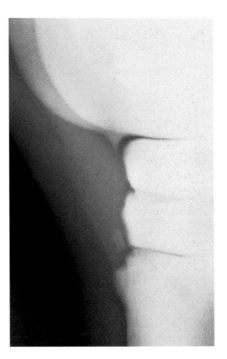 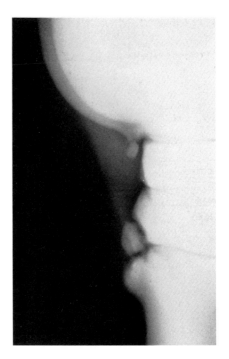

Figure 7.5(d) Lateromedial view of an adult hock. There is an active entheseophyte on the dorsoproximal aspect of the third metatarsal bone.

Figure 7.5(e) Lateromedial view of an adult hock. There is dystrophic mineralization in the cranial tibial tendon.

Figure 7.5(f) Fracture of a large entheseophyte on the dorsoproximal aspect of the third metatarsal bone. Note also the osseous opacity distal to the medial trochlea tali.

repeated, angling the x-ray beam 5–10° distally. Usually this 'opens up' the apparently narrowed side of the joint. Complete ankylosis of the centrodistal and/or tarsometatarsal joints, in the absence of subchondral bone lysis, is sometimes seen without associated lameness.

An exostosis on the proximolateral aspect of the third metatarsal bone is seen in some horses. This may have a heterogeneous opacity (see Figure 4.12, page 206), but is usually smoothly outlined. Such exostoses, despite invariably being associated with focal, intense increased radiopharmaceutical uptake, are generally of no clinical significance.

Dorsolateral-plantaromedial oblique view

This view (Figure 7.7) highlights the medial malleolus of the tibia, the medial trochlear tali and the dorsomedial aspects of the intertarsal joints. There is a variably sized and shaped lucent area in the proximal part of the tarsal groove which represents a synovial fossa. Similar areas in the corresponding articular surface of the tibia are not seen radiographically. The distal medial tuberosity of the talus is usually smoothly rounded; it may be smoothly irregular, reflecting previous tearing of the attachment of the medial short collateral ligament. The sinus tarsi, a non-articular area between the talus and calcaneus, is seen as a relatively lucent line or oval-shaped area between the two bones, and varies with the angle of projection.

There is a bony prominence on the dorsomedial aspect of the third tarsal bone at the site of attachment of one of the dorsal tarsal ligaments. The

[331]

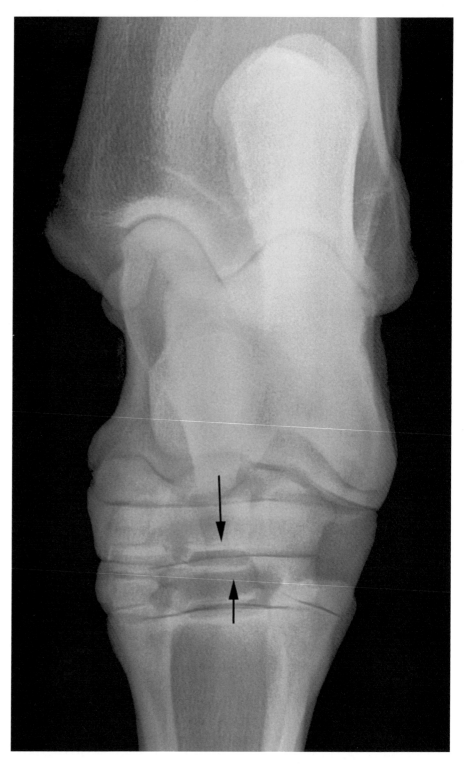

Figure 7.6(a) Dorsoplantar view and diagrams of a normal adult hock. Lateral is to the right. Note the relatively lucent areas in the central and third tarsal bones in the middle of the centrodistal joint (arrows), a normal finding.

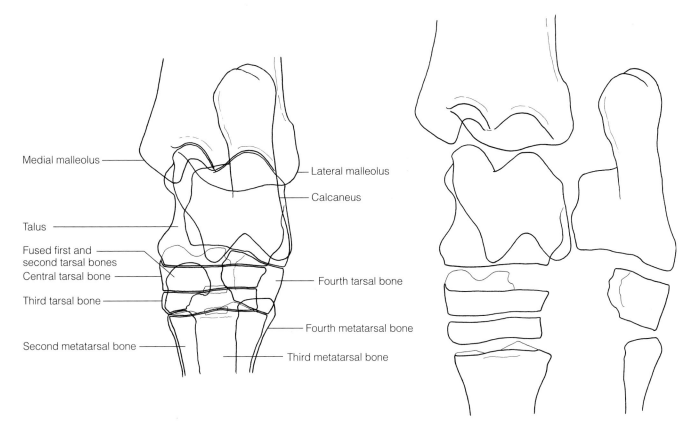

Medial malleolus
Lateral malleolus
Calcaneus
Talus
Fused first and second tarsal bones
Central tarsal bone
Third tarsal bone
Second metatarsal bone
Fourth tarsal bone
Fourth metatarsal bone
Third metatarsal bone

Figure 7.6(a) *Cont'd*

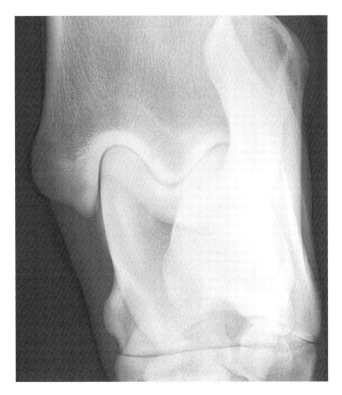

Figure 7.6(b) Dorsal 15° lateral-plantaromedial oblique radiographic view of a normal adult tarsus. This degree of obliquity allows assessment of the distal and axial aspects of the medial malleolus. Compare with Figures 7.6(a) and 7.12(b).

[333]

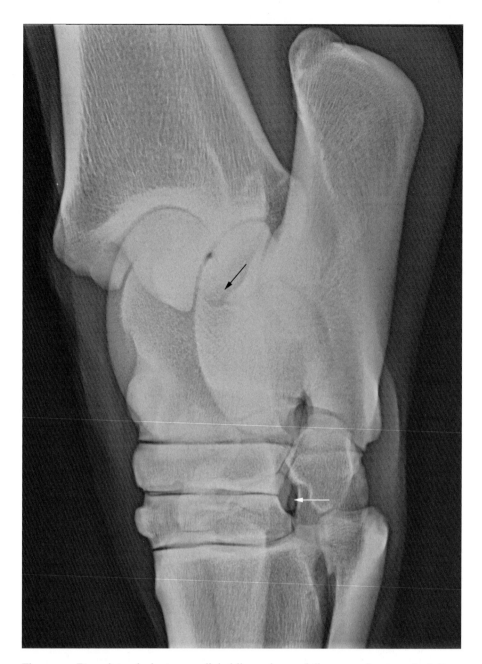

Figure 7.7 Dorsolateral-plantaromedial oblique view and diagrams of a normal adult hock. There is a radiolucent area (black arrow), a synovial fossa, in the intertrochlear groove of the talus. The third tarsal bone has a medial prominence. The dorsal opening of the tarsal canal is clearly outlined (white arrow). Note the relatively lucent areas in the central and third tarsal bones in the middle of the centrodistal joint, a normal finding.

subchondral bone of the distal talus, the central and third tarsal bones and the proximal aspect of the third metatarsal bone is relatively sclerotic. There are non-articular depressions on the opposing surfaces of the talus, central and third tarsal bones and third metatarsal bones that result in relatively lucent areas in the centre of the centrodistal and tarsometatarsal joints. These are sites of intertarsal ligaments.

In a well positioned dorsolateral-plantaromedial oblique view, the dorsal opening of the tarsal canal, through which passes the perforating tarsal

[334]

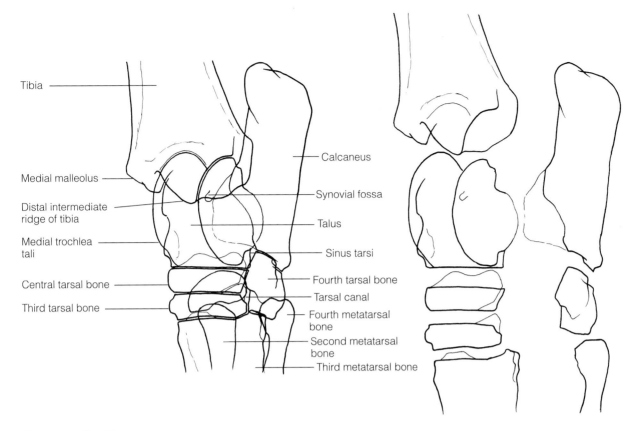

Labels on left figure:
- Tibia
- Medial malleolus
- Distal intermediate ridge of tibia
- Medial trochlea tali
- Central tarsal bone
- Third tarsal bone

Labels on right of left figure:
- Calcaneus
- Synovial fossa
- Talus
- Sinus tarsi
- Fourth tarsal bone
- Tarsal canal
- Fourth metatarsal bone
- Second metatarsal bone
- Third metatarsal bone

Figure 7.7 *Cont'd*

artery and a branch of the deep fibular (peroneal) nerve, is seen as a well defined lucent area. The canal is not in the sagittal plane but courses slightly obliquely; therefore, unless the x-ray beam is parallel with the long axis of the canal, its walls will be seen as bone encroaching into the canal. This must be differentiated from new bone on the lateral aspect of the centrodistal joint (see Figure 7.18a, page 350). This new bone can usually also be seen in a dorsoplantar view. The plantar opening of the tarsal canal appears as a relatively lucent area superimposed over the fourth tarsal bone.

Dorsomedial-plantarolateral oblique view

This view (Figure 7.8) highlights the sustentaculum tali, the lateral trochlea tali, the dorsolateral aspects of the intertarsal joints, and the plantar aspect of the sustentaculum tali and the central, first and second tarsal bones. Occasionally the distal end of an incompletely ossified fibula is seen. A separate bony fragment from the distal intermediate ridge of the tibia is often best seen in this view.

Dorsoplantar (flexed) view

The proximal parts of the medial trochlear ridge, the sustentaculum tali, the tarsal groove, the tuber calcanei and the talocalcaneal joint are highlighted in this view (Figure 7.9). Other structures are underexposed and cannot be assessed properly.

[335]

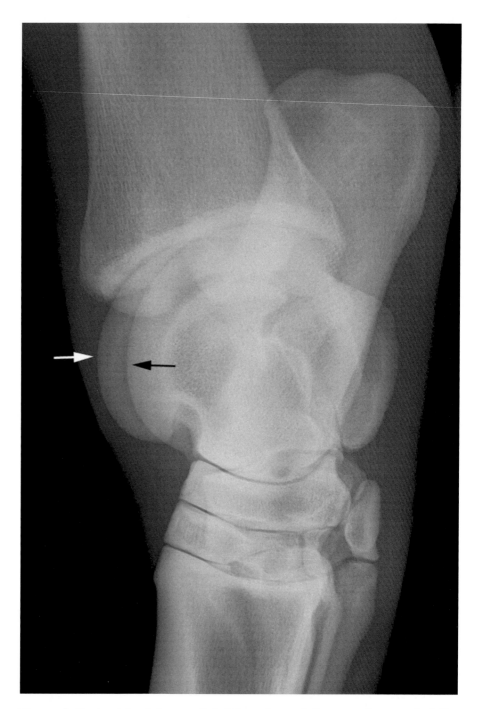

Figure 7.8 Plantarolateral-dorsomedial oblique view and diagrams of a normal adult hock. The medial trochlea tali (black arrow) and the lateral trochlea tali (white arrow) are clearly separated. The sustentaculum tali is highlighted on the plantar aspect of the talus. Note the inverted flask-shaped joint space between the third and fused first and second tarsal bones.

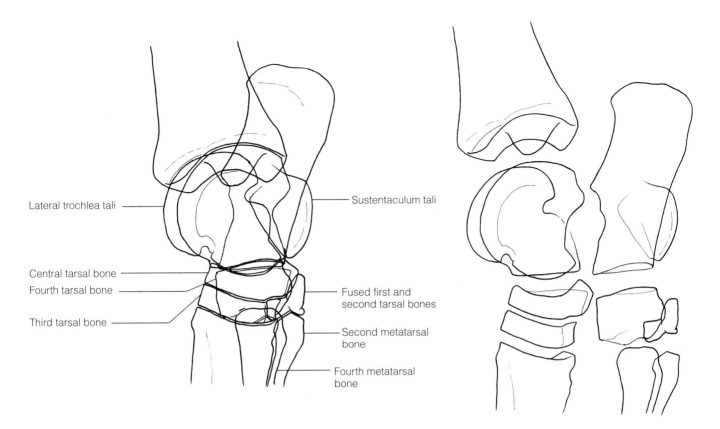

Lateral trochlea tali

Central tarsal bone
Fourth tarsal bone
Third tarsal bone

Sustentaculum tali

Fused first and
second tarsal bones

Second metatarsal
bone

Fourth metatarsal
bone

Figure 7.8 *Cont'd*

SIGNIFICANT RADIOLOGICAL ABNORMALITIES

Congenital abnormalities

Congenital malformation of the sustentaculum tali of the calcaneus (fibular tarsal bone) occurs in Saddlebreds and occasionally in Thoroughbreds (Figure 7.10). Flattening of the proximal aspect of the sustentaculum tali results in the deep digital flexor tendon slipping dorsally and medially. Clinically the plantar aspect of the tarsal region appears broader than usual and there is tarsal valgus. Radiographic abnormalities are detectable only in the dorsoplantar (flexed) view, in which the contour of the sustentaculum tali appears flattened.

Tarsal bone collapse

Tarsal bone collapse may be recognized radiographically in neonatal foals, in older foals or young adults. In a neonate the tarsal bones appear relatively immature; they are smaller and more rounded than usual due to incomplete ossification (Figure 7.11a). They may have a granular opacity (the bone is comprised of opaque granules). Clinically the neonatal foal shows excessive flexion of the hocks (sickled and curby hock conformation) and/or tarsal valgus deformities. The condition is most common in premature foals or those born one of a twin. Unless the limbs are supported from the first days of life in cylinder tube casts, until ossification has progressed

[337]

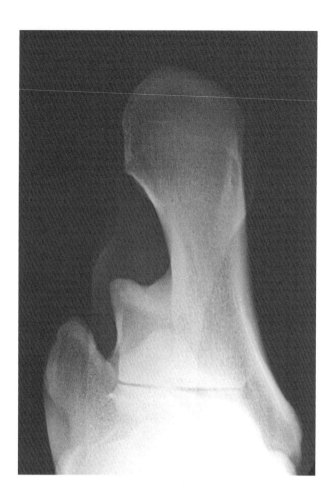

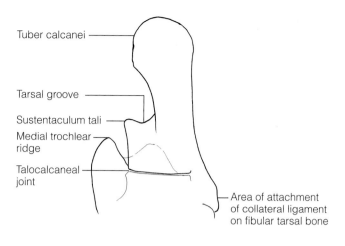

Figure 7.9 Dorsoplantar (flexed) view and diagram of a normal hock. Lateral is to the right.

further, normal weight bearing will result in compression of either or both the central and third tarsal bones. The compressed bones appear wedge shaped in both lateromedial and dorsoplantar views, and may show fragmentation with narrowing of the joint spaces. This condition has also been seen in association with osteomyelitis of the third and central tarsal bones, in which case the bone may have a mottled opacity due to lucent areas within the bone. Since tarsal collapse is often bilateral, both hocks should be examined radiographically.

Tarsal collapse may pass unrecognized until the horse starts work, when there may be an acute onset of unilateral or bilateral hindlimb lameness or stiffness. Radiographic examination reveals wedge-shaped central and/or third tarsal bones (Figures 7.11b and 7.11c) and evidence of secondary joint disease (e.g. collapse of the joint spaces and periarticular new bone). In less severe cases there may only be a slight wedge-shaped appearance of the third tarsal bone. Compare the height of the bone dorsally with the plantar aspect.

In the neonate, provision of external support to the limb permits endochondral ossification to proceed without deformation of the bones and, provided that treatment is started early, prognosis is fair to good. In the adult, the prognosis is usually poor for performance animals, although ankylosis of the bones may occur ultimately.

[338]

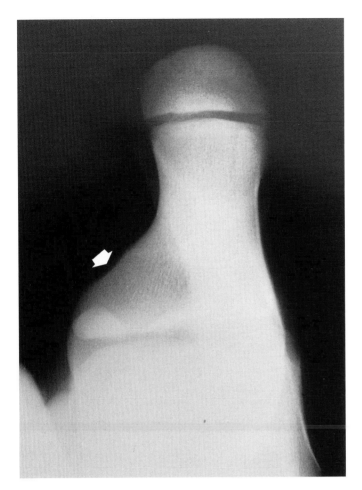

Figure 7.10 Dorsoplantar (flexed) oblique view of the hock of a 3-week-old Thoroughbred foal with a malformed hock. Lateral is to the right. There is flattening of the sustentaculum tali (arrow).

Osteochondrosis

Radiographic abnormalities which are thought to be a manifestation of osteochondrosis include: (a) separation of a bony fragment at either the medial (Figures 7.12a and 7.12b) or the lateral malleolus of the tibia, or the distal intermediate ridge of the tibia (Figure 7.13); (b) bony fragments at the distal end of the medial trochlear ridge of the talus (see Figure 7.4, page 328); (c) separation of a bony fragment from the medial proximal tubercle of the talus, and (d) an irregular, flattened contour of the medial and/or lateral ridges of the talus with or without radiolucent zones in the underlying subchondral bone (Figures 7.14a and 7.14b). Bony fragments of the medial and lateral malleoli of the tibia must be differentiated from avulsion fractures. Some medial malleolar articular fragments are not detectable in a dorsoplantar projection; a dorsal 15° lateral-plantaromedial oblique view may be required (Figure 7.12b). Fragments distal to the distal end of the trochlear ridges may have originated from the distal aspect of the tibia and have fallen distally. Lesions frequently occur bilaterally. Fragments at the distal intermediate ridge of the tibia are most common and can be detected

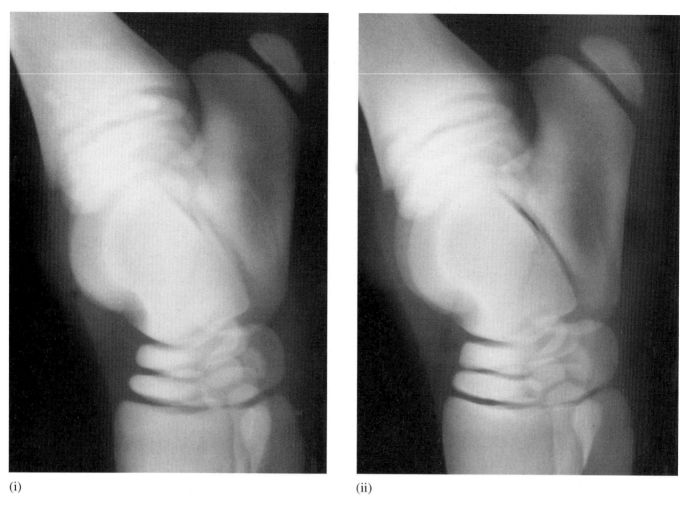

(i)   (ii)

Figure 7.11(a) Lateromedial views of a premature Thoroughbred foal born at a gestational age of 318 days. The radiographs were obtained (i) 6 days and (ii) 12 days post partum, i.e. at 324 and 330 days' gestation. Note the rounded edges of the incompletely ossified tarsal bones and the progressive enlargement of the bones.

at less than 3 months of age. They vary considerably in size, but are often bilaterally symmetrical. There may be an obvious lucent defect in the adjacent subchondral bone. The majority occur on the lateral aspect of the distal intermediate ridge of the tibia and are readily seen in plantarolateral-dorsomedial oblique views; however medial lesions occasionally occur and are seen in a slightly more plantar position in this oblique view and are easily missed. Osteochondritic lesions may cause release of inflammatory debris into the joint and resultant synovitis and distension of the tarsocrural joint.

The incidence of osteochondrosis in the tarsus is particularly high in certain breeds (e.g. Standardbreds, Warmbloods and some heavy horse breeds) and there may be a hereditary predisposition to the condition. In Dutch Warmbloods it has been shown that fragments at the distal intermediate ridge of the tibia are frequent (>65%) at 1 month of age, but in the majority (80%) the radiographic appearance is normal at 1 year of age. Lesions of the lateral trochlear ridge of the talus are less frequent (30%) at

[340]

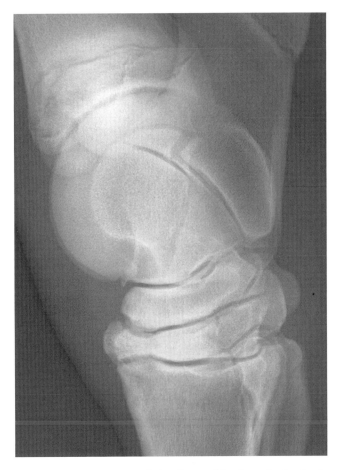

Figure 7.11(b) Lateromedial radiographic view of a hock of a 5-month-old Thoroughbred foal. The foal presented with lameness and swelling on the distal dorsal aspect of the hock. There is deformation of the third tarsal bone with narrowing of the height of the bone plantar to the dorsal articular margin. However despite mild joint space narrowing of the centrodistal and tarsometatarsal joints dorsally, there remains congruity between the articular margins of the central and third tarsal bones and the third metatarsal bone.

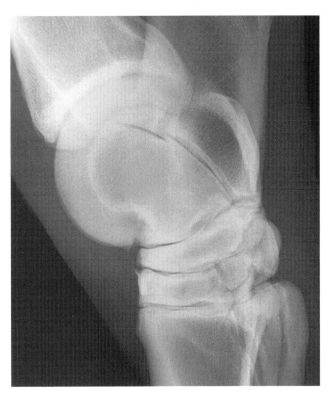

Figure 7.11(c) Lateromedial radiographic view of the left hock of a 9-year-old Thoroughbred cross with mild left hindlimb lameness, improved by intra-articular analgesia of the tarsometatarsal joint. The dorsal aspect of the central tarsal bone is narrow from proximally to distally and is sclerotic. There is mild modelling of the dorsal aspect of the central tarsal bone and a small osteophyte on the dorsoproximal aspect of the third tarsal bone. The dorsal aspect of the third tarsal bone is also sclerotic.

1 month of age, but the majority (97%) are normal at 1 year of age. A lesion present at 5 months of age in either location is likely to persist.

Lameness may or may not be present, or may develop at a later stage. Lameness is more likely in association with large or mobile fragments. Chronic distension of the tarsocrural joint capsule may lead to degenerative joint disease and ultimately lameness. In Standardbreds, these lesions have been associated with subtle hindlimb gait abnormalities at high speeds. In Warmbloods, performance at high levels may be compromised. Lesions of the trochlear ridges of the talus are more often associated with mild to moderate lameness, but not invariably so. The potential significance of osteochondritic lesions as a cause of lameness must be assessed carefully. Surgical treatment may be indicated and although the bog spavin may resolve, a good cosmetic result cannot be guaranteed, despite good functional results.

[341]

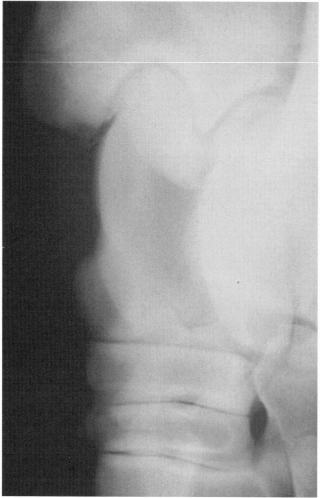

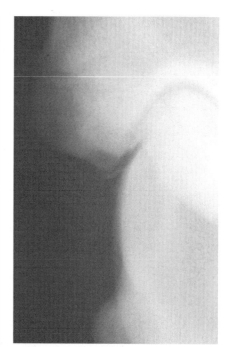

(a)

Figure 7.12(a) Dorsolateral-plantaromedial oblique view of a yearling Thoroughbred. There is a discrete osseous opacity distal to the medial malleolus of the tibia, a manifestation of osteochondrosis. Also see inset, top right.

Figure 7.12(b) Dorsal 15° lateral-plantaromedial oblique radiographic view of the right hock of a yearling Warmblood with marked distension of the tarsocrural joint, but no detectable lameness. There is an osteochondral fragment on the axial aspect of the medial malleolus (arrows), a manifestation of osteochondrosis.

(b)

Physitis or physeal dysplasia

Physitis or physeal dysplasia, which is possibly related to osteochondrosis, can cause enlargement of the distal end of the tibia, stiffness and sometimes an angular limb deformity. Radiographically the metaphysis of the bone is broadened and asymmetrical. There is sclerosis of the metaphysis adjacent to the physis, which may be more irregular in appearance than normal. The cortices of the metaphysis may be abnormally thick. Most cases resolve

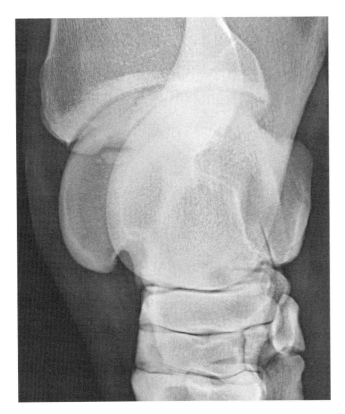

Figure 7.13 Dorsomedial-plantarolateral oblique radiographic view of the right hock of a 7-year-old Warmblood showjumper with distension of the tarsocrural joint, but no lameness. There appears to be a single large osteochondral fragment of the distal intermediate ridge of the tibia and a smaller fragment immediately dorsal to it. These osteochondrosis fragments were removed surgically and three pieces were found.

spontaneously with appropriate management of diet and exercise, although an angular limb deformity may persist in severe cases.

Degenerative joint disease

In many horses there is a poor correlation between pain associated with the distal joints of the hock and the radiographic abnormalities. There may be lameness and no detectable radiographic changes; alternatively there may be extensive radiographic changes and no associated lameness. In some horses the radiographic changes are quite advanced when clinical signs are first recognized. Radiographic examination of horses with obvious enlargements on the medial aspects of the distal joints of the hocks often reveals that this is caused primarily by soft-tissue swelling. Perineural and intra-articular anaesthesia are helpful to establish the significance of radiographic abnormalities and to define the source of pain if no lesions are detectable. This may be combined with anaesthesia of the cunean bursa in selected cases.

The centrodistal (distal intertarsal) and tarsometatarsal joints are affected most frequently, either alone or in combination. The condition

[343]

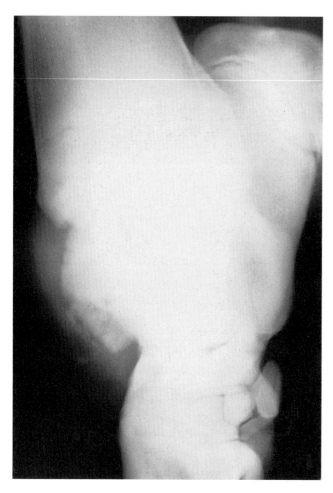

Figure 7.14(a) Plantarolateral-dorsomedial oblique view of a hock of a yearling Shire horse. There is a large osteochondritic lesion of the distal aspect of the lateral trochlea tali.

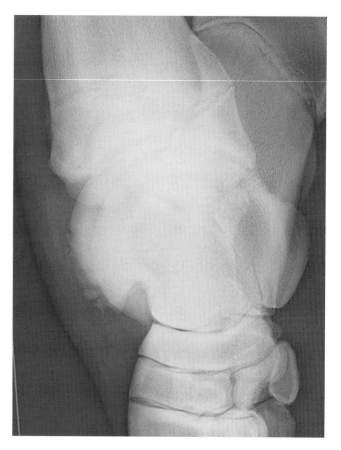

Figure 7.14(b) Dorsomedial-plantarolateral oblique view of the right hock of a weanling Thoroughbred with distension of the tarsocrural joint. There is an irregular outline of the lateral trochlea of the talus and multiple mineralized fragments, a manifestation of osteochondrosis.

often occurs bilaterally. The talocalcaneal–centroquartal (proximal intertarsal) joint is less commonly involved, but there is often associated distension of the tarsocrural joint capsule because of the communication between these two joints. Degenerative joint disease of the talocalcaneal joint occurs rarely.

There is considerable variation between horses in the type, extent and progression of radiographic abnormalities that develop. These changes include periarticular osteophytes (Figures 7.15a-d), periosteal new bone (Figure 7.16), subchondral bone lysis (Figures 7.17a-c) and/or sclerosis, decreased corticomedullary demarcation and narrowing or loss of the joint space (spaces) (Figures 7.18a and 7.18b). In the early stages of the disease the lesions may be subtle and only detectable in a single radiographic view; thus a complete radiographic examination is important. Even in more advanced cases the radiographic abnormalities are occasionally visible on only one of the four standard projections. Since small osteophytes and periosteal new bone are less opaque than the parent bone, they are easily overlooked. The radiographs should always be viewed over high-intensity illumination to study the bone margins, or if obtained digitally the images should be manipulated to permit evaluation of the bone margins. Both hocks should be examined radiographically if changes are found in one limb. It may be necessary to repeat a view at different exposures in order to evaluate both corticomedullary demarcation and trabecular pattern properly, and to identify marginal osteophytes.

Spur formation on the dorsoproximal aspect of the third metatarsal bone (see Figures 7.5a and 7.5b, page 330) may not reflect significant intra-articular disease and its significance must be interpreted with care. This may be an entheseophyte associated with the insertion of the cranial tibial tendon, fibularis (peroneus) tertius, or the dorsal tarsometatarsal ligament; however, an osteophyte may reflect degenerative joint disease. Osteophyte formation may also be associated with an incomplete or complete articular fracture of the dorsoproximal aspect of the third metatarsal bone (see Chapter 4, page 224). Osteophyte formation involving the dorsal aspects of the centrodistal joint (Figures 7.15b and 7.15c) or the lateral aspect of this joint (Figure 7.18a) is often associated with lameness. Osteophytes on the lateral aspect of the centrodistal joint are best seen in dorsoplantar and dorsolateral–plantaromedial oblique views, encroaching upon the tarsal canal (Figures 7.15d and 7.18a). Large osteophytes on the proximal aspect of the third metatarsal bone do occasionally fracture; a fracture piece (see Figure 7.5f, page 331) should not be confused with dystrophic mineralization in the cranial tibial tendon (see Figure 7.5e, page 331).

Irregular periosteal new bone occurs most commonly on the dorsome-dial aspects of the joints, and usually signifies degenerative joint disease. It may be seen alone or in combination with destructive lesions of bone. Destructive lesions may result in irregular margins of the central and third tarsal bones and the third metatarsal bone and/or lucent zones in the sub-chondral bone. If there are extensive lucent areas in the subchondral bone, lameness is usually persistent. There are sometimes discrete osseous cyst-like lesions in the subchondral bone.

Narrowing of the joint spaces (Figures 7.18a and 7.18b) can occur with any of these changes and is most accurately assessed on appropriately posi-tioned dorsoplantar views, but should be verified on other views. Care should be taken not to diagnose joint narrowing from poorly positioned radiographs. An additional view at a slightly different angle may show no evidence of narrowing. Occasionally, narrowing of the joint space is the only radiographic abnormality detectable. Conventional radiographs may under-estimate the degree of functional ankylosis. The joint spaces may become obliterated completely, resulting in ankylosis of the bones and resolution of lameness. Persistence of lameness may be due to continued subchondral bone pain, or to early changes in more proximal or distal joints. Nuclear scintigraphy is useful in determining active bone modelling. In other cases there is extensive extra-articular inactive bone bridging the joints with some loss of joint space.

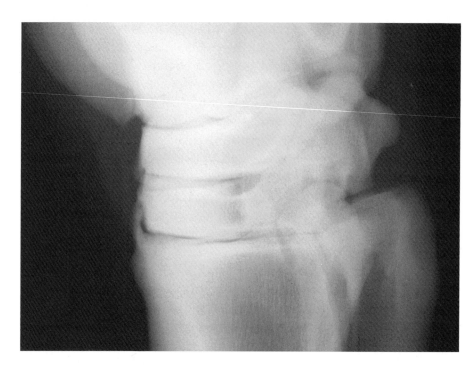

Figure 7.15(a) Slightly oblique lateromedial view of a hock of a 2-year-old Thoroughbred. There is a large, active osteophyte on the dorsoproximal aspect of the third metatarsal bone. Lameness was alleviated by intra-articular analgesia of the tarsometatarsal joint.

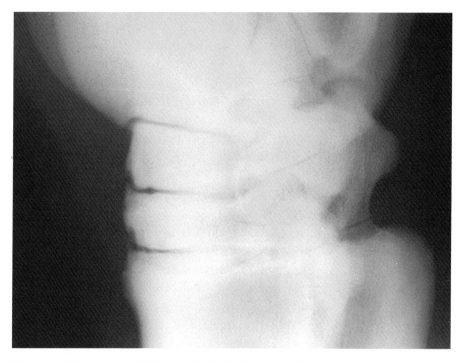

Figure 7.15(b) Lateromedial view of a hock of a mature horse with osteophyte formation involving the centrodistal and tarsometatarsal joints. The radiograph is underexposed to highlight the periarticular new bone.

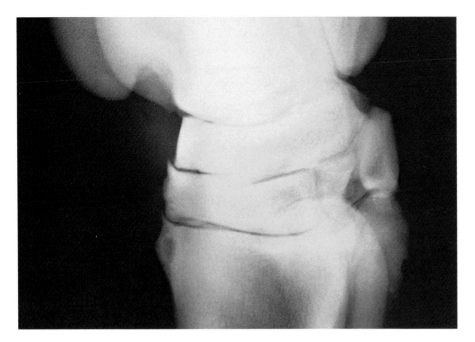

Figure 7.15(c) Plantarolateral-dorsomedial oblique view of a hock of a mature horse with osteophyte formation involving the centrodistal and tarsometatarsal joints. Note also the modelling of the dorsal aspect of the third tarsal bone and the irregular opacity of the proximodorsal aspect of the third metatarsal bone. The radiograph is underexposed to highlight the periarticular new bone.

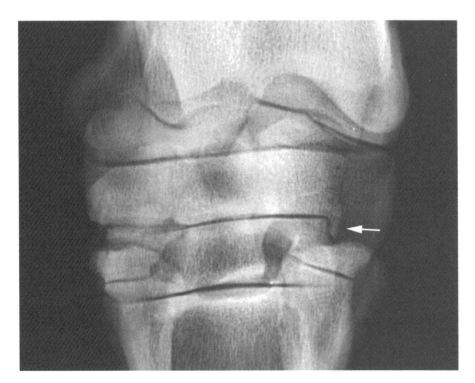

Figure 7.15(d) Dorsoplantar radiographic view of the left hock of a 7-year-old Arab cross Thoroughbred show horse. Lameness was improved by tibial and fibular nerve blocks or intra-articular analgesia of the tarsometatarsal joint. There is a periarticular osteophyte on the distal lateral aspect of the central tarsal bone (arrow).

[347]

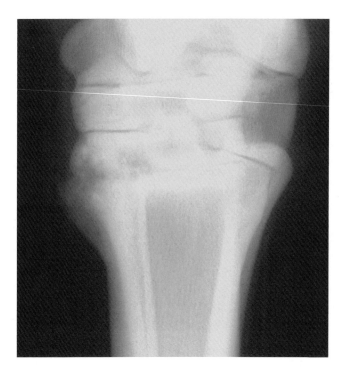

Figure 7.16 Dorsoplantar view of a hock of a mature riding pony with degenerative joint disease of the tarsometatarsal joint. Lateral is to the right. The radiograph is underexposed to highlight the extensive periosteal new bone on the medial aspect of the joint. There are ill defined subchondral lucent zones adjacent to the narrowed tarsometatarsal joint.

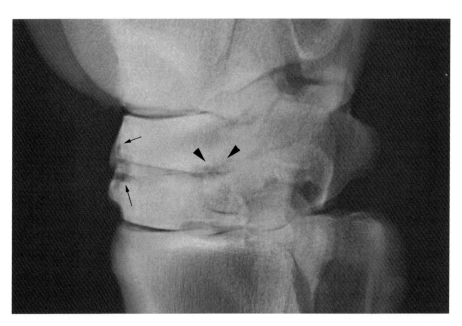

Figure 7.17(a) Lateromedial radiographic view of the left hock of a 7-year-old riding horse. There is narrowing of the centrodistal joint space. There are ill defined lucent zones on the distal dorsal aspect of the central tarsal bone and the proximodorsal aspect of the third tarsal bone (arrows). The region of the intertarsal ligament between the central and third tarsal bones is poorly defined (arrow heads).

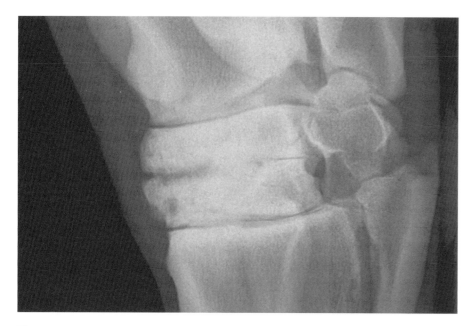

Figure 7.17(b) Dorsolateral-plantaromedial oblique view of the left hock of a 7-year-old Warmblood cross purchased 3 weeks previously. The horse showed mild lameness, markedly exacerbated by proximal limb flexion. There is partial obliteration of the centrodistal joint space, especially in the region of the intertarsal ligament, and extensive subchondral bone lysis adjacent to the joint dorsomedially. There is generalized sclerosis of the central and third tarsal bones and an ill defined lucent zone in the distal dorsal aspect of the third tarsal bone.

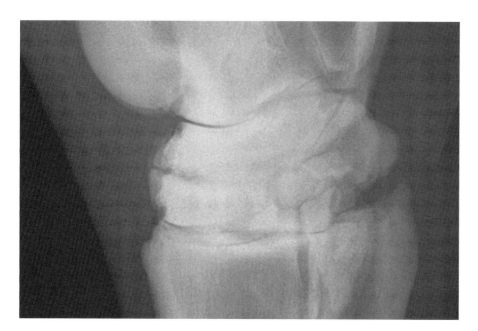

Figure 7.17(c) Lateromedial radiographic view of the same hock as in Figure 7.17(b). There is narrowing of the centrodistal joint space, subchondral bone lysis dorsally, extensive sclerosis of the central and third tarsal bones and modelling on the dorsal aspect of each bone.

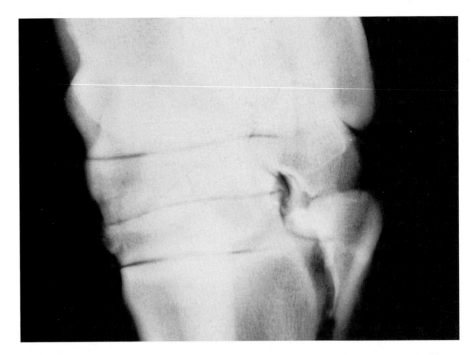

Figure 7.18(a) Dorsolateral-plantaromedial oblique view of a hock of a 3-year-old Thoroughbred. There is narrowing of the centrodistal joint space and osteophyte formation on its lateral aspect encroaching upon the tarsal canal.

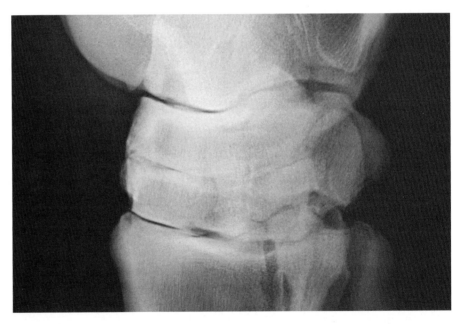

Figure 7.18(b) Lateromedial radiographic view of the right hock of a 9-year-old Warmblood dressage horse with lameness improved by intra-articular analgesia of the tarsometatarsal joint, and abolished by perineural analgesia of the fibular and tibial nerves. There is marked narrowing of the centrodistal joint space and some sclerosis of the dorsal aspect of the central and third tarsal bones.

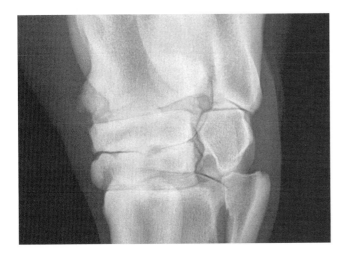

Figure 7.19(a) Dorsolateral-plantaromedial oblique radiographic view of the right hock of an 8-year-old Connemara cross with lameness of 4 months' duration and distension of the tarsocrural joint. Lameness was accentuated by proximal limb flexion. There is narrowing of the talocalcaneal-centroquartal joint, new bone on the distal medial tuberosity of the talus, modelling of the dorsomedial articular margins of the talocalcaneal-centroquartal joint and periarticular osteophyte formation on the distal dorsomedial aspect of the central tarsal bone.

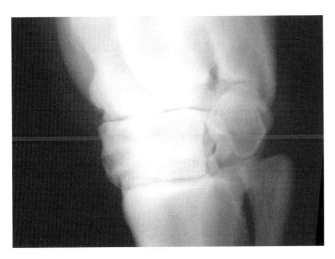

Figure 7.19(b) Dorsolateral-plantaromedial oblique view of a hock of a mature riding horse. There is modelling of the distal medial tuberosity of the talus and of the medial aspect of the talocalcaneal-centroquartal joint with osteophyte formation (barely discernible because it is relatively less opaque). The central and third tarsal bones are fused.

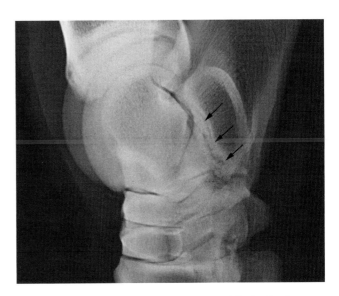

Figure 7.19(c) Lateromedial view of the right hock of a 15-year-old dressage horse with moderate lameness abolished by fibular and tibial nerve blocks and improved by intra-articular analgesia of the tarsocrural joint. There is narrowing of the talocalcaneal joint space and subchondral lysis (arrows) consistent with degenerative joint disease.

The shape of the central and third tarsal bones should be assessed carefully, in order to detect cases in which degenerative joint disease has developed secondarily to tarsal bone collapse (see page 337).

The speed of progression of changes is both variable and unpredictable, and it is unusual to be able to monitor progressive fusion of the joints radiographically. Some horses may be treated conservatively either by intra-articular medication or by administration of anti-inflammatory analgesics and corrective shoeing. Surgical or chemical arthrodesis of the affected joints can be an effective treatment, particularly for those with extensive lytic lesions. Involvement of the talocalcaneal–centroquartal (proximal

[351]

intertarsal) joint (Figures 7.19a and 7.19b) or the talocalcaneal joint (Figure 7.19c) warrants a guarded prognosis.

Periosteal proliferative reactions at the sites of attachment of ligaments and joint capsules

Twisting or wrenching the hock may result in a sprain of the soft-tissue structures of the hock and severe lameness. Radiographic examination is often unrewarding initially, but may be important to rule out a fracture. Diagnostic ultrasonography may be useful to evaluate the collateral ligaments of the tarsocrural joint. Nuclear scintigraphy may help to identify areas of increased bone metabolism or blood supply. After approximately 3–6 weeks, extensive periosteal reactions may develop at the sites of attachment of the joint capsules, collateral ligaments and intertarsal ligaments (Figure 7.20). The sites of periosteal reactions should be correlated carefully with the sites of soft-tissue attachments to confirm which structures may have been damaged. These changes may be progressive and follow-up examination after a further 6–8 weeks may give a better indication of the extent of the damage. Lameness often takes a considerable time to resolve and, if new bone involves the articulations of the hock, or if there is extensive fibrosis of the ligaments involved, may be persistent.

An avulsion fracture of either the medial or, more commonly, the lateral malleolus of the tibia (Figure 7.21a) may occur in association with sprain of the collateral ligaments of the tarsocrural joint. The fracture may be simple or comminuted. Fracture fragments may be displaced and rotated. It may be helpful to obtain a dorsal 15° medial-plantarolateral oblique view to highlight the fragment(s) (Figure 7.21b). In contrast to the osteochondral fragments of osteochondrosis, a recent fracture is more irregular in shape. Ultrasonography can be useful to identify the precise location of a fracture in the frontal plane and to assess the collateral ligaments. Periosteal new bone may develop on the distal cranial tibia, and entheseous new bone at the insertion of the collateral ligaments on the talus. Conservative treatment offers a moderate prognosis. However, surgical removal may facilitate recovery, especially if the fracture has a large articular component or is considerably displaced.

A fracture of the lateral malleolus of the tibia can also occur as a result of direct blunt trauma, for example a kick. The force of the injury may be translated across the distal tibia, resulting in the development of periosteal new bone medially.

Luxation

Luxation of the tarsus is not common but may occur at any of the joints. The horse shows a severe, non-weight-bearing lameness, a variable degree of soft-tissue swelling and obvious instability of the tarsus. Radiographic examination is performed to establish which joint is involved and the extent of concurrent damage (Figure 7.22). 'Stressed' views may be helpful (see

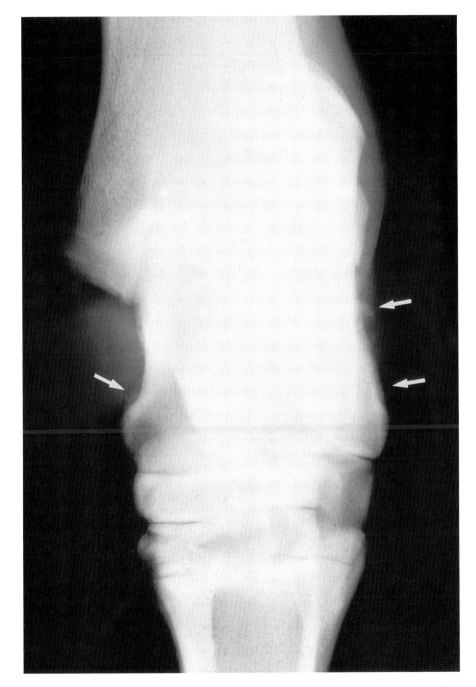

Figure 7.20 Dorsoplantar view of a hock of a 6-year-old steeplechaser several weeks after a severe fall. Lateral is to the right. There is extensive periosteal new bone (arrows) at the sites of insertion of the medial and lateral collateral ligaments of the tarsocrural joint. The radiograph is underexposed to highlight this new bone formation.

page 355). The majority of luxations are associated with fractures of one or more tarsal bones. The prognosis for luxation of the tarsocrural joint is poor, but closed reduction and external immobilization has been successful in treating luxations of the talocalcaneal–centroquartal (proximal intertarsal) or tarsometatarsal joints in horses which resumed light work, or were used for breeding.

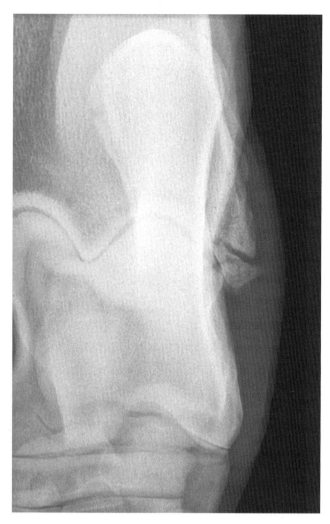

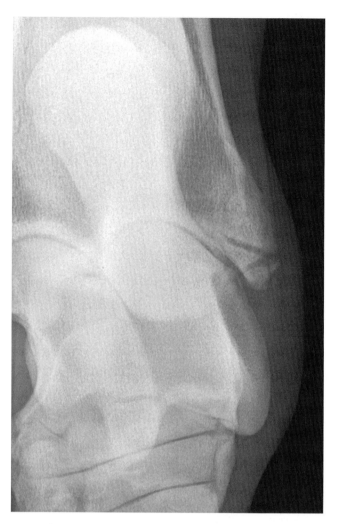

Figure 7.21(a) Dorsoplantar radiographic view of the left hock of a 6-year-old steeplechase horse. There are at least two osseous fragments of the lateral malleolus of the tibia. Compare with Figure 7.21(b).

Figure 7.21(b) Dorsal 15° medial-plantarolateral oblique view of the same hock as in Figure 7.21(a). Comminution of the fracture of the lateral malleolus is more easily seen.

Thoroughpin

Persistent lameness and swelling of the digital flexor tendon sheath (tarsal sheath) proximal to the hock (thoroughpin) may be associated with lesions of the sustentaculum tali of the calcaneus and/or mineralization in the soft tissues (Figure 7.23a). Although the latter may be identified in the standard radiographic views (particularly the plantarolateral-dorsomedial oblique view), lesions of the sustentaculum tali are often only visible in the dorso-plantar (flexed) view (Figure 7.23b). Contrast radiography and ultrasonography are additional techniques useful in the assessment of this condition. The presence of radiographic changes (e.g. lesions of the sustentaculum tali, mineralization within the sheath or filling defects in the sheath) associated with thoroughpin warrants a guarded prognosis.

[354]

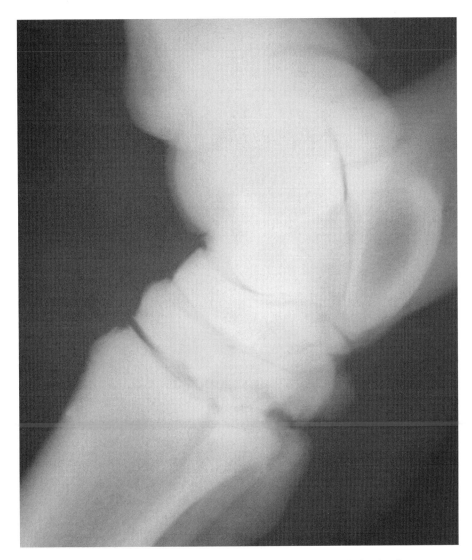

Figure 7.22 Flexed and stressed lateromedial radiograph of a right hock of a 7-year-old Cob with severe lameness. There is abnormal opening of the dorsal aspect of the tarsometatarsal joint reflecting subluxation.

Infectious arthritis and osteomyelitis

Infectious arthritis occurs most commonly in young foals, but may be a sequel to trauma in an adult, and occasionally develops without an apparent cause. The tarsocrural joint is most commonly affected, resulting in distension of the joint capsule and lameness. The lower joints may be involved alone or in combination and, especially in young foals, the central and third tarsal bones must be inspected carefully for evidence of lucent zones indicative of concurrent osteomyelitis (type T osteomyelitis, see page 32). In foals the distal tibial physis and epiphysis should also be evaluated with care, since in the majority of cases type P osteomyelitis is present.

Trauma in the region of the calcaneus may result in a chronically draining wound and severe lameness. Osteomyelitis of the tuber calcanei may be a sequel, but radiographic abnormalities may only be detectable in a dor-

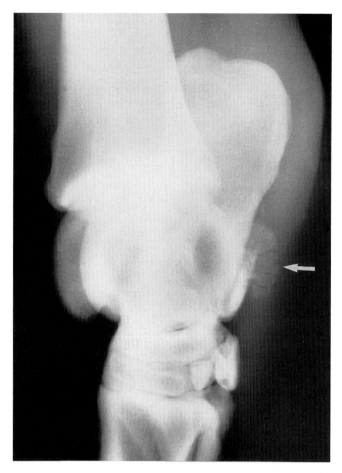

Figure 7.23(a) Plantarolateral-dorsomedial oblique view of a hock. There is considerable modelling of the sustentaculum tali (arrow) which was associated with distension of the tarsal sheath and severe lameness.

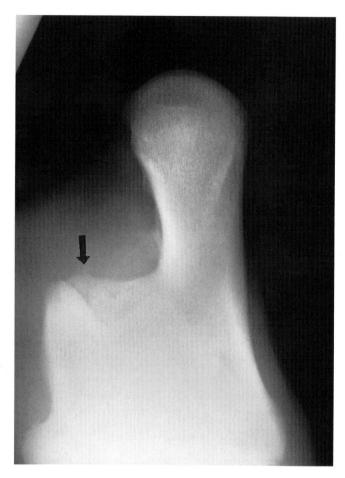

Figure 7.23(b) Dorsoplantar (flexed) view of the same hock as Figure 7.23a. Lateral is to the right. Note the irregular contour of the surface of the sustentaculum tali (arrow) over which the deep digital flexor tendon passes, and the poorly defined opacities in the soft tissues medial to the calcaneus.

soplantar (flexed) view. Sinography may be helpful to establish if a draining sinus communicates with the bone. Ultrasonography may permit identification of osseous lesions much earlier than radiography. A guarded prognosis is warranted even with surgical treatment.

Osseous cyst-like lesions

Single osseous cyst-like lesions occur occasionally, most commonly in the distal tibia, the talus, the calcaneus and the third metatarsal bone. They are generally, but not always, associated with lameness. They may occur either unilaterally or bilaterally. Although some are identifiable radiographically, some osseous cyst-like lesions in the distal aspect of the tibia (medial malleolus, lateral malleolus, distal intermediate ridge) or proximal aspect of the talus (intertrochlear groove of the talus) have only been seen using computed tomography and/or during arthroscopic surgery. They are invariably associated with focal increased radiopharmaceutical uptake. Osseous cyst-like lesions may also occur in the central and third tarsal bones in association with degenerative joint disease (see page 343).

Hypertrophic osteopathy

See Chapter 1 (page 22).

Fractures

Because of the complex radiographic anatomy of the tarsus, detection of fractures is sometimes difficult. The support afforded by the intertarsal ligaments and collateral ligaments often results in minimal distraction of the fracture fragments. A slab fracture of the central or the third tarsal bone may be completely overlooked unless follow-up radiographs are obtained 7–10 days after the onset of lameness, when rarefaction along the fracture line will make it more obvious (Figure 7.24). Many oblique views may be required in order to identify the fracture. In young Thoroughbred racehorses a wedge-shaped conformation of the dorsolateral aspect of the third tarsal bone may be a risk factor for fracture. Nuclear scintigraphy may be useful in acute cases in which a fracture is suspected. Increased uptake of technetium may demonstrate results of trauma to the central and third tarsal bones, but in some cases a fracture is not subsequently identifiable. Treatment of slab fractures by internal fixation offers the best prognosis for future soundness, although secondary degenerative joint disease may be a sequel.

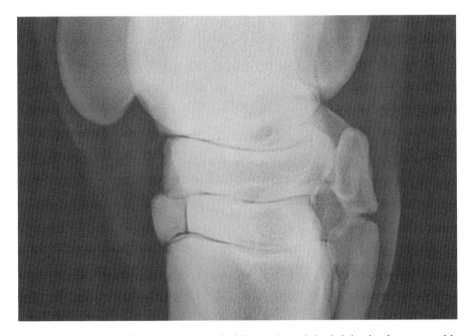

Figure 7.24 Dorsomedial-plantarolateral oblique view of the left hock of a 3-year-old Thoroughbred flat racehorse. There is a frontal plane slab fracture of the third tarsal bone. The fracture traverses the narrowest part of the bone. Note the sclerosis of the dorsal aspect of the central and third tarsal bones.

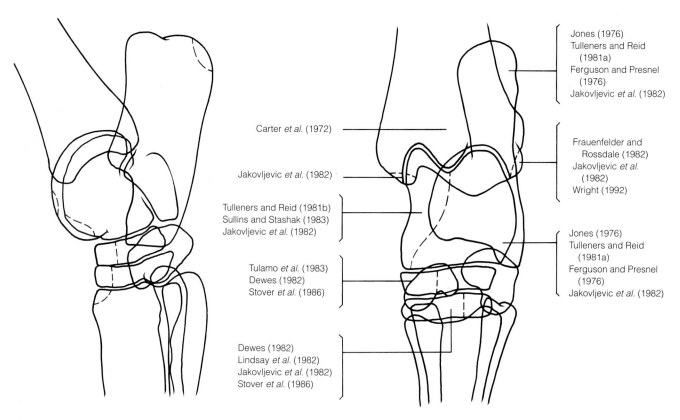

Jones (1976)
Tulleners and Reid
(1981a)
Ferguson and Presnel
(1976)
Jakovljevic et al. (1982)

Carter et al. (1972)

Frauenfelder and
Rossdale (1982)
Jakovljevic et al.
(1982)
Wright (1992)

Jakovljevic et al. (1982)

Tulleners and Reid (1981b)
Sullins and Stashak (1983)
Jakovljevic et al. (1982)

Jones (1976)
Tulleners and Reid
(1981a)
Ferguson and Presnel
(1976)
Jakovljevic et al. (1982)

Tulamo et al. (1983)
Dewes (1982)
Stover et al. (1986)

Dewes (1982)
Lindsay et al. (1982)
Jakovljevic et al. (1982)
Stover et al. (1986)

Figure 7.25 Location of common fracture sites in the hock and suggested references (see 'Further reading').

Sagittal fractures of the talus cause acute-onset severe lameness. They may be very difficult to detect in the acute stage. They are associated with focal intense increased radiopharmaceutical uptake in the talus. Sequential radiographic examinations may reveal the radiolucent fracture line in dorsopalmar or slightly oblique dorsopalmar radiographic views. The prognosis with conservative management is usually favourable.

There are many types of fractures within the tarsus (Figure 7.25). The prognosis depends on the site of the fracture and its configuration, but is generally guarded. However, large fractures involving the distal third of the lateral trochlea of the talus respond well to surgical removal of the fracture fragment because this part of the bone is not a major weight-bearing component of the joint. The dorsoplantar (flexed) view may be necessary to identify fractures of the sustentaculum tali. Readers are advised to consult the references given under 'Further reading' for additional information about specific fracture types (Figure 7.25).

Fractures of the distal tibial physis are quite common in foals and yearlings, Salter-Harris type II (see Chapter 1, page 25) occurring most frequently. Treatment either by immobilization in a cast or by internal fixation has been successful in some cases. Malleolar fractures of the distal tibia are discussed on page 352.

Axelsson, M., Bjornsdottir, S., Eksell, P., Haggstrom, J., Sigurdsson, H. and Carlsten, J. (2001) Risk factors associated with hindlimb lameness and degenerative joint disease in the distal tarsus of Icelandic horses. *Equine vet. J.*, **33**, 84–90

Baird, D. and Pilsworth, R. (2001) Wedge-shaped conformation of the dorsolateral aspect of the third tarsal bone in the Thoroughbred racehorse is associated with development of slab fractures in this site. *Equine vet. J.*, **33**, 617–620

Ball, M., Allen, D. and Parks, A. (1996) Surgical treatment of subchondral cyst-like lesions in the tibia of an adult pony. *J. Am. Vet. Med. Ass.*, **208**, 704–706

Barneveld, A. (1983) Equine bone spavin. *PhD Thesis*, University of Utrecht

Bassage, L., Garcia-Lopez, J. and Currid, E. (2000) Osteolytic lesions of the tuber calcanei in 2 horses. *J. Am. Vet. Med. Ass.*, **217**, 710–716

Beard, W., Bramlage, L., Schneider, R. and Embertson, R. (1994) Postoperative racing performance in Standardbreds and Thoroughbreds with osteochondrosis of the tarsocrural joint: 109 cases (1984–1990). *J. Am. Vet. Med. Ass.*, **204**, 1655–1659

Bjonsdottir, S., Axelsson, M., Eksell, P., Sigurdsson, H. and Carlsten, J. (2000) Radiographic and clinical survey of degenerative joint disease in the distal tarsal joints in Icelandic horses. *Equine vet. J.*, **32**, 263–267

Blaik, M., Hansen, R., Kincaid, S., Hathcock, J. *et al.* (2000) Low-field magnetic resonance imaging of the equine tarsus: normal anatomy *Vet. Radiol. and Ultrasound*, **41**, 131–141

Boero, M., Kneller, S., Baker, G., Metcalf, M. and Twardock, A. (1988) Clinical, radiographic and scintigraphic findings associated with enthesitis of the lateral collateral ligaments of the tarsocrural joint in Standardbred racehorses. *Equine vet. J.*, Suppl. **6**, 53–59

Carlsten, J., Sandgren, B. and Dalin, J. (1993) Development of osteochondrosis in the tarsocrural joints and osteochondral fragments in the fetlock joint in Standardbred trotters. I. A radiological survey. *Equine vet. J.*, Suppl. **16**, 42–47

Carter, E., Horney, F. and Pennock, P. (1972) Distal tibial fractures in the horse. *Mod. Vet. Pract.*, Jan., 41–43

Cohen, N., Carter, G., Watkins, J. and O'Conor, M. (2006) Association of racing performance with specific abnormal radiographic findings in Thoroughbred yearlings sold in Texas. *J. Equine Vet. Sci.*, **26**, 462–474

Courouce-Malblanc, A., Leleu, C., Bouchilloux, M. and Geffroy, O. (2006) Abnormal radiographic findings in 865 French Standardbred trotters and their relationship to racing performance. *Equine vet. J.*, Suppl., **36**, 417–422

Davison, E., Ross, M. and Parente, E. (2005) Incomplete sagittal fracture of the talus in 11 racehorses: outcome. *Equine vet. J.*, **37**, 457–461

De Moor, A., Verschooten, F., Desmet, P., Steenhaut, M., Hooreens, J. and Wolf, G. (1972) Osteochondritis dissecans of the tibiotarsal joint in the horse. *Equine vet. J.*, **4**, 139–143

Dewes, H. (1982) The onset and consequence of tarsal bone fractures in foals. *N.Z. Vet. J.*, **30**, 129–135

Dik, K. and Merkens, H. (1987) Unilateral distension of the tarsal sheath in the horse: a report of 11 cases. *Equine vet. J.*, **19**, 307–313

Dik, K. and Enzerink, E. (1998) The radiographic development of osteochondral abnormalities in the hock and stifle of Dutch Warmblood foals from 1 to 11 months of age. *Equine vet. J.*, Suppl., **31**, 9–15

Dusterdieck, K., May, K., Pleasant, S. and Howard, R. (2002) Distal intertarsal joint subluxation in a pony. *Equine vet. Educ.*, **14**, 12–15

Edwards, G. (1978) Changes in the sustentaculum tali associated with distension of the tarsal sheath (thoroughpin). *Equine vet. J.*, **10**, 97–100

Eksell, P., Uhlhorn, H. and Carlsten, J. (1999) Evaluation of different projections for radiographic detection of tarsal degenerative joint disease in Icelandic horses. *Vet. Radiol. and Ultrasound*, **40**, 228–232

Elce, Y., Ross, M., Woodford, A. and Arensberg, C. (2001) A review of central and third tarsal bone slab fractures in 57 horses. *Proc. Am. Assoc. Equine Pract.*, **47**, 488–490

Farrow, C., McNeel, S., Morgan, J. and Resch, R. (1976) Visualisation of the tuber calcis and sustentaculum in the horse. *Calif. Vet.*, **30**, 14–15

Ferguson, J. and Presnel, K. (1976) Tension band plating of a fractured equine fibular tarsal bone. *Can. Vet. J.*, **17**, 314–317

Firth, E., Dik, K., Goedegebuure, S., Hagens, F., Verberne, L., Merkens, H. and Kersjes, A. (1980) Polyarthritis and bone infection in foals. *Vet. Med.*, **B27**, 102–124

Firth, E., Goedegebuure, S., Dik, K. and Poulos, P. (1985) Tarsal osteomyelitis in foals. *Vet. Rec.*, **116**, 261–266

Frauenfelder, H. and Rossdale, P. (1982) What is your diagnosis? *J. Am. Vet. Med. Ass.*, **180**, 1109–1110

Fretz, P. (1980) Angular limb deformities in foals. *Vet. Clin. N. Am. Large Anim. Pract.*, **2**, 125–150

Gabel, A. (1980) Lameness caused by inflammation in the distal hock. *Vet. Clin. N. Am. Large Anim. Pract.*, **2**, 101–124

Garcia-Lopez, J. and Kirker-Head, C. (2004) Occult osseous cyst-like lesions of the equine tarsocrural joint. *Vet. Surg.*, **564**, 557–564

Grondahl, A., Jansen, J. and Terge, J. (1996) Accessory ossification centres associated with osteochondral fragments in the extremities of horses. *J. Comp. Path.*, **114**, 385–398

Grondahl, A. and Engeland, A. (1995) Progression and association with lameness and racing performance in Standardbred trotters. *Equine vet. J.*, **26**, 152–155

Gross, D. (1984) Tarsal luxation and fracture in a pony. *Mod. Vet. Pract.*, **45**, 68–69

Hand, D., Watkins, J. and Honnas, C. (2001) Osteomyelitis of the sustentaculum tali in horses: 10 cases (1992–1998). *J. Am. Vet. Med. Ass.*, **219**, 341–345

Hartung, K., Munzer, B. and Keller, H. (1983) Radiologic evaluation of spavin in young trotters. *Vet. Radiol.*, **24**, 153–155

Hoppe, F. (1984) Osteochondrosis in Swedish horses. *Thesis*, Sveriges Lantbruksuniversitet, Uppsala

Jakovljevic, S., Gibbs, C. and Yeats, J. (1982) Traumatic fractures of the equine hock: a report of 13 cases. *Equine vet. J.*, **14**, 62–68

Jenner, F., Solano, M., Gliatto, J., Lavallee, S. and Kirker-Head, C. (2003) Osteosarcoma of the tarsus in a horse. *Equine vet. J.*, **35**, 214–216

Jones, R. (1976) The diagnosis and treatment of avulsion fractures of the sustentaculum tali in a horse. *Can. Vet. J.*, **17**, 287–290

Kane, A., Park, D., McIlwraith, C., Rantanen, N., Morehead, J. and Bramlage, L. (2003a) Radiographic changes in Thoroughbred yearlings. Part 1: Prevalence at the time of sales. *Equine vet. J.*, **35**, 354–365

Kane, A., McIlwraith, C., Park, R., Rantanen, N., Morehead, J. and Bramlage, L. (2003b) Radiographic changes in Thoroughbred yearlings. Part 1: Association with racing performance. *Equine vet. J.*, **35**, 366–374

Labens, R., Innocent, G. and Voute, L. (2007) Repeatability of a quantitative rating scale for assessment of horses with distal tarsal osteoarthritis. *Vet. Radiol. and Ultrasound*, **48**, 204–211

Laws, E., Richardson, D., Ross, M. and Moyer, W. (1993) Racing performance of Standardbreds after conservative and surgical treatment for tarsocrural osteochondrosis. *Equine vet. J.*, **25**, 199–202

Lindsay, W., McMartin, R. and McClure, J. (1982) Management of slab fractures of the third tarsal bone in 5 horses. *Equine vet. J.*, **14**, 55–58

MacDonald, M., Honnas, C. and Meagher, D. (1989) Osteomyelitis of the calcaneus in horses: 28 cases (1972–1987). *J. Am. Vet. Med. Ass.*, **194**, 1317–1320

Martens, R. and Auer, J. (1980) Haematogenous septic arthritis and osteomyelitis in the foal. *Proc. Am. Ass. Equine Pract.*, **26**, 47–63

Moll, H., Slane, D., Humburg, J. and Jagar, J. (1987) Traumatic tarsal luxation repaired without internal fixation in three horses and three ponies. *J. Am. Vet. Med. Ass.*, **190**, 297–300

Moreau, H. and Denoix, J.-M. (1994) Calcification of the medial collateral ligament of the hock in a jumping horse. *Pract. Vet. Equine*, **26**, 219–220

Morgan, J. (1967) Necrosis of the third tarsal bone of the horse. *J. Am. Vet. Med. Ass.*, **151**, 1334–1342

Moyer, W. (1987) Bone spavin: a clinical review. *J. Equine Med. Surg.*, **2**, 362–371

Murphy, E., Schneider, R., Adams, S. *et al.* (2000) Long-term outcome on conservative management of tarsal slab fractures in 25 horses (1976–1999). *J. Am. Vet. Med. Ass.*, **216**, 1949–1954

Philips, T. (1986) Unusual hock problems. *Proc. Am. Ass. Equine Pract.*, **32**, 663–667

Pilsworth, R. (1992) Incomplete fracture of the dorsal aspect of the third metatarsal bone as a cause of hindlimb lameness in racing Thoroughbreds: a review of three cases. *Equine vet. J.*, **24**, 147–150

Post, E., Singer, E., Clegg, P. *et al.* (2003) Retrospective study of 24 cases of septic calcaneal bursitis in the horse. *Equine vet. J.*, **35**, 662–668

Rose, P. and Moore, I. (2003) Imaging diagnosis – avulsion of the medial collateral ligament of the tarsus in a horse. *Vet. Radiol. and Ultrasound*, **44**, 657–659

Ross, M., Sponseller, M., Gill, H. and Moyer, W. (1993) Articular fracture of the dorsoproximal aspect of the third metatarsal bone in five Standardbred racehorses. *J. Am. Vet. Med. Ass.*, **203**, 698–700

Sandgren, B. (1993) Osteochondrosis in the tarsocrural joint and osteochondral fragments in the metacarpo/metatarsophalangeal joints in young Standardbreds. *PhD Thesis*, University of Uppsala

Santschi, E., Adams, S., Fessler, J. *et al.* (1997) Treatment of bacterial tarsal tenosynovitis and osteitis of the sustentaculum tali of the calcaneus in 5 horses. *Equine vet. J.*, **29**, 244–247

Schougaard, H., Falk Ronne, J. and Philipson, J. (1990) A radiographic survey of tibio-tarsal osteochondrosis in a selected population of trotting horses in Denmark and its possible genetic significance. *Equine vet. J.*, **22**, 288–289

Shaver, J., Fretz, P., Doige, C. and Williams, D. (1979) Skeletal manifestations of suspected hypothyroidism in two foals. *J. Equine Med. Surg.*, **3**, 269–275

Shively, M. (1982) Correct anatomic nomenclature for the joints of the equine tarsus. *Equine Pract.*, **4**(4), 9–13

Shively, M. and Smallwood, J. (1980) Radiographic and xeroradiographic anatomy of the equine tarsus. *Equine Pract.*, **2**(4), 19–34

Smith, R., Dyson, S., Schramme, M., Head, M., Payne, R., Platt, D. and Walmsley, J. (2005) Osteoarthritis of the talocalcaneal joint in 18 horses. *Equine vet. J.*, **37**, 166–171

Storgaard, J., Jorgensen, H., Proschowsky, H., Falke-Ronne, J., Willeberg, P. and Hesselholt, M. (1997) The significance of routine radiographic findings with respect to racing performance and longevity in Standardbred trotters. *Equine vet. J.*, **29**, 55–59

Stover, S., Hornhof, W., Richardson, G. and Meagher, D. (1986) Bone scintigraphy as an aid to diagnosis of occult distal tarsal bone trauma in 3 horses. *J. Am. Vet. Med. Ass.*, **182**, 624–627

Stromberg, B. and Rejno, S. (1978) Osteochondritis in the horse: a clinical and radiological investigation of the knee and hock joints. *Acta Vet. Scand.*, Suppl. **358**, 139–152

Sullins, K. and Stashak, T. (1983) An unusual fracture of the tibiotarsal bone in a mare. *J. Am. Vet. Med. Ass.*, **182**, 1395–1396

Tomlinson, J., Redding, W., Berry, C. and Smallwood, J. (2003) Computed tomographic anatomy of the equine tarsus. *Vet. Radiol. and Ultrasound*, **44**, 174–178

Tulamo, R., Bramlage, L. and Gabel, A. (1983) Fractures of the central and third tarsal bones in horses. *J. Am. Vet. Med. Ass.*, **182**, 1234–1238

Tulleners, E. and Reid, C. (1981a) Osteomyelitis of the sustentaculum talus in a pony. *J. Am. Vet. Med. Ass.*, **178**, 290–291

Tulleners, E. and Reid, C. (1981b) An unusual fracture of the tarsus in two horses. *J. Am. Vet. Med. Ass.*, **178**, 291–294

Wheat, J. (1963) Trochlear fractures of the tibiotarsal bone. *Proc. Am. Ass. Equine Pract.*, **9**, 86–87

Wheat, J. and Rhode, E. (1964) Luxation and fracture of the hock of the horse. *J. Am. Vet. Med. Ass.*, **145**, 341–344

White, N. and Turner, T. (1980) Hock lameness associated with degeneration of the talocalcaneal articulation. *Vet. Med. Small Anim. Clin.*, **75**(4), 678–681

Wong, D., Scaratt, W., Maxwell, V. and Moon, M. (2003) Incomplete ossification of the carpal, tarsal and navicular bones in a dysmature foal. *Equine vet. Educ.*, **15**, 72–81

Wright, I. (1992) Fractures of the lateral malleolus of the tibia in 16 horses. *Equine vet. J.*, **24**, 424–429

Chapter 8
The stifle and tibia

Stifle

RADIOGRAPHIC TECHNIQUE

Four radiographic views are necessary for complete evaluation of the stifle joint:

1 Lateromedial and/or flexed lateromedial
2 Caudal 60° lateral-craniomedial oblique
3 Caudocranial
4 Cranioproximal-craniodistal oblique

In many cases sufficient information can be obtained using views (2) and (3). If low-output portable equipment is used, all four views may be best obtained with the horse under general anaesthesia.

Equipment

For caudocranial views of the stifle in mature horses, an x-ray machine with a minimum output of 90 kV and 20 mAs is required. Radiography should only be attempted with the horse standing if it is co-operative. A fractious horse may inflict serious damage to personnel and equipment, and will result in unacceptably high radiation hazards. If the horse cannot be calmed using sedation and/or a twitch, general anaesthesia should be used.

Digital systems or fast rare earth screens and films are recommended. Large cassettes (35 cm × 43 cm) are advisable in order to visualize an adequate length of the femur and tibia. A cassette holder should ideally be used; however, holders of this size are cumbersome and difficult to hold still. For this reason the cassette is often hand held. Using these large cassettes, and with adequate collimation of the x-ray beam, the holder's gloved hands should be well away from the primary beam. The difficulty in aligning the cassette and x-ray beam in the standing horse makes it advisable to dispense with the use of a grid. Under general anaesthesia, the quality of the radiographs can be enhanced by using a parallel grid.

The use of an aluminium wedge filter greatly improves the quality of the radiographs and enables the stifle joint to be examined using fewer exposures.

Positioning

Lateromedial view

A true lateromedial view may be required if osseous irregularities near the distal insertion of the cranial cruciate ligament are suspected. The limb to be examined should be positioned caudal to the contralateral limb, fully weight bearing. This facilitates positioning of the cassette on the medial aspect of the stifle. The cassette usually has to be hand held, as high in the groin region as possible. The x-ray beam should be centred on the femorotibial joint. Palpate the tibial crest and centre immediately proximal to it, approximately 10 cm caudal to the cranial aspect of the limb. To obtain lateromedial alignment, the beam should initially be aligned parallel to a tangent to the bulbs of the heel, but this may require alteration on subsequent films.

Flexion of the stifle, either with the limb lifted and retracted or with the horse resting the toe on the ground, 'drops' the stifle and facilitates obtaining a true lateromedial radiograph. Some horses will not tolerate a cassette on the medial aspect of the hindlimb with the limb weight bearing, but will accept it if the limb is flexed. This view requires an extra person to flex the limb.

A flexed lateromedial view (see Figure 8.7c, page 373) also potentially gives extra room in which to position the cassette. Other advantages of the flexed lateromedial view include better visualization of the proximal tibia in the region of the intercondylar eminences, assessment of the proximal aspect of the trochlear ridges of the femur, without superimposition of the patella, and a clearer view of the apex of the patella.

Caudolateral-craniomedial oblique view

A caudal 60° lateral-craniomedial oblique view is generally preferable to a straight lateromedial view for two reasons. Firstly, an oblique view prevents superimposition of the images of the trochlear ridges and the condyles of the femur. Secondly, the large adductor muscle mass on the medial aspect of the horse's thigh, together with the testicles in entire males, make accurate positioning of the cassette for a true lateromedial view difficult. With a caudal 60° lateral-craniomedial oblique view, the cassette can be positioned slightly more cranial to the joint (Figure 8.1).

Angling the x-ray beam 10–15° proximodistally (downwards) further facilitates alignment of the beam and the cassette. The x-ray beam should be centred approximately 10 cm caudal to the cranial aspect of the limb, at the level of the femorotibial joint, which is readily palpable immediately proximal to the tibial crest.

An alternative technique is to position the cassette lateral to the stifle, with the x-ray machine medial. The x-ray beam passes under the ventral aspect of the abdomen to obtain a cranial 60° medial 15° distal-caudolateral proximal oblique view of the stifle. This technique allows easier positioning

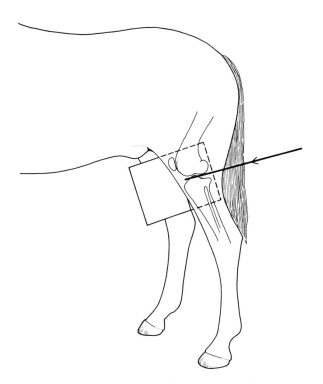

Figure 8.1 Positioning of the limb, cassette and x-ray beam to obtain a caudal 60° lateral-craniomedial oblique view of the stifle.

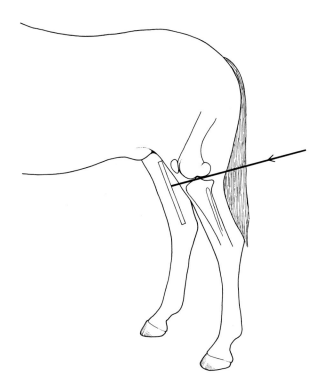

Figure 8.2 Positioning of the limb, cassette and x-ray beam to obtain a caudoproximal-craniodistal oblique view of the stifle.

of the cassette and is accepted more readily by a fractious horse. It is impracticable in a stallion or a horse with a low abdominal wall.

Further obliquity (Cd45°L-CrMO) gives better separation of the femoral condyles (see Figure 8.9, page 375).

Caudocranial view

The caudocranial view is preferred to a craniocaudal view, because positioning is easier. It does put the equipment and the radiographer at risk, but with experienced handlers, correct cassette positioning and sedation, these problems can be minimized. Positioning the horse with the limb positioned caudally and angling the x-ray beam 10–20° proximodistally, may facilitate positioning of the cassette. Make sure that the heel of the foot is on the ground, because slight elevation of the heel may result in apparent, artefactual narrowing of the femorotibial joint space. The cassette can be positioned without touching the flank, and this aids correct alignment of cassette and x-ray beam (Figure 8.2). The cassette should be slowly advanced medially until the radiographer can see the edge of the cassette between the hindlimbs. Care should be taken not to touch the sheath in male horses. The x-ray beam should be centred on a line bisecting the limb, i.e. approximately between the semimembranosus and semitendinosus muscles, at the level of the distal third of these muscles. Alternatively the exit point of the

[365]

beam from the cranial aspect of the joint should be at the level of the tibial crest.

An aluminium wedge filter is useful to attenuate the x-ray beam laterally and medially, to avoid overexposure of the edges of the joint, particularly if changes involving the periarticular structures are suspected. Overexposure of the fibula almost inevitably occurs, particularly in younger animals in which the fibula is predominantly cartilaginous.

Cranioproximal-craniodistal oblique view

This view is primarily employed to assess the patella and the trochleas and intertrochlear groove of the femur. It is indispensable in cases of patellar fractures.

With a standing horse, the limb should be held semi-flexed behind the horse (as if for shoeing), with the femorotibial joint at right angles and the tibia horizontal. The cassette is held approximately horizontal, with its caudal edge against the cranial aspect of the tibia, centred just proximal to the tibial crest (Figure 8.3a). It is not possible to align the x-ray beam perpendicular to the cassette, but satisfactory views are obtained by angling the x-ray beam in a cranial 45° proximal 10° lateral-distal medial oblique direction to avoid the abdominal wall. Adducting the flexed lame limb may facilitate positioning by rotating the stifle outwards.

The above view is sometimes more easily obtained with the horse under general anaesthesia. The horse is placed in dorsal recumbency with the limb fully flexed. The x-ray beam is directed in a craniodistal-cranioproximal direction and is centred on the femoropatellar articulation, i.e. approximately 8 cm distal to the profile of the flexed joint. The cassette is positioned along the cranial aspect of the femur (Figure 8.3b). An aluminium wedge filter is useful to avoid overexposure of the cranial aspect of the patella.

NORMAL ANATOMY, VARIATIONS AND INCIDENTAL FINDINGS

Immature horse

Important radiographic changes occur in the stifle during growth. Six centres of ossification are present at birth (Figures 8.4a and 8.4b): the metaphysis and distal epiphysis of the femur; the proximal epiphysis and metaphysis of the tibia; the tibial tuberosity (apophysis) and the patella.

At birth, the patella is a triangular shape, which becomes more complex with age. Initially it has an irregular contour and granular subchondral bone opacity due to incomplete ossification. The articular surface is concave. The patella is usually fully ossified by 4 months of age.

At birth, the lateral and the medial trochlear ridges of the femur are similar in size. The proximal parts of these ridges have an irregular contour and granular subchondral bone opacity. This appearance is normally present until 3 months of age but may persist until 5 months. It is caused by irregular subchondral ossification and should be differentiated from infectious

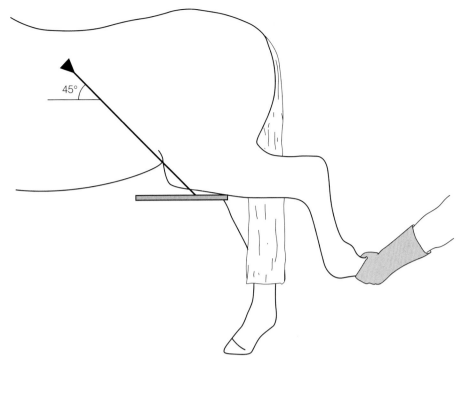

Figure 8.3(a) Positioning of the limb, cassette and x-ray beam to obtain a cranioproximal-craniodistal oblique view of the patella with the horse standing. It may be necessary to angle the x-ray beam slightly from lateral to medial.

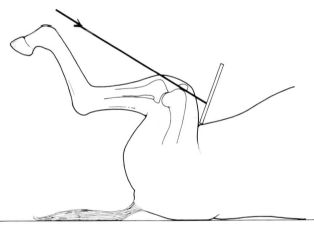

Figure 8.3(b) Positioning of the limb, cassette and x-ray beam to obtain a craniodistal-cranioproximal oblique view of the patella with the horse in dorsal recumbency.

arthritis (joint-ill), which can have a similar radiographic appearance (see Figure 8.25b, page 395). At approximately 2 months of age, the medial trochlear ridge becomes more prominent than the lateral ridge at its proximal part, becoming wider and rounder with a smoothly contoured shoulder (Figure 8.5).

The distal femoral physis is wavy and irregular in outline. It closes at 24–30 months of age. The femoral condyles are smoothly outlined. Irregularity of the condyles should be interpreted as pathological at any age. The femorotibial joint space appears wide at birth due to incomplete ossification of the epiphyses. This incomplete ossification results in apparent sloping of the tibial condyles (Figure 8.4b), which later become more horizontal. The intercondylar eminences (lateral and medial) of the tibia are also

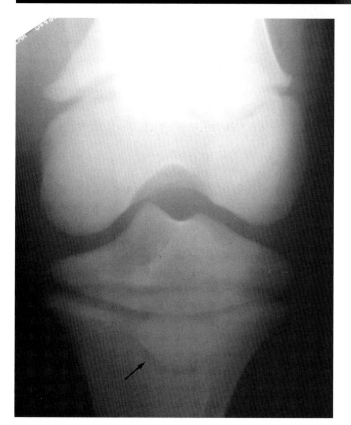

Figure 8.4(a) Flexed lateromedial view of a stifle of a normal 15-day-old foal. Note the irregular contour and granular subchondral opacity of the proximal part of the femoral trochlear and of the patella. The physes are relatively wide. The lateral and medial trochlear ridges of the femur are of similar size. There is an approximately triangular lucent area cranial to the femoropatellar joint representing fat. Note also the separate centre of ossification of the tibial crest (the tibial apophysis).

Figure 8.4(b) Caudocranial view of the stifle of a normal 3-week-old foal. Lateral is to the right. Incomplete ossification of the proximal tibial epiphysis gives the impression of slanting of the tibial condyles. The femorotibial joint space is wide compared with that of the adult. The tibial apophysis and its physis can be identified superimposed on the tibial metaphysis (arrow).

[368]

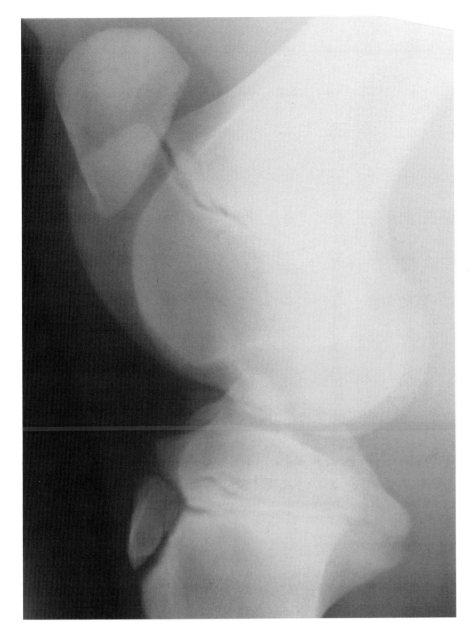

Figure 8.5 Lateromedial view of the stifle of a normal 2-month-old foal. The proximal part of the medial trochlear ridge of the femur and the patella are still incompletely ossified and therefore have an irregular outline. The shape of the trochlea of the femur and the patella, however, is more similar to an adult than to the neonatal foal (compare with Figure 8.4a).

incompletely developed, appearing small and blunted. The corresponding intercondylar fossa is shallow.

At birth, the apophysis (centre of ossification of the tibial tuberosity) is separated from the proximal tibial epiphysis as well as from the proximal tibial metaphysis. The apophyseal–metaphyseal physis is seen on lateromedial views as an oblique lucent line of irregular width, and on craniocaudal views as a V-shaped lucent line overlying the proximal tibial metaphysis. The apophyseal–epiphyseal physis closes between 9 and 12 months of age,

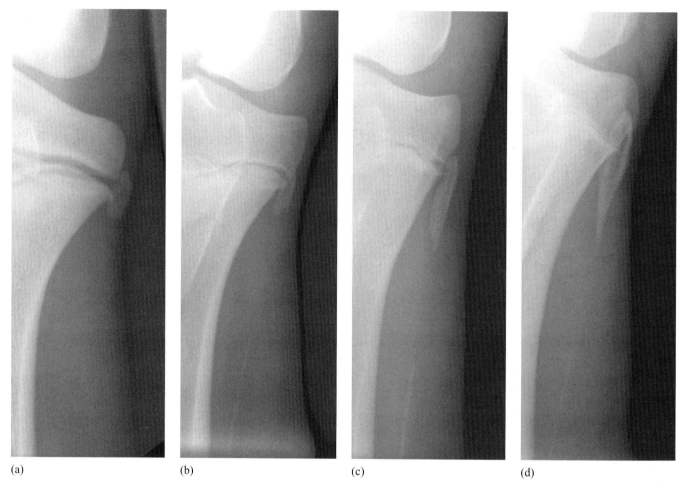

(a) (b) (c) (d)

Figure 8.6 Caudomedial-craniolateral oblique views of the fibulas of seven horses of variable age: (a)-(d) are skeletally immature horses and show progressive ossification occurring with increasing age; (e)-(g) are skeletally mature horses. Ossification often occurs from more than one centre of ossification which may never fuse, resulting in persistent lucent lines traversing the fibula (f and g).

and the apophyseal–metaphyseal physis closes at 30–36 months. The proximal tibial physis (epiphyseal–metaphyseal physis) closes at 24–30 months of age.

The fibula shows very little ossification until 1–2 months of age, at which time ossification occurs from one or more centres (Figures 8.6a-d). This ossification may remain incomplete, resulting in horizontal or oblique radiolucent lines in the fibula (Figures 8.6e-g). These should not be confused with fractures.

Skeletally mature horse

Lateromedial view

With the exception of a slight degree of obliquity, the principal radiographic features of the lateromedial view (Figure 8.7b) are the same as those described in detail below for the caudal 60° lateral-craniomedial oblique view.

[370]

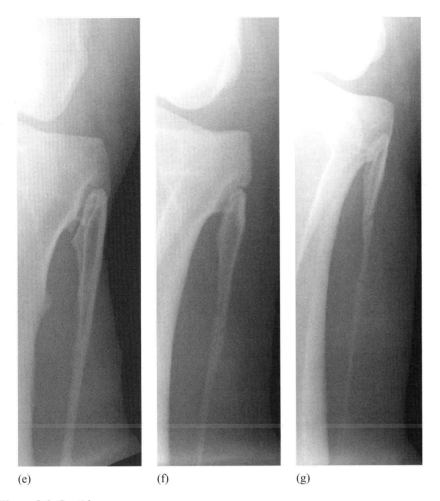

(e)   (f)   (g)

Figure 8.6 *Cont'd*

Caudal 60° lateral-craniomedial oblique view

The large medial trochlear ridge of the femur is positioned proximal and cranial to the smaller lateral trochlear ridge (Figure 8.7a). The trochlear ridges are smoothly curved in outline. Proximally the medial trochlear ridge has a small flattened area at its junction with the metaphysis of the femur. The distal two-thirds of the medial ridge are flatter than the lateral. There is a small notch where the medial trochlear ridge merges with the medial femoral condyle. From this notch an irregular sclerotic line traverses the condyles in a caudal and slightly proximal direction. This is the intercondylar fossa. Immediately above the notch, the convergence of two sclerotic lines indicates the extensor fossa. There is a sclerotic line parallel to the trochlear ridges, which represents the base of the intertrochlear groove. On the lateral trochlear ridge there is a flattened area at its transition into the lateral condyle. Neither this, nor the poorly developed area of decreased opacity immediately proximal to this area should be interpreted as an osteochondral defect. If the x-ray beam is angled from too far cranially, the lateral trochlear ridge may appear flattened. The most proximal part of the ridge may have an indistinct margin (Figure 8.8) which should not be confused with a manifestation of osteochondrosis. The femoral condyles have a

[371]

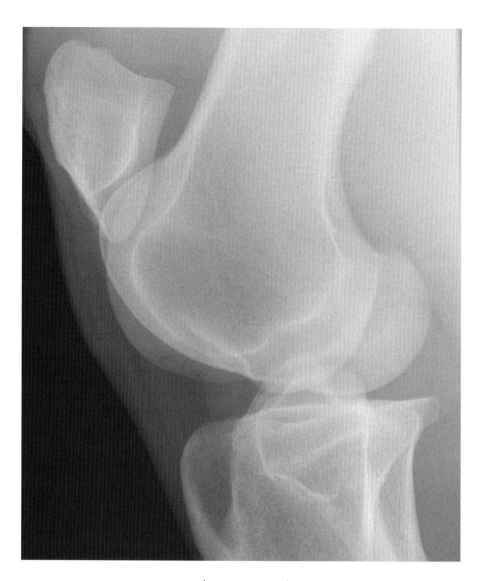

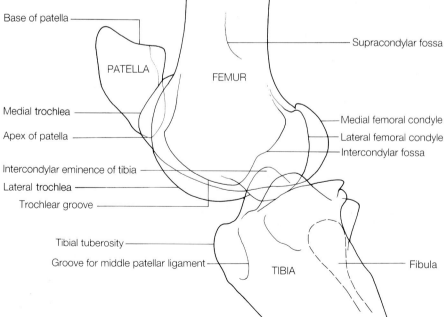

Base of patella

Medial trochlea

Apex of patella

Intercondylar eminence of tibia

Lateral trochlea

Trochlear groove

Tibial tuberosity

Groove for middle patellar ligament

PATELLA

FEMUR

TIBIA

Supracondylar fossa

Medial femoral condyle

Lateral femoral condyle

Intercondylar fossa

Fibula

Figure 8.7a Caudal 60° lateral-craniomedial oblique view and diagram of a normal adult stifle. Note the smooth curved contour of the lateral and medial trochlear ridges of the femur. The medial trochlea is larger than the lateral. Compare with Figure 8.9.

[372]

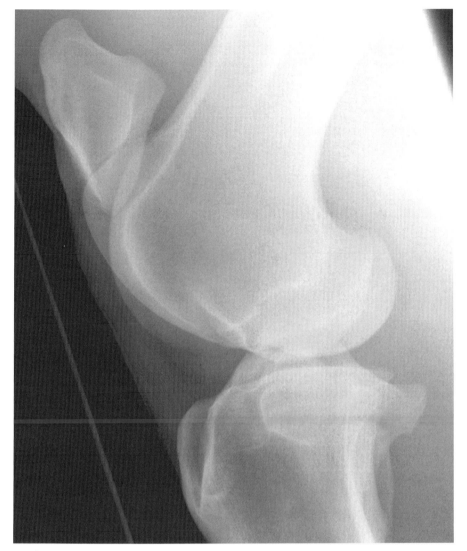

Figure 8.7b True lateromedial view of the stifle of a normal adult horse. The larger medial trochlea of the femur is projected cranial to the lateral trochlea.

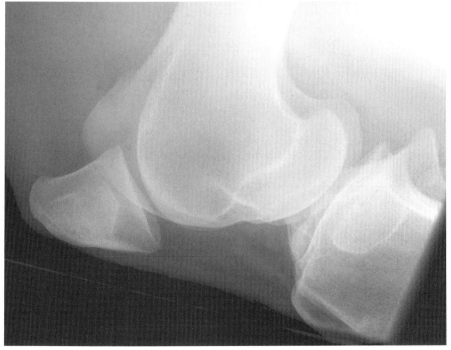

Figure 8.7c Flexed lateromedial view of the stifle of a normal adult horse. Compared with a weight-bearing view the patella has moved distally and the cranial aspect of the femorotibial joint is opened.

[373]

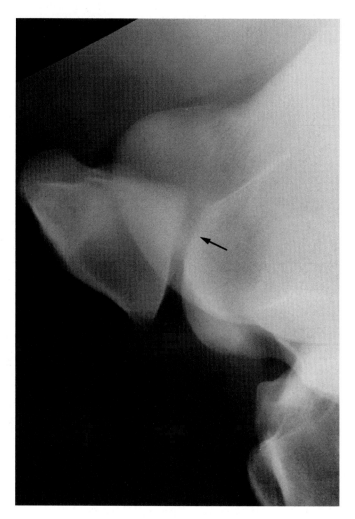

Figure 8.8 Lateromedial (flexed) view of the stifle of a normal adult horse. The contour of the proximal aspect of the lateral trochlea of the femur is slightly flattened and ill defined (arrow). This is the result of angulation of the x-ray beam from too far cranially and does not represent a pathological abnormality. Compare with Figures 8.7a (normal) and 8.15 (osteochondrosis).

smooth convex outline. On the 60° oblique view the condyles are partly superimposed, the medial condyle being projected slightly caudal to the lateral condyle. Fabellae occasionally occur proximal to the caudal aspect of the femoral condyles.

The position of the patella in relation to the distal femur changes with the degree of flexion/extension of the femorotibial joint. When the horse is bearing weight, the patella is positioned over the proximal aspect of the medial trochlear ridge. With flexion of the femorotibial joint, the patella moves distally which aids visualization of the proximal aspect of the trochlea. Softly exposed radiographs may demonstrate the patellar ligaments.

The femoral condyles and the intercondylar eminences of the tibia are superimposed on this view. The tibial tuberosity and tibial crest are recognized cranially.

A soft-tissue opacity is often seen at the cranial aspect of the femorotibial joint, cranial to the site of insertion of the cranial cruciate ligament.

[374]

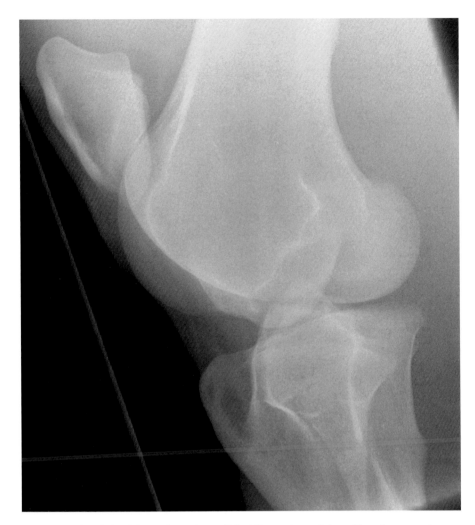

Figure 8.9 Caudal 45° lateral-craniomedial oblique view of the stifle of a normal mature horse. Compare with Figures 8.7a and 8.7b.

Caudal 45° lateral-craniomedial oblique view

The femoral condyles are further separated in the caudal 45° lateral-craniomedial oblique view (Figure 8.9), compared to a Cd60°L-CrMO view.

Caudocranial view

The patella is seen partly superimposed upon the lateral cortex of the diaphysis of the femur (Figure 8.10a). The medial ridge of the supracondylar fossa and the border of the extensor fossa on the lateral surface of the lateral femoral condyle can also be evaluated.

Deviations from a true caudocranial view may outline slight osseous irregularities along either the medial or the lateral femoral epicondyles. An oval area of decreased opacity is frequently seen at the proximolateral aspect of the intercondylar fossa of the femur, as is a flask-shaped lucent area distal and slightly lateral to the intercondylar eminences of the tibia. They occur as the result of superimposition, and should not be interpreted

[375]

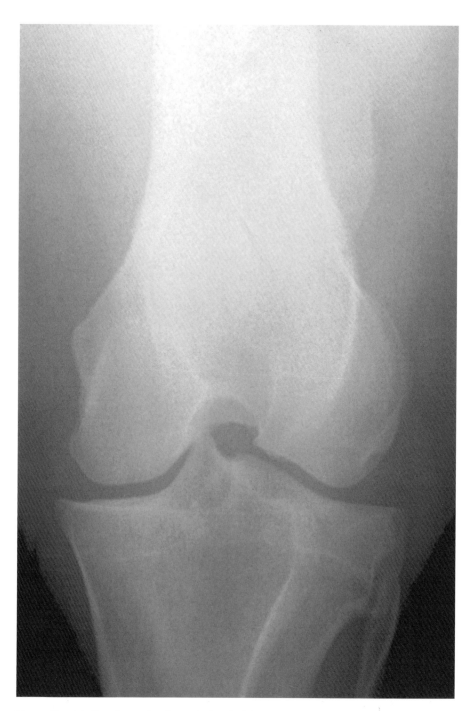

Figure 8.10(a) Caudoproximal-craniodistal oblique view and diagram of a normal adult stifle. Lateral is to the right. Note the different shapes of lateral and medial femoral condyles. The intercondylar fossa has a well defined margin. The medial intercondylar eminence is larger than the lateral and more sharply pointed. Note the poorly defined lucent area distal to it.

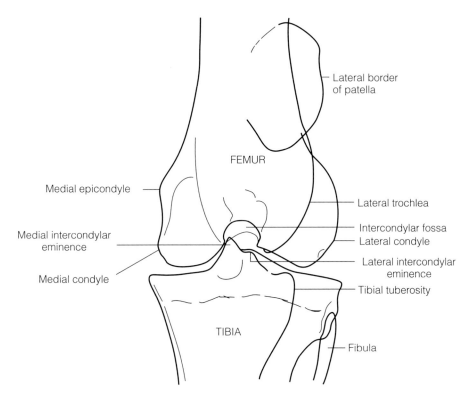

Figure 8.10(a) *Cont'd*

as cystic lesions in the bone. The border of the intercondylar fossa is relatively opaque.

The medial femoral condyle is rounder than the lateral, but slight flattening of the medial femoral condyle or slight concavity of bone outline (a 'dimple') (Figure 8.10b) are acceptable if the trabecular pattern of the subchondral bone is normal. The shape of the femoral condyles and the width of the femorotibial joint change with the angle of projection of the radiograph.

The lateral condyle of the femur has a proximomedial-distolateral inclination. The lateral joint space of the femorotibial joint is narrower than the medial space; this does not indicate collapse of the lateral meniscus. The femorotibial joint space width medially and laterally appears to vary depending on the way in which the horse is standing and narrowing should be interpreted with extreme caution unless it can be reproduced in several views.

The medial intercondylar eminence of the tibia is larger and more pointed than the lateral eminence (Figures 8.10a and 8.10c). The lateral condyle of the tibia has a proximomedial-distolateral inclination to mirror the outline of the lateral femoral condyle. Superimposed on the lateral condyle and metaphysis are the tibial tuberosity and tibial crest. There are focal areas of reduced opacity distal to the intercondylar eminences and

[377]

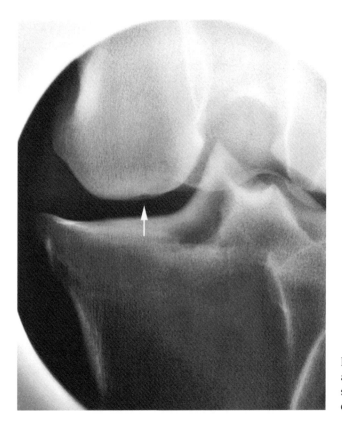

Figure 8.10(b) Caudocranial radiographic view of the left stifle of a 7-year-old Irish Sports Horse. Medial is to the left. There is a small concave radiolucent depression in the medial femoral condyle (arrow).

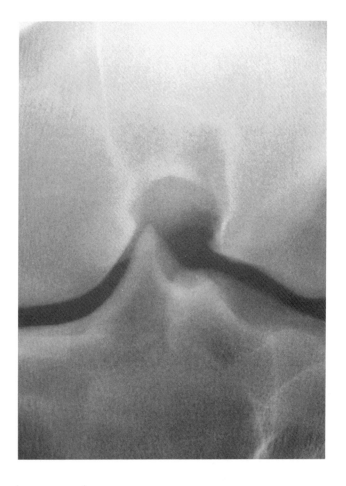

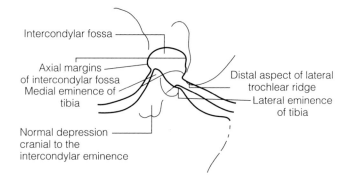

Intercondylar fossa

Axial margins of intercondylar fossa

Medial eminence of tibia

Distal aspect of lateral trochlear ridge

Lateral eminence of tibia

Normal depression cranial to the intercondylar eminence

Figure 8.10(c) Caudocranial radiographic view of the axial aspect of the femorotibial joint of a normal mature horse. Lateral is to the right.

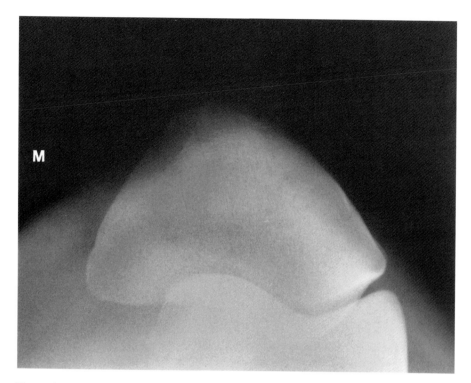

Figure 8.11 Cranioproximal-craniodistal oblique view of a patella and femoral trochleas of a normal adult horse. Note the larger medial trochlea of the femur (M = medial).

proximal to the tuberosity of the tibia. The fibula articulates with the lateral aspect of the tibia.

Cranioproximal-craniodistal oblique view

The medial trochlear ridge is larger than the lateral and is separated from it by the trochlear groove (Figure 8.11). The patella is approximately triangular and its medial angle is blunter than the lateral. The patella has a uniform opacity with a distinct subchondral bone plate and a smooth articular outline.

Other structures are poorly defined on this view.

Knowledge of the sites of soft tissue attachments in the stifle region is an important prerequisite for accurate radiographic interpretation (Figures 8.12, 8.13 and 8.14, Table 8.1).

SIGNIFICANT FINDINGS

Osteochondrosis

In this text, subchondral bone cysts (osseous cyst-like lesions) are regarded as a separate entity from osteochondrosis, although they are considered by some workers to be part of the same syndrome (see 'Osseous cyst-like lesions', page 385).

[379]

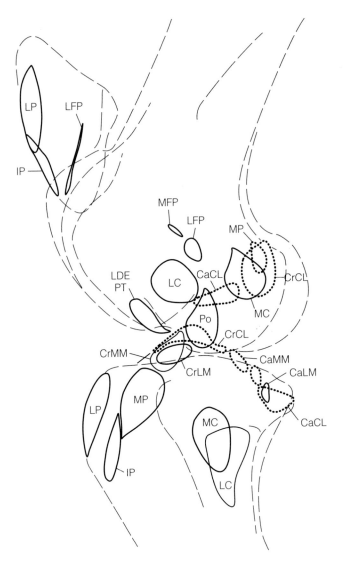

Figure 8.12(a) Diagram of a caudal 60° lateral-craniomedial oblique view of the stifle illustrating the sites of ligament and tendon attachments. The areas of attachment situated within the intercondylar area are marked with dotted lines. See Table 8.1. (Adapted figure courtesy of *Equine vet. J.*)

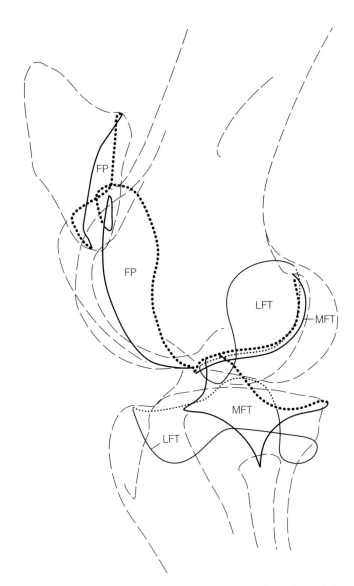

Figure 8.12(b) Diagram of a caudal 60° lateral-craniomedial oblique view of the stifle illustrating the sites of joint capsule attachments. The attachments situated on the medial aspect of the patella and femur are marked with dotted lines. See Table 8.1. (Adapted figure courtesy of *Equine vet. J.*)

In the stifle, osteochondrosis is most commonly recognized radiographically involving the lateral trochlear ridge of the femur. Lesions are also seen restricted to the articular surface of the patella. Less commonly, lesions may also involve the medial trochlear ridge and the trochlear groove. Osteochondrosis frequently occurs bilaterally and both stifles should be radiographed.

Radiographic indications of osteochondrosis of the lateral trochlear ridge are most easily detected on a caudal 60° lateral-craniomedial oblique view, and may include:

1 Flattening, especially of the middle third of the ridge (Figure 8.15).

2 An irregular contour of the ridge, usually limited to the middle third, but occasionally involving as much as two-thirds of the ridge. There may be

[380]

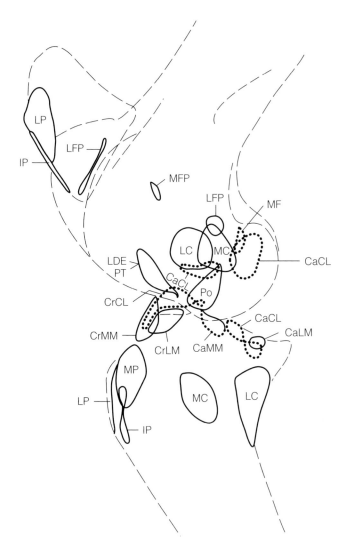

Figure 8.13(a) Diagram of a lateromedial view of the stifle illustrating the sites of ligament and tendon attachments. The areas of attachment situated within the intercondylar area are marked with dotted lines. See Table 8.1. (Adapted figure courtesy of *Equine vet. J.*)

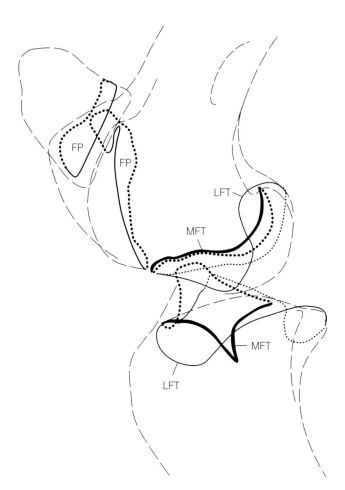

Figure 8.13(b) Diagram of a lateromedial view of the stifle illustrating the sites of joint capsule attachments. The attachments of the femoropatellar joint on the medial aspect and of the femorotibial joint within the intercondylar area are marked with dotted lines. See Table 8.1. (Adapted figure courtesy of *Equine vet. J.*)

one or more subchondral lucent defects extending for up to 2 cm into the ridge (Figures 8.16 and 8.17b). These may have a sclerotic margin and are easily demonstrated on slightly more oblique views.

3 Radiopaque fragments may be present within a defect in the ridge (Figure 8.17a).

4 In long-standing cases, the lateral trochlear ridge may be grossly undersized but have a regular outline (Figure 8.18). This is normally due to fragmentation and remodelling. There may be one or more rounded, radiopaque fragments within the femoropatellar joint or attached to the joint capsule. Occasionally similar changes are identified in the medial trochlea of the femur. Very severe undersizing of the lateral trochlea may predispose to secondary luxation of the patella.

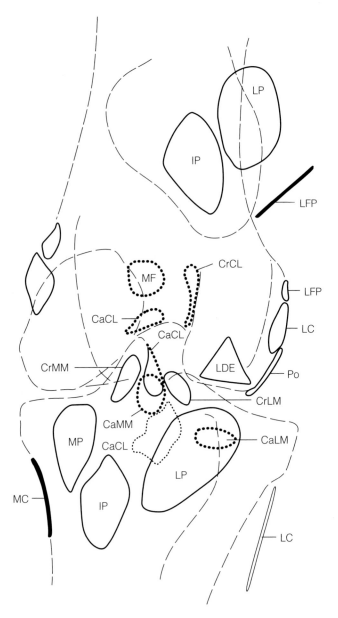

Figure 8.14(a) Diagram of a caudocranial view of the stifle illustrating the sites of ligament and tendon attachments. The areas of attachment situated on the caudal aspect of the femur and tibia are marked with dotted lines. See Table 8.1. (Adapted figure courtesy of *Equine vet. J.*)

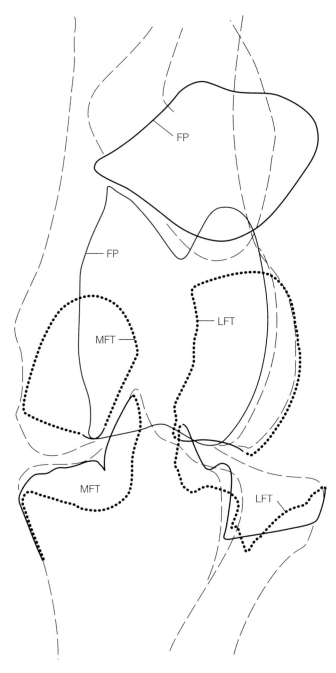

Figure 8.14(b) Diagram of a caudocranial view of the stifle illustrating the sites of joint capsule attachments. The areas of attachment situated on the caudal aspect of the femur and tibia are marked with dotted lines. See Table 8.1. (Adapted figure courtesy of *Equine vet. J.*)

Table 8.1 Legends for the soft tissue structures indicated in Figures 8.12, 8.13 and 8.14.

CHAPTER 8
The stifle and tibia

LP	Lateral patellar ligament
IP	Intermediate patellar ligament
MP	Medial patellar ligament
LFP	Lateral femoropatellar ligament
MFP	Medial femoropatellar ligament
LC	Lateral collateral ligament of the femorotibial joint
MC	Medial collateral ligament of the femorotibial joint
CrLM	Cranial tibial ligament of the lateral meniscus
CrMM	Cranial tibial ligament of the medial meniscus
CaLM	Caudal tibial ligament of the lateral meniscus
CaMM	Caudal tibial ligament of the medial meniscus
MF	Meniscofemoral ligament of the lateral meniscus
CrCL	Cranial cruciate ligament
CaCL	Caudal cruciate ligament
Po	Tendon of the popliteus muscle
PT	Tendon of origin of fibularis (peroneus) tertius
LDE	Tendon of origin of the long digital extensor muscle
FP	Femoropatellar joint capsule
LFT	Lateral sac of the femorotibial joint capsule
MFT	Medial sac of the femortibial joint capsule

5 The articular surface of the patella may be irregular (Figure 8.19), most commonly near the apex. Other patellar changes include subchondral lucent zones, with or without surrounding sclerosis. These changes are rare, and may occur alone or in association with lesions of the lateral trochlear ridge. A fragment occasionally occurs in isolation at the base of the patella at its articular margin. It is important to ensure that the whole of the patella is visualized on radiographs and the proximal part is not missed. The aetiology of these fragments has not been confirmed. Lesions of the patella may warrant a more guarded prognosis.

Simultaneous involvement of more than one structure in the joint has been suggested as indicative of a poor prognosis. Radiography tends to underestimate the degree of pathological abnormality which may be detected arthroscopically.

Osteochondrosis cannot be detected radiographically until a moderate degree of subchondral bone change is present. It is important that oblique views are included and care should be taken not to overlook subchondral lucencies on overexposed films. Slight flattening of the lateral trochlear ridge need not be accompanied by clinical symptoms, and is occasionally seen with sclerosis of the subchondral bone as an incidental finding in older horses.

In early and mild cases, conservative management may be adequate. Once distension of the joint capsule and lameness are present, surgical intervention is recommended. Post-operatively, there will be some modelling of the defect, but even in clinically successful cases the radiographic appearance will remain abnormal.

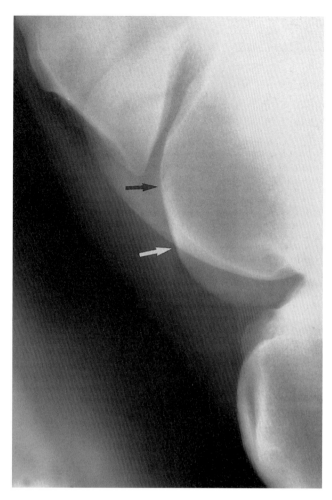

Figure 8.15 Lateromedial view of a stifle of an adult horse. There is flattening of the middle one-third of the lateral trochlear ridge of the femur (arrows) (compare with Figure 8.7a). There is sclerosis of the underlying subchondral bone. There were no associated clinical signs in this Grand Prix Showjumper.

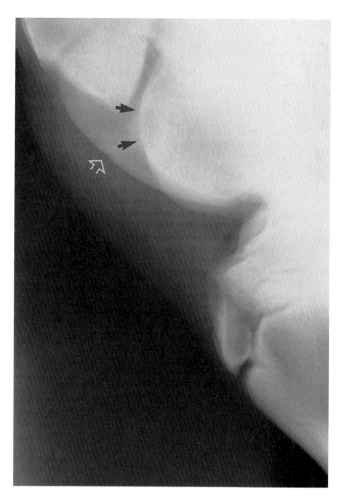

Figure 8.16 Lateromedial view of a stifle of an 8-month-old Thoroughbred foal. There is loss of the distinct osteochondral outline of the middle one-third of the lateral trochlear ridge of the femur (solid arrows). In the underlying subchondral bone there is an oval-shaped area of decreased opacity. In addition, there is a subtle depression in the outline of the middle of the medial trochlear ridge (open arrow). Similar changes were present in the contralateral limb. The foal showed only slight hindlimb stiffness, but experienced great difficulty in getting up. Grossly and histologically, the abnormalities extended into the subchondral bone. Note also the separate ossification centre of the apophysis of the tibia.

The disease may remain asymptomatic throughout the horse's life, or may become symptomatic late in life. In older horses there are usually discrete bony opacities in association with a shallow defect and subchondral sclerosis. In these cases the bony fragments must be removed in order to provide a congruent articulation and prevent the development of secondary degenerative joint disease.

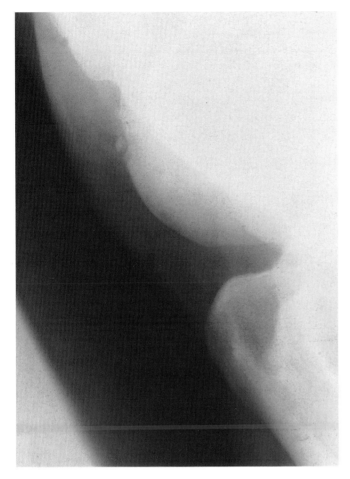

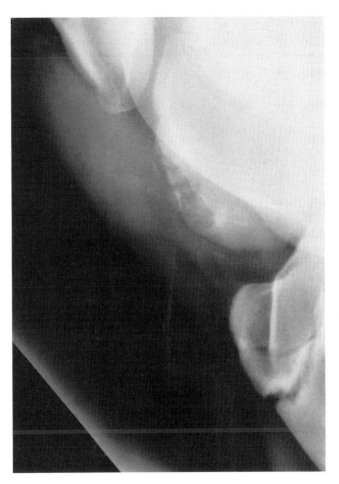

Figure 8.17(a) Caudal 60° lateral-craniomedial oblique view of a stifle of a 9-year-old horse. There is distension of the femoropatellar joint capsule and an irregularly outlined defect in the subchondral bone of the middle of the lateral trochlear ridge of the femur, within which are a number of radiopaque fragments. These represent mineralized cartilage and/or bone. The radiograph is exposed to highlight the lesions.

Figure 8.17(b) Caudal 60° lateral-craniomedial oblique view of a stifle of a 15-month-old Thoroughbred. There is distension of the femoropatella joint capsule and marked irregularity of the contour of the lateral trochlea of the femur due to fragmentation of the articular cartilage and resorption of the underlying bone. Mineralized debris is present in the femoropatellar joint and within the defect. There is also modelling of the apex of the patella.

Osseous cyst-like lesions

Subchondral bone cysts

Although subchondral bone cysts are considered by some authors to be part of the osteochondrosis syndrome, they are referred to in this text as a separate lesion. Experimental evidence has shown that an elliptical full-thickness cartilage plus subchondral bone defect, at the region of maximum weight bearing in the medial femoral condyle, will result in the development of an osseous cyst-like lesion within 3 weeks, which may progressively

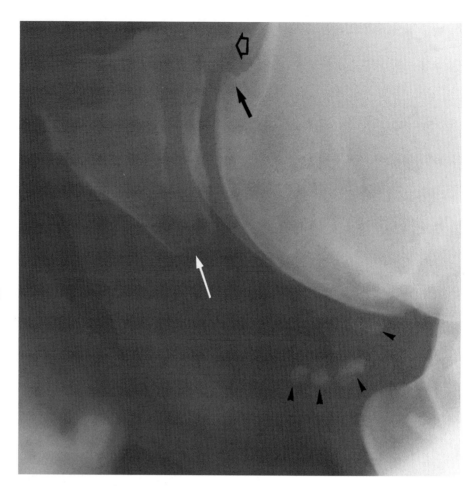

Figure 8.18 Caudal 60° lateral-craniomedial oblique view of a distal femur of an 8-year-old horse. There is considerable distension of the femoropatellar joint capsule. The lateral trochlear ridge, although relatively smoothly outlined, is undersized (compare with Figure 8.7a). There are several large, rounded mineralized fragments (arrow heads) within the femoropatellar joint ('joint mice'). Extensive modelling of the apex (white arrow) and base (open arrow) of the patella and the proximal aspect of the lateral trochlear ridge (black arrow) indicates secondary degenerative joint disease.

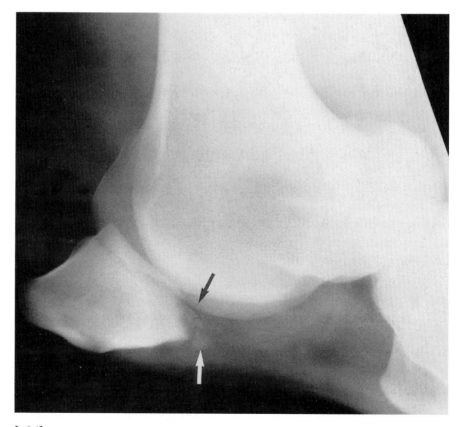

Figure 8.19 Flexed lateromedial view of a stifle of a 2-year-old Thoroughbred. The distal quarter of the articular surface of the patella is markedly irregular with extensive subchondral fragmentation towards the apex (arrows). These changes may be part of the osteochondrosis syndrome. Similar, usually less severe, changes may develop secondary to medial patellar desmotomy.

[386]

enlarge over the following 9 weeks. This supports clinical evidence of sub-chondral bone cysts developing in the medial femoral condyle of mature horses following known trauma.

Subchondral bone cysts in the stifle occur almost exclusively in the medial femoral condyle. They frequently develop bilaterally, although the horse may present with a unilateral lameness; therefore both hindlimbs should be examined radiographically. The fully developed subchondral bone cyst is seen as an almost circular lucent area within the subchondral bone. It is best seen on the caudocranial view and may be difficult to see on lateral or oblique views due to superimposition of the condyles. The cyst initially develops from a saucer-shaped radiolucent area proximal to the articular cartilage (Figure 8.20a). This lucent zone gradually enlarges to become dome shaped, with a flat base in close apposition to the articular surface (Figures 8.20b and 8.20c). If a cyst develops prior to skeletal maturity, continued growth and endochondral ossification of the epiphysis gives the impression that the cyst moves proximally into the condyle. The cyst becomes more rounded (Figure 8.21a) and a communicating lucent channel develops between the cyst and the medial femorotibial joint (Figure 8.21b). This channel is formed by infolding of the subchondral bone plate. An almost complete subchondral bone plate may become re-established at the medial femorotibial articulation.

Shallow saucer-shaped radiolucent lesions proximal to the articular cartilage do not necessarily develop into subchondral bone cysts. They need not cause pain, although many are believed to cause lameness at some time. A number of caudocranial views with varying proximodistal inclination of the x-ray beam are necessary to evaluate the subchondral trabecular pattern and the depth of the lesion. When a subchondral bone cyst is present in one limb, a shallow saucer-shaped lesion is occasionally present in the contralateral limb. This may remain quiescent or develop as discussed above.

Shallow saucer-shaped lesions when associated with lameness may respond to conservative treatment; surgical treatment has yielded inconsistent results. When well developed subchondral bone cysts are present, the radiographs should be carefully assessed for evidence of degenerative joint disease (see page 392), which may warrant a more guarded prognosis. Conservative treatment may restore clinical soundness in approximately 20–50% of horses, but there is little radiographic change except for the formation of a sclerotic rim of bone around the periphery of the cyst. Long-standing cysts may be seen radiographically when not causing lameness, but their future clinical significance is uncertain.

Surgical treatment of subchondral bone cysts results in up to 60% of cases returning to normal work. The prognosis is more favourable in horses up to 3 years of age compared with older horses. There is little correlation between clinical progress and the post-operative radiographic appearance of a cyst, although in some cases progressive enlargement of the cyst has been noted, associated with persistent lameness. Radiographic resolution of the lesion is not necessary for a satisfactory clinical outcome. Injection of the cyst lining with corticosteroids has produced favourable results in

[387]

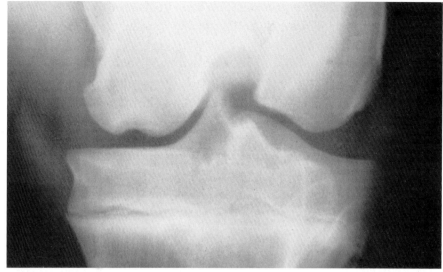

(a)

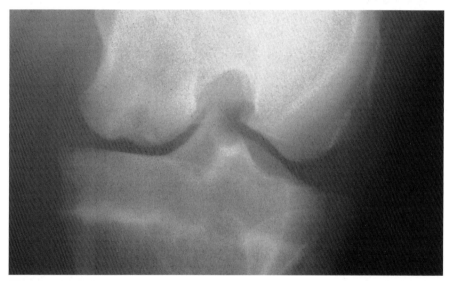

(b)

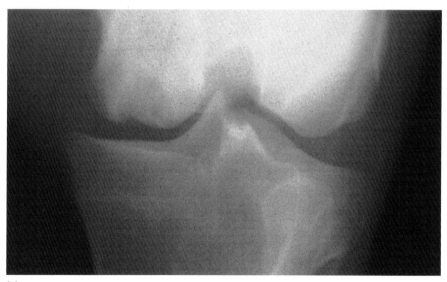

Figure 8.20 Caudocranial views of one stifle of an Arab horse, showing the development of a dome-shaped subchondral bone cyst in the medial femoral condyle from a crescent-shaped subchondral defect: (a) 12 months of age; (b) 18 months of age; (c) 21 months of age. Note the sclerotic rim surrounding the defect.

(c)

[388]

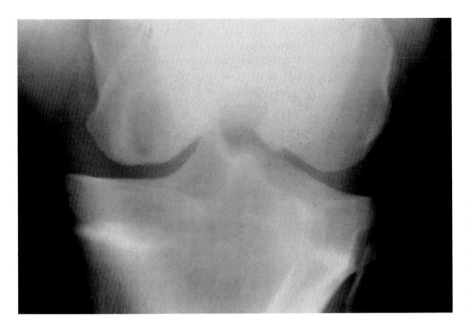

Figure 8.21(a) Caudocranial view of a stifle of a 2-year-old horse. There is a large oval subchondral bone cyst in the medial femoral condyle. There is a thin rim of sclerosis surrounding the cyst and apparent reformation of a subchondral bone plate between the cyst and the medial femorotibial joint.

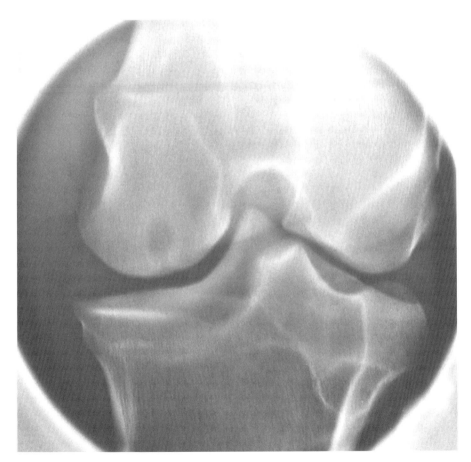

Figure 8.21(b) Caudocranial radiographic view of the left stifle of a 9-year-old Thoroughbred cross intermediate event horse, with intermittent lameness of variable severity. Medial is to the left. There is a subchondral bone cyst in the medial femoral condyle, with a clearly defined 'neck' through the subchondral bone. The subchondral bone cyst has a mildly sclerotic rim.

horses of all ages, with approximately 60% returning to full athletic function.

Focal flattening of the subchondral bone of the medial femoral condyle is a frequent finding in yearling Thoroughbreds, but is believed not to influence performance. Focal flattening or mild concavity of the subchondral bone of the medial femoral condyle, with or without altered trabecular architecture or an underlying semicircular sclerotic zone, has been seen in some older horses with pain associated with the medial femorotibial joint (Figure 8.22). Arthroscopic evaluation usually reveals abnormalities of the overlying articular cartilage.

Other osseous cyst-like lesions

Osseous cyst-like lesions may occur in the lateral femoral condyle and the proximal epiphysis of the tibia (Figure 8.23a). Osseous cyst-like lesions in the proximal tibia may be surrounded by a marked sclerotic rim. These have been identified in both the medial and lateral condyles of the tibia either alone (in immature horses) or in conjunction with other signs of degenerative joint disease (in mature horses) (Figure 8.23b). Medical or surgical treatment has been successful in some young horses, but the prognosis in adult horses is guarded. Osseous cyst-like lesions distal to the intercondylar

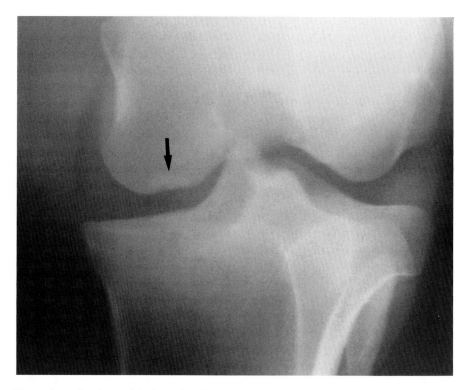

Figure 8.22 Caudocranial view of a stifle of a 7-year-old dressage horse, with pain associated with the medial femorotibial joint. There is flattening of the centre of the articular margin of the medial femoral condyle, with underlying subchondral sclerosis (arrow). The overlying articular cartilage was abnormal.

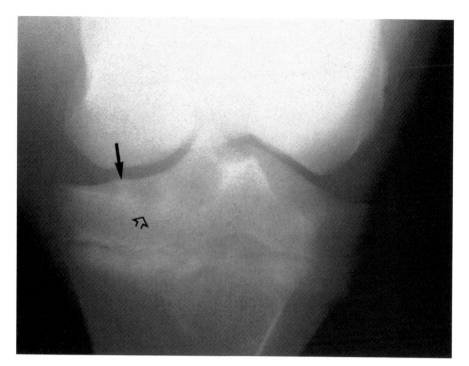

Figure 8.23(a) Caudocranial view of a stifle of a 1-year-old Thoroughbred. The osteochondral outline of the medial tibial condyle is slightly irregular (black arrow). There is a well circumscribed osseous cyst-like lesion in the subchondral bone, surrounded by a broad rim of sclerosis (open arrow). There is also a suggestion of slight flattening of the opposing medial femoral condyle.

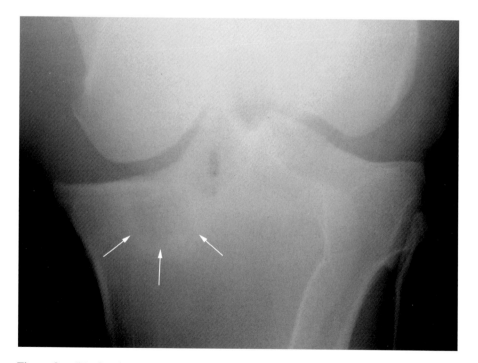

Figure 8.23(b) Caudocranial radiographic view of the left stifle of a 12-year-old Grand Prix showjumper. Lameness was partially improved by intra-articular analgesia of the medial femorotibial joint. Medial is to the left. There is a large osseous cyst-like lesion in the proximomedial aspect of the tibia, surrounded by a broad rim of sclerosis (arrows). There is modelling of the distal medial aspect of the femur and the proximomedial aspect of the tibia consistent with degenerative joint disease.

eminences may be associated with cruciate ligament injuries (see Figure 8.27, page 397) or tearing of cranial meniscal ligaments.

Physitis

Physitis is associated with irregular widening of the physis, usually involving the distal femoral physis. The incidence in the stifle is very low. Bilateral physitis may result in an upright hindlimb stance and a stiff and stilted gait. The differential diagnosis should include osteochondrosis.

Degenerative joint disease

Degenerative joint disease of the femorotibial joint is best recognized radiographically on a caudocranial view (Figures 8.24a-c). The lateromedial view is more useful for the femoropatellar joint. Changes include:

- Periarticular osteophyte formation
- Flattening of the articular surfaces
- Sclerosis of the subchondral bone
- Lucent zones in the subchondral bone
- Narrowing of the femorotibial joint space

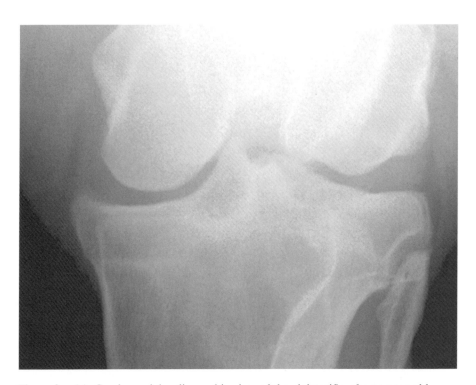

Figure 8.24(a) Caudocranial radiographic view of the right stifle of a 14-year-old Welsh Cob cross Thoroughbred with lameness of 9 months' duration. Medial is to the left. There is marked modelling of the proximomedial aspect of the tibia and a large periarticular osteophyte, consistent with degenerative joint disease. Surgical exploration revealed a tear of the cranial aspect of the medial meniscus and extensive fibrillation of the cranial meniscal ligament of the medial meniscus.

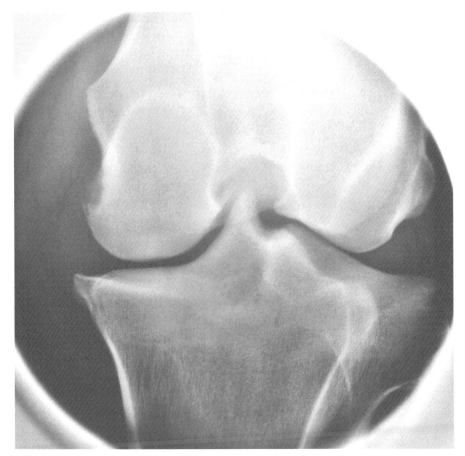

Figure 8.24(b) Caudocranial radiographic view of the left stifle of a 12-year-old Welsh Cob mare with sudden onset, severe lameness, markedly improved by intra-articular analgesia of the medial femorotibial joint. Medial is to the left. There is modelling of the distal medial aspect of the femur and the proximomedial aspect of the tibia consistent with degenerative joint disease. There was intense increased radiopharmaceutical uptake in the medial femoral condyle. Surgical exploration revealed profound widespread degeneration of the articular cartilage. There was only temporary response to intra-articular medication. Follow-up radiography 3 months later revealed no change. However post-mortem examination revealed extensive subchondral bone necrosis in the medial femoral condyle.

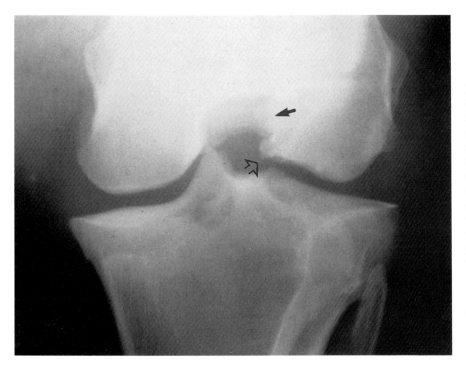

Figure 8.24(c) Caudocranial view of a stifle of an 8-year-old horse. Lateral is to the right. There is irregularity in the contour of the lateral aspect of the intercondylar fossa (black arrow) and new bone formation on the most axial aspect of the lateral femoral condyle (open arrow). There is a suggestion of a discrete mineralized opacity proximal to the medial intercondylar eminence of the tibia. The circular lucent zone with a more opaque centre, distal to the medial intercondylar eminence, is abnormal (compare with Figure 8.10). These changes are indicative of degenerative joint disease and probably result from trauma to either the cruciate ligament and/or a cranial meniscal ligament (see Figure 8.26).

[393]

Osteophytes on the tibial condyles, best seen on caudocranial views, are not necessarily a cause of lameness, although they may reflect the presence of joint disease. They occur most often on the medial tibial condyle. It is helpful to compare the radiographs of suspected lesions with radiographs of the contralateral joint. Degenerative joint disease may develop secondarily to trauma to other structures of the stifle, and the radiographs should be inspected carefully for evidence of meniscal damage, cruciate ligament injury or collateral ligament injury (see below). Diagnostic ultrasonography is essential for evaluating soft-tissue pathology, including damage of the meniscal cartilages, the patellar ligaments and the collateral ligaments of the joint, and is also more sensitive for detection of periarticular osteophytes than radiography. If the degree of lameness and the extent of radiographic and ultrasonographic abnormalities are not well correlated, exploratory arthroscopy is indicated. There may be widespread articular cartilage and associated intra-articular soft-tissue pathology in association with relatively minor radiographic abnormalities.

A poor prognosis is warranted for advanced degenerative joint disease of the stifle, although in early disease intra-articular medication with corticosteroids or polysulphated glycosaminoglycans may provide short-term, and in some cases permanent, resolution of lameness.

Infection

Septic arthritis (type S) and osteomyelitis in foals (types E and P) frequently affect the femorotibial joint and the femoral condyles (the medial condyle being most commonly affected; Figure 8.25a). Lateromedial radiographs may reveal patchy lucencies in the subchondral bone due to destruction and collapse of the cartilage and the subchondral bone. An irregular joint surface is therefore seen (Figure 8.25b). This should not be confused with the radiographic appearance of incomplete ossification normally seen in the trochlear ridges of the femur and the patella in young foals (see Figure 8.4, page 368). Changes may also be recognized within the tibial epiphysis and are usually best demonstrated on caudocranial views.

Osteomyelitis of the patella may occur in horses of any age. It is usually the result of direct trauma to the region and is often associated with a draining sinus. Although radiographic changes may be seen in a lateromedial view, a cranioproximal-craniodistal oblique view may be required. Contrast radiography of cases with a discharging sinus may be useful.

Miscellaneous soft-tissue injuries

In addition to the collateral ligaments common to most joints, the femorotibial joint includes lateral and medial menisci and associated ligaments, as well as cranial and caudal cruciate ligaments.

Collateral ligaments

The collateral ligaments of the femorotibial joint originate from the femoral epicondyles. In most normal horses, the outline of the epicondyles may be

[394]

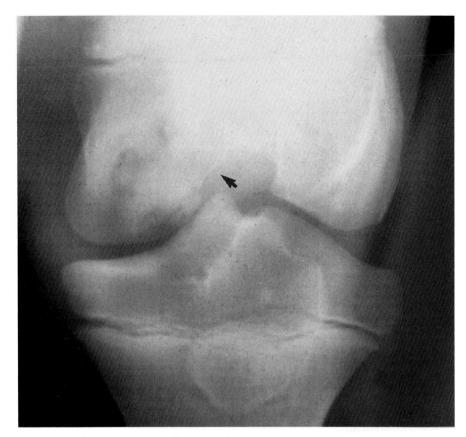

Figure 8.25(a) Caudoproximal-craniodistal oblique view of a stifle of a 3-month-old foal. Lateral is to the right. There are poorly defined lucent zones in the medial femoral condyle, surrounded by more sclerotic bone. There is a suggestion of a discrete fragment (arrow) extending from the medial aspect of the intercondylar fossa medially, which may represent a sequestrum or a pathological fracture. These radiographic abnormalities are consistent with severe type E osteomyelitis.

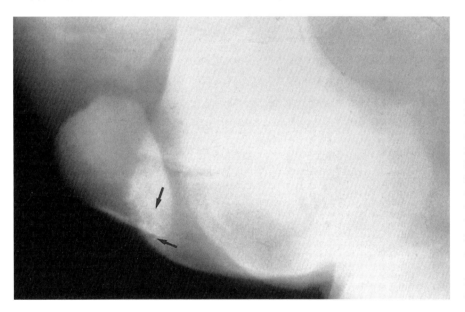

Figure 8.25(b) Slightly oblique lateromedial view of a stifle of an approximately 4-week-old Thoroughbred foal. The foal had distension of the femoropatellar joint capsule and synovial fluid analysis confirmed a diagnosis of septic arthritis. The apex of the patella and the trochlear ridges of the femur are incompletely ossified, as is normal for a foal of this age. There are also poorly defined lucent zones (arrows) in the subchondral bone of the medial trochlea ridge indicative of osteomyelitis.

irregular on caudocranial radiographs. Sprain of these ligaments may result in increased irregularity due to new bone production. There may also be entheseophyte formation at their insertions on the proximal tibia. Occasionally avulsion fractures occur. Further information may be obtained from ultrasonographic examination. If rupture of a collateral ligament is suspected, radiographs should be obtained with the joint under lateromedial stress, in order to confirm unilateral widening of the femorotibial joint space.

Meniscal damage

The true incidence of damage to the medial or lateral meniscus, or the supporting cranial and caudal ligaments, is unknown, but with the development of both ultrasonography and exploratory arthroscopy an increasing number of injuries are being identified, frequently unassociated with any detectable radiological abnormality. Some cases of degenerative joint disease (see page 392) develop secondarily to meniscal instability or meniscal tears. Traumatic injuries severe enough to damage the menisci may also result in damage to other structures, such as the collateral and meniscal ligaments. Plain and contrast radiographs are of limited value in outlining a meniscal tear, but meniscal damage may result in narrowing of the joint space. This is best assessed on caudocranial weight-bearing radiographs which may be difficult to obtain, as resting pain is often present. It is helpful to compare the width of the joint space with that of the contralateral stifle, but exact replication of the images is essential. Mineralization, with or without slight displacement, of a damaged meniscus has been recognized. Lucent zones distal to the intercondylar eminences of the proximal tibia may be seen in association with tears of the cranial meniscal ligaments.

Surgical debridement of tears of the axial aspect of a meniscus may have favourable results, but prognosis for other meniscal injuries is poor.

Cruciate ligaments

Rupture of the cranial and caudal cruciate ligaments has been described and has a poor prognosis.

Sprain of the cruciate ligaments with or without partial detachment of the distal insertion of the cranial cruciate ligament occurs more frequently. This ligament inserts with the cranial ligaments of the menisci immediately cranial to the intercondylar eminences. A discrete soft-tissue radiopacity immediately cranial and proximal to the site of insertion may indicate damage to the cruciate ligament. If seen on a lateromedial view, it should not be confused with the area of increased opacity seen on the cranial aspect of the normal femorotibial joint. In chronic cases there may be bony proliferative changes (Figure 8.26), often best seen on a flexed lateromedial view. Osseous cyst-like lesions may occur at the sites of origin and insertion of the cruciate ligaments. They are seen proximal to the intercondylar fossa, superimposed on the femoral condyles and/or distal to the intercondylar eminences of the tibia (Figure 8.27). Apparently detached osseous fragments may be evident in the intercondylar fossa, often in association with irregularities in the contour of the intercondylar eminences. All of these lesions are considered to have a guarded prognosis. A fracture of the medial intercondylar eminence may be seen in association with cruciate ligament injury, but is not synonymous with it. A fracture may be seen in isolation, with surgical removal resulting in a satisfactory outcome.

[396]

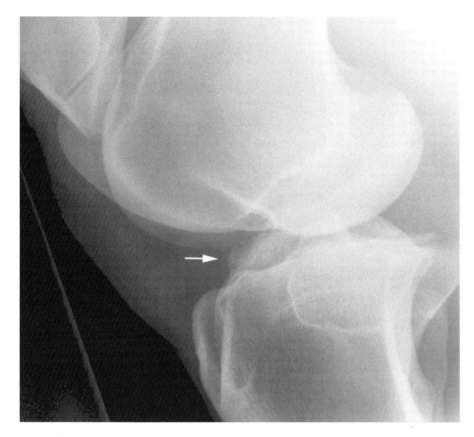

Figure 8.26 Lateromedial radiographic view of the right stifle of a 7-year-old polo pony with distension of the femoropatellar joint and moderate lameness. There is entheseous new bone on the cranioproximal aspect of the tibia at the insertion of the cranial ligament of the medial meniscus (arrow).

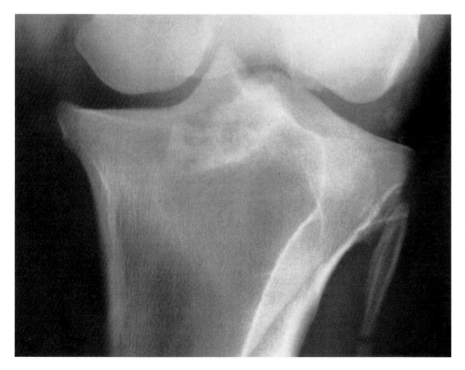

Figure 8.27 Caudocranial view of a proximal tibia of an 11-year-old Thoroughbred cross horse. Lateral is to the right. There is a poorly defined area of reduced radiopacity immediately distal to the intercondylar eminences. The area is circumscribed by a thick rim of sclerosis. Osseous cyst-like lesions occurring at this site have been associated with damage to the insertion of the cruciate ligament or a cranial meniscal ligament. There is slight modelling of the medial aspect of the medial tibial condyle. The circular opacity on the lateral aspect of the femorotibial joint is a screen artefact.

Other soft-tissue injuries

Caudal 60° lateral-craniomedial oblique radiographs, obtained with low kilovoltage, may reveal increased opacity of the patellar ligaments, especially on digital images. New bone formation near the proximal ligament insertions on the patella may also occur. These changes normally follow injury to the patella. The prognosis for this type of injury is good following rest. Ultrasonography is indicated to assess the integrity of the patellar ligaments.

Periosteal proliferation may be seen on the cranial aspect of the tibia, close to the distal aspect of the tibial crest, with or without cortical lucency. Sometimes a lucent line parallel to the cortical surface is seen, with or without a radiopaque fragment (Figure 8.28). These changes have been seen in young Thoroughbreds, with focal pain on pressure to the area, and probably reflect an insertional enthesopathy of semitendinosus. However,

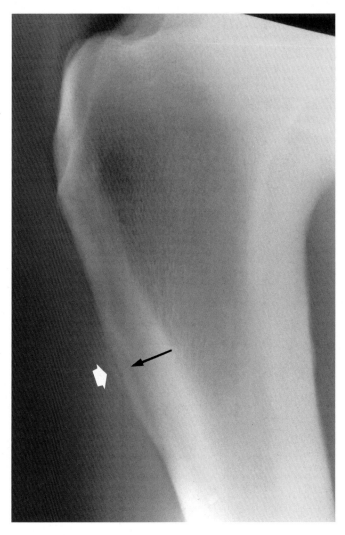

Figure 8.28 Lateromedial view of a proximal tibia of 3-year-old Thoroughbred racehorse. There is an osseous fragment (white arrow) at the tibial site of insertion of semitendinosus. The cranial cortex has a slightly irregular outline and there is a parallel lucent line in the cortical bone (black arrow).

[398]

such changes are occasionally seen as incidental abnormalities in older horses.

Desmitis of the middle patellar ligament may be associated with increased radiopharmaceutical uptake at the insertion on the tibial crest, however there are usually no associated radiographic abnormalities.

Injury of the origin of the gastrocnemius muscle on the caudal distal diaphyseal region of the femur occasionally results in focal periosteal new bone formation.

Modelling of the apex of the patella

Modelling of the apex of the patella may develop within weeks of performing a medial patellar desmotomy to treat intermittent upward fixation of the patella. Radiographic changes include spur formation at the apex of the patella, an irregular outline or fragmentation. Lameness may resolve with surgical debridement.

Calcinosis circumscripta

Calcinosis circumscripta (tumoral calcinosis) is a condition characterized by the formation of one or more hard, circumscribed subcutaneous swellings, typically formed at the lateral aspect of the femorotibial joint. Lameness is not usually present. Caudocranial radiographs demonstrate the lesion as a distinctly outlined mass of soft-tissue opacity irregularly infiltrated with small, highly opaque, amorphous granules (Figure 8.29). If lameness is present, surgery may be necessary.

Patellar luxation

Lateral luxation of the patella occurs occasionally in foals, but rarely in adults other than miniature breeds (including Shetlands), except secondary to severe osteochondrosis and subnormal size of the lateral trochlear ridge. Radiography may help to diagnose this condition. The radiographs should be inspected carefully to determine if there is primary hypoplasia of the trochlear ridges of the femur. The position and orientation of the patella are assessed most accurately on caudocranial views. Surgical treatment may be successful.

Upward fixation of the patella is a common condition, in which radiography is of little value. Lameness sometimes develops secondarily to medial patellar desmotomy for this condition. It is associated with remodelling of the apex and cranial distal surface of the patella, best seen in caudal 60° lateral-craniomedial oblique or flexed lateromedial views.

Infectious osteitis of the patella

Infectious osteitis of the patella usually follows known trauma and a penetrating wound. There may be a detectable radiolucent tract running from the skin surface to the cranial aspect of the patella, which develops both

[399]

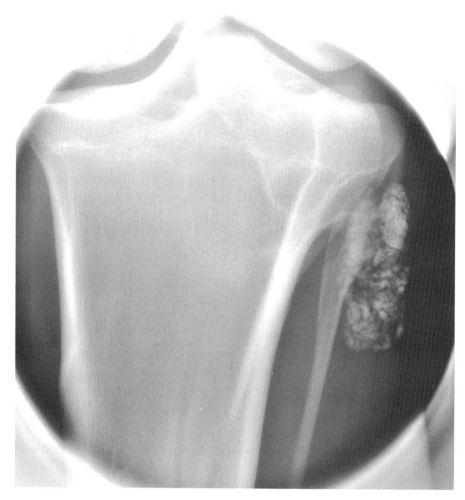

Figure 8.29 Caudocranial radiographic view of the proximal tibia of a 9-year-old Thoroughbred cross intermediate event horse (the same horse as in Figure 8.21(b)). Medial is to the left. There is an approximately rectangular area of heterogeneous opacity laterally, partially overlying the fibula. This is the typical appearance and location of calcinosis circumscripta.

lytic lesions and some new bone formation. A sequestrum and involucrum may develop. Diagnostic ultrasonography may be a more sensitive diagnostic technique early in the disease process.

Fractures

The presence of bone fragments in the joint may indicate the presence of a fracture or fractures, but it is not always possible to identify where the fragments have originated from. They should not be confused with fragments associated with osteochondrosis.

Patella

Patellar fractures may be recognized or suspected on lateromedial views (Figure 8.30a), but a flexed cranioproximal-craniodistal oblique view is

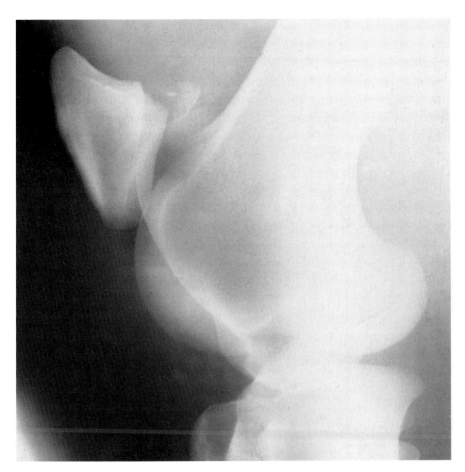

Figure 8.30(a) Caudal 60° lateral-craniomedial oblique view of a stifle of a 7-year-old horse which hit a fixed cross-country fence. There is a fracture of the base of the patella. A cranioproximal-craniodistal oblique view should be obtained to evaluate the patella more fully (see Figure 8.30b).

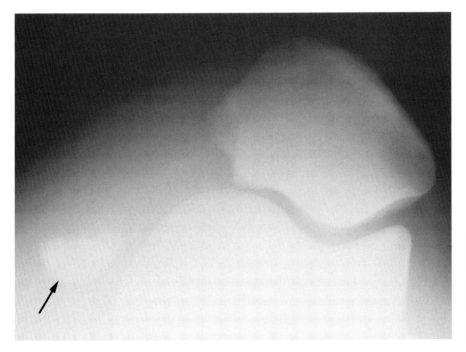

Figure 8.30(b) Cranioproximal-craniodistal oblique view of a patella of a 6-year-old eventer. Lateral is to the right. There is a displaced articular fracture of the medial aspect of the patella (arrow). The horse was treated by surgical removal of the fragment and made a complete recovery.

essential to ascertain the location and extent of a fracture and to determine if comminution is present (Figure 8.30b).

Small fragments separated from the base of the patella are often slightly displaced proximally and are best seen on lateromedial views. They are usually avulsion fractures at the insertion of the quadriceps muscle and seldom cause persistent lameness. Some persist radiographically, whereas others disappear.

Avulsion fractures of the medial angle of the patella (Figure 8.30b) are sometimes displaced proximally or medially. Lateromedial and cranioproximal-craniodistal oblique views are required to determine the location and extent of these fractures. Surgical removal of the avulsed fragment, sometimes together with the attached fibrocartilage, normally ensures a satisfactory clinical outcome, provided that there is no evidence of degenerative joint disease.

Sagittal patellar fractures involving the medial pole are sometimes seen in association with fractures of the lateral trochlear ridge of the femur (Figure 8.32) and this may affect the prognosis, unless recognized and treated accordingly.

Sagittal fractures of the patella involving more than the medial one-third of the bone carry a much poorer prognosis. Transverse fractures of the patella occur less commonly and are readily identifiable in lateromedial views. Treatment by internal fixation offers the best prognosis.

Occasionally an articular chip fracture occurs, which may only be detectable in cranioproximal-craniodistal oblique views (Figures 8.31a and 8.31b).

Femur

Fractures of the trochlear ridges and the caudal aspect of the femoral condyles can be demonstrated on caudal 60° lateral-craniomedial oblique views (Figure 8.32). They may be accompanied by fractures of the patella.

Fractures of the caudal aspect of the femoral condyles can be demonstrated on lateromedial oblique views, and usually occur with other injuries to the joint, which may seriously affect the prognosis. Care must be taken not to mistake fabellae (which are occasionally present at this location) for fractures.

Salter-Harris fractures of the distal femoral physis occur occasionally. Lateromedial and caudocranial views should be obtained. These fractures have a guarded prognosis, although internal fixation may be possible in younger animals.

Avulsion of the origin of fibularis (peroneus) tertius from the lateral extensor fossa of the femur occurs occasionally, usually in foals and rarely in adult horses, resulting in loss of function of the reciprocal apparatus of the hindlimb and lameness. One or more fragments may be avulsed and are usually displaced cranially and distally. The prognosis is poor in adults and guarded in foals, although removal of the fragments and prolonged rest have been successful in some horses. Avulsion of the origin of the gastrocnemius tendon on the distal caudal aspect of the femur occasionally occurs

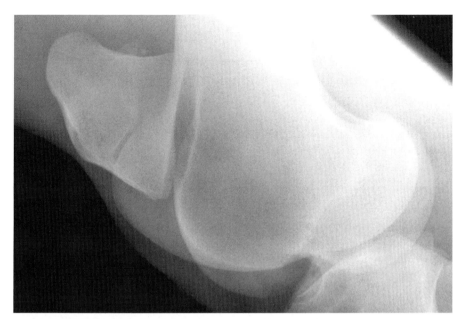

Figure 8.31(a) Lateromedial radiographic view of the left stifle of a 10-year-old Thoroughbred event horse with sudden onset lameness 3 days previously after hitting a cross-country fence. There was effusion in the femoropatellar joint. There are two mineralized opacities, fracture fragments, partially superimposed over the proximal aspect of the patella. Compare with Figure 8.31(b).

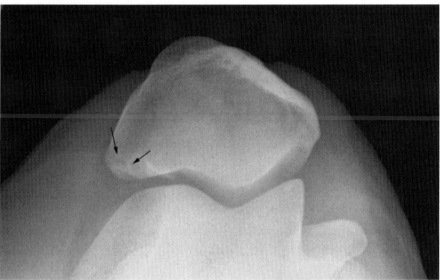

Figure 8.31(b) Cranioproximal-craniodistal oblique view of the same stifle as in Figure 8.31(a). Medial is to the left. There is a small articular fracture of the medial pole of the patella (arrows).

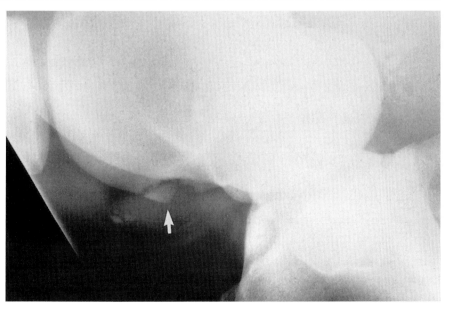

Figure 8.32 Flexed lateromedial view of a stifle of an adult horse with a fracture of the distal aspect of the lateral trochlear ridge (arrow). Note the more distal location of this fracture compared with the typical site of osteochondrosis. Cranioproximal-craniodistal oblique views also demonstrated a slightly displaced avulsion fracture of the medial aspect of the patella.

in foals; in adult horses muscle failure is more common. It results in inability to bear weight on the limb and dropping of the hock with partial weight bearing.

Tibia

Fractures of the tibial tuberosity or fractures of the tibial crest are best seen on a caudolateral-craniomedial oblique view (Figure 8.33). They are frequently the result of direct trauma, e.g. hitting a fixed fence. Care must be taken in horses less than 3 years of age to differentiate fractures from the normal apophyseal–metaphyseal physis (see page 366). The radiographs should be inspected carefully to determine the presence of comminution and to relate the precise fracture location to the insertion of the patellar ligaments. Conservative treatment of non-displaced fractures may be ade-

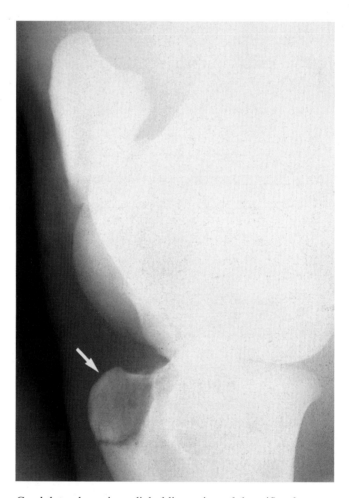

Figure 8.33 Caudolateral-craniomedial oblique view of the stifle of a 12-year-old Thoroughbred, 7 days after the onset of lameness. There is a slightly displaced avulsion fracture of the tibial tuberosity (arrow). The fracture is traversed by many poorly defined lucent lines. The horse was treated conservatively and made a complete recovery.

quate, although healing may be prolonged. If there is significant separation of the fracture, surgical repair or fragment removal may be required.

Fractures of the medial intercondylar eminence may be associated with damage to the cranial cruciate ligament (see page 396), but not necessarily so. In the absence of cruciate ligament injury, surgical removal of the fragment warrants a fair prognosis.

Fractures of the proximal physis of the tibia are rare.

Fibula

Fractures of the fibula may give rise to lameness (Figure 8.34). Care should be taken not to interpret normal lucent lines across the fibula as fractures (see pages 370–371). Fracture lines tend to run obliquely across the fibula and are normally associated with both resorption and callus.

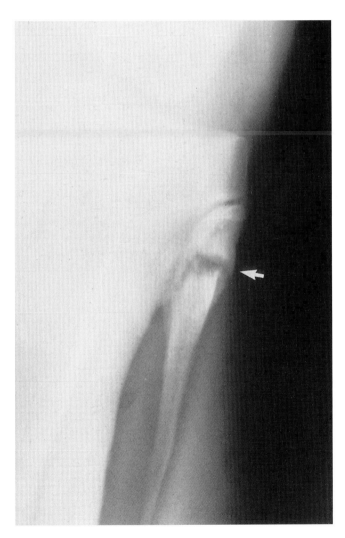

Figure 8.34 Caudocranial view of a stifle of a 10-year-old Thoroughbred. There is a slightly displaced fracture of the head of the fibula. External callus is present (arrow). This fracture became a non-union fracture and required pulsating electromagnetic field treatment to stimulate osseous healing.

Tibia

RADIOGRAPHIC TECHNIQUE

Good-quality radiographs of the tibia may be obtained using a portable x-ray machine and either rare earth or high-definition screens with appropriate film. Large cassettes are useful but it may be necessary to obtain radiographs of the proximal and distal halves of the tibia separately.

There is less muscle surrounding the distal half of the tibia, so exposure factors should be reduced accordingly. A complete assessment requires four views: lateromedial, caudocranial (or craniocaudal), craniolateral-caudomedial oblique and caudolateral-craniomedial oblique. The caudocranial view is best obtained by holding the cassette parallel to the cranial aspect of the bone and directing the x-ray beam perpendicularly to the cassette, i.e. obliquely downward. This is therefore more correctly termed a caudoproximal-craniodistal oblique view.

NORMAL ANATOMY, VARIATIONS AND INCIDENTAL FINDINGS

The proximal and distal aspects of the tibia are described on pages 366–379 and in Chapter 7 (pages 323–335). In the caudocranial view the tibial crest is superimposed over the lateral aspect of the proximal tibia, and in an immature horse the lucent line of the open physis should not be confused with a fracture. Lateral to the tibial crest is an obliquely orientated narrow or broad lucent line, the nutrient canal, which extends through the metaphysis and proximal diaphysis (Figure 8.35). There is a prominent ridge on the medial aspect of the proximal tibial metaphysis and this may be outlined in a caudocranial projection as a smooth irregularity of the medial cortex. Its outline will depend upon the angle of projection.

SIGNIFICANT RADIOLOGICAL ABNORMALITIES

Enostosis-like lesions and other focal opacities

Enostosis is defined as a mass of proliferating bone within a bone and is a general term used synonymously with bone islands in man and panosteitis in the dog. Equine enostosis-like lesions have been characterized radiographically as focal or multifocal intramedullary sclerosis in the diaphyseal region of long bones, near the nutrient foramen, often along the endosteal surface of the bone. In the horse they have been recognized most commonly in the tibia (Figure 8.36), humerus, radius and the third metacarpal and metatarsal bones. Their clinical significance is unclear, although in some horses they are associated with lameness that generally resolves with time. They should not be confused with endosteal callus secondary to a fatigue or stress fracture.

Small focal rounded radiopacities (Figure 8.37) have been seen in the proximal tibia. Their aetiology and clinical significance are unknown.

[406]

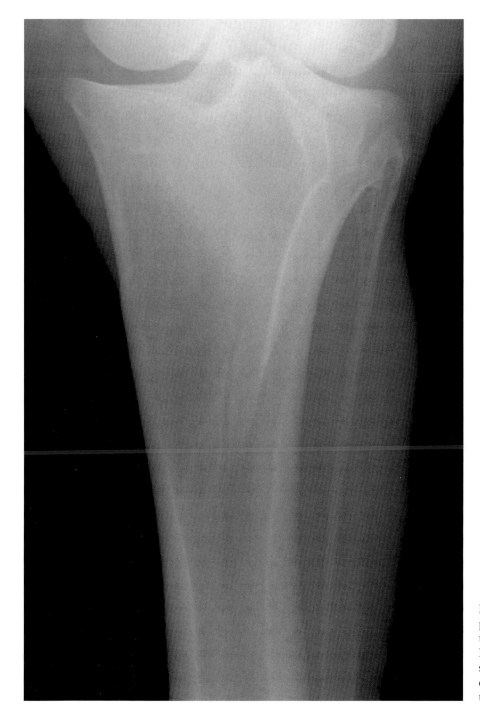

Figure 8.35 Caudocranial view of the proximal two-thirds of a normal adult tibia and fibula. Lateral is to the right. Note the oblique broad lucent line surrounded by mild sclerosis in the diaphysis of the tibia which represents the principal nutrient foramen.

Fractures

Proximal and distal physeal fractures are considered on page 405 and in Chapter 7 (page 358).

Complete diaphyseal fractures of the tibia are usually either mid-shaft oblique fractures or spiral fractures, and result in severe, non-weight-bearing lameness, soft-tissue swelling and crepitus. A complete radiographic examination should be performed if surgical repair is contemplated, in order to determine if the fracture is single or comminuted and to determine its

[407]

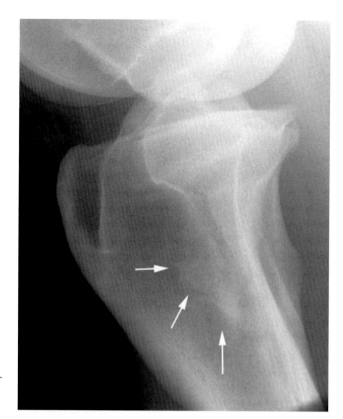

Figure 8.36 Lateromedial view of the proximal aspect of the tibia. There is an ill defined radiopaque area in the caudal aspect of the tibia (arrows), an enostosis-like lesion. This was not associated with lameness.

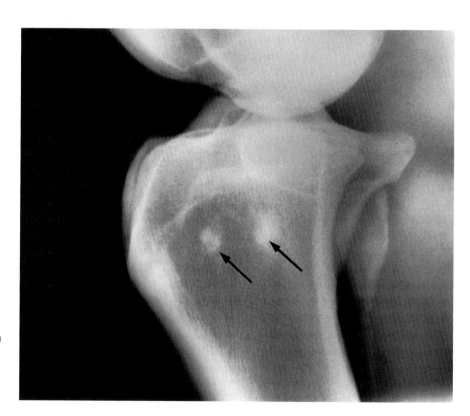

Figure 8.37 Lateromedial view of the proximal tibia of a 6-year-old Welsh Section A pony. There are two irregularly outlined opacities (arrows) in the medulla of the proximal tibia. Their aetiology is unknown. Note also the separate centres of ossification of the fibula.

precise orientation. Surgical repair may be successful in foals, but in older horses the prognosis is very poor.

Incomplete metaphyseal and diaphyseal stress fractures occur most commonly in young Thoroughbred horses and Standardbreds, and are associated with an acute onset of lameness, which may resolve rapidly. Careful palpation of the medial aspect of the tibia, where there is a minimum of overlying soft tissues, may identify a focus of pain. Swelling is often minimal and clinical diagnosis may be extremely difficult in the acute stage, without the use of nuclear scintigraphy. Radiographic examination in the acute stage may be similarly unrewarding. Repeat radiographic examination after 7–10 days may reveal a fracture line and slight callus formation may be evident where the fracture passes through the cortex (Figure 8.38). Alternatively endosteal sclerosis may be the only radiographic abnormality. However, in some horses radiographic abnormalities are never detectable. In the

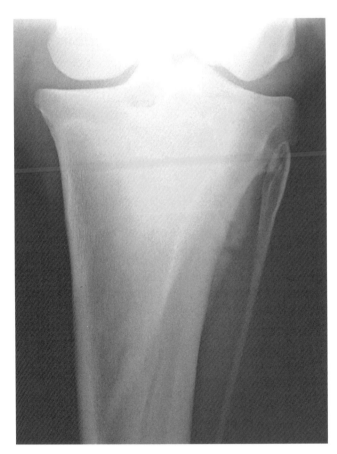

Figure 8.38(a) Caudocranial radiographic view of the proximal aspect of the right tibia of a 3-year-old Thoroughbred flat racehorse with sudden onset bilateral hindlimb lameness, which improved rapidly with rest. Medial is to the left. The radiograph was obtained 14 days after the recognition of lameness. There was focal intense increased radiopharmaceutical uptake in the proximocaudal aspect of the tibia. There is extensive periosteal callus associated with an incomplete proximocaudal stress fracture. Compare with Figure 8.38(b).

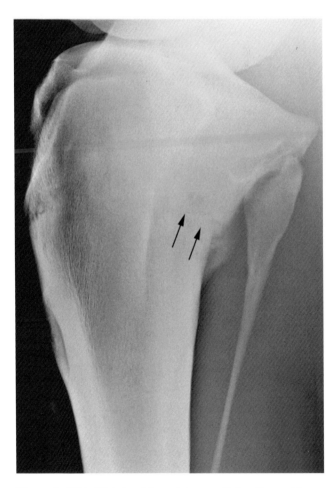

Figure 8.38(b) Slightly oblique lateromedial radiographic view of the proximal tibia of the same horse as Figure 8.38(a). There is an ill defined approximately horizontal fracture (arrows) of the proximocaudal aspect of the tibia, with extensive periosteal callus. Note also that the cranial aspect of the physis of the apophysis of the tibia is not fully closed.

Thoroughbred the proximolateral or proximocaudal aspects of the tibia are the most common sites for these fractures, which may spiral distally. Fractures also occur on the mid-caudal diaphysis and the distal metaphyseal region of the tibia in Thoroughbreds. In Standardbreds oblique mid-diaphyseal fractures are most common, with no tendency to spiral. Nuclear scintigraphy is generally a more sensitive indicator of trauma to the bone than radiography and increased radiopharmaceutical may be detected bilaterally, despite unilateral lameness. Most incomplete fractures heal satisfactorily if treated conservatively, although internal fixation has been used in selected cases to minimize the risk of the fracture becoming complete and possibly compound.

FURTHER READING

Adams, W.M. and Thilstead, J.P. (1985) Radiographic appearance of the equine stifle from birth to 6 months. *Vet. Radiol.*, **26**, 126–132

Arnold, C., Schaer, T., Baird, D. and Martin, B. (2003) Conservative management of 17 horses with nonarticular fractures of the tibial tuberosity. *Equine vet. J.*, **35**, 202–208

Baker, G., Moustafa, M., Boero, M., Foreman, J. and Wilson, O. (1987) Caudal cruciate ligament function and injury in the horse. *Vet. Rec.*, **121**, 131–321

Barr, E., Pinchbeck, G., Clegg, P. and Singer, E. (2006) Accuracy of diagnostic techniques used in the investigation of stifle lameness in horses – 40 cases. *Equine vet. Educ.*, **18**, 326–332

Bassage, L. and Ross, M. (1998) Enostosis-like lesions in the long bones of 10 horses: scintigraphic and radiographic findings. *Equine vet. J.*, **30**, 35–42

Bergman, E. (2007) Computed tomography and computed tomography arthrography of the equine stifle: technique and preliminary results in 16 clinical cases. *Proc. Amer. Assoc. Equine Pract.*, **53**, 46–55

Colbern, G. and Moore, J. (1984) Surgical management of proximal articular fracture of the patella in a horse. *J. Am. Vet. Med. Ass.*, **185**(5), 543–546

De Moor, A. and Verschooten, F. (1983) Subchondrale Knochenzysten und verwandte Läsionen beim Pferd. In *Orthopädie bei Huf- und Klauentieren* (edited by P.F. Knezevic), Schlutersche, Hannover, West Germany, pp. 244–250

Dik, K.J. and Nemeth, F. (1983) Traumatic patellar fractures in the horse. *Equine vet. J.*, **15**, 244–247

Dyson, S., Wright, I., Kold, S. and Vatistas, N. (1992) Clinical and radiographic features, treatment and outcome in 15 horses with fracture of the medial aspect of the patella. *Equine vet. J.*, **24**, 264–268

Embertson, R., Bramlage, L. and Gabel, A. (1986a) Physeal fractures in the horse 2. Management and outcome. *Vet. Surg.*, **15**(3), 230–236

Embertson, R., Bramlage, L., Herring, W. and Gabel, A. (1986b) Physeal fractures in the horse 1. Classification and incidence. *Vet. Surg.*, **15**(3), 223–229

Firth, E.C. (1983) Studies of the morphology of the immature equine radius and metacarpus, and its relationship to chondro-osseous disease. *PhD Thesis*, University of Utrecht

Foerner, J., Juzwiak, J., Watt, B. *et al.* (2006) Injection of equine subchondral bone cysts with triamcinolone: 73 horses (1999–2005). *Proc. Am. Assoc. Equine Pract.*, **52**, 412–413

Goulden, B.E. and O'Callaghan, M.K. (1980) Tumoral calcinosis in the horse. *N.Z. Vet. J.*, **27**, 217–219

Haynes, P., Watters, J., McClure, R. and French, W. (1980) Incomplete tibial fractures in three horses. *J. Am. Vet. Med. Ass.*, **177**, 1143–1145

Hermans, P., Kersjes, A., Van der Mey, G. and Dik, K. (1987) Investigation into the heredity of congenital lateral patellar subluxation in the Shetland pony. *Vet. Qtly.*, **9**(1), 1–8

Hertsch, B. (1980) Die Ossifikationsvorgänge am Kniegelenk beim jungen Pferde. *Zbl. Vet. Med. A*, **27**, 279–289

Chapter 9
The head

RADIOGRAPHIC TECHNIQUE

The head is a difficult area to radiograph, because it is mobile and high off the ground. A technique is described for obtaining radiographs of all parts of the head, but details on positioning, anatomy and significant findings are given under headings for individual areas. The use of tranquillizers (e.g. xylazine, romifidine or detomidine) may be beneficial, both for their sedative action and also because the head will be lowered, making the examination physically easier.

Because of the complex three-dimensional anatomy of the head there are some lesions that cannot be detected radiographically, but can be visualized using either computed tomography or magnetic resonance imaging. Computed tomography is probably most useful for assessment of osseous pathology, whereas magnetic resonance imaging is better for the evaluation of soft tissues, although it can also be used for bone.

Equipment

It is quite possible to obtain satisfactory radiographs with portable equipment. Because the head is anatomically complex, large cassettes (35 cm × 43 cm) should be used in order to maintain spatial relationships when evaluating the radiograph. It is often helpful to use both right and left projections in order to take advantage of both image sharpness and magnification in the localization of a lesion.

When obtaining radiographs of the head of a standing horse it is important to recognize that the holder of the horse is potentially close to the primary x-ray beam. It is essential to cone the beam down as much as possible. The horse holder should wear lead gloves and a thyroid protector in addition to a lead gown. A leather headcollar and its buckles may be superimposed over an area of interest, so the use of a rope halter may be preferable. With digital systems, even a rope halter may result in confusing artefacts. The x-ray cassette must be held by some mechanical device to reduce the radiation hazard to personnel and to minimize movement. A plate holder can easily be fixed to a wall, using vertical runners to allow adjustment for height, or it can be hung from a drip stand. This also to some extent restricts lateral movement of the head.

Usually only straight lateral and oblique views can be obtained in the conscious patient. Occasionally a dorsoventral view of the rostral portion of the head may be obtained. To obtain diagnostic films with correctly aligned ventrodorsal and occlusal views of the head of the horse, general anaesthesia is usually required.

[413]

A grid may be beneficial in all views of the head, except occlusal views. With portable x-ray machines, it is best to use either digital systems or standard rate rare earth screens and compatible film.

Positioning

Lateral view

A lateral view is normally obtained with the horse standing. The position for centring and the exposure factors depend on the area to be examined, e.g. the paranasal sinuses or the mandibular cheek teeth. If the horse is in lateral recumbency it is necessary to support the rostral end of the head to keep the midline of the head parallel with the cassette. Care must be taken that the head does not rotate along a rostral–caudal axis (i.e. turn sideways), and some support under the angle of the jaw may be required.

Ventrodorsal view

This view of the skull can only safely be obtained under general anaesthesia and it is difficult to obtain correctly positioned views. The horse is placed in dorsal recumbency and the head extended. It is generally not possible to bring the dorsal surface of the head to a horizontal position. For this reason, if the cassette is to be placed against the dorsal surface of the head (the preferred position), and not oblique to the head, a pad may be necessary under the cassette at the rostral end of the head to hold the cassette in position. If the cassette is to be placed far enough caudally to visualize the occipital bone, it may be necessary to raise the poll on a small radiolucent pad, or allow the head to become oblique to the cassette. The x-ray beam is aligned from the ventral aspect, in the midline, and perpendicular to the cassette. It is centred over the point of interest (Figure 9.1). The dorsoventral plane of the skull must be maintained vertical, as any degree of obliquity results in loss of information on the radiograph. It may be helpful to withdraw the endotracheal tube, if one is used, as this can mask abnormalities.

Oblique views

Oblique views are essential for evaluation of teeth roots, some fractures and for separation of the temporomandibular joints. The horse should be sedated and the head allowed to rest on a stand to minimize movement. If the horse is anaesthetized risk to personnel is minimized, the angle of obliquity can be more carefully controlled and repeat views can be accurately reproduced. The horse is positioned in lateral recumbency and the x-ray beam is angled relative to the head. In a standing patient, oblique views may be obtained by angling the x-ray beam and the cassette while keeping the head and neck of the horse straight. Alternatively rotate the horse's head towards a vertical

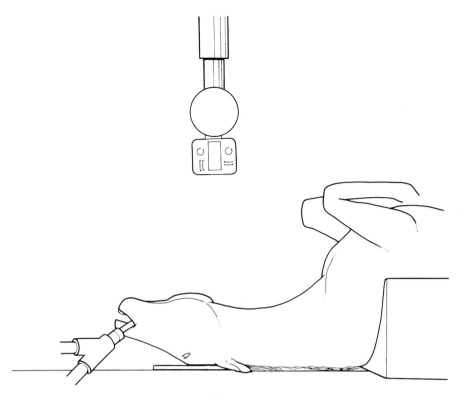

Figure 9.1 Positioning of the horse and cassette to obtain a ventrodorsal view of the head.

cassette, using a horizontal x-ray beam. The latter technique makes it more difficult to reproduce positioning accurately.

Cranium

This section covers the bony structures at the base of the skull which can all be visualized on one radiograph. It includes the cranial vault and the bony skull caudal to it. Also included are the ethmoid bones, part of the frontal bones, part of the vertical rami of the mandibles, and the atlas. The general positioning of the horse and equipment has been discussed above.

RADIOGRAPHIC TECHNIQUE

Lateral view

The x-ray beam is centred approximately 5 cm caudal to the orbit, and aligned at right angles to the midline of the head (and the cassette). When obtaining radiographs of the occiput it may be useful to pull the ears forwards to avoid their superimposition over the region of insertion of the nuchal ligament (see Figure 9.8b, page 429). This is easily done in a sedated horse by attaching sticky tape to the ears in order to pull them forwards.

[415]

Ventrodorsal view

The x-ray beam is centred on the larynx and aligned at right angles to the cassette.

Oblique views

There are no oblique views recommended as essential for examining this part of the head. They may be needed to examine the temporomandibular joints and the temporohyoid joints, as well as parts of the skull which are superimposed over the vertical ramus of the mandible, or that are masked by the very dense petrous temporal bone. They can also be used to determine on which side of the skull a lesion is present.

NORMAL ANATOMY, VARIATIONS AND INCIDENTAL FINDINGS

Immature horse

The skull is a complex structure; at birth a number of bones are not fully formed and many sutures are not fused. The ages at which these bones fuse and sutures are obliterated are given in Table 9.1.

Table 9.1 Fusion times for bones of skull.

Bone	Ossification centres at birth	Fusion of suture	Obliteration of suture
Occipital			
Parieto-occipital	1. Squamous	2 and 3 by 4 months	5 years
Spheno-occipital	2. Lateral	2/3 with 1, 12–24	5 years
Occipitomastoid	3. Basilar	months	Aged
Sphenoid			
Spheno-occipital	1. Presphenoid	Uncertain, but as foal	5 years
	2. Postsphenoid		
Ethmoid	1. Perpendicular	Uncertain, soon after	
	2. Cribriform	birth	
Parietal			
Parietal suture	One centre		4 years
Parieto-occipital			5 years
Premaxilla			
Left and right	One centre		4th year
Nasal			
Left and right	One centre		Do not fuse
Nasofrontal			1 year
Mandible			
Left and right	Two halves		3 months

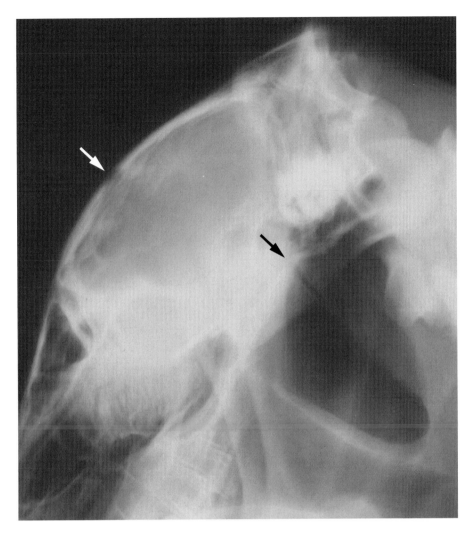

Figure 9.2 Lateral view of the cranium of a 1-month-old Thoroughbred. Note the radiolucency in the cortex of the frontal bones, an open fontanelle (white arrow). This normal feature closes by 3–4 months of age. Note also the clearly demarcated spheno-occipital suture line between the basioccipital and basisphenoid bones (black arrow). This is usually closed by approximately 5 years of age.

At birth, the cranium is rather more domed than in the adult and on a lateral radiograph a 'fontanelle' is evident as a radiolucency between the frontal bones at the rostral third of the cranial vault (Figure 9.2). This closes at 3–4 months. Also evident at birth is the nasofrontal suture, which becomes less evident over the first 6 months of life.

The spheno-occipital suture at the base of the cranium is seen on radiographs until about 5 years of age (Figure 9.2). It becomes a progressively less prominent feature as the foal ages. The position of the teeth in the maxillary sinus is different from that in an adult (see Figures 9.25(a) and 9.25(b), pages 462–463).

Skeletally mature horse

Figures 9.3a, 9.3b and 9.4 show normal lateral and dorsoventral views of the cranium of an adult horse.

[417]

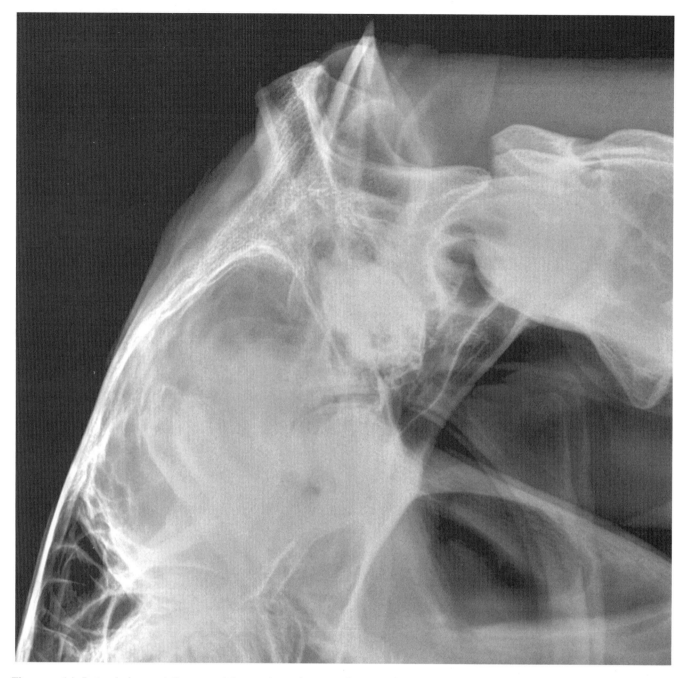

Figure 9.3(a) Lateral view and diagram of the cranium of a normal mature horse. There is slight rotation of the mandible resulting in separation of the right and left condylar and coronoid processes.

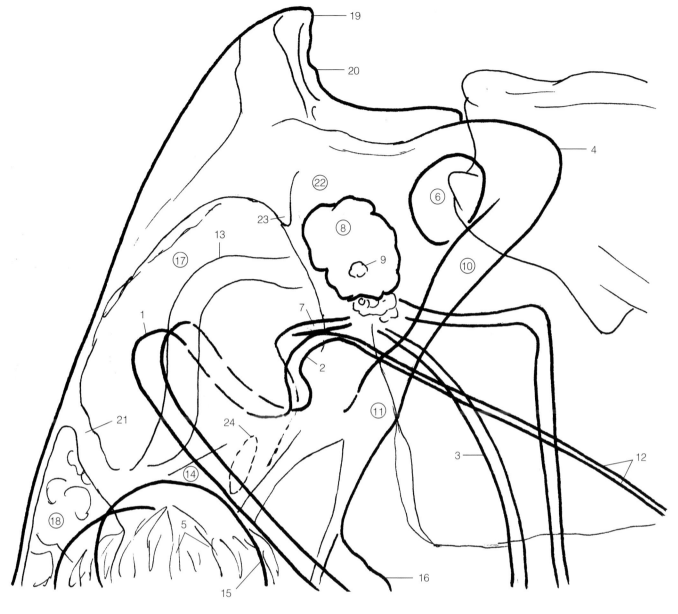

Figure 9.3(a) *Cont'd* 1 = coronoid process, 2 = condyloid process, 3 = stylohyoid, 4 = occipital condyle, 5 = ethmoid turbinates, 6 = hypoglossal foramen, 7 = temporomandibular articulation, 8 = petrous temporal bone, 9 = external acoustic meatus, 10 = basioccipital bone, 11 = body of basisphenoid, 12 = rami of mandibles, 13 = zygomatic process of temporal bone, 14 = zygomatic process of frontal bone, 15 = orbit, 16 = pterygoid process, 17 = cranium, 18 = frontal sinus, 19 = external occipital protuberance, 20 = external occipital crest, 21 = internal plate of frontal bone, 22 = caudal fossa of cranium, 23 = osseous temporal process, 24 = site of sphenopalatine sinus.

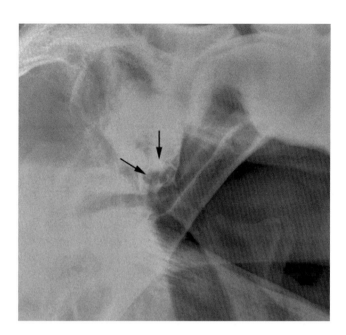

Figure 9.3(b) Close-up slightly oblique lateral radiographic view of the caudal aspect of the cranium centred on the temporostylohyoid articulation (arrows).

On lateral radiographs the cranial cavity is evident as a large oval structure. The dorsal aspect has a rather irregular appearance. Ventrally the base of the cranial cavity is superimposed on the dense articulations of the mandibles, the coronoid processes and the zygomatic arch, and is difficult to identify. At the caudal aspect of the cranial cavity, the two petrous temporal bones are evident as very opaque, irregular, roughly spherical bony masses.

The nuchal crest is a well defined structure on the caudal aspect of the squamous part of the occipital bone, the latter having a well defined medulla and smooth opaque cortices. New bone formation at the site of attachment of the nuchal ligament may be seen as an incidental abnormality, but may be associated with clinical signs (see page 425). Ventral to the temporal bones the basilar part of the occipital bone also has a well defined medulla, extending caudally to form the occipital condyles. The condyles have a smooth oval outline. Slightly oblique radiographs may reveal a small smooth depression in the caudal aspect of the condyles. This is a normal finding.

Rostral to the cranial cavity are the ethmoid turbinates which have a 'brush-like' appearance. Their caudal aspect is denser, roughly circular and surrounded by rather more opaque bone, the ethmoid plate. The rostral aspect of the ethmoid bones is superimposed over the maxillary sinus and additional radiographs may be required for satisfactory visualization.

Dorsal to the ethmoid turbinates are the frontal sinus and overlying frontal bones.

Ventral to the occipital and sphenoid bones are the lucent Eustachian tube diverticula (guttural pouches, see page 482), partly superimposed on the vertical rami of the mandibles. The outline of the trachea, pharynx, larynx and hyoid apparatus may also be seen (see page 482).

SIGNIFICANT FINDINGS

Dentigerous cysts

Dentigerous cysts (or temporal teratomata) of variable shape and size may be found in many positions (Figure 9.5). They frequently have an opaque core, composed of dental tissue, but may have less dense tissue surrounding it. They are frequently found around the base of the ear and in close apposition to the petrous temporal bones.

These cysts are usually only identified clinically after a mass is noted or a discharging sinus has formed. The introduction of a probe or contrast medium into the sinus is helpful in locating them. Dentigerous cysts can normally be removed surgically, the difficulty of the operation depending upon their position.

Choanal restriction

The choanae form the junction between the nasal and nasopharyngeal airways. Choanal restriction is relatively uncommon. Congenital total obstruction of the choanae may occur unilaterally or bilaterally, due to a bony or membranous septum, resulting in an abnormal respiratory noise, severe dyspnoea or death in a neonatal foal. A bony septum may be visible in a ventrodorsal radiographic view. If an obstructive membranous septum is suspected from endoscopic examination, it can be confirmed radiographically by observing blockage of positive radiographic contrast agent placed in the nasal cavities.

Narrowing of the caudal aspect of one or both nasal airways can occur, with or without deviation of the nasal septum, resulting in respiratory noise. Carefully positioned ventrodorsal radiographic views are required to document narrowing, with comparisons made between the two sides of the head, and between horses of similar breed, age and size.

Abnormalities of the nasal septum

Deviation of the nasal septum may be congenital, but is more commonly acquired and results in respiratory compromise. Acquired deformity is usually the result of an adjacent space-occupying mass and is usually readily identifiable in a well positioned dorsoventral or ventrodorsal radiograph. In a young horse with septal malformation, much of the distortion may be due to abnormalities of the soft tissues overlying the bone and may not be detectable radiographically, but can be visualized using magnetic resonance imaging.

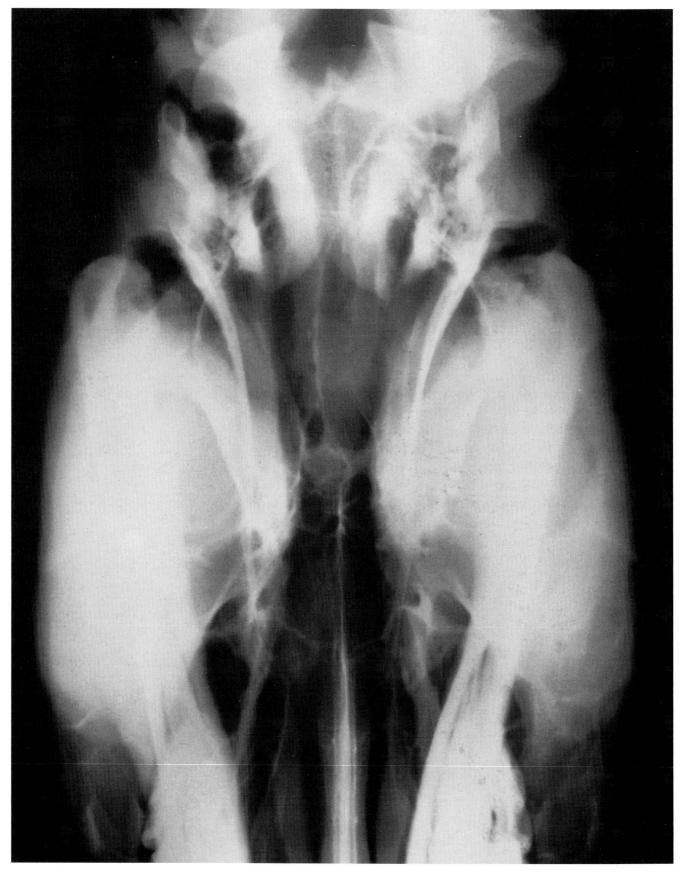

Figure 9.4 Ventrodorsal view and diagram of the cranium of a normal mature horse.

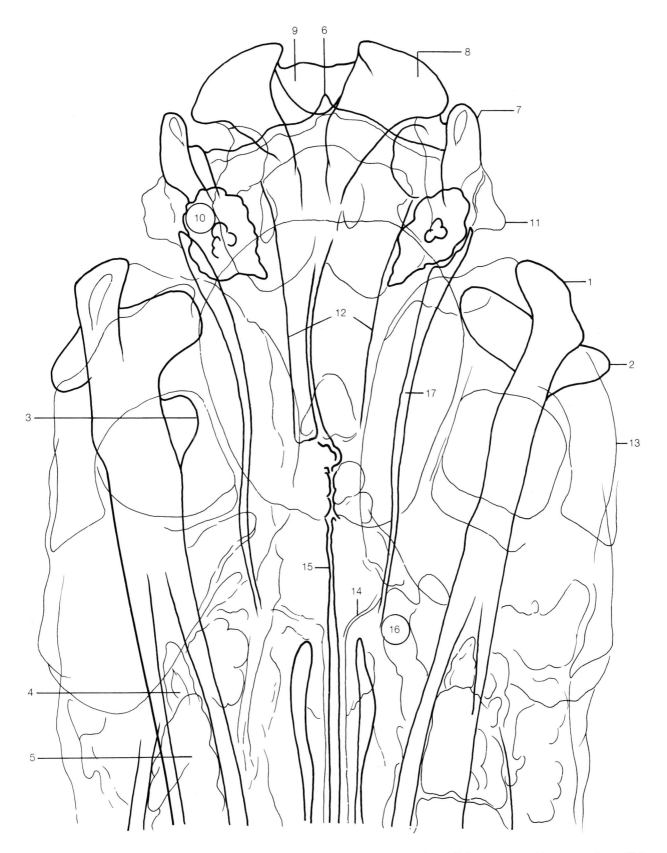

Figure 9.4 *Cont'd* 1 = caudal border of ramus of mandible, 2 = condylar process of mandible, 3 = coronoid process of mandible, 4 = third lower molar tooth, 5 = third upper molar tooth, 6 = nuchal crest, 7 = jugular process, 8 = occipital condyle, 9 = foramen magnum, 10 = tympanic bulla, 11 = mastoid process, 12 = basilar part of occipital bone, 13 = zygomatic arch, 14 = rostral border of choanae, 15 = vomer, 16 = ethmoid turbinate region, 17 = stylohyoid.

[423]

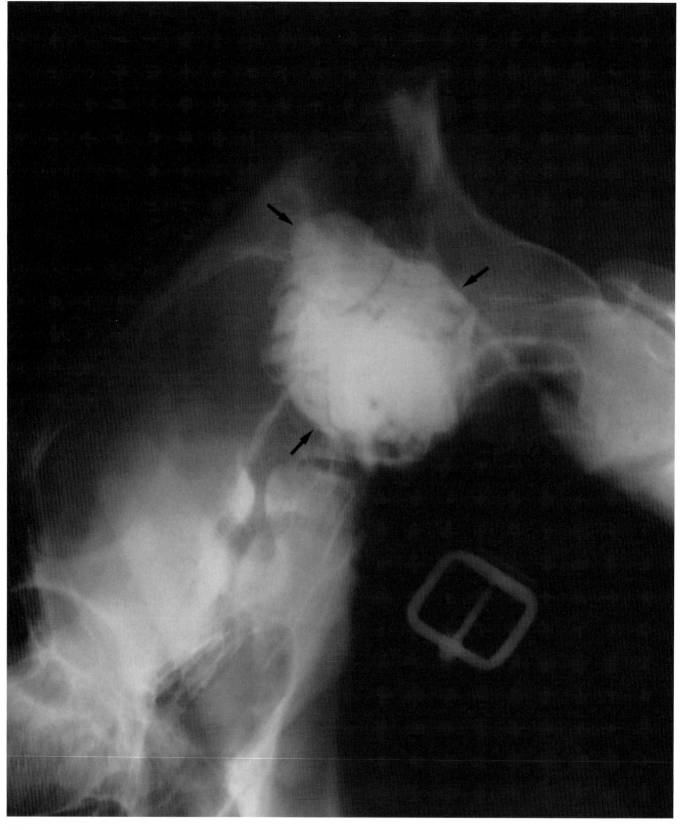

Figure 9.5 Lateral view of the occipital region of a 5-year-old Thoroughbred with a firm swelling distal to the ear. There is a large well circumscribed opaque mass (arrows) superimposed over the petrous temporal bone. In the dorsal part of the mass, a tooth-like structure can be seen. This mass is a dentigerous cyst.

Ethmoid haematoma and diseases of the Eustachian tube diverticulum

See pages 443 and 488–492.

Bony proliferation at the temporohyoid joint: 'otitis media'

So-called 'otitis media' in the horse may in fact be a misnomer. Clinical signs typical of peripheral vestibular disease and facial nerve paralysis are sometimes associated with specific radiographic changes, including an irregular increased opacity in the region of the acoustic meatus and articulation of the hyoid and petrous temporal bones, with or without fracture of the stylohyoid bone. Bony proliferation in the region of the temporohyoid joint may be visualized in an oblique projection (Figures 9.6a and 9.6b). The aetiology of these changes is not clear, although it is probably traumatic. Once the changes have developed, normal movement of the stylohyoid bone may result in haemorrhage into the middle and inner ear, giving recurrence or exacerbation of clinical signs. Surgical resection of part of the hyoid may give resolution of clinical signs and regression of the radiological changes.

Nasal polyps

Nasal polyps are soft-tissue masses that may partially occlude the airway and result in abnormal respiratory noise and/or nasal discharge. They appear radiographically as smoothly marginated soft-tissue opacities (Figure 9.7). They should be distinguished from soft-tissue opacities within a sinus, or an ethmoid haematoma, which may extend into the nasal cavities.

Hydrocephalus

Hydrocephalus in the horse is usually a clinical diagnosis, but may be confirmed by radiography. The cranial vault has a domed appearance, the overlying bones being thin. The cranial cavity has a homogeneous appearance. This condition is more common in the miniature breeds.

Entheseophyte formation on the occiput associated with the nuchal ligament

New bone formation may occur in the region of insertion of the nuchal ligament on the occiput (Figures 9.8a and 9.8b), also extending slightly dorsal and ventral to the site of insertion. This may be seen as an incidental finding, most commonly in Warmbloods. Clinically affected horses tend to resist the reins, find difficulty in flexion at the poll and may rear or head shake. The significance of the bony abnormality is determined by local infiltration of local anaesthetic solution. Treatment by local infiltration of corticosteroids and local anaesthetic solution, combined with modification of the training programme, has variable results.

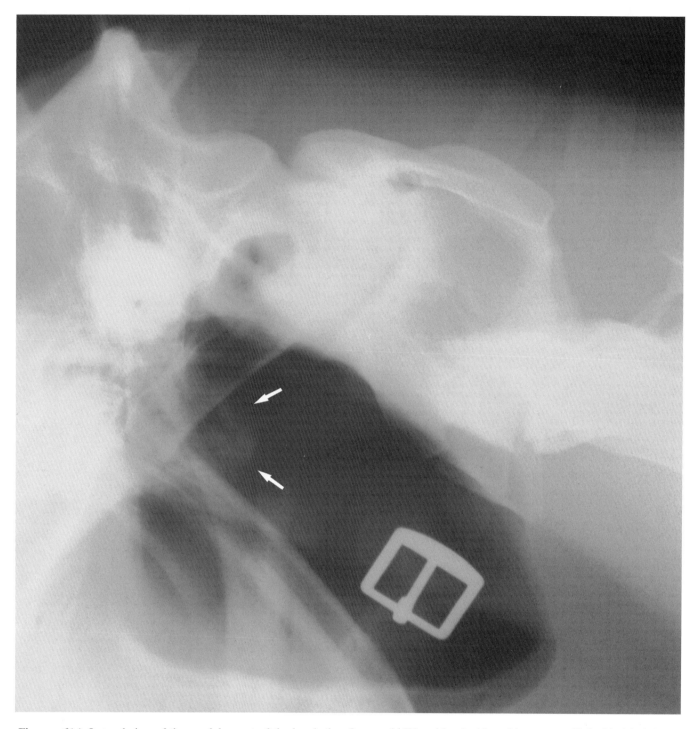

Figure 9.6(a) Lateral view of the caudal aspect of the head of an 8-year-old Warmblood with sudden onset of left-sided facial nerve paralysis, peripheral vestibular signs and keratoconjunctivitis sicca. There is a poorly defined area of increased opacity (arrows) in the region of the temporohyoid joint. See also Figure 9.6(b).

[426]

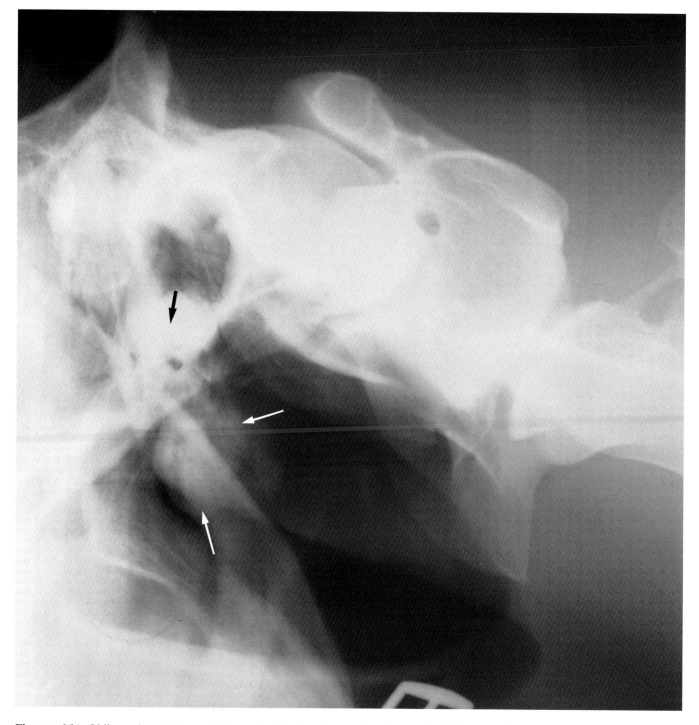

Figure 9.6(b) Oblique view of the caudal aspect of the head, separating the two hyoid bones and the rami of the mandibles. The opaque mass, new bone formation (white arrows), is much more easily seen than in the lateral view (compare with Figure 9.6a), and should be differentiated from the more dorsal acoustic meatus (black arrow). A piece of the stylohyoid bones was removed surgically. The bony mass regressed considerably and the horse made a complete functional recovery.

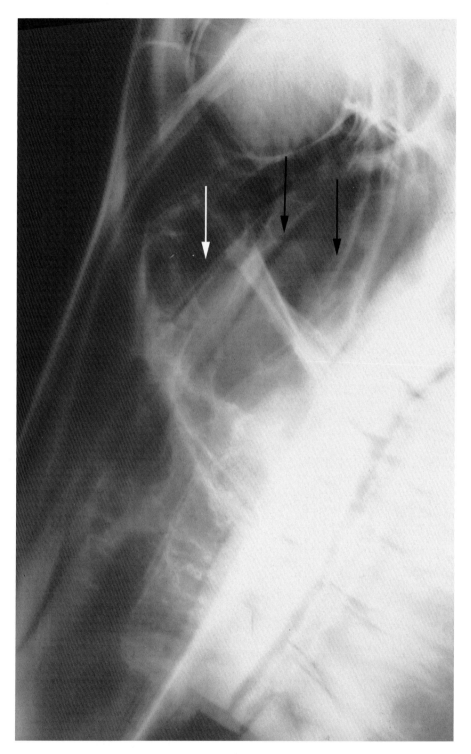

Figure 9.7 Lateral radiograph of the head of a 4-year-old horse with a 10-week history of a bilateral nasal discharge. Within the nasal cavity are several (at least three) well circumscribed soft-tissue opacities (arrows). These are nasal polyps. The paranasal sinuses are normal.

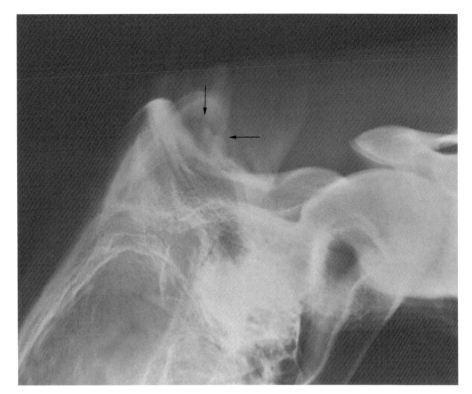

Figure 9.8(a) Lateral radiographic view of the caudal aspect of the head of a 7-year-old dressage horse. When ridden the horse would episodically throw its head in the air almost vertically. There is entheseous new bone on the caudal aspect of the occiput (arrows) at the insertion of the nuchal ligament. The horse's behaviour when ridden was markedly improved by infiltration of local anaesthetic solution around this entheseous new bone. Note that the opacity of the ears is superimposed over this entheseous new bone. Compare with Figure 9.8(b). Entheseous new bone at this site can also be seen as an incidental abnormality.

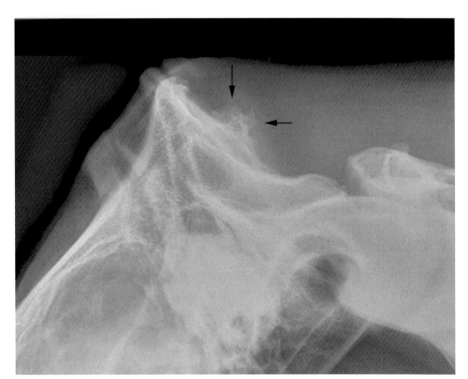

Figure 9.8(b) Lateral radiographic view of the caudal aspect of the head of a 7-year-old Irish Sports Horse event horse. The ears have been pulled forwards and taped. There is irregularly outlined entheseous new bone on the caudal aspect of the occiput (arrows). Compare with Figure 9.8(a). The horse had a recent onset of headshaking behaviour coinciding with the onset of sunny weather. The entheseous new bone is probably an incidental abnormality.

Fractures

Frontal bone

Depression fractures of the frontal bone are relatively common after trauma to the head. They can be seen on lateral or slightly oblique lateral views, and are best visualized when the exposure is made for the sinuses (page 433). They are evident, in an acute case, as an area of bone pushed ventrally relative to the remainder of the dorsal surface of the face. It is important to check for possible sequestra in more chronic cases. These cases should also be assessed for concurrent sinusitis and possible involvement of the bony orbit and lacrimal duct.

If treated conservatively, there is generally good functional healing, provided that sequestra do not form. It is possible to raise these fractures surgically to give more aesthetically pleasing healing.

Nasofrontal suture separation

This is a relatively common finding in young horses (Figures 9.9a and 9.9b). There is frequently no history of trauma, but a hard swelling forms across the dorsal aspect of the head, level with the rostral aspect of the orbits. On radiographs this is apparent on lateral views as a radiopaque protuberance of callus forming in the region of the nasofrontal suture. Typically the bone shows increased opacity either side of the suture, and initially a radiolucent suture line may be evident traversing the new bone. There may be concurrent involvement of the nasolacrimal suture and occasionally bleeding into the maxillary sinus is evident as a fluid line within the sinus. A degree of epiphora may be present temporarily, or permanently, if the area of suture affected involves the nasolacrimal duct. This lesion is of little clinical significance, but occasionally results in permanent disfiguration of the head.

Basioccipito–basisphenoid suture separation

This fracture usually occurs after direct trauma, typically a horse falling over backwards and hitting its head on the ground. It is most commonly seen in young horses, when the suture is not closed, and radiological confirmation of separation may therefore be very difficult. It is generally best visualized on good lateral and oblique views. Signs of separation include widening of the suture or the formation of a step deformity, however fractures with minimal displacement may not be detectable. In chronic injuries callus can occasionally be detected. Computed tomography may be a more sensitive means of detection.

Clinical signs reflect cranial nerve involvement and may include blindness, incoordination and slight nasal haemorrhage. The condition carries a very guarded prognosis, depending on the degree of clinical signs seen.

[430]

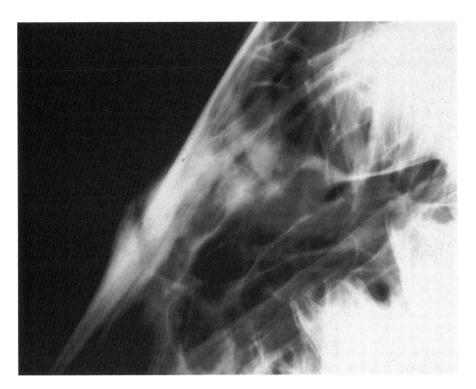

Figure 9.9(a) Oblique view of the nasofrontal region of a 6-year-old Thoroughbred. The history is of the development, over the past 2 weeks, of a firm swelling on the dorsal midline of the head, distal to the eyes. There is separation at the nasofrontal suture and associated incomplete bridging callus. The underlying sinus is of normal lucency.

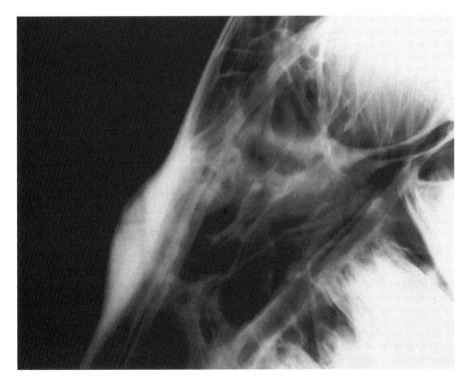

Figure 9.9(b) Oblique view of the nasofrontral region of the same horse as in Figure 9.9a, 6 weeks later. The callus is much more extensive and has a relatively smooth outline.

[431]

Avulsion fracture of the rectus capitis ventralis major and minor muscles from the basioccipital and basisphenoid bones

This is an unusual fracture that may occur if a horse falls over backwards and hits the poll, with the ventral neck muscles in tension. This results in traction forces being applied to the base of the skull by the paired rectus capitis ventralis major muscles, that insert on tubercles at the junction between the basioccipital and basisphenoid bones. There is usually associated haemorrhage, which may result in haematoma formation in the retropharyngeal space. Bone fragments may be seen ventral to the basisphenoid bone, sometimes close to the stylohyoid bone. There may be a step deformity at the sphenoccipital suture. Bone fragments may puncture the guttural pouch and haemorrhage may pool in the pouch. Increased soft-tissue opacity in the retropharyngeal region and guttural pouch area may obliterate the normal air-filled guttural pouches seen radiographically. Gas can accumulate in the subarachnoid and epidural spaces. In some horses fracture fragments cannot be identified, but a presumptive diagnosis can be made based upon the other radiological abnormalities.

Avulsion fracture of the nuchal crest

This is an unusual finding. It is associated with trauma and results in stiffness of the neck. A small radiopaque fragment may be seen caudal to the nuchal crest on lateral radiographs. A hopeful prognosis can be given with conservative treatment.

Fractures involving the orbit

Fractures involving the zygomatic arch occur as the result of trauma to the region of the eye. They are generally difficult to visualize on radiographs, but are most easily seen on lateral views of the cranial region. Slight obliquity of the view, to separate the two arches, may be helpful. Fractures may be simple or comminuted, with varying degrees of displacement. Although the prognosis for simple undisplaced fractures is quite good, displacement and comminution, causing remodelling of the orbit, often causes chronic ophthalmitis. Surgery to reduce displacement and remove sequestra may therefore be required.

Fracture of the mandible

Fractures of the vertical ramus of the mandible are usually visualized on lateral or slightly oblique lateral views (see Figure 9.37b, page 483). As the ramus of the mandible is relatively thin, fractures may be difficult to delineate and require several different exposures for complete visualization. The prognosis varies depending on the configuration of the fracture and the age of the horse (see page 480). Fractures of the horizontal ramus are discussed on pages 480–481 (Figure 9.37a).

RADIOGRAPHIC TECHNIQUE

Lateral view

The x-ray beam is centred midway between the orbit and the lateral opening of the infraorbital canal, about 2.5 cm dorsal to the facial crest. It is aligned at right angles to the midline of the head and the cassette.

Ventrodorsal view

The x-ray beam is centred in the midline between the horizontal rami of the mandible, approximately one-third of the distance from the caudal aspect of the rami towards the rostral aspect of the mandible. It is aligned at right angles to the cassette.

Dorsoventral views can be obtained in a well sedated horse, but careful collimation of the x-ray beam is essential to ensure safety of personnel. The x-ray tube is positioned in front of the head, with the beam angled obliquely downwards, perpendicular to the cassette. The cassette is held ventral to the mandible and parallel to it. It is not possible to evaluate the more caudal structures of the head (caudal to the maxillary sinuses) using this technique, and it is difficult to obtain true dorsoventral views without some degree of obliquity.

Oblique views

There are no oblique views recommended as essential for examining the sinuses themselves, although they may be helpful to separate overlying images. They are frequently required to determine the primary cause of sinusitis, especially to evaluate the teeth roots.

NORMAL ANATOMY, VARIATIONS AND INCIDENTAL FINDINGS

The lateral view allows visualization of lesions involving the frontal sinus, maxillary sinus and nasal cavity (Figure 9.10).

The frontal sinus appears triangular on lateral radiographs and is seen dorsal to the turbinate bones and rostral to the cranial vault. There are normally two distinct septa positioned in a dorsoventral direction across the sinus.

The maxillary sinus is immediately dorsal to the cheek teeth, which form the ventral border of the sinus. The appearance of this varies with the stage of development of the teeth. The sinus extends from the orbit caudally to include the last three or four cheek teeth rostrally (depending partly on the age of the animal). The dorsal border of the sinus is difficult to visualize on radiographs, but runs parallel to the facial crest, along a line roughly level

[433]

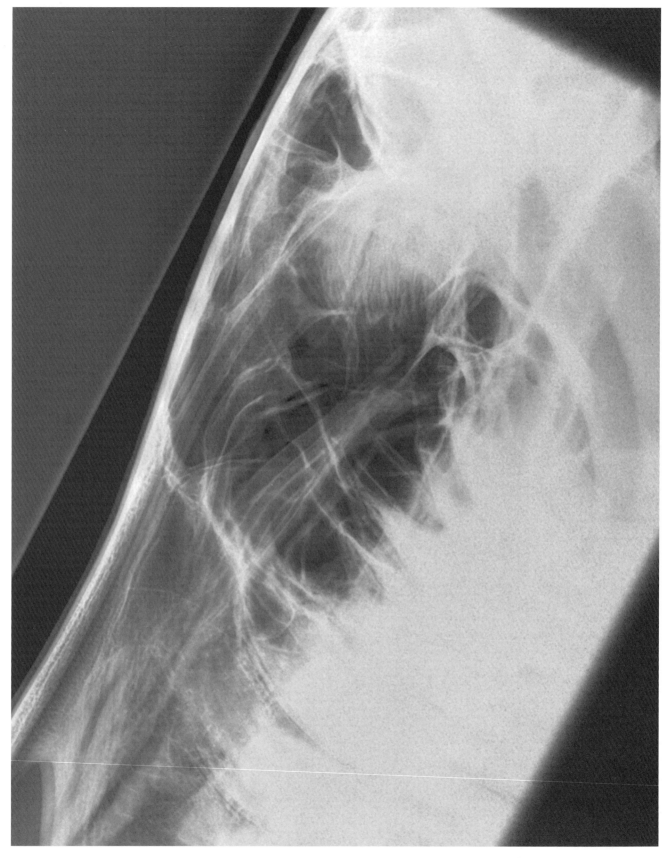

Figure 9.10 Lateral view and diagram of the nasofrontal region of a normal adult horse, exposed to evaluate the paranasal sinuses rather than the tooth roots.

[434]

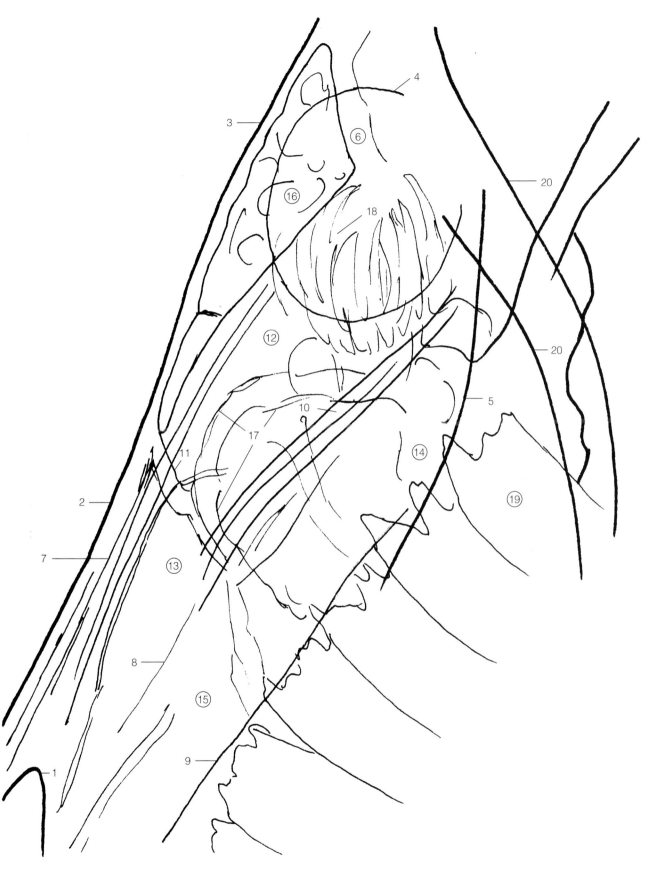

Figure 9.10 *Cont'd* 1 = nasomaxillary notch, 2 = nasal bone, 3 = frontal bone, 4 = orbit, 5 = facial crest, 6 = internal plate of frontal bone, 7 = dorsal nasal meatus, 8 = middle nasal meatus, 9 = ventral nasal meatus, 10 = infraorbital canal, 11 = conchal sinus septum, 12 = conchofrontal sinus, 13 = recess of dorsal nasal concha, 14 = sinus of ventral nasal concha, 15 = recess of ventral nasal concha, 16 = frontal sinus, 17 = margin of maxillary sinus, 18 = ethmoid turbinates, 19 = third upper molar tooth, 20 = cranial aspect of ramus of mandible.

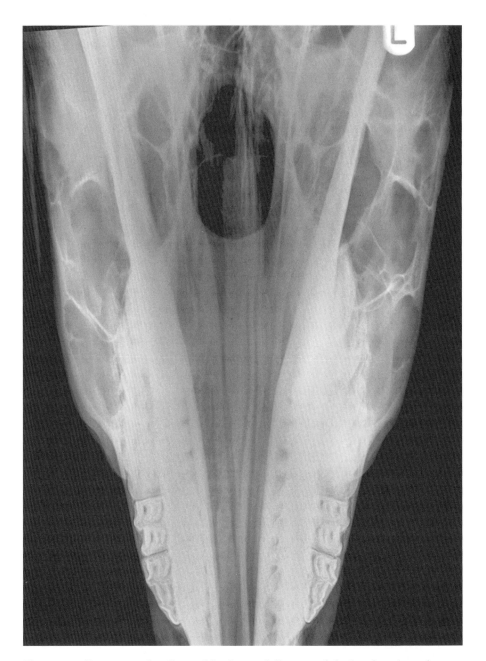

Figure 9.11 Dorsoventral radiographic view and diagram of the head to show the paranasal sinuses to the left and to the right, the rami of the mandibles and the nasal septum of a clinically normal adult horse. The well circumscribed radiolucent area represents air in the pharynx, rostral to the ethmoid turbinates, demarcated rostrally by the caudal aspect of the hard palate. Rostral to this radiolucent area the nasal septum is deviated slightly to the right of the image.

with the infraorbital foramen. The sinus is divided into rostral and caudal parts by a septum lying obliquely across the centre of the sinus.

The nasal cavities are medial and dorsal to the maxillary sinus.

On ventrodorsal or dorsoventral (Figure 9.11) views, the two horizontal rami of the mandible and the cheek teeth are the dominant features. The narrow nasal septum runs a straight course in the midline, between the two rami. The nasal cavity and turbinates are located on either side of the

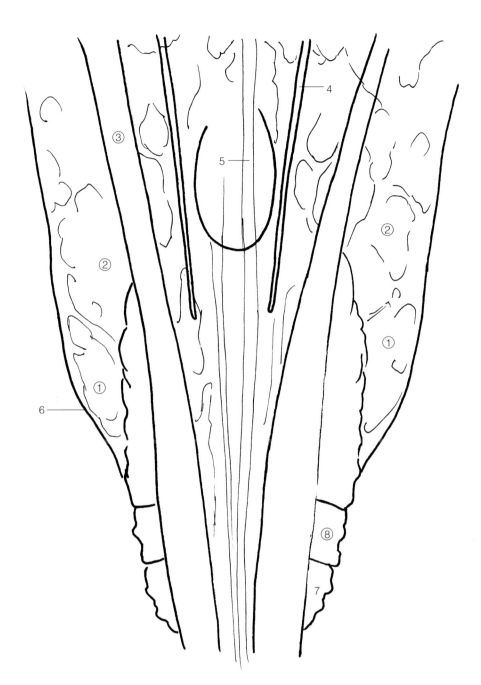

Figure 9.11 *Cont'd* 1 = rostral maxillary sinus, 2 = caudal maxillary sinus, 3 = mandible, 4 = stylohyoid, 5 = nasal septum, 6 = facial crest, 7 = second left upper premolar, 8 = third left upper premolar.

septum. A small portion of the maxillary sinus can be seen lateral to the mandible and cheek teeth.

SIGNIFICANT FINDINGS

Sinusitis

Sinusitis in the maxillary (Figures 9.12a and 9.12b) or frontal sinuses will usually give rise to increased opacity of the sinus on lateral radiographs. The

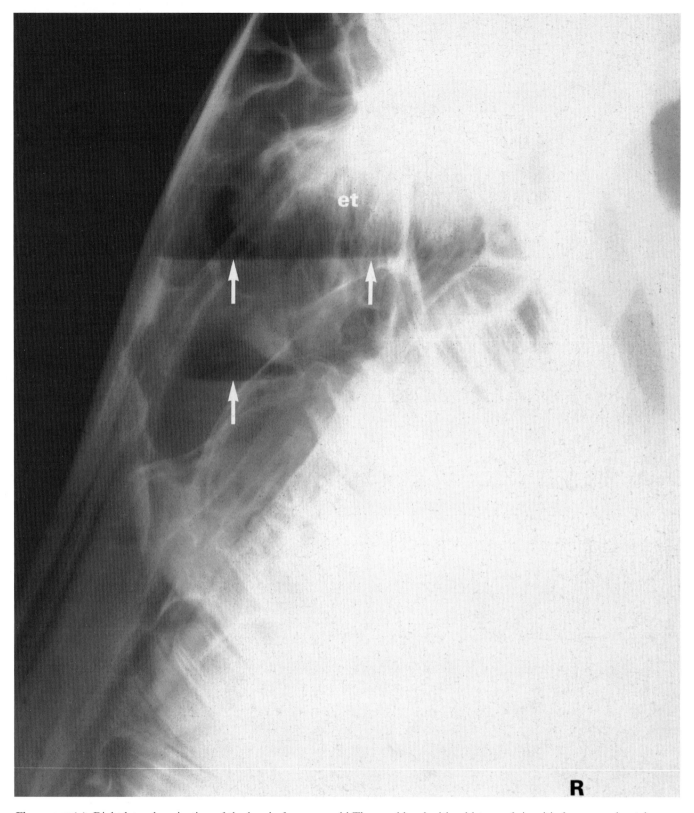

Figure 9.12(a) Right lateral projection of the head of a 2-year-old Thoroughbred with a history of sinusitis for approximately 12 months. There are fluid lines (arrows) in both the frontal and maxillary sinuses. In the right lateral projection the fluid lines were smaller and sharper than in the left lateral projection, indicating right-sided involvement. Note the position of the proximal fluid line relative to the ethmoid turbinates (et).

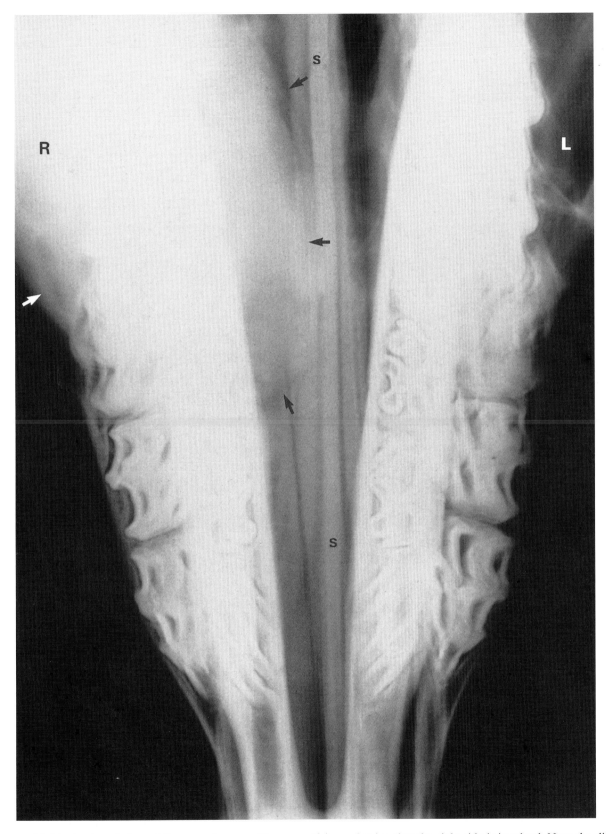

Figure 9.12(b) Ventrodorsal view of the same horse as Figure 9.12(a), confirming that the right side is involved. Note the diffuse soft-tissue opacity (arrows) in the right maxillary sinus (R) and the relatively more lucent left maxillary sinus (L). There is minimal deviation of the nasal septum (s).

radiograph must be correctly exposed, otherwise this increase in opacity may be missed. On standing radiographs, one or more horizontal fluid lines are generally visible in the sinuses (Figure 9.12a). When viewing the radiographs they should be positioned at the same angle as when exposed, if the fluid lines are to be horizontal. The radiograph should be carefully evaluated to determine if there is more than one fluid line, reflecting involvement of more than one sinus cavity. The fluid is generally of uniform opacity, unless there is inspissated pus, when it may be heterogeneous. The increased opacity should be distinguished from other causes such as a maxillary cyst or dental tumour (see pages 443–446).

It should be remembered that sinusitis in the horse is frequently secondary to other conditions, e.g. tooth root abscess, ethmoid haematoma, maxillary sinus cysts, or fracture. The radiographs should be carefully examined for possible causative conditions. It may be necessary to drain the sinus and obtain further radiographs before the primary cause can be identified.

Clinically, sinusitis is usually associated with a unilateral nasal discharge, frequently of a purulent and malodorous nature. Although some cases of sinusitis will respond to treatment with antibiotics, surgical drainage and correction of the underlying cause are often required.

Submucosal cyst

A submucosal cyst may result in deformity of the facial bones and new bone production. A soft-tissue mass is identifiable radiographically (Figure 9.13). Clinically the facial deformity should be differentiated from that due to a previous fracture, a sinus cyst or a tumour. The soft-tissue opacity should be distinguished from an ethmoid haematoma, sinusitis, or other causes of sinus opacity. In contrast to sinusitis a horizontal fluid line cannot usually be identified.

Maxillary sinus cyst

This condition is not uncommon, but can be difficult to diagnose with certainty, especially in the early stages. It usually occurs in young horses (up to 5 years old), but is occasionally seen in older animals. The presenting signs are usually facial swelling, respiratory noise or unilateral nasal discharge. A secretory lining is present in the sinus and this is fluid filled. In the early stages this may pass undetected on lateral radiographs, causing only a slight increase in the opacity of the sinus. The cyst may be loculated, facilitating differentiation from sinusitis, and may completely fill the sinus. The cyst may gradually enlarge and may cause distortion of the surrounding bone. Usually the medial wall of the sinus is gradually pushed towards the midline (mesially), and this may cause gradual progressive obstruction of the nasal passages and obstruction of the airway – this can be seen on ventrodorsal views (Figure 9.14). This view will also allow the opacity of the parts of the sinus seen lateral to the mandibular rami to be compared. In more advanced cases, there may also be dorsolateral displacement of the maxilla, causing a

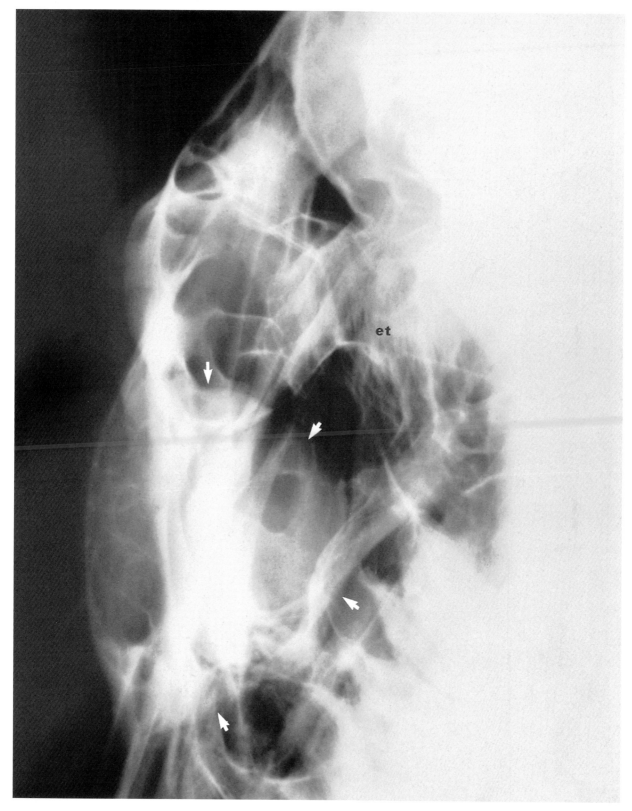

Figure 9.13 Right oblique view of the frontal area of a 10-year-old Quarterhorse with a history of a slowly progressive deformity of the facial bones on the right side. There is a well circumscribed soft-tissue mass (arrows) rostral to the ethmoid turbinates (et), extending dorsally and deforming the nasal and maxillary bones. This soft-tissue mass is a submucosal cyst. The sinuses appear otherwise normal.

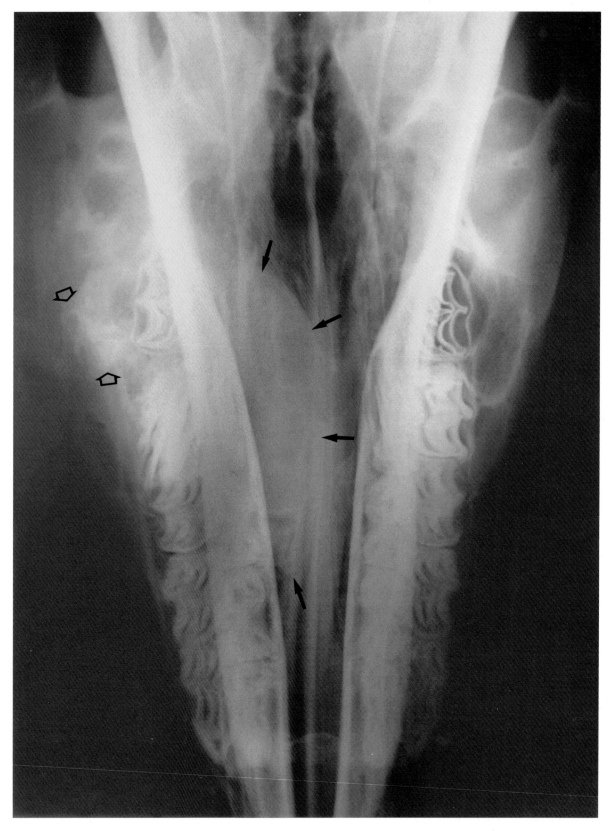

Figure 9.14 Ventrodorsal view of the head of a yearling Thoroughbred with stertorous breathing and an intermittent right-sided nasal discharge. Right is to the left. There is a large, well circumscribed radiopacity in the right maxillary sinus (solid arrows), axial to the molar teeth. Note the deviation of the nasal septum to the left. There is also an ill defined opacity (open arrows) abaxial to the molar teeth (compare with the left side). Diagnosis: maxillary sinus cyst.

gradual 'swelling' of the face of the horse. Treatment is by surgical resection of the cyst, including its lining.

Maxillary cysts

Multiple cystic lesions of the maxilla, usually involving the tooth roots, sometimes occur in young foals. Their origin is uncertain. This lesion may be seen on lateromedial views, but ventrodorsal views are also useful to visualize the extent of involvement of the maxilla hidden radiographically by the superimposition of the very opaque outline of the teeth. Multiple radiolucent, sometimes lobulate cystic lesions are present, often with enlargement in size of the maxilla. In extensive cases there may be little bone surrounding the cysts. Treatment is by surgical drainage, but the prognosis is guarded, depending on the extent of the lesion.

Ethmoid haematoma

This condition is usually characterized clinically by intermittent nasal haemorrhage, usually unilateral. Strictly speaking it is a condition of the nasal chamber and will only affect the sinuses in advanced cases. It is most easily diagnosed endoscopically, but it may be visualized on radiographs, and these may help ascertain the size and involvement of the lesion (Figures 9.15a and 9.15b). The lesion is of soft tissues and is therefore only seen as a slight increase in radiopacity. In early cases the lesion is seen on lateral views overlying the maxillary sinus immediately rostral to the ethmoid bone. It may be more easily seen on ventrodorsal views, where the opacity of the two sides of the head can be compared. In advanced cases there may be remodelling of the turbinate bones and nasal septum. The lesion may also invade the sinuses in some cases.

The condition is treated by surgical resection of the lesion and carries a fair to guarded prognosis. More recently, treatment by repeated injection of formaldehyde into the lesion has shown promising results.

Other causes of opacity of the maxillary sinus

The most common cause of opacity of the maxillary sinus is undoubtedly sinusitis. Frequently this is associated with tooth disease. In some cases, however, the tooth root may become surrounded by fibrous tissue, and this has been seen to extend into the maxillary sinus and may completely fill the sinus on one side. In rare cases this fibrous reaction may mineralize, giving discrete areas of radiopaque material within the sinus (Figure 9.16). These changes can be seen on lateral radiographs, but ventrodorsal views are needed to determine the extent of the lesion. These lesions require surgical treatment.

Although neoplasia is rare in the horse, tumours are more common in the head than elsewhere in the horse. Squamous cell carcinoma,

[443]

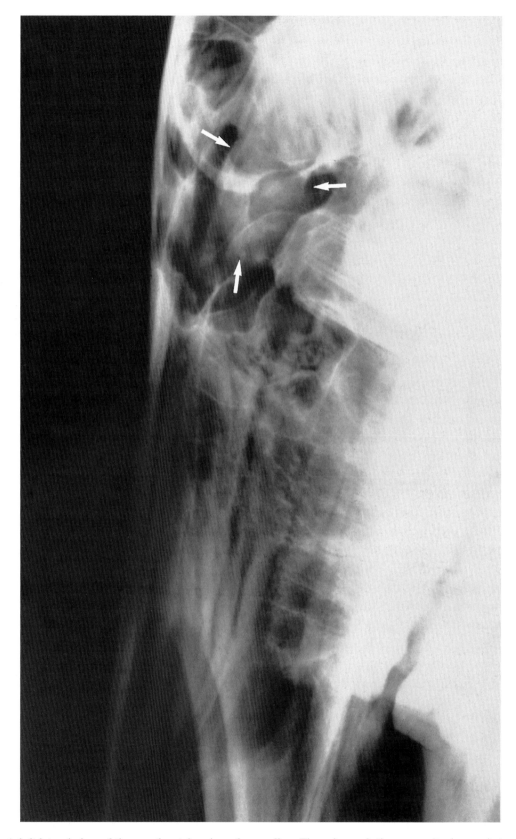

Figure 9.15(a) A left lateral view of the nasofrontal region of a yearling. There is a soft-tissue opacity (arrows) dorsal to the most caudal upper cheek tooth, adjacent to, and summating with, the ethmoid turbinates. The mass is an ethmoid haematoma. Note that this projection is slightly oblique: the cheek teeth are at different levels.

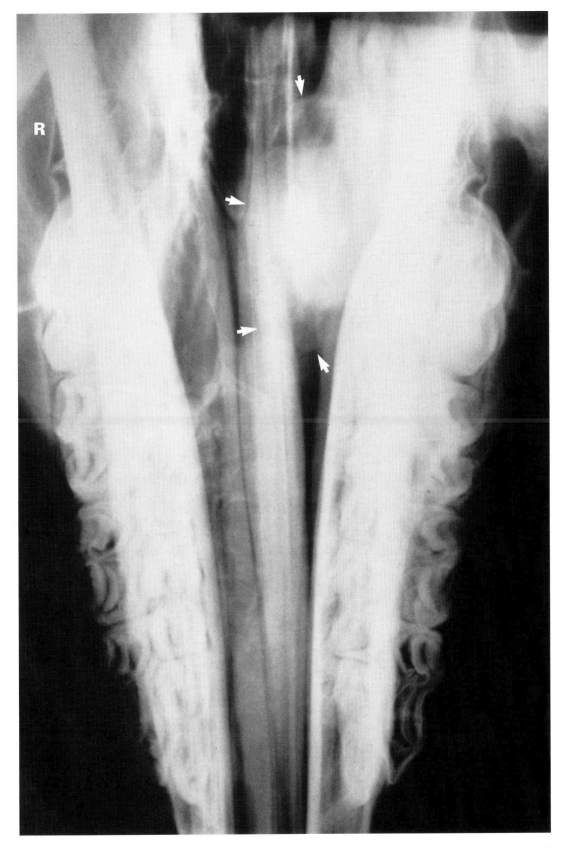

Figure 9.15(b) Ventrodorsal view of the same horse as in Figure 9.15(a) demonstrating much more clearly the soft-tissue opacity (arrows) axial to the most caudal left cheek tooth. There is slight deviation of the nasal septum towards the right (R). The mass is an ethmoid haematoma.

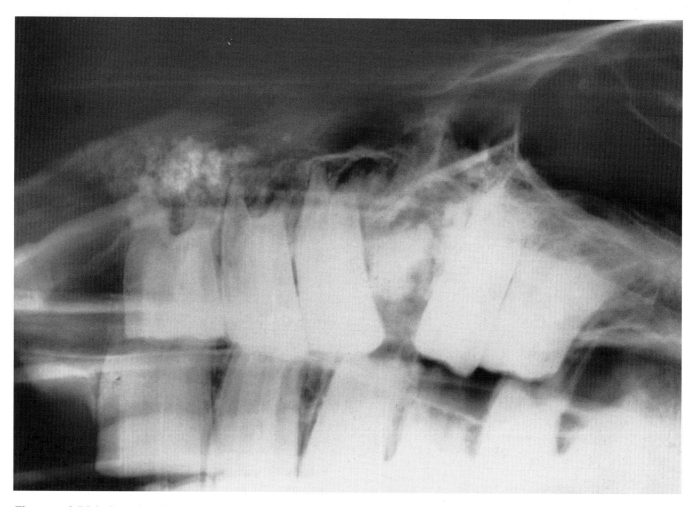

Figure 9.16 Right lateral oblique view of the maxillary region of a 10-year-old Standardbred. The horse had previously had the bulk of the fourth upper right cheek tooth removed, but a piece remains. There is periapical lysis (rarefaction) around the caudal root of the third upper cheek tooth. Dorsal to the first upper right cheek tooth is an area of dystrophic mineralization within the conchal sinus. The rostral maxillary sinus and the ventral conchal sinus communicate via the conchomaxillary opening. Such dystrophic mineralization ('coral') is invariably the result of chronic infection (usually dental in origin).

osteosarcoma (Figure 9.17), odontoma and melanoma may occur in this region, and have the characteristic appearance of neoplasia, as described in Chapter 1 (page 21).

Adamantinomas and ameloblastic odontomas are tumours derived from the enamel organ (the embryological precursor of a tooth), and are seen in young horses. Radiographically they appear as lesions of the maxilla or mandible and have a variable appearance. An adamantinoma remains as primarily soft tissue and has a septate configuration, resulting in a 'foamy' appearance. An odontoma is derived from dental residues and tends to have a more opaque tooth-like structure (Figures 9.18a and 9.18b).

Osteomas are benign, smoothly outlined, opaque tumours. They may become very large before being detected, as they grow slowly and cause few clinical signs. They have been associated with head shaking.

[446]

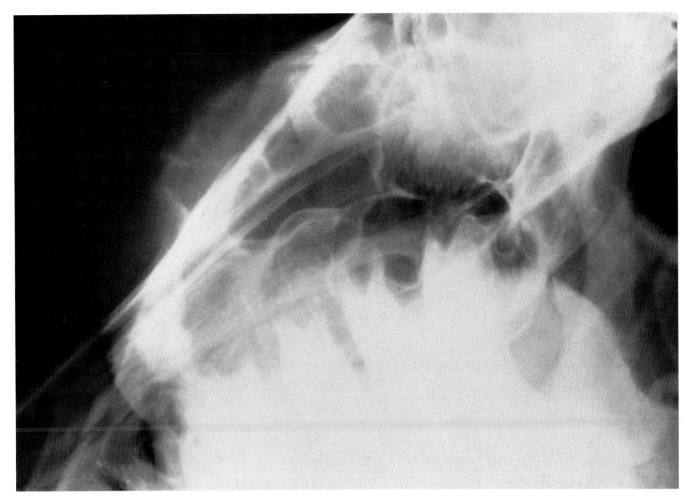

Figure 9.17 Lateral view of the nasofrontal region of an aged Thoroughbred with facial swelling. There is a large opaque mass occupying the region of the frontal and maxillary sinuses and distorting the frontal and nasal bones. The mass was identified as an osteosarcoma at post-mortem examination.

Adenocarcinomas occur in the frontal sinus and the nasal cavity. They occur in older animals and are very destructive. They are rapid growing and tend to be ill defined. There is usually an associated unilateral nasal discharge.

Increased lucency of the maxillary sinus

Increased lucency of the bone surrounding the maxillary sinus has been seen associated with neoplasia (see page 446) and maxillary cysts (see page 443).

Cyst-like lesions of the incisive bone (premaxilla)

Cyst-like lesions occasionally develop in the incisive bone (premaxilla). These are expansile lesions that usually result in distortion of the facial contour and thinning of the overlying cortex (Figures 9.19a and 9.19b).

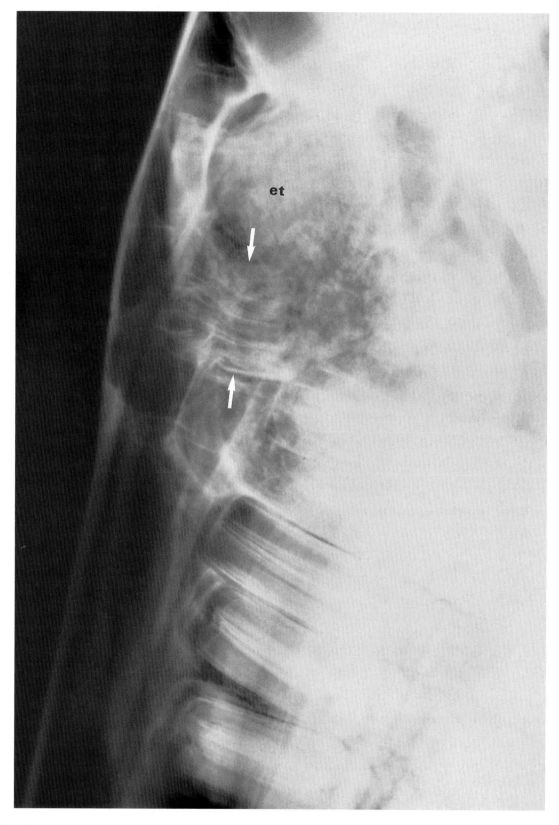

Figure 9.18(a) Slightly oblique left lateral view of the nasofrontal region of a 3-year-old Thoroughbred with a recent history of swelling below the left eye, left-sided mucoid nasal discharge and dyspnoea. There is a large mass of irregular opacity in the region of the most caudal upper cheek tooth. Within the mass are several opacities resembling teeth (arrows); et = ethmoid turbinates.

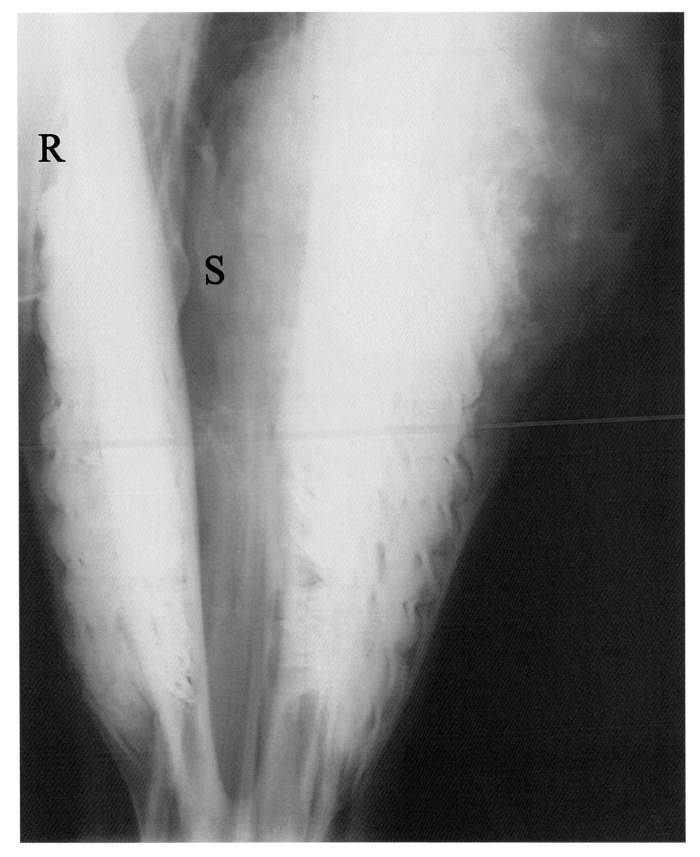

Figure 9.18(b) Ventrodorsal view of the same horse as in Figure 9.18(a), clearly demonstrating the mass and showing marked distortion of the nasal septum (S) towards the right (R) and narrowing of the nasal passage. Post-mortem examination confirmed that the mass was an ameloblastic odontoma.

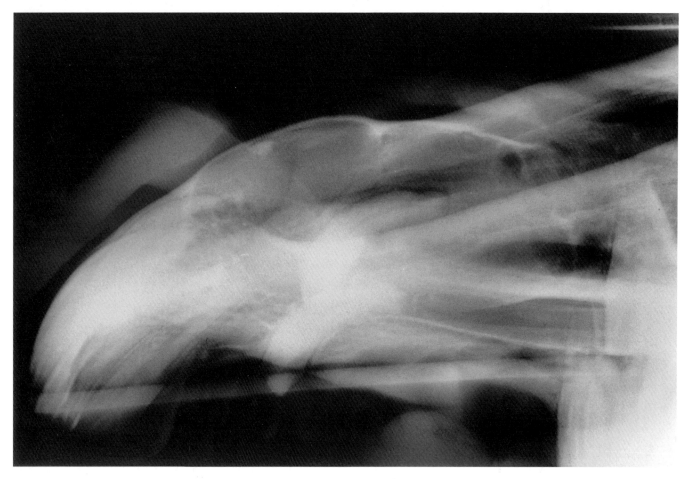

Figure 9.19(a) Right oblique view of the rostral head region of an aged pony with a slowly enlarging facial swelling. There is a cyst-like lesion in the incisive bone (premaxilla), distorting its dorsal contour. The overlying cortex is thinned and has a slightly scalloped appearance caudally.

Teeth and mandible

Indications for evaluation of the teeth include quidding, weight loss, facial swelling, unilateral nasal discharge, oral malodour, difficulties in eating, oral discomfort, reluctance to accept the bit and head shaking.

The Triadan system of tooth numbering has been adopted by veterinarians dealing with dentistry, thus replacing the terms incisor, canine, premolar and molar (cheek) teeth. This can be confusing to the uninformed. The teeth are numbered sequentially 0–11 from the central incisor caudally; the right maxillary teeth are prefixed 1, the left maxillary cheek teeth are prefixed 2, the left mandibular teeth are prefixed 3 and the right mandibular teeth are prefixed 4 (Table 9.2). We have maintained traditional terminology in this text, but provide this table as a reference source.

[450]

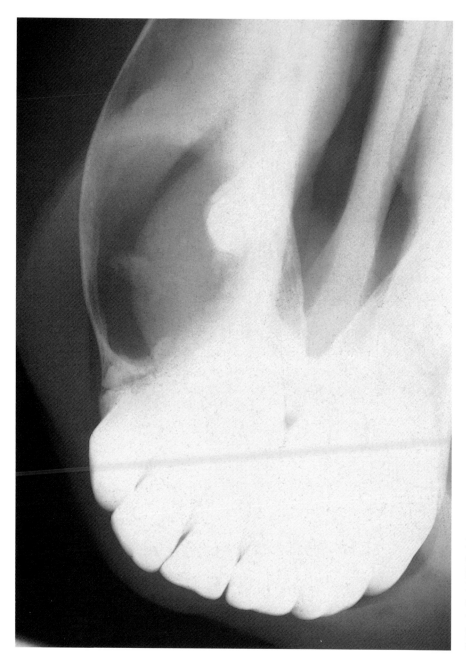

Figure 9.19(b) Slightly oblique dorsoventral, occlusal view of the incisive region (the same horse as in Figure 9.19a). The cyst-like lesion is well defined. There are ill defined opacities within it. The right canine tooth is partially superimposed over the axial aspect of the cyst-like lesion.

Table 9.2 The Triadan method of tooth numbering.

Tooth	Maxillary teeth		Mandibular teeth	
	Right	Left	Right	Left
Central incisor	101	201	401	301
Middle incisor	102	202	402	302
Corner incisor	103	203	403	303
Canine (tush)	104	204	404	304
Vestigial 1st premolar/wolf tooth	105	205	(405)	(305)
2nd premolar/1st cheek tooth	106	206	406	306
3rd premolar/2nd cheek tooth	107	207	407	307
4th premolar/3rd cheek tooth	108	208	408	308
1st molar/4th cheek tooth	109	209	409	309
2nd molar/5th cheek tooth	110	210	410	310
3rd molar/6th cheek tooth	111	211	411	311

Mandible

The views described below for the teeth, and on page 415 for the cranium, are also used to visualize the mandible. The exposure factors required for teeth and bone, however, are very different, and several radiographs may be needed of each area to acquire all the available information.

Temporomandibular joint

The temporomandibular joint can be examined using lateromedial views obtained with the head in the sagittal plane or rotated to facilitate separation of the left and right sides. However, to avoid superimposition, a skyline view can be used to assess the left and right joints independently. The horse's head is supported on a stand with adjustable height so that the poll is extended and the muzzle is almost horizontal (Figure 9.20). The x-ray tube is positioned below and to the side of the head to be examined, directed caudally. The x-ray beam is directed at an angle of 35° to the long axis of the head and 50° proximally. A cassette is positioned horizontally above the poll, held in a cassette holder. The x-ray beam should be well collimated and

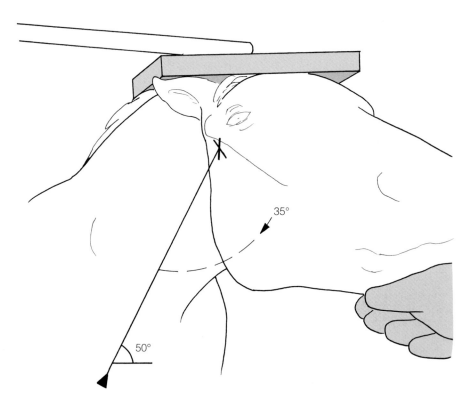

Figure 9.20 Positioning of the horse, x-ray beam and imaging plate to obtain a rostral 35° lateral 50° ventral-caudodorsal oblique view of the temporomandibular joint.

personnel should wear lead gloves. This rostral 35° lateral 50° proximal-caudal oblique view allows good visualization of the lateral aspect of the temporomandibular joint (Figure 9.27, page 465).

Cheek teeth

Lateral view

Satisfactory lateral views can usually be obtained with the horse standing. The x-ray beam is centred at the point where the first molars (fourth cheek teeth) of the upper and lower jaws meet. The x-ray beam is aligned at right angles to the midline of the head and the cassette.

Ventrodorsal view

A ventrodorsal view is best and most safely obtained with the horse in dorsal recumbency under general anaesthesia. It is important to ensure that the midline of the head is positioned vertically, to avoid oblique views. The x-ray beam is centred in the midline between the horizontal rami of the two mandibles, at the level of the first molars. In a standing horse dorsoventral radiographic views of adequate quality can be obtained in a co-operative patient, using the technique described on page 433. It is more difficult to evaluate the most caudal cheek teeth using this method.

Oblique views

Oblique views are essential to view the roots of the teeth satisfactorily, since their density precludes examination of one tooth superimposed over another. Radiographs are most easily obtained with the horse in lateral recumbency, with the head resting on the cassette, but can also be obtained in a standing horse (see below). The best radiographs are obtained with the teeth of interest against the cassette, although for clinical reasons it is often more practicable to have these teeth uppermost. To view the teeth against the cassette, the x-ray beam is then angled dorsally 30° to visualize the maxillary roots or ventrally 30° to visualize the mandibular roots (Figure 9.21). The x-ray beam should be centred on the root to be examined. If the tooth of interest is uppermost, then the angulation of the x-ray beam is reversed.

It is possible to separate the left and right tooth arcades with the horse standing. For maximum safety the x-ray beam should be collimated as tightly as possible. It is usually easiest to rotate the horse's head towards or away from the cassette, which is positioned vertically, using a horizontal x-ray beam. If the head is turned towards the cassette, the maxillary cheek teeth nearest the x-ray tube and the mandibular cheek teeth roots nearest the cassette will be visualized.

Alternatively, the head can be maintained in a neutral position. The tooth roots to be examined are positioned closest to the cassette, which is

[453]

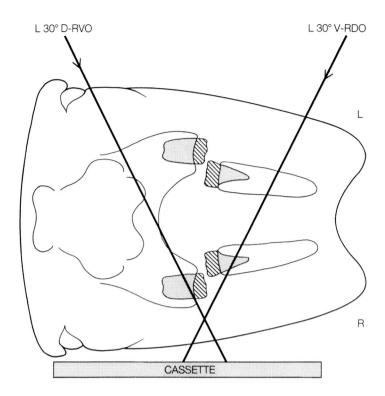

L 30° D-RVO   L 30° V-RDO

L

R

CASSETTE

Figure 9.21 Diagrammatic transverse section of head to show angulation of the x-ray beam to obtain views of the right maxillary (L30°D-RVO) and mandibular (L30°V-RDO) cheek teeth roots with the horse in right lateral recumbency under general anaesthesia.

positioned perpendicular to the angle of the x-ray beam. To examine the roots of the maxillary cheek teeth, the x-ray beam is angled obliquely from midline in front of the head, 60° to the side away from the cassette, 30° proximal towards the cassette (Figure 9.22). For the roots of the mandibular cheek teeth, the obliquity of the x-ray beam is reversed. Using this second technique it is easier to reproduce the angle of projection accurately. The precise angle of the x-ray beam needed to evaluate the mandibular cheek teeth varies depending on the intermandibular width; a more horizontal x-ray beam is required for a broad head and a more vertical x-ray beam for a narrow head.

Open-mouth oblique views

Open-mouth oblique views are necessary to view the erupted crowns of the maxillary and mandibular cheek teeth. The horse is sedated, and the mouth is held open using a Butler's gag, or preferably a non-radiopaque object such as a PVC cylinder or a piece of wood placed between the incisors. The degree to which the mouth is opened will depend on the size of the pony or horse. The head is held straight and the cassette, supported in a cassette holder, is positioned parallel to the long axis of the horse's head. The x-ray beam is carefully collimated and is directed perpendicular to the long axis of the horse's head, centred at the rostral extremity of the facial crest, at the level of the occlusal surfaces of the cheek teeth (Figure 9.23). Angling the

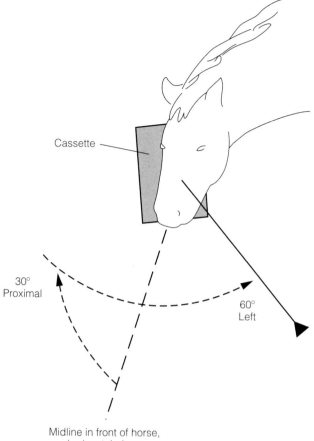

Cassette

30°
Proximal

60°
Left

Midline in front of horse,
horizontal plane

Figure 9.22 Positioning to obtain oblique views of the upper cheek teeth in a standing horse, with the head in a neutral position. The teeth to be examined are closest to the cassette. The x-ray beam must be tightly collimated to ensure safety of personnel.

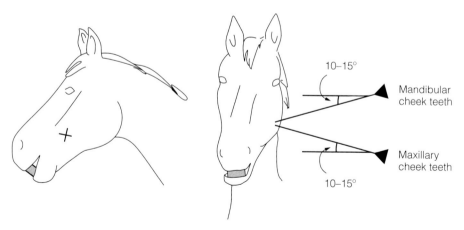

10–15°

Mandibular
cheek teeth

Maxillary
cheek teeth

10–15°

Figure 9.23 Technique for obtaining open-mouth oblique views of the teeth. The mouth is held open as far as possible. The imaging plate is positioned parallel to the long axis of the horse's head. The x-ray beam is directed 10–15° to evaluate the contralateral mandibular or maxillary cheek teeth.

[455]

beam 10–15° dorsal or ventral projects the occlusal surfaces clear of the bulk of the teeth (Figure 9.26, page 465). A lateral 15° proximal view is used to evaluate the contralateral maxillary cheek teeth and a lateral 10° distal view is used to image the contralateral mandibular cheek teeth. The precise angles for optimal evaluation of the cheek teeth crowns are variable depending on a number of factors such as mandibular width and tooth wear. It is frequently not possible to view all the tooth surfaces on one view, and a number of views of slightly differing obliquity may be needed. Angulation depends upon the absolute size of the skull, the length of the erupted crown, the presence of abnormalities of wear and the degree of angulation of the curve of Spee (the dorsal curvature of the occlusal surface of the caudal three cheek teeth). If the x-ray beam is not perpendicular to the long axis of the horse's head this may result in distortion and overlapping of the cheek teeth crowns.

Incisors

Lateral view

The x-ray beam is centred at the rostral aspect of the head, on the occlusal surfaces of the incisor teeth. It is aligned at right angles to the midline of the head and the cassette.

Ventrodorsal view

In an anaesthetized horse a ventrodorsal view is obtained with the x-ray beam centred on the ventral aspect of the muzzle of the horse, and the x-ray cassette against the dorsal aspect of the head. It is also possible to obtain occlusal films of the incisor teeth, placing the cassette in the oral cavity, so that only the upper or lower teeth are visualized on the film. In a standing patient a dorsoventral view is more practicable. Occlusal films are rarely possible in a conscious patient.

Oblique views

Oblique views are not essential for routine examination of the incisor teeth, because the occlusal films give excellent visualization. They are, however, sometimes beneficial for examination of specific lesions, especially in conscious patients.

NORMAL ANATOMY AND VARIATIONS

In the rostral part of the rostral mandible there is an oval-shaped relatively lucent area, at the caudal aspect of which is an irregular opacity

(Figure 9.24a). This region of the mandibular symphysis is variable in appearance and should not be confused with a lesion. The horse has four premolars and three molars (Figures 9.25a-c). The first premolar (the wolf tooth) is frequently absent or is vestigial. Enamel is the most radiodense material in the body, making examination of the structure within the teeth impossible. The teeth develop and erupt from the gums as shown in Table 9.3. The developing tooth is first seen as a lucent area within the mandible or maxilla. As the enamel is laid down, the tooth itself becomes evident, the enamel gradually becoming folded, so that the tooth has its typical structure by the time it erupts from the gum. As the tooth erupts, the lamina dura develops a cystic and distended appearance. This should not be confused with a tooth root abscess, which has a similar appearance (see page 466). The lamina dura of the erupting tooth is more regular in outline and is not associated with any periosteal reaction or sclerosis of the surrounding bone. Anatomically the roots do not form until the tooth has erupted, when the base of the tooth becomes narrowed and more distinctly outlined. The roots of the premolars are aligned roughly at right angles to the long axis of the horizontal ramus of the mandible. The molars show progressive angulation, the roots being more caudal than the crowns towards the caudal aspect of the jaw.

As the teeth develop, the appearance of the mandible changes considerably. In the young horse the teeth are deeply embedded in the bone, which

Table 9.3 Tooth development.

Tooth	Precursor present	Erupt from gum	Come into wear	Tooth lost
Deciduous				
1st incisor	N/A	1st week	1 month	2½ years
2nd incisor	At birth	4–6 weeks	By 3 months	3½ years
3rd incisor	?	6–9 months	By 1 year	4½ years
Canine: inconsistent and do not erupt				
1st cheek tooth	N/A	0–2 weeks	By 1 year	2½ years
2nd cheek tooth	N/A	0–2 weeks	By 1 year	3 years
3rd cheek tooth	N/A	0–2 weeks	By 1 year	4 years
Permanent				
1st incisor	Approx. 20 months	2½ years	3 years	
2nd incisor	Approx. 30 months	3½ years	4 years	
3rd incisor	Approx. 42 months	4½ years	5 years	
Canine?	4–5 yr – inconsistent			
1st premolar (wolf tooth)	Inconsistent			
2nd premolar	Approx. 15 months	2½ years		
3rd premolar				
Upper	Approx. 17 months	3 years		
Lower	Approx. 15 months	2½ years		
4th premolar				
Upper	Approx. 25 months	4 years		
Lower	Approx. 25 months	3½ years		
1st molar	Approx. 3 months	9–12 months		
2nd molar	Approx. 10 months	2 years		
3rd molar	Approx. 30 months	4 years		

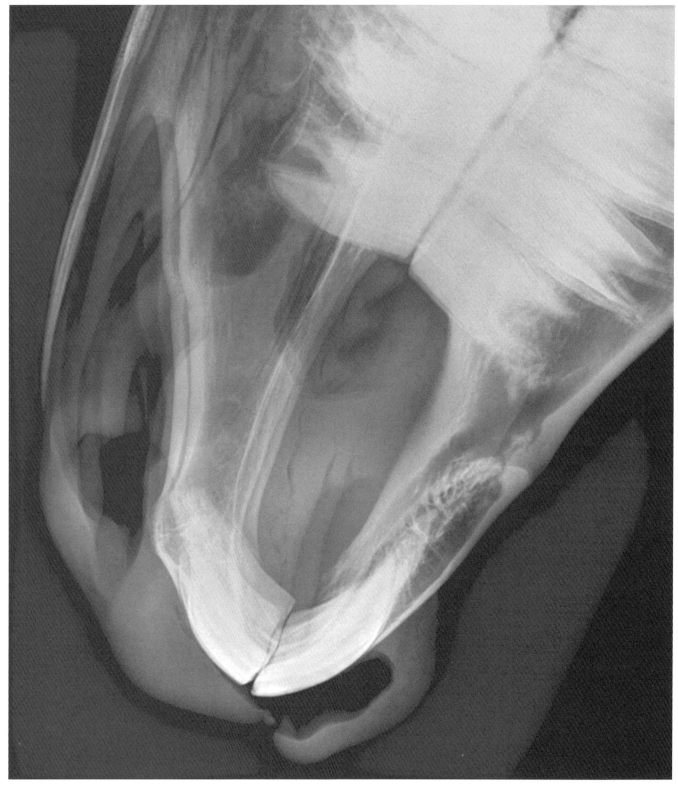

Figure 9.24(a) Lateral view and diagram of the rostral head of a normal mature horse.

[458]

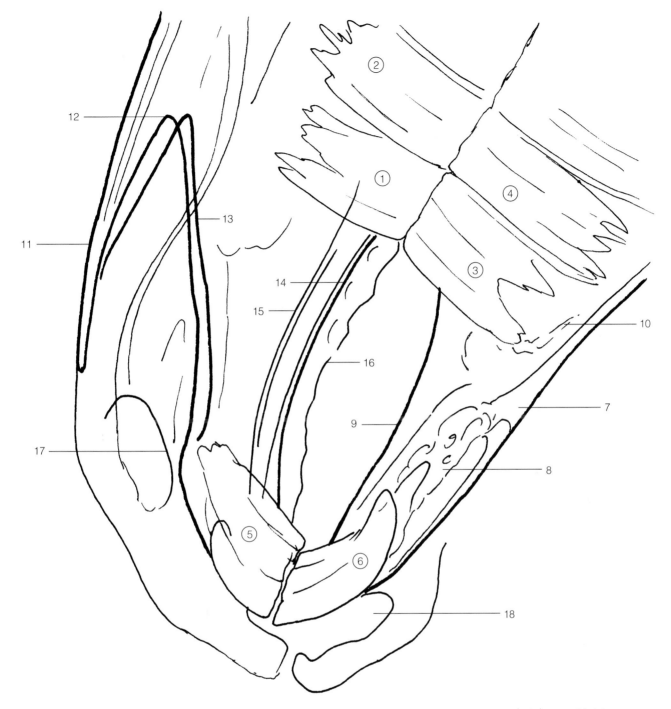

Figure 9.24(a) *Cont'd* 1 = second upper premolars, 2 = third upper premolars, 3 = second lower premolars, 4 = third lower premolars, 5 = upper incisor teeth, 6 = lower incisor teeth, 7 = body of mandible, 8 = area of mandibular symphysis, 9 = interalveolar margin of mandible, 10 = mandibular canal, 11 = nasal process, 12 = nasomaxillary notch, 13 = dorsal border of nasal process of incisive bone, 14 = interalveolar border of incisive bone, 15 = palatine process of incisive bone, 16 = ridge of hard palate, 17 = nostril, 18 = vestibulum oris.

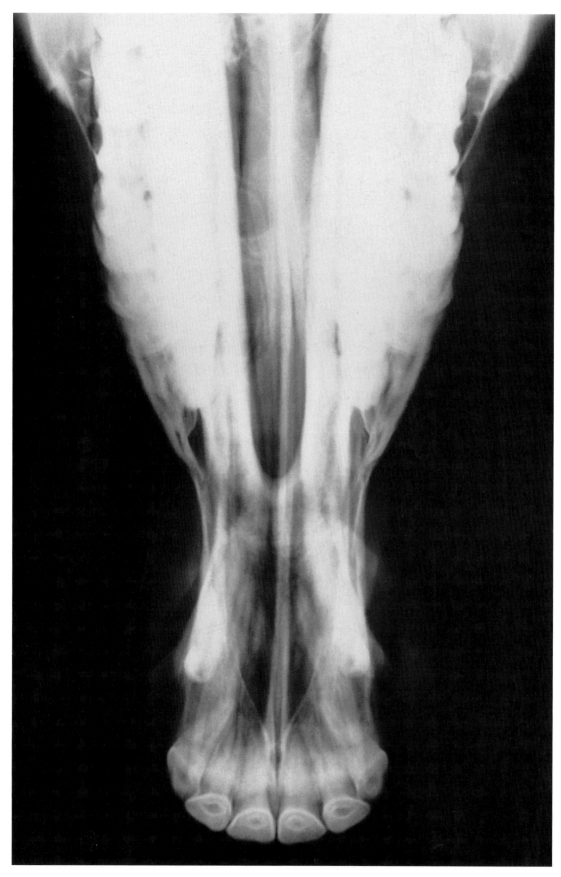

Figure 9.24(b) Ventrodorsal view and diagram of the rostral head of a normal mature horse.

[460]

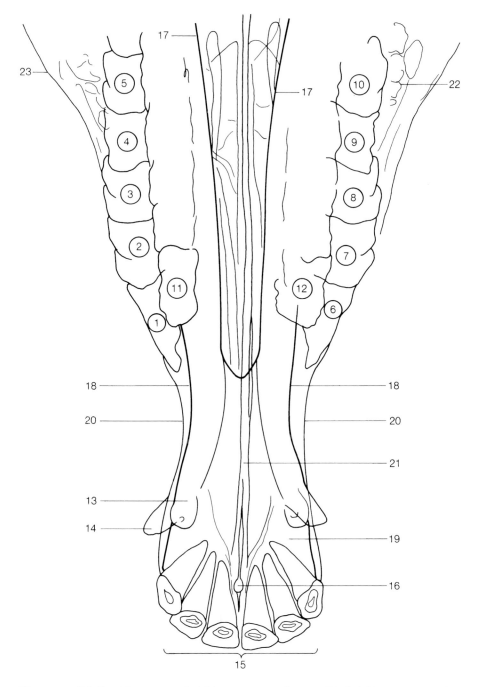

Figure 9.24(b) *Cont'd* 1 = second right upper premolar, 2 = third right upper premolar, 3 = fourth right upper premolar, 4 = first right upper molar, 5 = second right upper molar, 6 = second left upper premolar, 7 = third left upper premolar, 8 = fourth left upper premolar, 9 = first left upper molar, 10 = second left upper molar, 11 = second right lower premolar, 12 = second left lower premolar, 13 = incisive canine tooth, 14 = mandibular canine tooth, 15 = incisor teeth, 16 = interincisive canal, 17 = medial border of molar part of mandible, 18 = lateral border of body of mandible, 19 = body of incisive bone, 20 = lateral border of nasal process of incisive bone, 21 = vomer, 22 = maxillary sinus, 23 = facial crest.

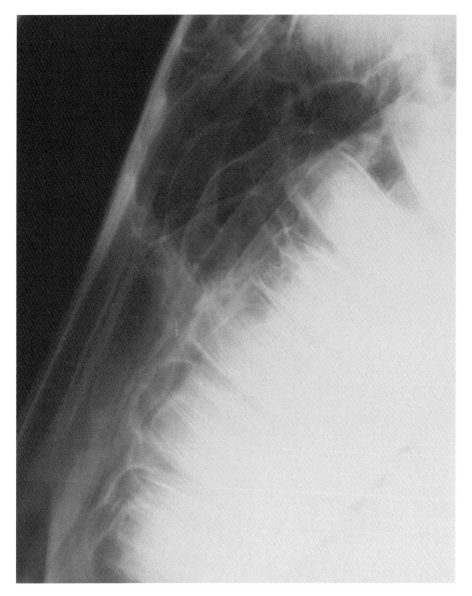

Figure 9.25(a) Right oblique view of the maxillary region of a normal 3-year-old Thoroughbred. Note the well defined periapical lucent zones which represent the normal dental sacs. The lamina dura are well delineated (compare with Figures 9.15a and 9.29).

is accordingly rather thick. At about 2 years of age the ventral aspect is often somewhat irregular, as the roots of the cheek teeth cause 'swellings' along the horizontal ramus. In the adult horse the ventral surface of the mandible is smooth and the bone is somewhat thinner, as the teeth are extruded from the bone.

In a normal horse the erupted crowns of the maxillary and mandibular cheek teeth are closely apposed (Figure 9.26).

The incisor teeth gradually change their angle throughout life, the occlusal surfaces becoming more rostral with age (Figures 9.24a and 9.24b, pages 458–461).

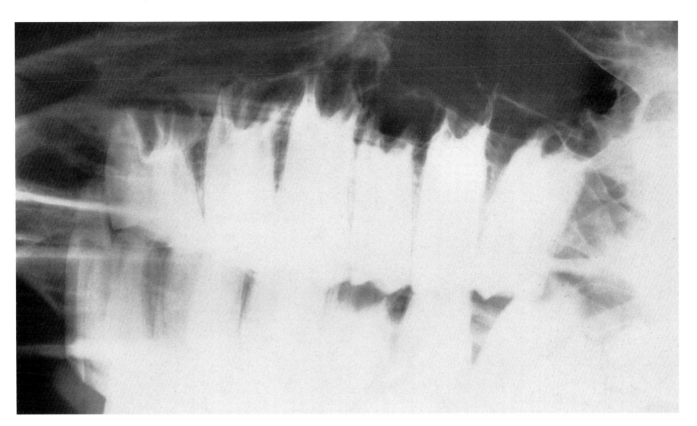

Figure 9.25(b) Right oblique view and diagram of the maxillary region of a normal 10-year-old Thoroughbred. The exposure was selected to highlight the detail of the tooth roots.

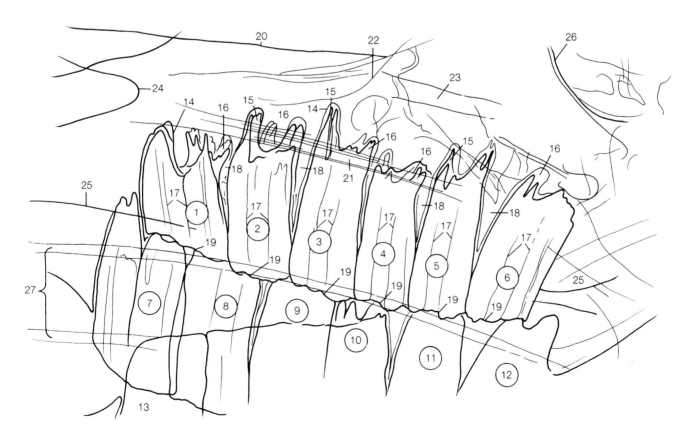

Figure 9.25(b) *Cont'd* 1 = second right upper premolar, 2 = third right upper premolar, 3 = fourth right upper premolar, 4 = first right upper molar, 5 = second right upper molar, 6 = third right upper molar, 7 = second left upper premolar, 8 = third left upper premolar, 9 = fourth left upper premolar, 10 = first left upper molar, 11 = second left upper molar, 12 = third left upper molar, 13 = second right lower premolar, 14 = socket, 15 = buccal root, 16 = lingual root, 17 = buccal longitudinal crest and folds of peripheral enamel, 18 = interalveolar septum, 19 = masticatory surface, 20 = dorsal nasal meatus, 21 = middle nasal meatus, 22 = sinus of nasal turbinate, 23 = infraorbital canal, 24 = nasomaxillary notch, 25 = hard palate, 26 = orbit, 27 = endotracheal tube.

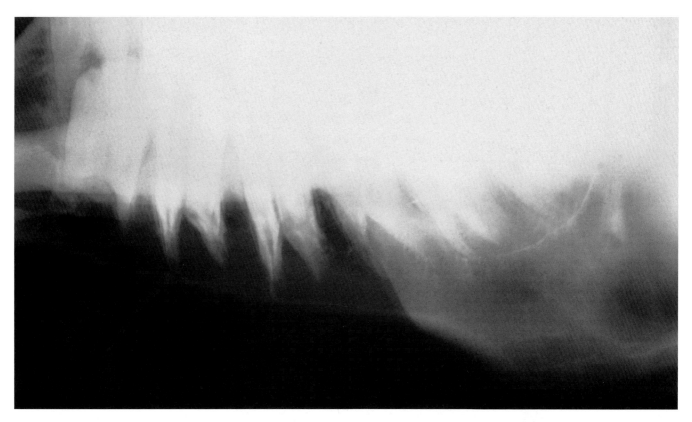

Figure 9.25(c) Right oblique view of the mandible of a normal 10-year-old Thoroughbred, to show the tooth roots.

The canine teeth (tushes or false wolf teeth) may be vestigial or absent, but are more common in geldings and stallions than in mares. They generally erupt at about 4–5 years of age, approximately in the middle of the interdental space (the gap between the incisors and premolars).

'Wolf teeth' are vestigial remnants of the first premolars. They are frequently absent or there may be up to four present. They tend to be placed close to the rostral aspect of the second premolar and generally have a roughly conical crown. There may be little or no apparent root to these teeth, or they may have a root penetrating variable depths into the bone. In many cases the teeth never penetrate the gum and can only be detected on x-ray or by palpation.

The rostral 35° lateral 50° proximal-caudal oblique view of the temporomandibular joint permits visualization of the lateral aspect of the joint (Figure 9.27). Structures axial to the plane of the coronoid process are superimposed with the calvarium. The temporal condyle of the squamous temporal bone has a flat or slightly concave ventral border and is confluent dorsally with the superimposed opacity of the zygomatic arch. The

[464]

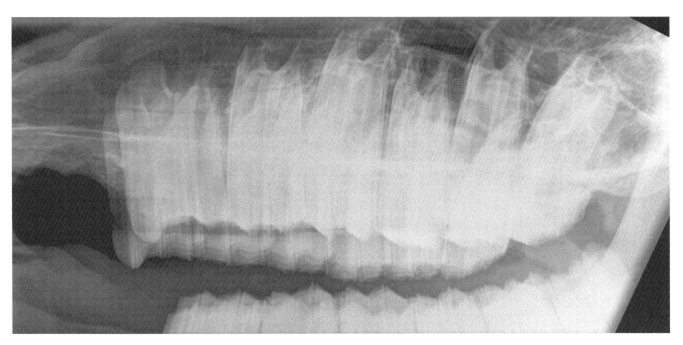

Figure 9.26 Open-mouth oblique view of the maxillary cheek teeth of an adult horse with no history of medical problems. Rostral is to the left. There are hooks on the rostral aspect of the first upper cheek teeth.

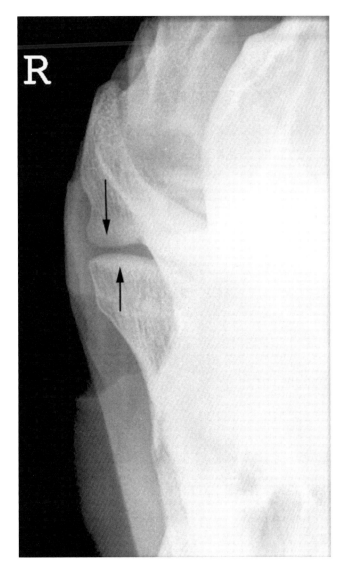

Figure 9.27 Rostal 35° lateral 50° ventral-caudodorsal oblique view of the lateral aspect of the right tempormandibular joint (arrows) of a normal adult horse.

mandibular condyle is a shelf of bone slightly convex dorsally, especially axially. The joint space is clearly seen between these structures.

SIGNIFICANT FINDINGS

Brachygnathia and prognathia

These conditions are generally congenital and can be seen on lateral radiographs. While it is not necessary to radiograph patients to make this diagnosis, radiographs of the cheek teeth may be valuable to check for sharp points where there is irregular wear, e.g. in brachygnathia the lower jaw is shorter than the upper, and there tend to be sharp points on the rostral aspect of the upper second premolar and caudal aspect of the lower third molar teeth.

Polydontia

Polydontia is the presence of teeth in excess of the normal dental formula. It most commonly results from persistence of the temporary dentition, particularly the incisors. Incisors are usually displaced labially or lingually and cause little trouble, although they may result in ulceration of the gum or lip. With the cheek teeth, the demand made for additional space by supernumerary teeth tends to result in teeth being rotated or adjacent teeth being displaced. This results in disturbance of the wear patterns, resulting in sharp spikes on the teeth and resultant damage to soft tissues.

Radiography is not really necessary to diagnose this condition, but it may be helpful in differentiating between deciduous and permanent teeth, the permanent teeth having longer roots.

Oligodontia

The congenital absence of a tooth is of little clinical significance, although it may lead to sharp points on teeth, caused by uneven wear.

Tumours of dental origin

Adamantinomas and ameloblastic odontomas are tumours derived from the enamel organ (the embryological precursor of a tooth). They are generally recognized in young horses. They may occur in the maxilla or the mandible and have a variable appearance. An adamantinoma remains primarily of soft tissue and has a septate, 'foamy' appearance. An odontoma usually has a more opaque tooth-like structure (Figures 9.18a and 9.18b, pages 448–449).

Tooth root infection

Infections of the tooth roots vary in their appearance and can be difficult to distinguish on radiographs. They show a number of changes progressing through: loss of detail of the lamina dura; lysis of the periapical bone, possibly with sclerosis of the surrounding bone; destruction of the apex of the tooth root, giving it an irregular margin or marked change in shape. Computed tomography is a very accurate means of identifying infected teeth. Nuclear scintigraphy is sometimes helpful for identification of the affected tooth (teeth). Ultrasonography is useful in the evaluation of soft-tissue swellings associated with mandibular teeth infections.

Infections of the teeth in the mandible tend to present clinically as swellings on the lower jaw (Figure 9.28). These may be very slow to develop and eventually a discharging sinus may occur at the ventral aspect of the swelling.

Infections of the upper teeth may develop similarly (Figures 9.29a-d), with swelling and discharge from the maxilla or periorbital area. More

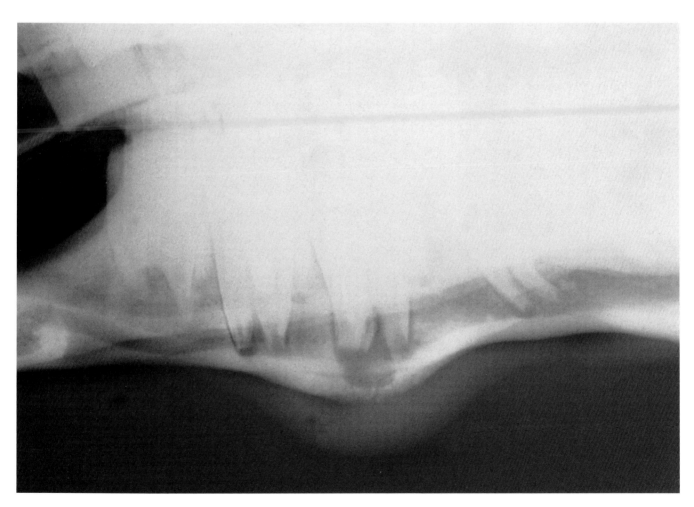

Figure 9.28 Left oblique view of the mandible of an 8-year-old Thoroughbred with a history of a swelling developing in the left mandibular region over the previous 4 weeks. There is distortion of the cortex of the mandible with overlying soft-tissue swelling. Note the radiating poorly bordered, active periosteal new bone formation covering the ventral aspect of the alveolus. There is loss of detail of the lamina dura and a suggestion of blunting of the tooth roots of the third lower cheek tooth with considerable lysis of the periapical bone. There is a suggestion of slight sclerosis of the surrounding bone rostrally and caudally. These abnormalities are typical of tooth root infection.

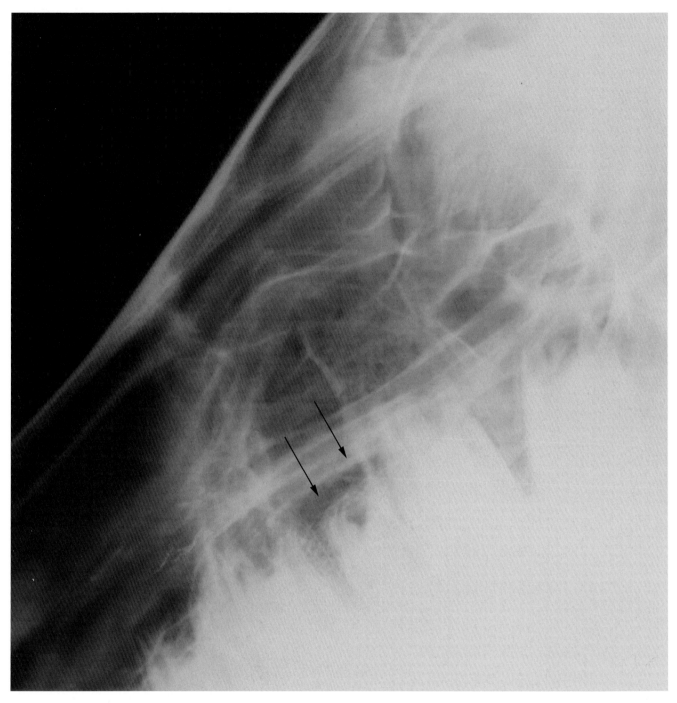

Figure 9.29(a) Lateral view of the upper cheek teeth of a 7-year-old Thoroughbred with headshaking behaviour of several months' duration and recent onset of left-sided, foul-smelling nasal discharge. The tooth roots of one of the fourth upper cheek teeth (arrows) are poorly defined. There is a reticular radiopacity superimposed over some of the tooth roots, which represents a rope halter. There is also diffuse heterogeneous opacity within the maxillary sinus.

[468]

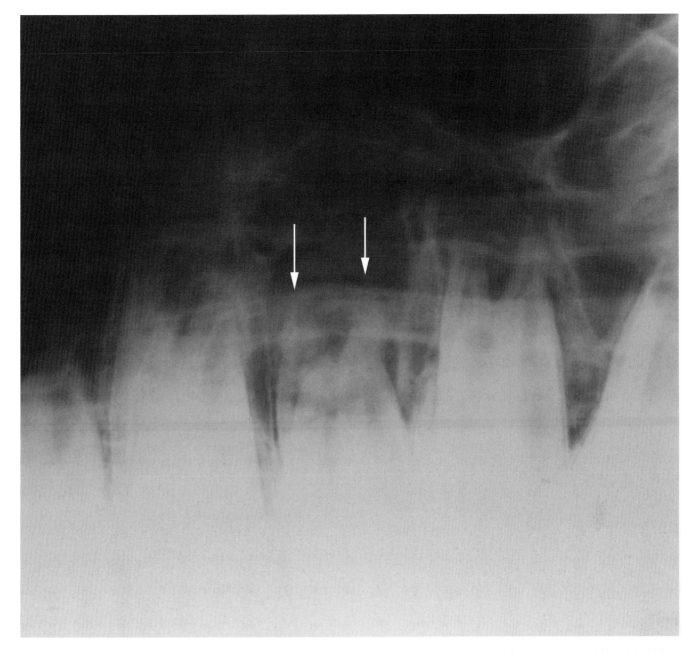

Figure 9.29(b) Left oblique view of the upper tooth arcade of the same horse as in Figure 9.29(a). The abnormalities of the left fourth upper cheek tooth are much more clearly defined (arrows). There is loss of the lamina dura and the tooth roots are reduced in opacity. The roots also have an abnormal shape. Rostral is to the left.

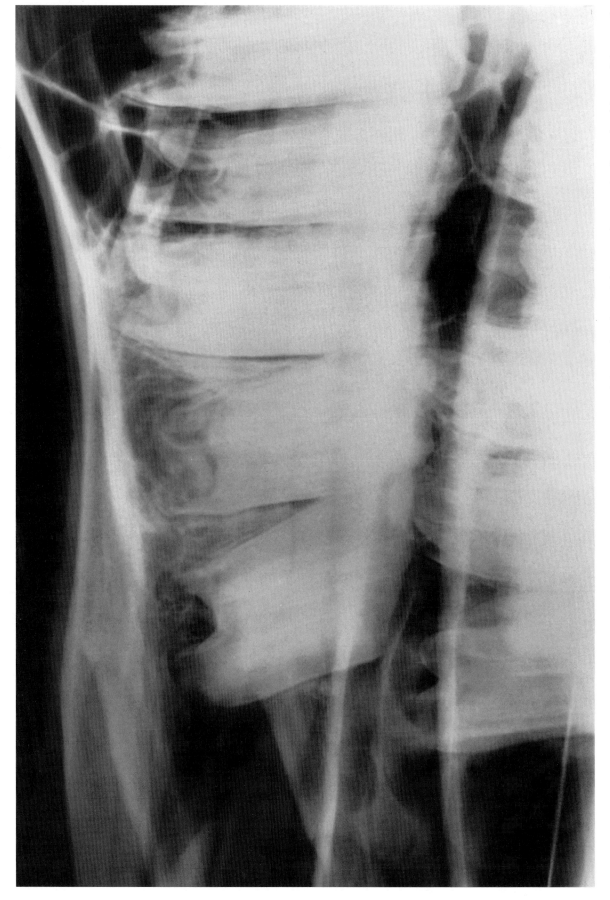

Figure 9.29(c) Oblique view of the right upper cheek tooth arcade. There is loss of definition of the lamina dura of the second upper cheek tooth, with a nodular opacity dorsal to it within an area of increased opacity. This is a more unusual finding associated with chronic tooth root infection. Compare with Figures 9.29(a) and 9.29(b).

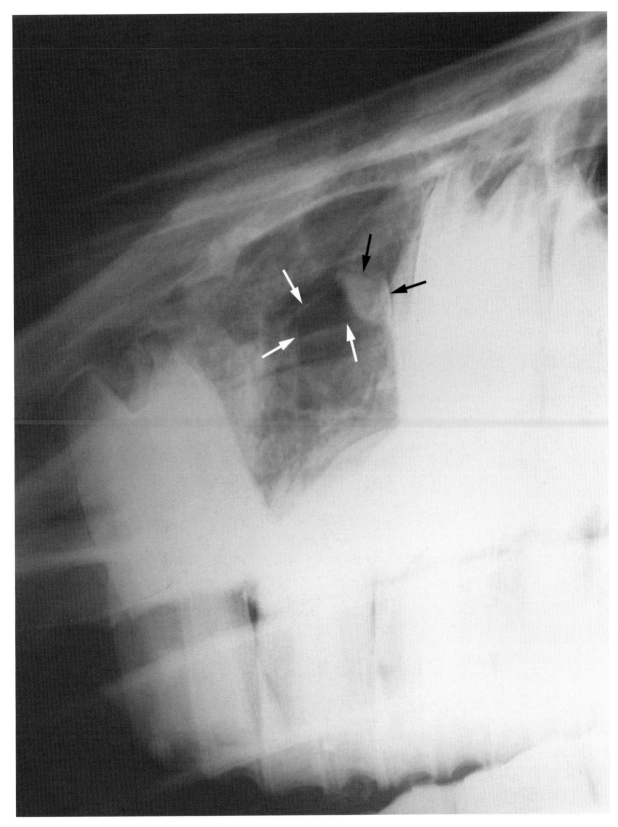

Figure 9.29(d) Left oblique view of the rostral upper cheek teeth 2 months after removal of the left third upper premolar. A chronic nasal discharge has persisted. There is a fragment of tooth (black arrows) rostral to which is a radiolucent area, surrounded by a more radiopaque rim (white arrows). Note also the diffuse, somewhat reticular opacity in the remainder of the space formerly occupied by the tooth. See inset.

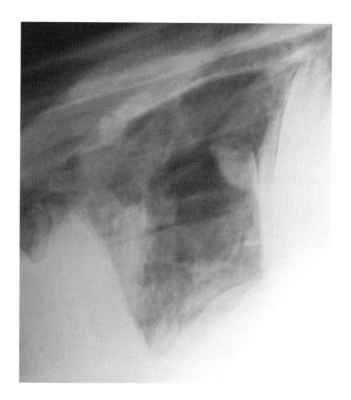

Figure 9.29(d) *Cont'd*

usually, if the upper molars (and occasionally fourth premolar) are involved, there will be either a nasal discharge or a purulent sinusitis (see 'Sinusitis', page 437). Infection of the maxillary teeth is sometimes accompanied by quite extensive fibrous reactions in the maxillary sinus, possibly including areas of local mineralization. If such changes are found in the maxillary sinus, tooth root infection or periodontal disease should always be considered a likely cause (see Figure 9.16, page 446).

By the time these infections have been diagnosed it is usually necessary to extract the affected teeth. Although attempts have been made to drain these infections and operate on or fill the tooth roots, this is generally unsuccessful, uneconomic and, in view of the reasonable prognosis for conventional treatment, unnecessary.

Periodontal disease

Periodontal disease is more common in the maxillary teeth than in the mandibular teeth. The radiographic signs are similar to those for root infections, but there tends to be more reaction on the alveolar bone. Although periodontal disease is frequently accompanied by, or the result of, food material packing around the teeth, and even passing up into the maxillary sinus, it may be accompanied by little detectable oral discomfort.

Disorders of the erupted crowns

A diastema is a space between two adjacent teeth which may be congenital or acquired, due to tooth loss or a fracture. It can result in impeded mastica-

[472]

tion of food, which becomes trapped, putrefied and leads to gingivitis, gingival recession and ultimately to periodontal disease and pain.

Diastemata can occur in young horses due to insufficient angulation of the rostral and caudal cheek teeth, or when the tooth buds develop too far apart. In older horses multiple diastemata may develop because the cheek teeth narrow towards their apices and therefore the rostrocaudal width of the exposed crown decreases. Diastemata are difficult to detect clinically and cannot be seen in standard oblique views. Open-mouth oblique views are essential for diagnosis (Figure 9.30a). Treatment of a single diastema causing severe periodontal pain may require removal of a single tooth on one side of the diastema. Conservative treatment should be attempted initially, particularly if multiple diastemata are present.

Other abnormalities of the erupted crowns include traumatic or idiopathic fractures, abnormalities of wear such as exaggerated transverse ridges, wavemouth (Figure 9.30b) or stepmouth, supernumerary or reduced number of cheek teeth and the presence of retained and impacted deciduous cheek tooth remnants which may be confirmed on oblique open-mouth views. They may however be better detected by clinical examination.

Mandibular periostitis

Periostitis of the mandible is characterized radiologically as periosteal new bone formation, usually on the ventral surface of the mandible. It can be the result of trauma, with an incomplete fracture of the cortex of the mandible, or develop subsequent to chronic bruising, e.g. as a result of tight-fitting tack or repeated contusion from looking over a high door. The soreness will resolve once the inciting factor is removed, although some change in contour of the mandible is likely to remain. This condition should be differentiated from tooth root abscess and tumour of the mandible.

Osteomyelitis

Osteomyelitis of the mandible is not uncommon and is characterized radiographically by destruction of bone with or without new bone formation (Figure 9.31). It is sometimes difficult to distinguish radiographically extensive infection from a tumour. Small lesions may be treated surgically, but extensive lesions carry a guarded prognosis.

Mandibular cysts

Multiple cystic lesions of the mandible, usually involving the tooth roots, are not uncommon in young foals (Figure 9.32). They generally involve the rostral half or two-thirds of the horizontal ramus. Their origin is uncertain. This lesion is easily recognized on lateral radiographs as multiple radiolucent cystic lesions in the mandible, often with enlargement in size of the mandible. In extensive cases there may be little bone surrounding the cysts.

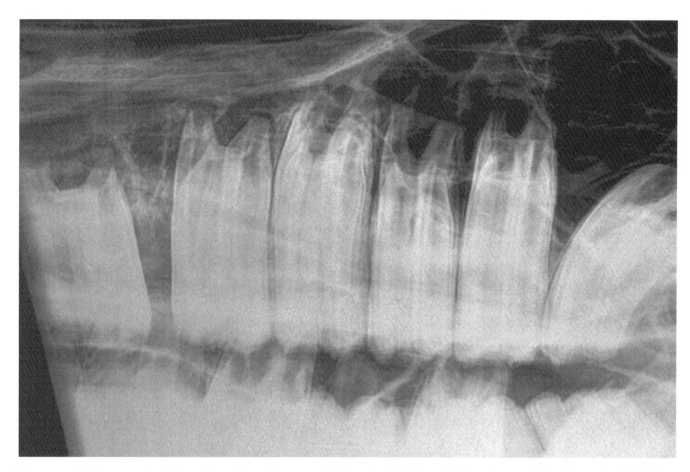

Figure 9.30(a) Open-mouth oblique view of the right upper cheek teeth of a 6-year-old Appaloosa which presented with facial swelling and marked gingivitis. Rostral is to the left. There is a space, a diastema, between the rostral two cheek teeth.

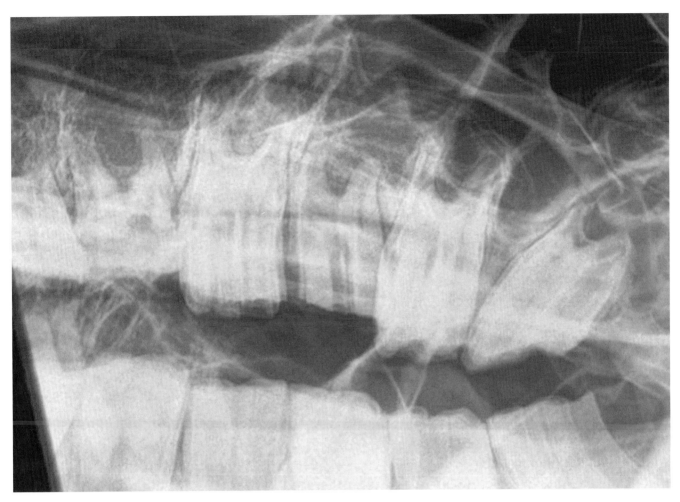

Figure 9.30(b) Open-mouth oblique view of the right cheek teeth of an 11-year-old Welsh pony. Two maxillary cheek teeth had previously been removed from the left side, but nasal discharge persisted. There is a very irregular alignment of the ventral aspect of the maxillary cheek teeth.

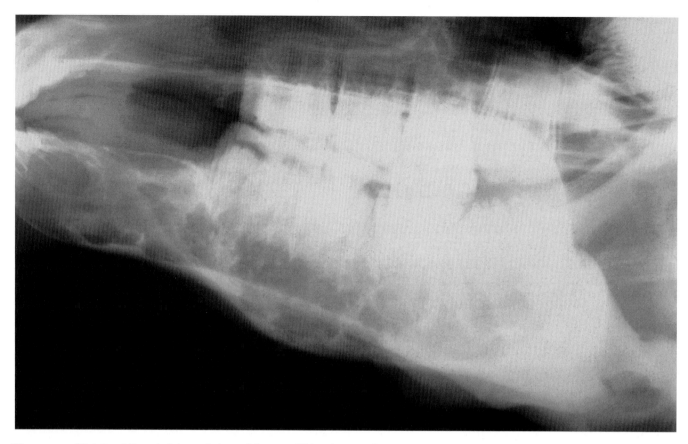

Figure 9.31 Slightly oblique left lateral view of the mandible of a weanling Morgan with a history of a small mass developing on the mandible 6 weeks previously and enlarging progressively despite antimicrobial therapy. There is a large expansile lesion of the mandible that has a reticulate or 'foamy' appearance. Post-mortem examination confirmed that this was the result of osteomyelitis, although its radiographic appearance was similar to that of an odontoma, a reparative granuloma or an aneurysmal bone cyst.

Clinically there is swelling of the mandible, often with a rather bulbous or even lobulate appearance. The teeth may be loose in the jaw in extensive cases and the horse may have difficulty eating. Differential diagnosis includes ameloblastoma, cystic fibrosis and infection. Treatment is by surgical drainage, but the prognosis is guarded, depending on the extent of the lesion.

Craniomandibular osteopathy

A condition resembling craniomandibular osteopathy in the dog has been recognized in the horse, resulting in large firm non-painful swellings on the ventral aspect of the rami of the mandibles of a young horse. Radiographically this is due to extensive periosteal new bone formation extending from the ventral cortices of the bones (Figure 9.33). Bone biopsies show similar histological changes to craniomandibular osteopathy in the dog. There is some degree of spontaneous regression of the lesions over 1 year. The lesions do not interfere with mastication.

[476]

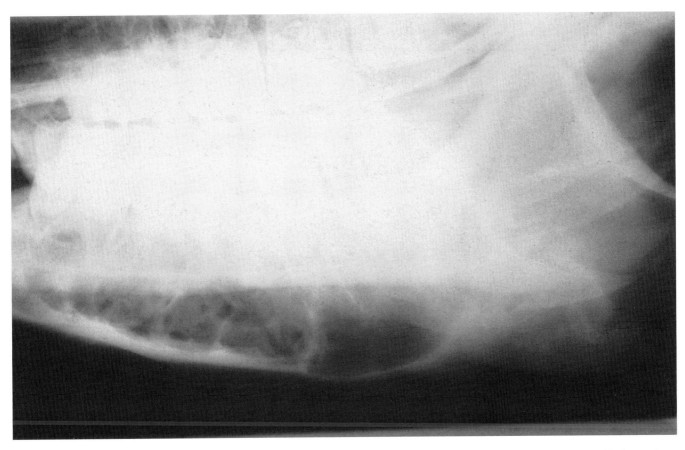

Figure 9.32 Left oblique view of the mandible of a 3-month-old Thoroughbred with diffuse swelling in the left mandibular region. There is a multiloculated cyst-like lesion involving the rostral half of the left mandible. The cortex of the bone is smoothly irregular and appears to be of variable width. The cyst-like structures extend as far as the tooth roots. The swelling resolved following surgical curettage.

Tumours

The mandible is one of the more common sites for a tumour in bone in the horse, including osteosarcomas, adamantinomas and ossifying fibromas. Most tumours result in widespread destruction of bone (Figures 9.34 and 9.35) and carry a poor prognosis. It is usually not possible to identify a specific tumour type by its radiographic appearance. Tumours must be differentiated from osteomyelitis (see Figure 9.31, page 476).

Tumour-like lesions are also seen, including osseous cyst-like lesions, mycetoma and an intraosseous epidermoid cyst.

Temporomandibular joint arthritis

This is a rare condition, and may be infectious or more usually traumatic in origin. The radiographic changes seen are similar to those seen in any other joint (see Chapter 1, page 34); for example proliferative new bone around the joint accompanied in infectious cases by bone lysis. The oblique anatomy of the joint may conceal early lesions. Ultrasonography may be more sensitive for detection of early periarticular osteophyte formation and

[477]

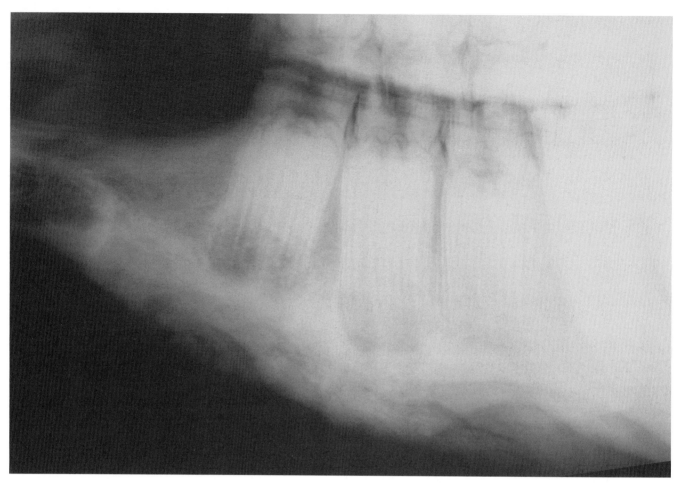

Figure 9.33 Lateral view of the head of a 3-year-old Thoroughbred colt with a rapidly expanding mass on the cranial aspect of the ramus of the left and right mandibles. There is extensive new bone on the ventral aspect of the mandible and loss of the cortex. The rami of the mandible have a heterogeneous radiopacity. The lesions progressively resolved with time and non-steroidal anti-inflammatory treatment. Diagnosis: craniomandibular osteopathy.

for assessment of the meniscal cartilage. The condition is very painful when advanced, resulting in dysphagia and weight loss. Arthroscopic surgery may be useful in early cases. The prognosis for advanced cases is poor, although condylectomy has been described and may be beneficial.

Luxation of the temporomandibular joint

Temporomandibular joint luxation is usually the result of trauma and may occur unilaterally or bilaterally. There may be associated fractures. Oblique radiographic views may be required to separate the two joints. There is usually associated malocclusion of the molars. The radiographs should be inspected carefully for the presence of concurrent fractures.

[478]

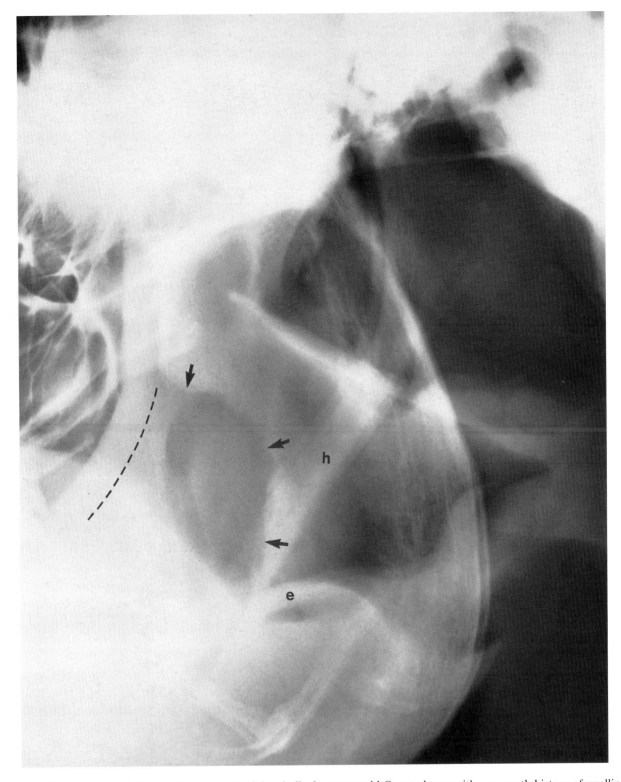

Figure 9.34 Slightly oblique left lateral radiograph of the skull of a 7-year-old Quarterhorse with a 3-month history of swelling in the region of the left mandible and difficulty in chewing. There is a large lucent area (arrows) in the cranial angle of the left mandible. The bone adjacent to the margins of the defect appears lytic and irregular. The left stylohyoid bone (h) cannot be evaluated totally, but appears to be involved in the process. The approximate location of the normal cranial angle of the mandible is marked with a dotted line. The epiglottis (e) is normal. Post-mortem examination confirmed the presence of a squamous cell carcinoma.

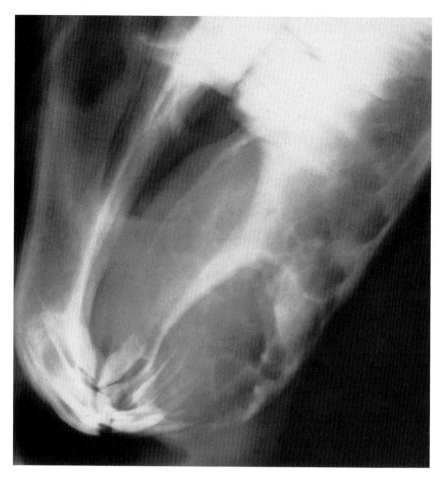

Figure 9.35 Left lateral view of the rostral maxilla and mandible of a yearling Thoroughbred. A firm lump was noted on the left rostral mandible 2 months previously. There is a large multiloculated expansile mass in the left mandible which is displacing the incisor teeth. The mass was excised surgically and histological examination revealed that this was fibrous dysplasia with reactive new bone, but no evidence of malignancy.

Fractures

Fractures of the rostral aspect of the mandible are common, especially in foals and young horses. They frequently involve a fracture at, or immediately caudal to, the third incisor (Figure 9.36). They may result in one or more teeth being broken or torn from the body of the mandible, usually with some associated bone. Injuries may involve only one side, or both mandibles may be fractured. These fractures generally require surgical intervention, either to remove loose fragments or to stabilize the fracture by internal fixation or intra-oral fixation using cerclage wire. They carry a good prognosis with surgical treatment, although some brachygnathia may result or develop with growth.

Fractures of the horizontal ramus (Figure 9.37a) occur at any point, although they frequently involve the interdental space. They may respond to conservative treatment if unilateral, or may benefit from internal fixation. Internal fixation may be impracticable if the tooth roots are too closely

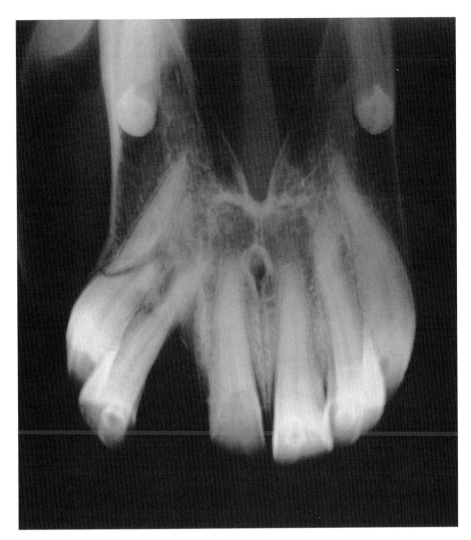

Figure 9.36 Intra-oral ventrodorsal view of the rostral mandible of a show pony. There is a displaced fracture of the mandible involving the tooth roots of the corner and intermediate incisors. Note that the root of the corner incisor is fractured.

involved with the fracture line, and in some cases in young horses the tooth roots may involve too much of the bone for fixation to be possible, although wiring adjacent teeth together may help give some increased stability to the jaw. Fractures of the horizontal ramus of the mandible often open into the oral cavity, with some risk of developing osteomyelitis.

Fractures of the vertical ramus (Figure 9.37b) of the mandible are often best visualized on the view described on page 415 for examination of the cranium. They are usually unilateral and may be difficult to delineate. They may require several different exposures for complete evaluation. Internal fixation is not generally practicable or necessary, because if the horse can feed adequately the fractures usually heal with conservative treatment. The prognosis is good, provided that the fracture does not enter the temporomandibular joint.

The radiographs should be carefully examined to exclude concurrent dislocation of the temporomandibular joint.

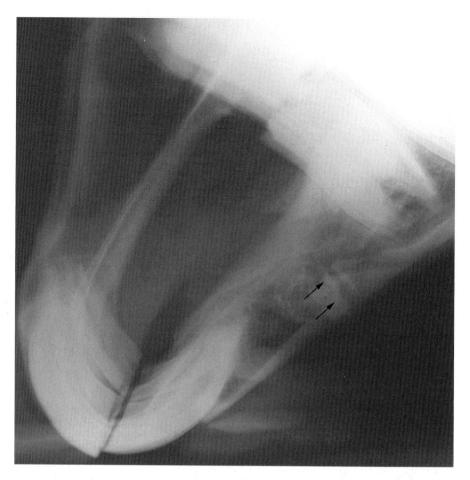

Figure 9.37(a) Lateral view of the rostral aspect of the head of a pony found salivating in the field with multiple small external wounds and a painful swelling of the right mandibular area caudal to the mandibular symphysis. There is a chronic fracture of the horizontal ramus of the mandible (arrows), with sclerosis adjacent to the fracture.

Sequestrum of the interdental space

The mandibular interdental space is relatively poorly covered by soft tissues and is potentially at risk to trauma from the bit. This may predispose it to sequestrum formation. Radiographically there are typical signs of sequestrum formation (see Chapter 1, page 22), usually immediately rostral to the first premolar (Figure 9.38). Oblique views are necessary to separate the two horizontal rami of the mandible. This can be achieved by turning the horse's head slightly towards or away from the x-ray machine.

Clinical signs include depressed appetite, oral discomfort, slight swelling on the ventral and lateral aspects of the mandible, and sometimes a draining sinus. Surgical treatment carries a good prognosis.

Pharynx, larynx and Eustachian tube diverticulum

This area includes structures that are an integral part of the respiratory system and the reader may also want to refer to Chapter 12. Radiographs

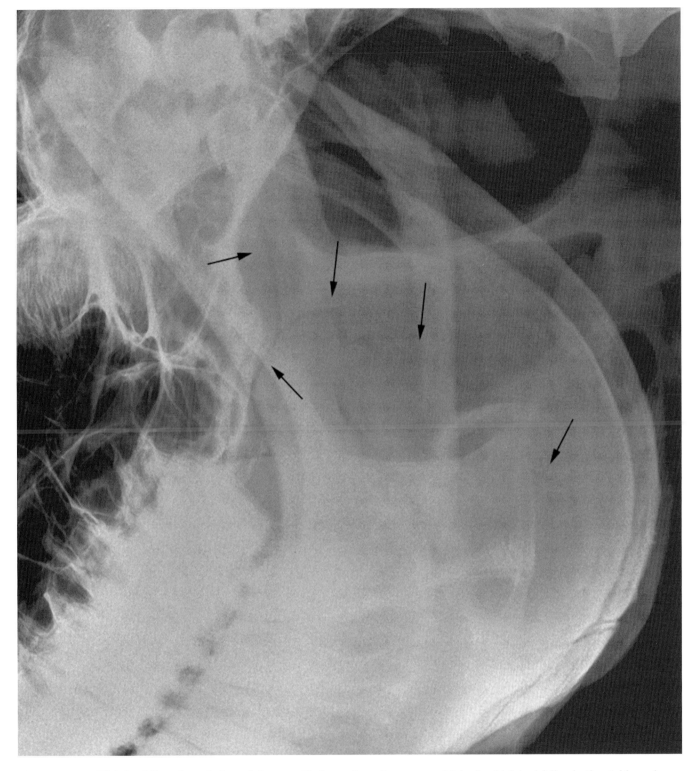

Figure 9.37(b) Slightly oblique lateral view of the mandibular region of a 14-year-old Arab which had fallen in the stable and showed bleeding from the mouth and nose. There is a comminuted fracture of the vertical ramus of the mandible (arrows).

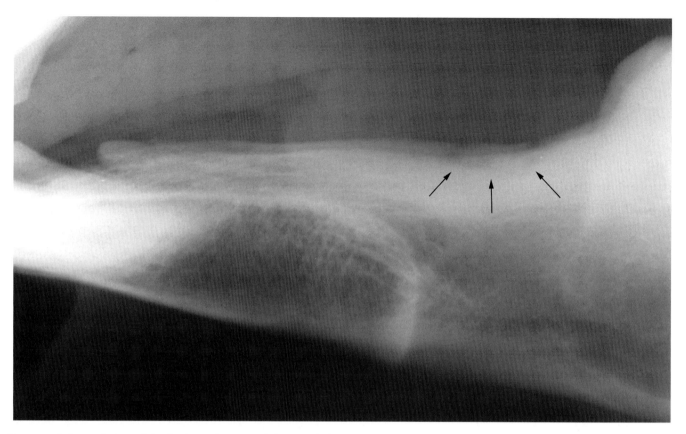

Figure 9.38 Lateral view of the horizontal ramus of the mandible of a 12-year-old Hunter with a history of bleeding from the mouth during exercise. There was gingival ulceration rostral to the first lower cheek tooth. Rostral is to the left. There is a sequestrum (arrows) in the interdental space.

of this area give visualization of the soft palate, epiglottis, hyoid apparatus, nasopharynx and Eustachian tube diverticulum (guttural pouch).

RADIOGRAPHIC TECHNIQUE

Lateral view

Evaluation of this area is almost always limited to lateral views, normally obtained with the horse standing. The x-ray beam is centred between the base of the ear and the angle of the mandible, and aligned at right angles to the midline of the head and the cassette. When the Eustachian tube diverticulum (guttural pouch) is being evaluated, it is often advantageous to obtain both right and left lateral radiographs in order to determine the side of involvement (see page 413). Exposures appropriate for soft tissues should be used.

Ventrodorsal view

This view is obtained under general anaesthesia and is difficult to obtain without some degree of rotation. The horse is placed in dorsal recumbency and the head extended. The poll is placed on a small pad, so that the x-ray

[484]

cassette can be placed in contact with the dorsal aspect of the skull, and be placed far enough caudally to visualize the Eustachian tube diverticulum and pharynx. The dorsoventral plane of the skull must be maintained vertical, in order that diagnostic radiographs are obtained. It may be necessary to reposition the head to obtain straight ventrodorsal views, as any obliquity results in loss of information on the radiograph. It may also be helpful in some cases to withdraw the endotracheal tube, if one is used, as this can mask abnormalities.

NORMAL ANATOMY, VARIATIONS AND INCIDENTAL FINDINGS

When examining radiographs of this area it is important to remember that the soft-tissue structures are constantly moving. Radiographs only indicate the position of the structure for a fraction of a second in the life of the patient, and must be interpreted on this basis. For this reason, assessment of the relationship of structures such as the soft palate or epiglottis to other structures must be interpreted with care (Figures 9.39a and 9.39b).

The most obvious structures on this view are the radiolucent Eustachian tube diverticula (guttural pouches) (Figure 9.39b). The dorsal aspect is in contact with the base of the skull and the atlas. The caudal border lies

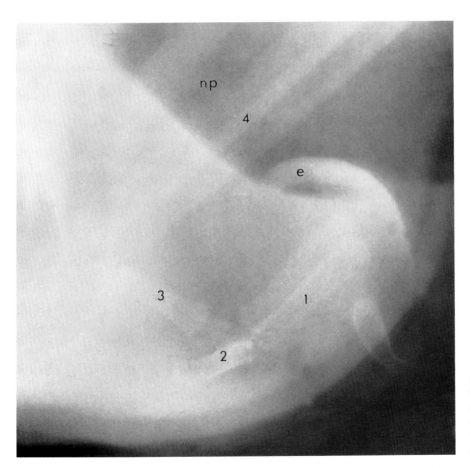

Figure 9.39(a) Well collimated slightly oblique lateral view of a normal pharynx of an immature horse. The nasopharynx (np) contains air. Note the epiglottis (e), thyrohyoid (1), basihyoid (2), ceratohyoid (3) and stylohyoid (4).

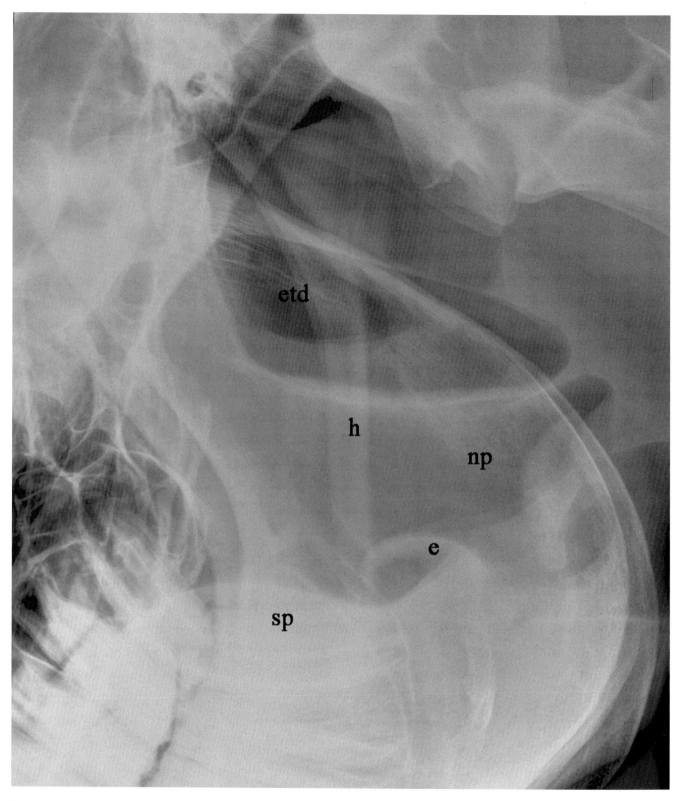

Figure 9.39(b) Slightly oblique view and diagram of the pharyngeal region of a normal adult horse. Note that the cranial angles of the left and right mandibles are slightly separated, indicating slight obliquity. There is gas in the Eustachian tube diverticulum (etd) and the nasopharynx (np). The epiglottis (e), soft palate (sp) and stylohyoid bones (h) are clearly demarcated.

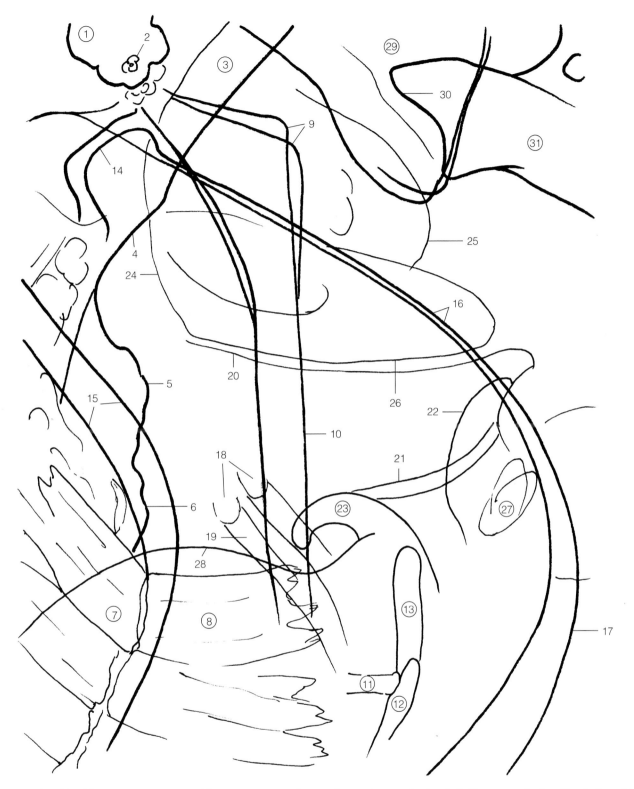

Figure 9.39(b) *Cont'd* 1 = petrous temporal bone, 2 = external acoustic meatus, 3 = basioccipital bone, 4 = body of basisphenoid bone, 5 = pterygoid process, 6 = maxillary tuberosity, 7 = third upper molar tooth, 8 = third lower molar tooth, 9 = stylohyoid angle, 10 = stylohyoid, 11 = ceratohyoid, 12 = basihyoid, 13 = thyrohyoid, 14 = condyloid process of mandible, 15 = ramus of mandible, cranial edge, 16 = ramus of mandible, caudal edge, 17 = angle of mandible, 18 = mandibular foramen, 19 = mandibular canal, 20 = dorsal wall of pharynx, 21 = aryepiglottic fold, 22 = arytenoid cartilage, 23 = epiglottis, 24 = cranial wall of Eustachian tube diverticulum (guttural pouch), 25 = caudal wall of Eustachian tube diverticulum (guttural pouch), 26 = plica salpingopharyngea, 27 = laryngeal ventricles, 28 = soft palate, 29 = atlas (first cervical vertebra), 30 = dens, 31 = axis (second cervical vertebra).

approximately below the articulation of the atlas and axis. The ventral border forms the roof of the pharynx, and lies approximately level with the dorsal aspect of the arytenoid cartilages and the rostral aspect of the ethmoid bone. The ventral cranial third of the Eustachian tube diverticulum lies between the vertical rami of the mandible. The caudal and ventral borders of each Eustachian tube diverticulum are apparent as double lines, as the two pouches seldom lie exactly over one another. The greater cornua of the stylohyoid bones cross the diverticulum between the medial and lateral compartments.

The soft palate is at the rostral aspect of the pharynx. Rostrally it is seen caudal to the last upper molars, generally positioned about midway between the crown and root of the tooth. It follows a smooth S-shaped course over the back of the tongue, to lie under the epiglottis caudally. There is sometimes a small triangular area of air between the soft palate and the base of the tongue.

The epiglottis is clearly seen caudal to the last lower molar, the opening formed by the epiglottis and arytenoid cartilages forming a smooth continuation of the tracheal lumen into the nasopharynx. The epiglottis is markedly curved (dorsally convex), nearly forming a complete semicircle. Its base is approximately vertical, while the tip lies nearly at a right angle to the dorsal surface of the soft palate.

A small lucent gas shadow may be seen at the base of the epiglottis, in the trachea (the middle ventricle of the larynx), and two further lucent crescents are seen below the base of the arytenoid cartilages (the lateral ventricles).

The tracheal rings are clearly delineated. Dorsal to the trachea, immediately caudal to the tip of the arytenoid cartilage, a small lucent linear air shadow may occasionally be seen in the cranial part of the oesophagus. This should not extend more than 2–5 cm in length in a normal horse.

Mineralization of the laryngeal cartilages, hyoid apparatus and tracheal rings may occur as a normal variation in some older horses.

SIGNIFICANT FINDINGS

Eustachian tube diverticulum empyema

Although probably becoming a less common condition, this may be seen in areas with a large population of horses. It usually follows a streptococcal infection, particularly *Streptococcus equi*. Clinically there is usually a unilateral offensive purulent nasal discharge.

Empyema may fill one or both pouches (Figure 9.40), giving an increase in radiopacity of the diverticulum. There is normally a fluid line in the diverticulum, which aids differentiation from a soft-tissue mass. It is possible to determine if the condition involves one or both pouches by obtaining ventrodorsal views. It may be easier, however, to obtain radiographs from the left and right sides. The radiographs are compared for magnification and sharpness of the fluid line. The air cap appears larger and less sharp when away from the cassette. It is often possible to obtain a further radiograph

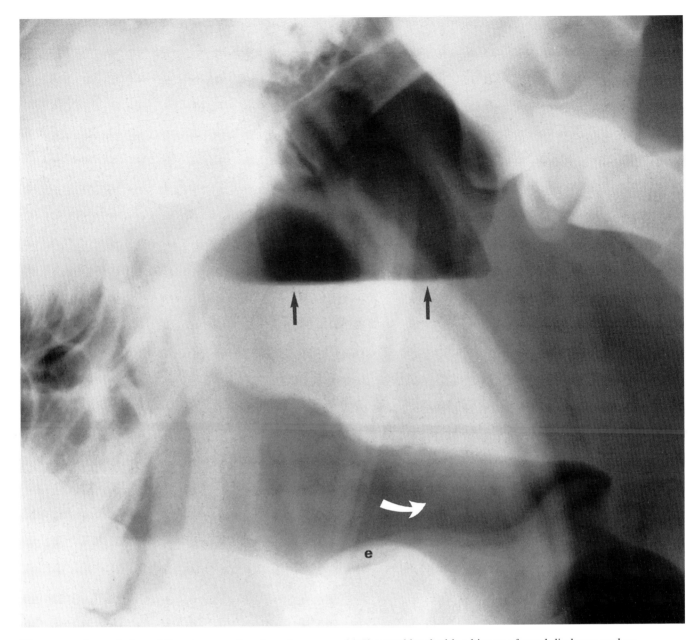

Figure 9.40 Lateral view of the pharyngeal region of a 2-year-old Thoroughbred with a history of nasal discharge and an occasional cough. There is a fluid line (straight arrows) in one or both Eustachian tube diverticula. The ventral half of the diverticulum is uniformly opaque due to the accumulation of pus, i.e. empyema. Note also the irregular outline of the dorsal pharyngeal wall and the fine mottled opacities (curved arrow) in the dorsal nasal pharynx. This represents pharyngeal lymphoid hyperplasia. The epiglottis (e) is normal.

with the nose of the horse elevated. This moves the fluid within the diverticulum and allows assessment of the thickness of the cranial ventral margins. The thickness of the diverticular walls at this point gives some indication of the nature of the fluid and the chronicity of the condition.

The condition should initially be treated conservatively, but surgical drainage may be needed. A reasonable prognosis can be given for early cases, but if surgery is required the prognosis is guarded.

[489]

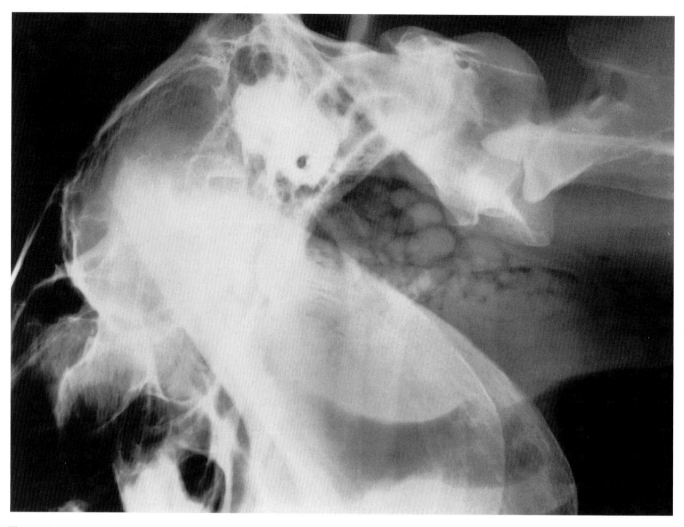

Figure 9.41 Lateral view of the pharyngeal region of an 8-year-old pony. There are many well circumscribed opaque masses within the Eustachian tube diverticulum. These are chondroids, a sequel to *Streptococcus equi* infection.

Eustachian tube diverticulum chondrosis

Eustachian tube diverticulum chondrosis normally results from chronic empyema that has been inadequately treated. If it occurs as a sequel to strangles, the horse may be a permanent carrier and potential shedder of *Streptococcus equi*. The chondroids seen on radiographs are smooth, irregularly shaped radiopaque masses within the diverticula (Figure 9.41). Although some cases are asymptomatic, removal of the chondroids may be indicated, especially if *Streptococcus equi* is cultured.

Eustachian tube diverticulum tympany

Tympany of the Eustachian tube diverticulum is most commonly seen in young animals. It generally presents clinically as a soft fluctuant swelling in the parotid area. In severe cases it may cause respiratory distress.

Radiographically it presents as a grossly enlarged Eustachian tube diverticulum, extending caudal to the atlas (Figure 9.42). There is some rounding

[490]

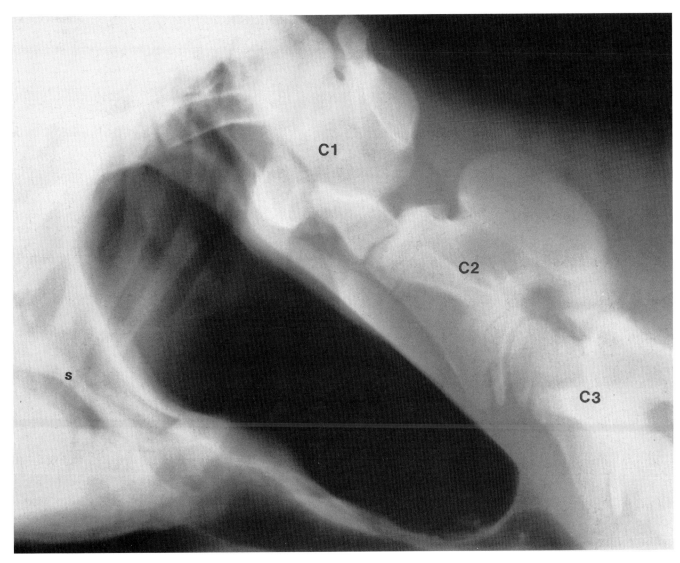

Figure 9.42 Right lateral view of the pharyngeal region of a 1-month-old Arab. The soft tissues in the parotid region were noted to be enlarged soon after birth and progressively enlarged and became more fluctuant. Both Eustachian tube diverticula are markedly distended with gas (air) and extend caudally to the level of the middle of the third cervical vertebra. This is consistent with bilateral Eustachian tube diverticula tympany. Note also gas in the oesophagus just caudal to the distended diverticula. The soft palate (s) is delineated by air in the oropharynx. The epiglottis is flat against the soft palate.

of the outline of the diverticulum and often narrowing of the nasopharynx. Generally the condition is unilateral so that two distinct diverticular outlines can be seen. Occasionally bilateral cases occur.

The condition may arise from the presence of excessive soft tissue at the pharyngeal orifice, which acts as a valve and allows air into the pouch during deglutition but does not allow for the exit of air. As a sequel to the condition, there may be respiratory distress due to narrowing of the pharynx, and in some cases aspiration pneumonia. For this reason, radiographs of the thorax should also be obtained. Cases may resolve spontaneously as the horse ages, but usually require surgical treatment.

Eustachian tube diverticulum mycosis

Plain radiographs of the guttural pouch are generally unrewarding for the diagnosis of mycosis. Fluid lines may be seen in the Eustachian tube diverticulum, or there may be no radiological abnormality on plain radiographs. This is a life-threatening condition, and angiography of the carotid tree may be useful in diagnosis and treatment (see page 687).

The condition can present as slight or massive spontaneous epistaxis, usually when at rest. In a minority of cases it may present as difficulty in deglutition, Horner's syndrome, or as other signs of damage to the cranial nerves. The condition is thought to result from mycotic infection of an aneurysm, generally but not always involving the internal carotid artery.

Eustachian tube diverticulum masses

A number of masses are seen in association with the Eustachian tube diverticulum. The most common is enlargement of the parotid or retropharyngeal lymph nodes (Figure 9.43), which may impinge on the wall of the diverticulum and give the appearance of a mass involving the Eustachian tube diverticulum. Similarly, cysts and abscesses may give this appearance.

Tumours of the pouch have been recorded, the most common being a squamous cell carcinoma.

Pharyngeal lymphoid hyperplasia

This condition is seen radiographically as a diffuse mottled increase in soft-tissue opacity of the pharyngeal wall (see Figure 9.40, page 489). This is frequently recognized in the racing Thoroughbred, but may be a normal phenomenon in the development of all young horses. It may cause some respiratory noise and respiratory obstruction, but its effect on performance is uncertain. Treatment is by conservative management and it has a good long-term prognosis.

Fracture and osteomyelitis of the stylohyoid bone

It is thought that osteomyelitis of the stylohyoid bone may be followed by pathological fracture, and for this reason these two apparently separate conditions are treated here as one. The condition can be seen on lateral radiographs, although slightly oblique views may be necessary to determine whether the left or right bone is involved. Fracture of the stylohyoid bone can also be seen in isolation (Figure 9.44).

Epiglottic entrapment

In this condition the apex and lateral margins of the epiglottis become enveloped by the ventral mucosa and aryepiglottic folds (Figure 9.45). The radiographic appearance is varied, but the epiglottis always appears blunted and shortened. It should be confirmed by endoscopy and must be

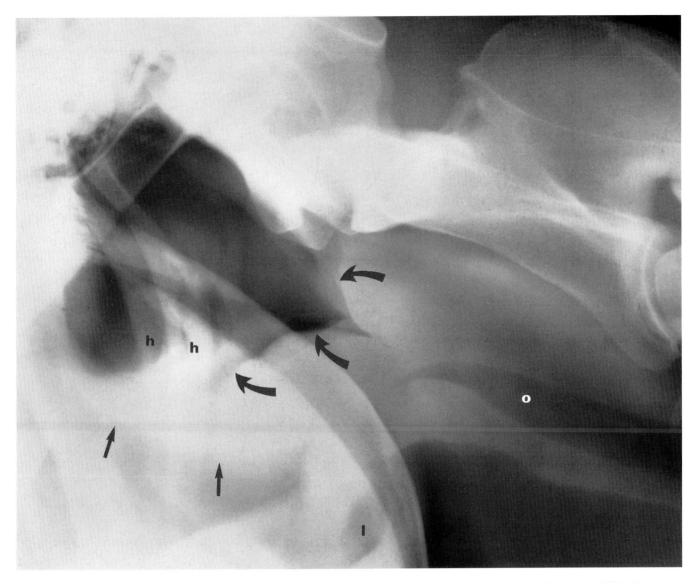

Figure 9.43 Lateral view of the pharyngeal region of a 4-year-old Quarterhorse with a 3-day history of dysphagia. Clinical examination revealed eighth and ninth cranial nerve deficits and bilateral nasal discharge containing food. The ventral margins of the Eustachian tube diverticula (ETD) are irregular (straight arrows) and there is soft-tissue swelling in the retropharyngeal area impinging on the ventral caudal aspect of the ETD (curved arrows). There is air in the oesophagus (o) and the lateral saccules (1). The stylohyoid bones (h) are normal. The caudal ventral soft-tissue mass is due to retropharyngeal lymphadenopathy and local inflammation, caused by infection with *Streptococcus equi*. Compare with Figure 9.41.

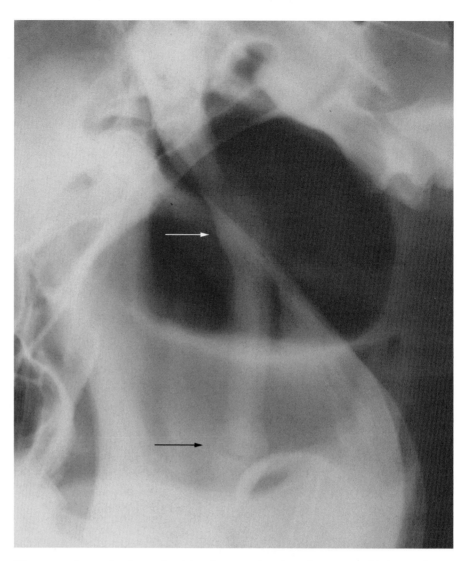

Figure 9.44 Lateral radiograph of the pharyngeal region of a 15-year-old Quarterhorse. The mare had exhibited transient facial nerve paralysis 12 months previously, which had recently recurred. There is osteitis of the temporohyoid joint, with bony proliferation on the stylohyoid (arrow 1). Such bony proliferation may be visible endoscopically via the guttural pouch. There is also a pathological, delayed union fracture with callus further distally (arrow 2), which is unable to heal due to constant movement of the stylohyoid. Note the flaring of the ends of the bone at the fracture site (black arrow) and slight sclerosis along the fracture margins, typical of a delayed union. A normal epiglottis is partially superimposed over the distal fracture piece.

differentiated from epiglottic shortening (see below). There may be concurrent dorsal displacement of the soft palate but this is inconsistent.

Clinically the horse shows exercise intolerance and abnormal respiratory sounds at high speeds, but is asymptomatic at rest. Treatment is surgical and carries a reasonable prognosis.

Epiglottic shortening

Abnormal shortness of the epiglottis may predispose to dorsal displacement of the soft palate or entrapment of the epiglottis by the aryepiglottic folds. The length of the epiglottis can only be assessed objectively on radiographs

[494]

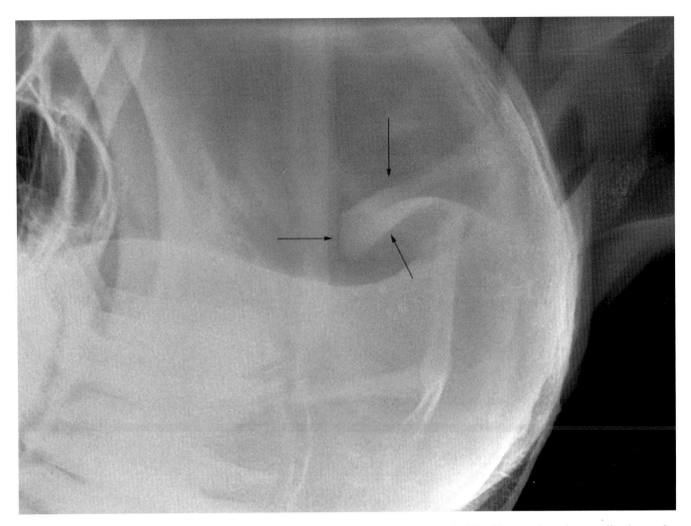

Figure 9.45 Lateral radiographic view of the pharynx of an 11-year-old Thoroughbred with a history of persistent salivation and food reflux. Rostral is to the left. There is entrapment of the epiglottis by the aryepiglottic folds (arrows). Endoscopic examination revealed marked thickening and ulceration of the aryepiglottic folds, and confirmed entrapment of the epiglottis. There was also moderate, diffuse pharyngitis.

by taking magnification into account. Radiopaque markers of known length (A*l* and A*r)* must be taped to the right and left sides of the horse's neck. The length of these markers on a lateral radiograph should be measured (R*l* and R*r)*, together with the distance between the tip of the epiglottis and the thyroid cartilage (R*e)*. The formula for correction for magnification to determine the actual epiglottic length (A*e)* is as follows:

$$A e / R e = (A l / R l + A r / R r) / 2$$

Normal values have been recorded for the Thoroughbred (8.76 ± 0.44 cm) and Standardbred (8.74 ± 0.38 cm).

A horse with an abnormally short epiglottis is usually asymptomatic at rest, but may show exercise intolerance and make an abnormal respiratory noise at high-speed exercise.

Sub-epiglottic cysts

Sub-epiglottic cysts are believed to arise from remnants of the thyroglossal duct (Figures 9.46a and 9.46b). They are visualized as well circumscribed radiopaque (soft-tissue) masses under the ventral aspect of the base of the epiglottis. They displace the epiglottis in a caudodorsal direction. Treatment is surgical and carries a reasonable prognosis.

Arytenoid chondritis

Arytenoid chondritis causes exercise intolerance and abnormal respiratory noise. The arytenoid cartilages may have a mottled increase in opacity or an irregular outline, particularly of the cranial margin of the cartilage (Figure 9.47). They may also have some mineralization, which may occasionally be seen incidentally in old animals, where there is more generalized involvement throughout the laryngeal cartilages (Figure 9.48). If the condition is unilateral in a breeding horse it may be treated conservatively, but surgery is usually required to return a horse to athletic function or if the condition is bilateral.

Dorsal displacement of the soft palate

Dorsal displacement of the soft palate may be intermittent or persistent, with the soft palate located dorsal to the epiglottis (Figure 9.49). The

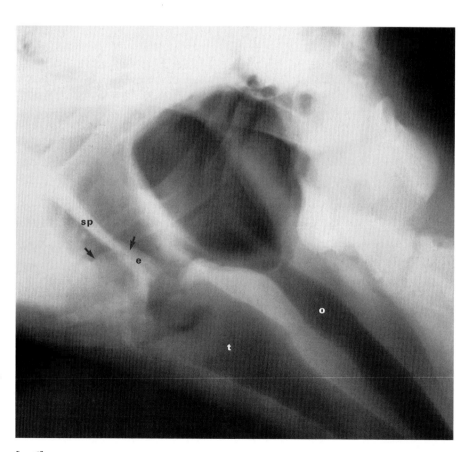

Figure 9.46(a) Lateral view of the pharyngeal region of a 1-month-old Standardbred colt, with a history of dyspnoea following suckling or strenuous exercise. There is a smoothly outlined soft-tissue opacity (arrows), ventral to the epiglottis (e), in the oropharynx. The mass, a subepiglottic cyst, appears to displace the soft palate (sp) dorsally above the epiglottis, but the area between the soft palate, epiglottis and subepiglottic cyst cannot be defined. Note air in the oesophagus (o) and the trachea (t).

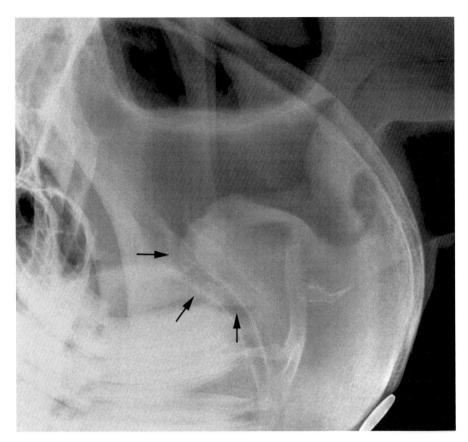

Figure 9.46b Lateral radiographic view of the pharynx of a 6-year-old Thoroughbred cross Cob with a 4-month history of coughing and reflux of food. There is a large radiopaque mass (arrows) ventral to the epiglottis, a subepiglottic cyst.

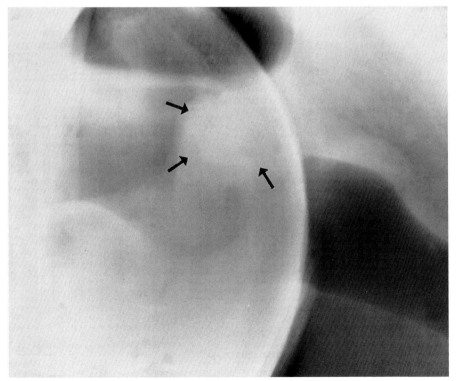

Figure 9.47 Lateral view of the pharyngeal region of an 11-year-old hunter with a history of exercise intolerance and an abnormal respiratory noise. Endoscopic examination of the larynx revealed distortion in shape of the arytenoid cartilages, i.e. arytenoid chondropathy (chondritis). Radiographically there is extensive well defined soft-tissue swelling (arrows) on the craniodorsal aspect of the larynx (in some cases there may also be ill defined mineralization within the arytenoid cartilages).

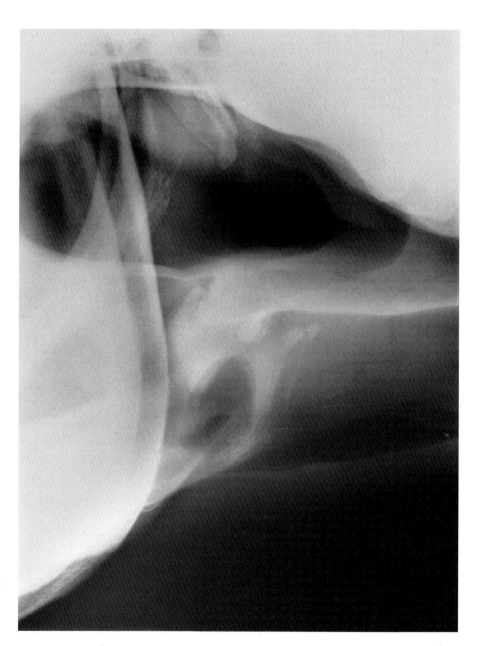

Figure 9.48 Lateral view of the pharyngeal region of an aged Thoroughbred. The head is slightly extended to improve visualization of this area. There is partial mineralization of the laryngeal cartilages. This was an incidental radiological finding.

presence of air between the tongue and soft palate is usually the first radiographic abnormality noticed. Careful examination of the radiograph may show the caudal part of the soft palate lying over the epiglottis. This is a dynamic condition and so may not be seen on plain radiographs. It is most likely to be demonstrated immediately after the horse swallows and may be more easily confirmed by endoscopy or radiographic screening. This condition has been reported in horses that have shown no clinical signs of exercise intolerance.

Cleft palate

This condition is most commonly seen in foals, but may not be diagnosed in some animals until quite late in life. Careful evaluation of lateral

[498]

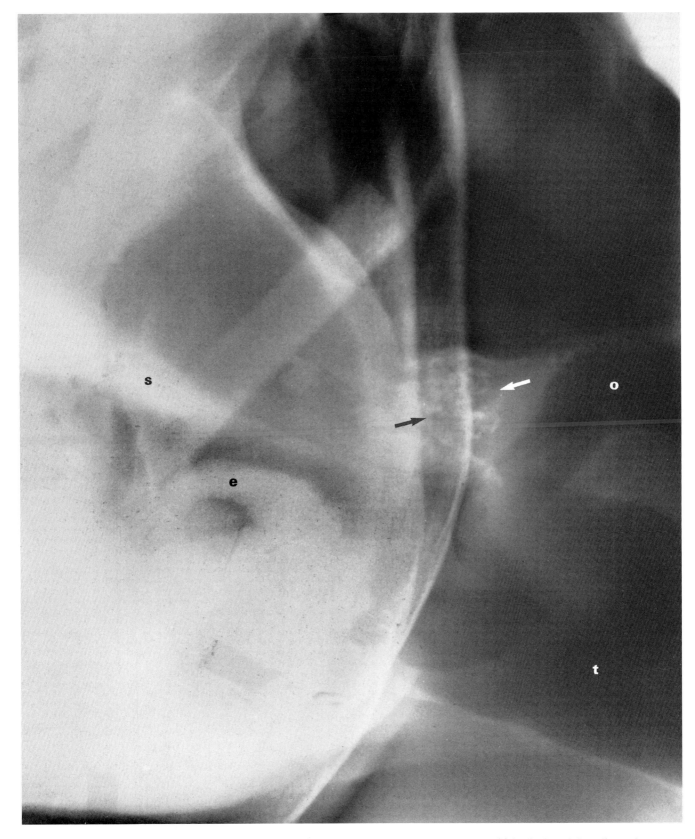

Figure 9.49 Lateral view of the pharyngeal region of an aged Thoroughbred. The soft palate (s) is displaced dorsally to the epiglottis (e). There is an area of diffuse mineralization (arrows) in the dorsocaudal nasopharynx. Note gas in both the trachea (t) and the oesophagus (o).

radiographs may reveal the presence of a double soft palate shadow. Positive contrast studies (barium swallows, see page 658) may reveal the presence of contrast agent dorsal to the soft palate. If clinically significant, these cases frequently develop aspiration pneumonia, so assessment of the thorax should be carried out.

Confirmation of the diagnosis by endoscopy is necessary to determine the extent of the cleft. In mild cases, conservative treatment is often sufficient. In more extensive cases, surgery may be necessary but does carry a very guarded prognosis.

Multilobular osteoma (chondroma rodens)

Multilobular osteoma is not common, but has a characteristic radiographic appearance. It is a well defined mass with clearly demarcated undulating borders and a homogeneous stippled internal radiopacity. Clinical signs depend on the location of the mass in the skull. The mass usually enlarges slowly. Surgical removal is indicated.

Aneurysmal bone cyst

Aneurysmal bone cysts are rare in the horse, but have been reported in the mandible and the long bones. The lesion is characterized radiographically by an expansile relatively lucent lesion, traversed by opaque incomplete septa. The overlying cortex is thinned and there is usually extensive periosteal new bone formation. Surgical debridement and bone grafting can be attempted.

Luxation of the temporomandibular joint

Temporomandibular joint luxation is usually the result of trauma, and may occur unilaterally or bilaterally. There may be associated fractures. Oblique radiographic views may be required to separate the two joints. There is usually associated malocclusion of the molars. The radiographs should be inspected carefully for the presence of concurrent fractures.

FURTHER READING

Ackerman, N., Coffman, J. and Corley, E.A. (1974) The spheno-occipital suture of the horse: its normal radiographic appearance. *J. Am. Vet. Rad. Soc.*, **15**, 79–81

Acland, H.M., Orsini, J.A., Elkins, S., Lee, J.W., Lein, D.H. and Morris, D.D. (1984) Congenital ethmoid carcinoma in a foal. *J. Am. Vet. Med. Ass.*, **184**, 979–981

Arenchibia, A., Vazquez, J., Jaber, R., Gib, F., Ramirez, J. *et al.* (2000) Magnetic resonance imaging and cross-sectional anatomy of the normal equine sinuses and nasal passages. *Vet. Radiol. and Ultrasound*, **41**, 313–319

Barakzai, S. and Dixon, P. (2003) A study of open-mouthed oblique radiographic projections for evaluating lesions of the erupted (clinical) crown. *Equine vet. Educ.*, **15**, 143–148

Beard, W. and Hardy, J. (2001) Diagnosis of conditions of the paranasal sinuses in the horse. *Equine vet. J.*, **13**, 265

Beard, W., Robertson, J. and Leeth, B. (1990) Bilateral congenital cysts in the frontal sinuses of a horse. *J. Am. Vet. Med. Ass.*, **196**, 453–454

Behrens, E., Schumacher, J. and Morris, E. (1991) Contrast paranasal sinusography for evaluation of disease of the paranasal sinuses of five horses. *Vet. Radiol.*, **32**, 105–109

Blythe, L., Watrous, B., Schmitz, J. and Kaneps, A. (1984) Vestibular syndrome associated with temporohyoid joint fusion and temporal bone fracture in three horses. *J. Am. Vet. Med. Ass.*, **185**, 775–781

Boles, C.L. (1975) Epiglottic entrapment and follicular pharyngitis: diagnosis and treatment. *Proc. Am. Ass. Equine Pract.*, **21**, 29–34

Boles, C.L., Raker, C.W. and Wheat, J.D. (1978) Epiglottic entrapment by aryteno-epiglottic folds in the horse. *J. Am. Vet. Med. Ass.*, **172**, 338–342

Caldwell, L. (2006) A review of diagnosis, treatment and sequelae of incisor-luxation fractures in horses (from a dentist's point of view). *Proc. Am. Ass. Equine Pract.*, **52**, 559–564

Camus, A., Burba, D., Valdes, M. and Taylor, H. (1996) Intraosseous epidermoid cyst in a horse. *J. Am. Vet. Med. Ass.*, **209**, 632–633

Carmult, J. (2003) Understanding the equine diastema. *Equine vet. Educ.*, **15**, 34–37

Cook, W. (1973) The auditory tube diverticulum (guttural pouch) in the horse. Its radiographic examination. *J. Am. Vet. Rad. Ass.*, **14**, 51–71

Dacre, I., Kempson, S. and Dixon, P. (2007) Equine idiopathic cheek tooth fractures. Part 1: Pathological studies on 35 fractured cheek teeth. *Equine vet. J.*, **39**, 310–321

Dixon, P., Tremaine, H., Pickles, K., Kuhns, L. *et al.* (1999a) Equine dental disease Part 1: a long-term study of 400 cases: disorders of incisor, canine and first premolar teeth. *Equine vet. J.*, **31**, 369–377

Dixon, P., Tremaine, H., Pickles, K., Kuhns, L. *et al.* (1999b) Equine dental disease Part 2: a long-term study of 400 cases: disorders of development and eruption and variations in position of the cheek teeth. *Equine vet. J.*, **31**, 519–528

Dixon, P., Tremaine, H., Pickles, K., Kuhns, L. *et al.* (2000a) Equine dental disease Part 3: a long-term study of 400 cases: disorders of wear, traumatic damage and idiopathic fractures, tumours and miscellaneous disorders of the cheek teeth. *Equine vet. J.*, **32**, 9–18

Dixon, P., Tremaine, H., Pickles, K., Kuhns, L. *et al.* (2000b) Equine dental disease Part 4: a long-term study of 400 cases: apical infections of cheek teeth. *Equine vet. J.*, **32**, 182–194

Dixon, P., McGorum, B., Railton, D., Hawe, C. *et al.* (2001) Laryngeal paralysis: a study of 375 cases in a mixed-breed population of horses. *Equine vet. J.*, **33**, 452–458

Dixon, P., Dacre, I., Tremaine, H., McCann, J. and Barakzai, S. (2005) Standing oral extraction of cheek teeth in 100 horses (1998–2003). *Equine vet. J.*, **37**, 105–112

Dixon, P., Bararzai, S., Collins, N. and Yates, J. (2007) Equine idiopathic cheek tooth fractures: Part 3. *Equine vet. J.*, **39**, 327–333

Evans, L.H. (1981) Entrapment of the epiglottis. *Proc. Am. Ass. Equine Pract.*, **27**, 61–62

Ferraro, G.L. (1981) Equine follicular pharyngitis. *Proc. Am. Ass. Equine Pract.*, **27**, 55–56

Ferrell, E., Gavin, P., Tucker, R., Sellon, D. and Hines, M. (2002) Magnetic resonance for evaluation of neurologic disease in 12 horses. *Vet. Radiol. and Ultrasound*, **43**, 510–517

Frame, E., Riihimaki, M., Berger, M., Vatne, M. and McEvoy, F. (2005) Scintigraphic findings in a case of temporohyoid osteoarthropathy in a horse. *Eqine vet. Educ.*, **17**, 11–13

Freeman, D. (2006) Guttural pouch tympany – a rare and difficult disease. *Equine vet. Educ.*, **18**, 234–238

Gasser, A., Love, N. and Tate, L. (2000) Ethmoid haematoma. *Vet. Radiol. and Ultrasound*, **41**, 247–249

Gayle, J., Redding, W., Vacek, J. and Bowman, K. (1999) Diagnosis and surgical treatment of periapical infection of the third mandibular molar in five horses. *J. Am. Vet. Med. Ass.*, **215**, 829–832

Gibbs, C. and Lane, J.G. (1987) Radiographic examinations of the facial, nasal and paranasal sinus regions of the horse. (ii) Radiological findings. *Equine vet. J.*, **19**, 474–482

Gibbs, C., Lane, J.G., Meynink, S.E. and Steele, F.C. (1987) Radiographic examinations of the facial, nasal and paranasal sinus regions of the horse. (i) Indications and procedures in 235 cases. *Equine vet. J.*, **19**, 466–473

Gibb, S. (2000) Dental imaging. In: *Equine dentistry*. Eds. Baker, G. and Easley, J., pp. 220–249 W.B. Saunders, Philadelphia

Gift, L., DeBowes, R., Clem, M., Rasmir-Raven, A. and Nyrop, K. (1992) Brachygnathia in horses: 20 cases (1979–1989). *J. Am. Vet. Med. Ass.*, **200**, 715–719

Haynes, P.F. (1981) Persistent dorsal displacement of the soft palate associated with epiglottic shortening in two horses. *J. Am. Vet. Med. Ass.*, **197**, 677–681

Haynes, P.F., Snider, T.G., McClure, J.R. and McClure, J.J. (1980) Chronic chondritis of the equine arytenoid cartilage. *J. Am. Vet. Med. Ass.*, **177**, 1135–1142

Henninger, R., Beard, W., Schneider, R., Bramlage, L. and Burkhardt, H. (1999) Fractures of the rostral portion of the mandible in horses: 89 cases (1979–1997), *J. Am. Vet. Med. Ass.*, **214**, 1648–1652

Henninger, W., Frame, E., Willman, M., Simhofer, H. *et al.* (2003) CT features of alveolitis and sinusitis in horses. *Vet. Radiol. and Ultrasound*, **44**, 269–276

Jackman, B. and Baxter, G. (1992) Treatment of a mandibular bone cyst by use of a corticancellous bone graft in a horse. *J. Am. Vet. Med. Ass.*, **201**, 892–894

Jubb, K.V.F., Kennedy, P.C. and Palmer, N. (1985) *Pathology of Domestic Animals*, 3rd edn, Academic Press, Orlando

Kiper, M., Wrigley, R., Traub-Dragatz, J. and Bennett, D. (1992) Metallic foreign bodies in the mouth or pharynx of horses: seven cases (1983–1989). *J. Am. Vet. Med. Ass.*, **200**, 91–93

Lamb, C. and Schelling, S. (1989) Congenital aneurysmal bone cyst in the mandible of a foal. *Equine vet. J.*, **21**, 130–132

Lane, J.G. (1989) The management of guttural pouch mycosis. *Equine vet. J.*, **21**, 321–324

Lane, J., Gibbs, C., Meynink, S. and Steele, F. (1987) Radiographic examination of the facial, nasal and paranasal regions of the horse: I. Indications and procedures in 235 cases. *Equine vet. J.*, **19**, 466–473

Lane, J., Longstaff, J. and Gibbs, C. (1987) Equine paranasal sinus cysts: a report of 15 cases. *Equine vet. J.*, **19**, 537–544

Latimer, C., Wyman, C., Dresem, C. and Burt, J. (1984) Radiographic and gross anatomy of the nasolacrimal duct of the horse. *Am. J. Vet. Res.*, **46**, 451–458

Latimer, C. and Wyman, C. (1984) Atresia of the nasolacrimal duct in three horses. *J. Am. Vet. Med. Ass.*, **184**, 989–992

Lavach, J.D. and Severin, G.A. (1977) Neoplasia of the equine eye, adnexa and orbit: a review of 68 cases. *J. Am. Vet. Med. Ass.*, **170**, 202–203

Linford, R., O'Brien, T., Wheat, J. *et al.* (1983) Radiographic assessment of epiglottic length and pharyngeal and laryngeal diameters in the Thoroughbred. *Am. J. Vet. Res.*, **44**, 1660–1666

Lischer, C., Walliser, U., Witzmann, P., Wehrlieser, M. and Ohlerth, S. (2005) Fracture of the paracondylar process in four horses: advantages of CT imaging. *Equine vet. J.*, **37**, 483–487

Morgan, J.P. and Silverman, S. (1993) *Techniques of Veterinary Radiography*, 5th edn, Iowa State University Press

Morrow, K., Park, R., Spurgeon, T., Stashak, T. and Arceneaux, B. (2000) Computed tomographic imaging of the equine head. *Vet. Radiol. and Ultrasound*, **41**, 491–498

Nykamp, S., Scrivani, P. and Pease, A. (2004) Computed tomography dacrocystography evaluation of the nasolacrimal apparatus. *Vet. Radiol. And Ultrasound*, **45**, 23–28

Orsini, J., Baird, D. and Ruggles, A. (2004) Radiotherapy of a recurrent ossifying fibroma in the paranasal sinuses of a horse. *J. Am. Vet. Med. Ass.*, **224**, 1483–1486

Quinn, G., Tremaine, H. and Lane, J. (2005) Supernumerary cheek teeth (n = 24): clinical features, diagnosis, treatment and outcome in 15 horses. *Equine vet. J.*, **37**, 505–509

Prichard, M., Hackett, R. and Erb, H. (1992) Long-term outcome of tooth repulsion in horses – a retrospective study of 61 cases. *Vet. Surg.*, **21**, 145–149

Ramirez, O., Jorgensen, J. and Thrall, D. (1998) Imaging basilar skull fractures in the horse: a review. *Vet. Radiol. and Ultrasound*, **39**, 391–395

Ramzan, P., Marr, C., Meehan J. and Thompson, A. (2008) A novel oblique radiographic projection of the equine temporomandibular joint. *Vet. Rec.* In press

Richardson, J., Lane, J.G. and Day, M. (1994) Congenital choanal restriction in 3 horses. *Equine vet. J.*, **26**, 162–165

Robert, M.C., Groenendyk, S.L. and Kelly, W.R. (1978) Ameloblastic odontoma in a foal. *Equine vet. J.*, **10**, 91–93

Schambourg, M., Marcoux, M. and Celeste, C. (2006) Salingoscopy for the treatment of recurrent guttural pouch tympany in a filly. *Equine vet. Educ.*, **18**, 231–233

Schmotzer, W.B., Haltgren, B.D., Watrous, B.J., Wagner, P.C. and Kaneps, A.J. (1987) Nasomaxillary fibrosarcomas in three young horses. *J. Am. Vet. Med. Ass.*, **191**, 437–439

Schumacher, J., Smith, B. and Morgan, S. (1988) Osteoma of paranasal sinuses of a horse. *J. Am. Vet. Med. Ass.*, **192**, 1449–1450

Smallwood, J., Wood, B., Taylor, W. and Tate, L. (2002) Anatomic reference for computed tomography of the head of a foal. *Vet. Radiol and Ultrasound*, **43**, 99–117

Stephenson, R. (2005) An unusual case of headshaking caused by a premaxillary bone cyst *Equine vet. Educ.*, **17**, 79–82

Stilson, A.E., Hening, D.S. and Robertson, J.T. (1985) Contribution of the nasal septum to the radiographic anatomy of the equine nasal cavity. *J. Am. Vet. Med. Ass.*, **186**, 590–592

Taylor, D., Wisner, E., Kuesis, B., Smith, S. and O'Brien, T. (1993) Gas accumulation in the subarachnoid space resulting from blunt trauma to the occipital region of a horse. *Vet. Radiol. and Ultrasound*, **34**, 191–193

Taylor, L. and Dixon, P. (2007) Equine idiopathic cheek teeth fractures: Part 2: A practice based survey of 147 affected horses in Britain and Ireland. *Equine vet. J.*, **39**, 322–326

Thrall, D.E. (2007) *Textbook of Veterinary Diagnostic Radiology*, 5th edn. Saunders, Elsevier, St. Louis

Tremaine, H. and Dixon, P. (2001a) A long-term study of 277 cases of equine sinonasal disease. Part 1: Details of horses, historical, clinical and ancillary diagnostic findings. *Equine vet. J.*, **33**, 274–282

Tremaine, H. and Dixon, P. (2001b) A long-term study of 277 cases of equine sinonasal disease. Part 2: Treatment and results of treatment. *Equine vet. J.*, **33**, 283–289

Trostle, S., Rantanen, N., Andersen, M., Taylor, S. and Vrono, D. (2005) Juvenile ossifying fibroma in a 12 week old foal. *Equine vet. Educ.*, **17**, 284–286

Tudor, R., Ramiriz, O., Tate, L. and Gerard, M. (1999) A congenital malformation of the maxilla of a horse. *Vet. Radiol. and Ultrasound*, **40**, 353–356

Tulleners, E. (1991) Correlation of performance with endoscopic and radiographic assessment of epiglottic hypoplasia in racehorses with epiglottic entrapment corrected by use of contact neodymium: ytrium aluminum laser. *J. Am. Vet. Med. Ass.*, **198**, 621–626

Walker, M., Schumacher, J., Schmitz, D., McMullen, W. *et al.* (1998) Cobalt 60 radiotherapy for treatment of squamous cell carcinoma of the nasal cavity and paranasal sinuses in three horses. *J. Am. Vet. Med. Ass.*, **212**, 848–851

Walker, M., Sellon, D., Cornelisse, C., Hines, M., Ragle, C. and Schott, H. (2002) Temporohyoid osteoarthropathy in 33 horses (1993–2000). *J. Vet. Intern. Med.*, **16**, 697–703

Weller, R., Taylor, S., Maierl, J., Cauvin, E. and May, S. (1999) Ultrasonographic anatomy of the equine temporomandibular joint. *Equine vet. J.*, **31**, 529–532

Weller, R., Livesey, L., Maierl, J., Bowen, I. *et al.* (2001) Comparison of radiography and scintigraphy in the diagnosis of dental disorders in the horse. *Equine vet. J.*, **33**, 49–58

Woodford, N. and Lane, J. (2006) Long-term retrospective study of 52 horses with sinunasal cysts. *Equine vet. J.*, **38**, 198–202

Chapter 10
The spine

Cervical spine

Indications for radiographic examination of the cervical vertebrae include abnormal head and/or neck posture, swelling, stiffness or pain of the neck or back, trauma to the neck, ataxia, inability to stand and, occasionally, forelimb lameness. Radiographic assessment of such cases requires at least lateral radiographs of the occipital bone, all cervical vertebrae and the first thoracic vertebra. Lateral radiographs are best obtained with the horse standing, but can be obtained with the horse in lateral recumbency, under general anaesthesia. Ventrodorsal views can only be obtained in the recumbent horse. As in man, relating radiographic findings in the spine to clinical symptoms may be extremely difficult.

RADIOGRAPHIC TECHNIQUE

Equipment

Good-quality views of the cranial and mid-neck regions are within the capability of portable x-ray machines, but views of the seventh cervical (C7) and first thoracic (T1) vertebrae require more powerful equipment in all but the smallest horses. Digital systems or fast rare earth screens and appropriate film are recommended. A grid, although beneficial, is not essential for the cranial part of the neck, but is necessary for the caudal one-third.

In order to assess the relative alignment of the cervical vertebrae it is helpful to use large cassettes (35 cm × 43 cm) so that part of at least three vertebrae is projected on each film. The cassette should be supported in a cassette holder, which is mounted on a wall or mobile stand. If the cassette holder is not linked to the x-ray machine, alignment can be difficult, and it is helpful to mark the neck on both sides at the sites where the x-ray beam is to be centred. This is easily done using sticky tape.

Positioning

Radiography of the head and neck in the standing horse renders the handler particularly at risk to exposure to radiation, and appropriate precautions including wearing lead gloves are important. If the area to be radiographed involves the occipito-atlantal articulation, a rope halter should be used rather than a head collar with metal buckles, in order to avoid artefacts.

[505]

The standing horse

Slightly oblique radiographic views are difficult to interpret, and in most circumstances true lateral views are essential, especially if measurements of vertebral dimensions are to be obtained. It may be helpful if the horse handler pulls gently forwards on the halter, but this may result in changes in the alignment of the cervical vertebrae. Many horses are apprehensive of the x-ray machine and the cassette, especially when these are close to the head. To minimize movement of the horse it may be helpful to restrain it in stocks; sedation may be helpful, not only to reduce movement, but also because it causes the horse to lower its head and neck. However, when examining the caudal cervical vertebrae it may be necessary to raise the head and neck to avoid superimposition of the seventh cervical and first thoracic vertebrae and the scapula or shoulder joint.

Sedation of an ataxic horse should be carried out with care because it is likely that the ataxia will be exacerbated. A sedated horse usually moves less and it is more likely to hold the head and neck in the sagittal plane. It has the disadvantage that the neck may be flexed relative to the normal standing position; thus the alignment of the vertebrae is altered. In some horses it is not possible to obtain true lateral projections of all the cervical vertebrae, despite appropriate positioning. This usually reflects either abnormal muscle tone in the neck associated with pain or is the result of abnormal modelling of the caudal synovial facet joints, which results in a permanent slight rotation of the more cranial vertebrae.

Lead markers placed on the skin of the neck above the level of the vertebrae can be helpful for orientation when taking and interpreting radiographs. Complete radiographic assessment of the cervical vertebrae (C1–C7) of an adult horse usually requires at least four views: the occiput and C1 (atlas); C1–C3; C3–C5; and C5–T1. In most cases a fifth view is required to evaluate the seventh cervical vertebra and its articulation with the first thoracic vertebra. Radiographs are obtained with the horse standing square with its head and neck in the sagittal plane. The x-ray beam is aligned perpendicular to the neck. In the caudal half of the neck the cervical vertebrae are situated ventrally and the x-ray beam should be centred accordingly. It is usually easiest to radiograph the mid-neck region first and then the more caudal area, before examining the cranial part. This allows the horse to become familiar with the equipment before it is placed close to the head.

It is sometimes helpful to obtain both left to right and right to left projections in order to establish on which side of the neck a lesion is situated. The lesion is smaller and more clearly defined when closer to the cassette.

When obtaining radiographs of the occiput it may be useful to pull the ears forwards to avoid superimposition of the cartilages of the ears over the region of insertion of the nuchal ligament (see Figure 9.8b, page 429). This is easily achieved in a sedated horse by attaching sticky tape to the ears in order to pull them cranially.

In order to obtain true lateral projections when the horse is in lateral recumbency, it is necessary to support the head and neck, using radiolucent cushions, so that it is horizontal from the shoulder to the head. Aligning the x-ray machine and the cassette with the horse in this position may be difficult, but longer exposure times can be used. The neck may be flexed passively in order to accentuate a subluxation seen in a lateral view, but care must be taken neither to kink the endotracheal tube, to displace a fracture nor exacerbate a potential spinal cord compression.

Ventrodorsal views can only be obtained safely in a recumbent horse. Even with high-output x-ray machines it is difficult to get good-quality radiographs caudal to the fifth cervical vertebra because of the surrounding muscle mass. Myelography is discussed in Chapter 14 (page 694).

NORMAL ANATOMY, VARIATIONS AND INCIDENTAL FINDINGS

There are seven cervical vertebrae (C1–C7). In the resting position the neck is S-shaped with a smooth transition of angulation between the vertebrae, from slight flexion (dorsal convexity) cranially, to slight extension (dorsal concavity) caudally. This is particularly obvious in foals and small ponies. Apparent hyperflexion/subluxation at the articulation between the second and third or third and fourth (see Figure 10.13a, page 521) vertebrae may occur without clinical signs, in horses with a wide dorsoventral diameter of the vertebral foramen (minimum sagittal diameter).

The cervical vertebrae, other than the atlas, have a similar basic shape. The two sides of the vertebral arch (pedicles), its roof (lamina) and the body of each vertebra form the vertebral foramen in which lies the spinal cord (Figure 10.1). The series of vertebral foramina together constitute the vertebral canal. Within each vertebra the vertebral foramen appears approximately rectangular in shape (Figure 10.2). The minimum sagittal diameter (MSD) can be measured directly from a radiograph (Figure 10.2b). This is useful for comparison between vertebrae, but comparison between horses can be unreliable due to variable magnification. Comparison should only be made between horses of similar size (Table 10.1). In horses with severe stenosis of the vertebral canal, MSD measurements are sufficiently accurate to differentiate between normal and affected horses, but in less severe cases diagnosis can be difficult, unless combined with other subjective criteria.

The problem of variable magnification between horses, due to differences in object–film distance, can be eliminated by use of a sagittal ratio method, rather than absolute measurements, which thereby standardizes the assessment of MSD between horses. The intravertebral sagittal ratio is obtained by dividing the MSD value by the dorsoventral height of the corresponding vertebral body at the cranial aspect of its widest point (Figure 10.3a). Alternatively a corrected MSD can be used: the absolute MSD is

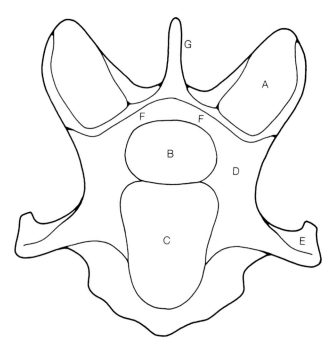

Figure 10.1 Craniocaudal view of the seventh cervical vertebra of an adult horse. A = facet of cranial articular process, B = vertebral foramen, C = head of vertebral body, D = lateral vertebral arch or pedicle, E = transverse process, F = dorsal laminae, forming dorsal arch, G = spinous process.

Table 10.1 Minimum sagittal diameter (mm) of the vertebral foramen, measured from radiographs of clinically normal horses. (From Mayhew *et al.*, 1978, with permission).

	Less than 320 kg body weight					
	C2	C3	C4	C5	C6	C7
Mean	23.8	19.8	18.7	19.7	21.1	22.9
Standard deviation	1.5	0.9	1.0	1.2	1.5	1.6
Reference	20.8	18.1	16.7	17.3	18.3	19.8
limits*	26.8	21.5	20.7	22.1	23.9	26.1

	More than 320 kg body weight					
	C2	C3	C4	C5	C6	C7
Mean	26.7	22.2	21.3	22.4	24.1	27.4
Standard deviation	2.3	1.8	1.8	1.8	2.5	2.6
Reference	22.1	18.5	17.7	18.7	19.0	22.6
limits*	31.3	25.9	24.9	26.1	29.1	32.6

*Minimum and maximum sagittal diameter which can be considered normal.

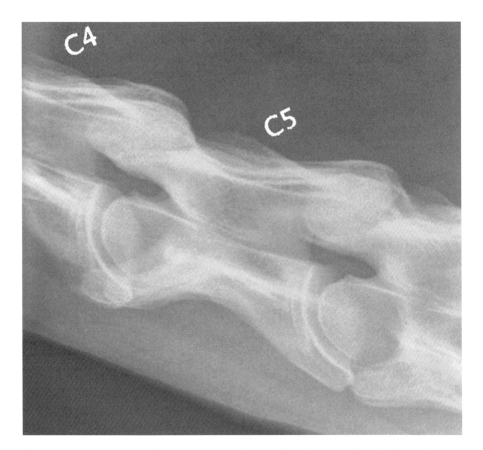

Figure 10.2(a) Lateral radiographic view of the mid-neck region (cervical vertebrae C4–C6) of a normal mature horse. Cranial is to the left.

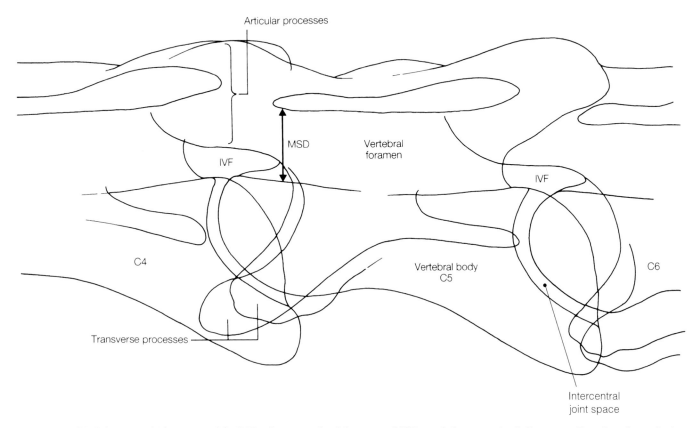

Figure 10.2(b) Diagram of Figure 10.2(a). IVF = intervertebral foramen, MSD = minimum sagittal diameter, C4 = fourth cervical vertebra, C5 = fifth cervical vertebra, C6 = sixth cervical vertebra.

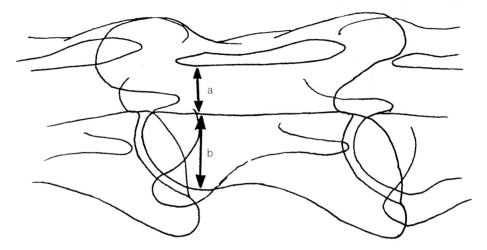

Figure 10.3(a) Method to obtain the sagittal ratio of the vertebral foramen. Divide the minimum sagittal diameter (MSD) (a) by the dorsoventral height (b) of the corresponding vertebral body at biggest point of its cranial aspect.

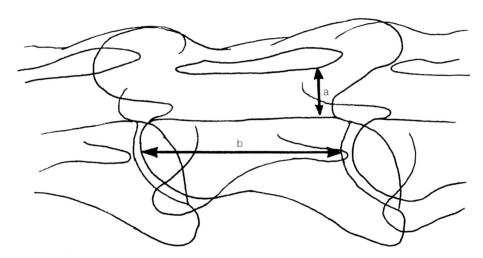

Figure 10.3(b) Method to obtain a corrected minimum sagittal diameter (cMSD). The absolute (measured) MSD (a) is divided by the length (b) of the corresponding vertebral body.

divided by the length of the vertebral body (Figure 10.3b; Table 10.2). Although these techniques are more objective methods of assessment of horses with generalized narrowing of the vertebral canal (see page 519), they are not on their own reliable for identification of potential sites of spinal cord compression, giving false-positive diagnoses. The sagittal diameter of the vertebral canal tends to be slightly smaller in the mid-cervical region compared with more cranial and caudal levels. Use of the intervertebral sagittal ratio provides additional accuracy for identification of a site of spinal cord compression. The intervertebral sagittal ratio is the minimum intervertebral distance between the proximocranial aspect of the cranial

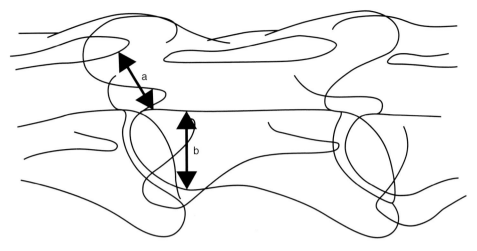

Figure 10.3(c) Measurement of the intervertebral diameter, the distance between the cranioproximal aspect of the physis of the cranial aspect of the vertebral body and the ventrocaudal aspect of the lamina of the immediately cranial vertebra (a). The height of the widest part of the cranial aspect of the vertebral head (b) is also measured. The intervertebral sagittal ratio is calculated by dividing the minimum intervertebral distance by the maximum height.

Table 10.2 Normal values for radiographic minimum sagittal diameter (MSD) (mm) and corrected MSD (cMSD) (%) for Thoroughbred foals, 3–7 months of age (From Mayhew *et al.*, 1993, with permission).

	Cervical vertebral site										
	C2	C2–C3	C3	C3–C4	C4	C4–C5	C5	C5–C6	C6	C6–C7	C7
MSD	23	28	20	25	20	25	21	26	21	31	23
Standard deviation	1	4	1	2	1	2	1	3	1	5	1
cMSD	18	33	24	30	24	31	25	34	27	46	35
Standard deviation	1	2	2	2	2	2	2	3	2	5	2

vertebral body physis and the caudoventral aspect of the lamina of the immediately cranial vertebra, divided by the maximal height of the cranial vertebral physis (Figure 10.3c).

The third, fourth and fifth cervical vertebrae are similar in shape (Figure 10.2), but the rest have distinctive characteristics.

The atlas (C1) has no body or articular process. It develops in two lateral halves which gradually ossify. In a ventrodorsal view of a neonate there is a longitudinal lucent line between the two halves.

The axis (C2) has separate centres of ossification for the dens (odontoid peg), head, body and caudal epiphysis (Figure 10.4). The dens fuses with the head at approximately 7 months (Figure 10.5). The cranial arch of C2 bears lateral vertebral foramina, the cranial borders of which are incomplete in young horses (Figure 10.7, page 514), and may remain as a notch in the adult. The dorsal spine usually has a smooth contour, but its cranial and caudal

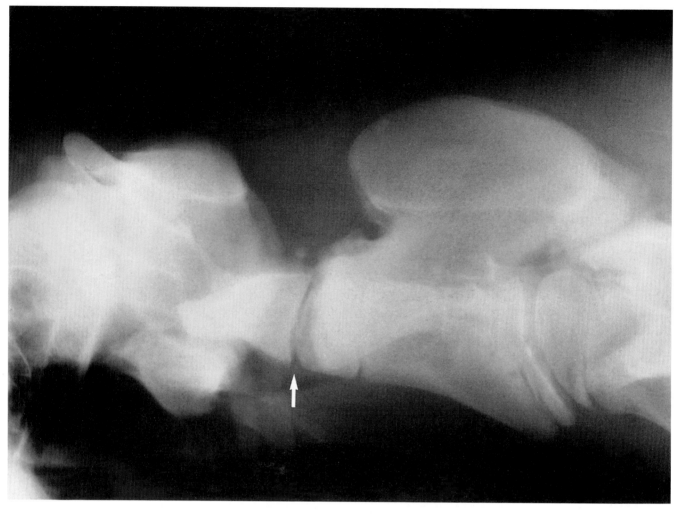

Figure 10.4 Lateral view of the cranial cervical vertebrae (C1–C3) of a 6-week-old Thoroughbred foal. Note the separate centre of ossification (arrowed) of the dens of the axis (C2). The cranial and caudal physes of C2 and C3 are open.

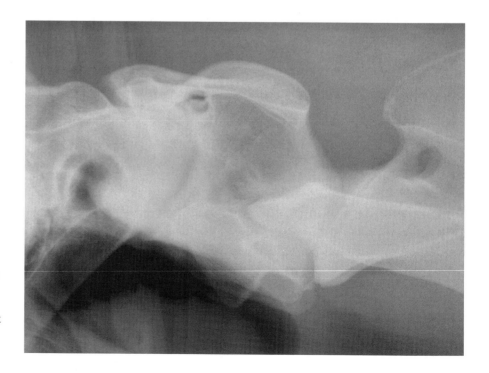

Figure 10.5 Lateral view of the occiput and cranial cervical vertebrae (C1 and C2) of a normal adult horse. Note the complete foramina in the cranial aspect of the axis (compare with Figure 10.7). There is slight rotation of the atlas.

edges may be slightly irregular. Occasionally a small bony spur is seen on the dorsal aspect of the caudal epiphysis (Figure 10.6) projecting into the vertebral canal.

The vertebral bodies of the third to seventh vertebrae have cranial and caudal epiphyses. Closure of the physes occurs gradually, the time varying between individuals. Closure of the cranial physes starts ventrally (Figure 10.7) and is complete by approximately 2 years after birth. The caudal physes remain open until 4–5 years of age, closure starting dorsally (Figure 10.7). The ventral processes of C6, and occasionally of other vertebrae, have small centres of ossification at their caudal limits that should not be confused with fractures (see Figure 10.12, page 520). The convex cranial articular surface of each vertebral body is usually smoothly curved or slightly flattened, and reasonably congruous with the concave caudal articular surface of the adjacent vertebra. The latter has a relatively sclerotic subchondral bone plate. Flattening of the joint surfaces or irregularity in width of an intercentral articulation should be regarded as abnormal (see page 530). It is helpful to compare the shape of adjacent vertebrae.

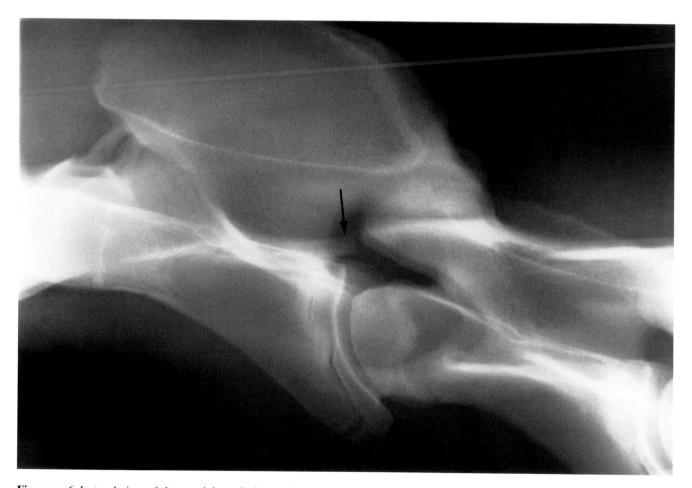

Figure 10.6 Lateral view of the cranial cervical vertebrae of a normal adult horse. There is a large spur (arrow) on the dorsocaudal aspect of the vertebral body of the axis (C2), protruding into the vertebral canal. This is a common incidental radiological finding. The large vertebral canal at this level makes it unlikely that the spur will impinge on the spinal cord.

[513]

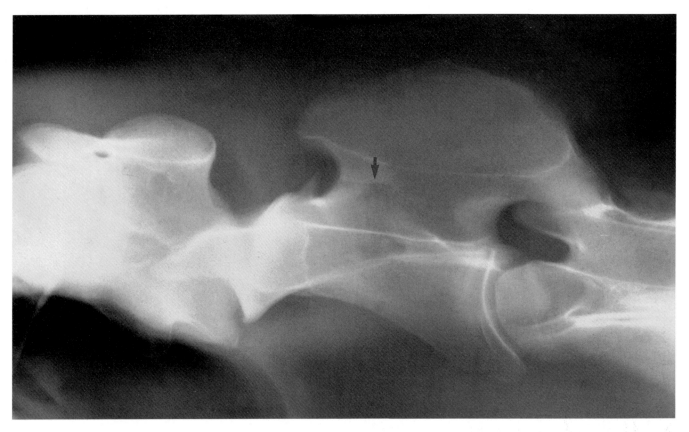

Figure 10.7 Lateral view of the cranial cervical vertebrae (C1–C3) of a normal Thoroughbred yearling. The cranial borders of the vertebral foramina of the axis (C2) are incomplete. The physes of C2 and C3 are not fully closed. The star-shaped lucent area (arrowed) in the vertebral arch of C2 is normal.

The third to seventh cervical vertebrae each have pairs of cranial and caudal articular processes projecting from the borders of the vertebral arch. The extremities of these processes carry articular surfaces (facets), which articulate with those of adjacent vertebrae, forming the cervical synovial articulations. The sixth cervical vertebra is different from C5; it is slightly shorter and it has a trifid transverse process. An extra ventral lamina or process projects caudally and ventrally (Figure 10.8). Sometimes one or both of these processes may be transposed on to the ventral surface of C7 (see Figures 10.15 and 10.16, pages 524–525) or very rarely onto C5. When this transposition on to C7 occurs bilaterally, the ventral aspect of C6 has the same profile as C5. C7 is shorter than C6 and usually has a small dorsal spinous process. This may be superimposed over the synovial articulation between C6 and C7, and should not be confused with new bone associated with degenerative joint disease. The first thoracic vertebra has a larger dorsal spinous process (Figure 10.9).

In older horses, small spondylitic spurs are sometimes seen as incidental findings on the ventral surface of the vertebral bodies adjacent to one or more intercentral articulations. Modelling of the synovial joints of the dorsal articular process of the fifth and sixth and the sixth and seventh cervical vertebrae occurs commonly (see Figure 10.15, page 524) and is considered in more detail below ('Modelling of the cervical synovial articulations', page 523).

[514]

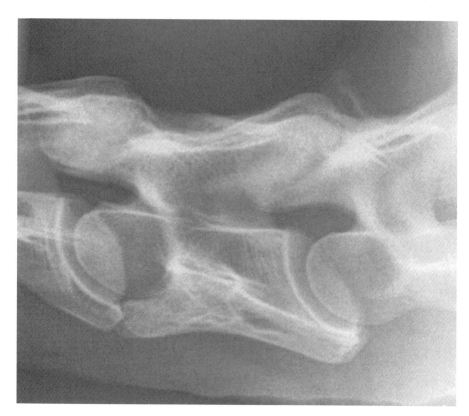

Figure 10.8 Lateral view of the caudal cervical vertebrae (C5–C7) of a normal adult horse. Cranial is to the left. The synovial intervertebral articulations between the sixth and seventh cervical vertebrae are larger than those of the fifth and sixth cervical vertebrae, but are within the normal range. There is a small dorsal spinous process on the dorsal aspect of the seventh cervical vertebra.

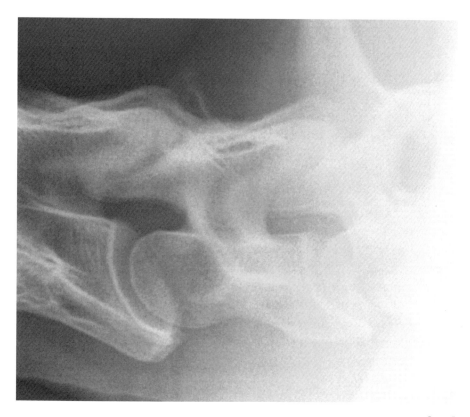

Figure 10.9 Lateral radiographic view of the cervicothoracic junction of a normal adult horse. Cranial is to the left. Note the smooth ventral aspect of the vertebral body of the seventh cervical vertebra and the large dorsal spinous process of the first thoracic vertebra.

SIGNIFICANT RADIOGRAPHIC ABNORMALITIES

When assessing radiographs of the neck it is important not only to examine each vertebra, but also to consider the neck as a whole and to evaluate the shape of the vertebral canal, the alignment of the vertebral bodies, the shape and size of the epiphyses, the regularity of both the intercentral and synovial articulations, and the size of the intervertebral foramina. Comparison with radiographs of a normal horse of similar age, and with bone specimens, is often helpful. When the results of lateral survey radiographs are negative or equivocal it may be necessary to obtain ventrodorsal (or, less commonly, dorsoventral) views and/or to perform myelography (see Chapter 14, page 694).

Congenital abnormalities

Vertebral malformations are rare and, although neck stiffness, distortion of the neck and/or ataxia may be seen soon after birth, some lesions are not clinically apparent until the spinal cord becomes compromised.

Occipito-atlanto-axial malformation (OAAM)

Occipito-atlanto-axial malformation is the most common congenital abnormality, and is most often seen in Arab horses, in which it is thought to be familial. The vertebral defects may be symmetrical or asymmetrical and include fusion and a variety of distorted shapes (Figure 10.10). Lateral and ventrodorsal radiographic views are needed for proper assessment of this abnormality.

Vertebral fusion

Vertebral fusion may involve two or more vertebrae (Figure 10.11). Absence of irregular bony callus helps to distinguish congenital fusion from fusion following a fracture in a foal, but in an older horse the two may be indistinguishable once the callus has modelled.

Developmental abnormalities

The cervical vertebrae can undergo modelling during growth, influenced by the biomechanical stresses placed upon them and the rate of bone turnover. The cause and time of onset of these changes are uncertain, but they result in one or more of a variety of cervical abnormalities, considered together as developmental abnormalities. These may predispose to, or cause, compression of the spinal cord and thus ataxia. Some of the changes described may be related to osteochondrosis. These changes may in part be reversed in foals by restriction of feed intake and exercise. It should be noted that any of these variants, alone or in combination, can be seen in clinically normal horses. The greater both the number of abnormal variants and their severity, the more likely there are to be associated clinical signs. Vertebral

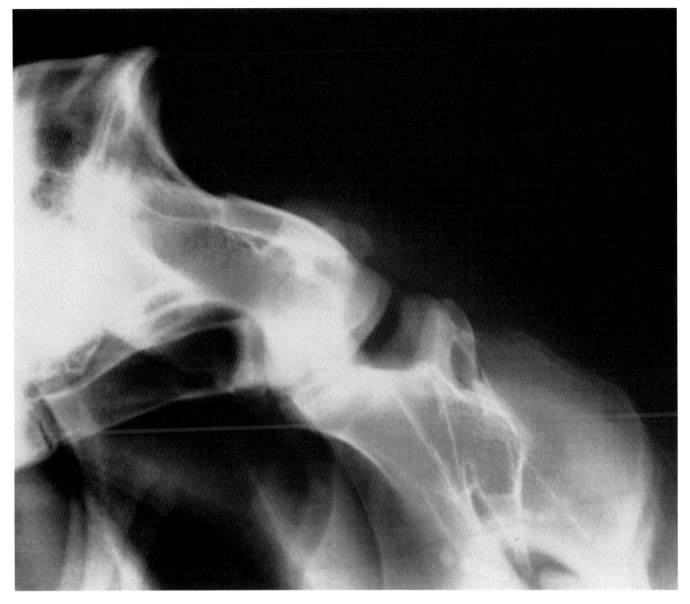

Figure 10.10 Lateral view of the occiput and the cranial cervical vertebrae (C1 and C2) of a yearling Arab filly exhibiting ataxia and abnormal prominence of the wings of the atlas. The atlas (C1) is fused to the occiput and the axis (C2) is misshapen – an occipito-atlanto-axial malformation. Note that the axis is slightly rotated. Compare with Figure 10.5.

stenosis and vertebral angulation are most likely to be associated with spinal cord compression, followed by enlargement of a caudal epiphysis and caudal extension of the arch of the vertebral canal over the cranial aspect of the next vertebra.

A semiquantitative method of assessing cervical radiographs includes documentation of encroachment of the caudal epiphyses dorsally into the vertebral canal ('ski jumps') (Figure 10.14, page 523), caudal extension of the dorsal aspect of the arch of the vertebral canal, intervertebral malalignment, abnormal ossification of the articular processes and degenerative joint disease of the articular processes (see below).

A recent study compared subjective assessment of plain radiographs, semiquantitative scoring of plain radiographs and myelography (positive

[517]

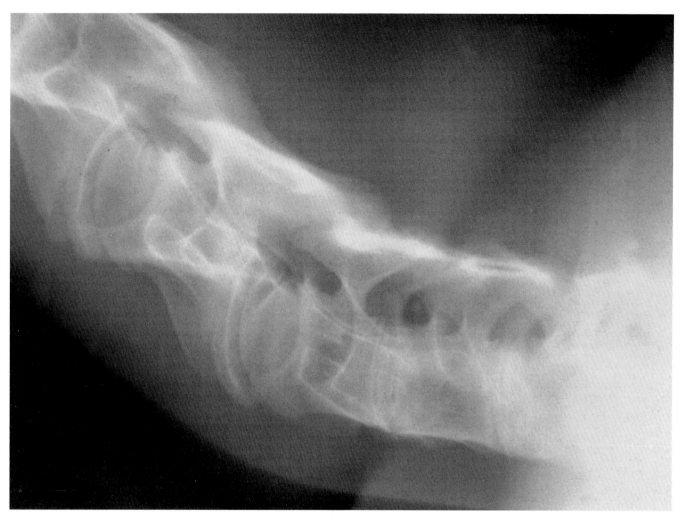

Figure 10.11 Lateral view of the caudal neck (C5–T1) of a 5-month-old Thoroughbred colt with forelimb and hindlimb ataxia. The sixth and seventh cervical and first thoracic vertebrae are misshapen and fused (a synostosis). This was a congenital abnormality. Note the absence of callus. Post-mortem examination revealed a small ventral meningomyelocele passing into a cleft in the vertebral bodies of C7 and T1.

results defined as ≥50% reduction in dorsal dye column) in a group of horses with histologically confirmed spinal cord disease due to cervical vertebral malformation and a second group with other causes of spinal cord disease. The semiquantitative method was most accurate (Tables 10.3 and 10.4). Semiquantitative measurements resulted in a higher sensitivity (87%) and specificity (94%) and more powerful positive predictive value (95%) and negative predictive value (84%) than either of the other techniques for identification of horses with spinal cord compression due to cervical vertebral malformation.

Enlargement of the caudal epiphyses

The caudal epiphyses of C2–C7 form the most caudal part of the floor of each vertebral foramen. Dorsal enlargement of one or more of the caudal epiphyses (a 'ski jump') can reduce the sagittal diameter of the vertebral

Table 10.3 Accuracy parameters for diagnosing cervical vertebral malformation from radiographs (From Mayhew and Green, 2000, with permission).

Parameter	Plain films (*n* = 77)	Scored films (*n* = 77)	Myelograms (*n* = 50)
Sensitivity	0.59	0.87	0.56
Positive predictive value	0.79	0.95	0.86
Negative predictive value	0.56	0.84	0.52

77 cases of histologically confirmed CVM and 31 cases of pathologically confirmed 'other than CVM' were analysed. Techniques used were subjective analysis (plain films), semi-quantitative scoring including minimum sagittal diameter measurements (scored films) and ≥50% reduction of the dorsal dye column (myelograms).

Table 10.4 Cervical intervertebral and intravertebral sagittal ratio measurements for18 horses with spinal cord disease determined histologically not to be due to cervical vertebral malformation (From Mayhew and Green, 2000, with permission).

	C2	C2–3	C3	C3–4	C4	C4–5	C5	C5–6	C6	C6–7*	C7
Median	73	93	60	71	58	73	60	81	58	71	62
Mean	72	90	61	71	59	73	61	80	60	70	63
Standard deviation (SD)	8	12	5	9	6	11	6	10	6	9	5
Mean −2 SD	56	66	51	53	47	51	49	60	48	52	53
Maximum	83	108	70	92	83	90	75	100	75	86	72
Minimum	55	63	52	60	49	56	52	63	54	58	55

*Measured in reverse from dorsocaudal aspect of the body of C6 to the cranial aspect of the dorsal lamina of the vertebral arch of C7.
Note that in some horses the intravertebral minimal sagittal ratio was <50%, but the intervertebral sagittal ratio was within the normal range.

foramen (see Figure 10.14, page 523), resulting in compression of the spinal cord and ataxia. This usually develops within the first year of life.

Vertebral stenosis

Short vertebral pedicles (the lateral walls of the vertebral foramen) result in reduction of the sagittal diameter of the vertebral foramen. The articular processes show only marginal clearance of the intervertebral foramina (Figure 10.12), which therefore appear reduced in size. The stenosis is usually more pronounced towards the cranial aspect of the vertebra, resulting in a triangular vertebral foramen. The condition is the basis for many cases of spinal cord compression and occurs most commonly in young male Thoroughbreds. Intravertebral and intervertebral sagittal ratio measurements or corrected MSD values may be more accurate than absolute MSD values for

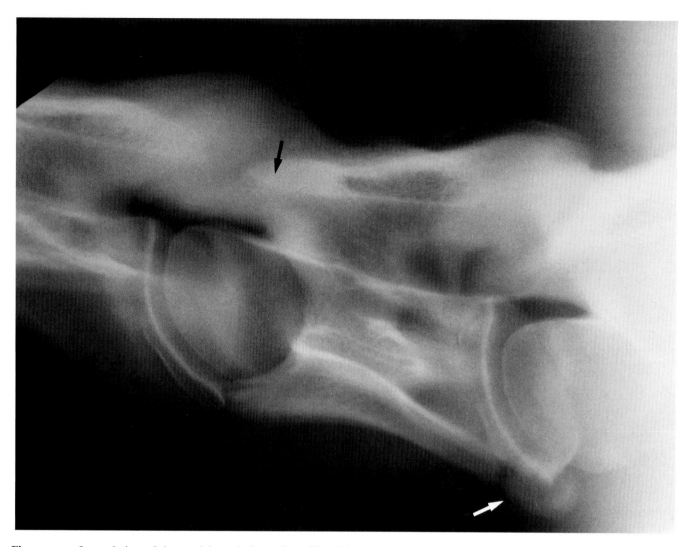

Figure 10.12 Lateral view of the caudal cervical vertebrae (C5–C7) of an ataxic yearling Thoroughbred colt. There is stenosis of the cranial orifice of C6 (black arrow) due to short vertebral pedicles. This causes the vertebral foramen to assume a triangular shape (compare with Figure 10.8) and causes a reduction in size of the intervertebral foramina. Note the separate centres of ossification (white arrow) on the caudal aspect of the ventral processes of C6. This is normal and should not be confused with a fracture.

detection of generalized vertebral stenosis (see pages 507–511). An intra-vertebral sagittal ratio at any vertebra from C4 to C6 of ≤50% (≤52% at C7) is a good predictor (26.1–41.5 times more likely) of the horse having cervical vertebral malformation. However, a small number of clinically normal horses and those with ataxia unrelated to cervical vertebral malformation have intravertebral sagittal ratios of <50% (Table 10.4). If both the intervertebral and intravertebral minimum sagittal ratios are calculated the results are more likely to predict accurately a site of spinal cord compression due to cervical vertebral malformation.

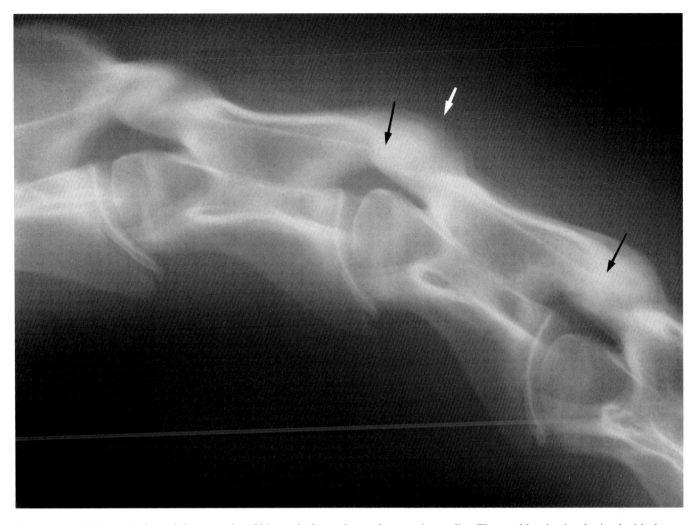

Figure 10.13(a) Lateral view of the second to fifth cervical vertebrae of an ataxic yearling Thoroughbred colt, obtained with the colt standing normally. There is subluxation of the third and fourth cervical vertebrae (white arrow) with narrowing of the minimal sagittal diameter of the vertebral canal. Spinal cord compression was confirmed at this level. Note also the caudal extension of the vertebral arch of the third and fourth cervical vertebrae (black arrows).

Vertebral instability, subluxation or angulation

Vertebral instability, subluxation or angulation occurs most commonly at the C3–C4 articulation (Figure 10.13a). The apparent subluxation is often present in the resting position and is exaggerated by flexion. Other developmental abnormalities (see 'OAAM', page 516, 'Vertebral stenosis', page 519, and 'Modelling of the cervical synovial articulations', page 523) are often present concurrently, resulting in narrowing of the sagittal diameter of the vertebral foramen and spinal cord compression, possibly at more than one site. Occasionally there is reciprocal hyperextension at a more caudal articulation, resulting in a 'zig-zag' orientation of the cervical vertebrae (Figure 10.13b). Slight malalignment of two adjacent vertebrae occurs commonly and may have no clinical significance. If the minimum sagittal

[521]

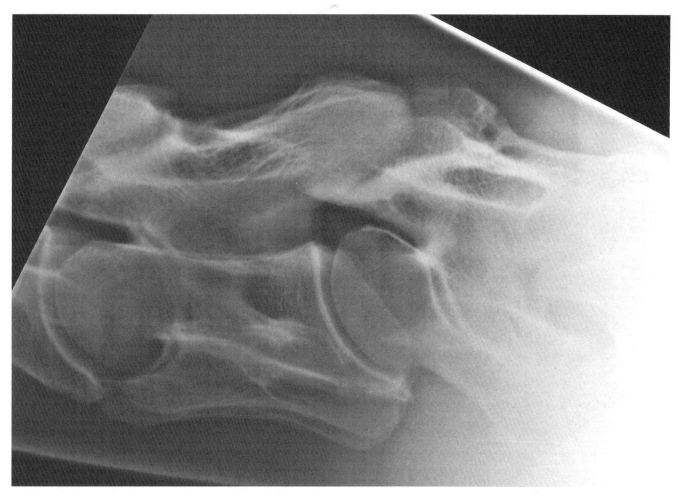

Figure 10.13(b) Lateral view of the caudal cervical vertebrae (C5–C7) of a 6-year-old Thoroughbred novice event horse presented because of difficult behaviour and poor performance. Clinical examination revealed mild hindlimb ataxia and weakness. Cranial is to the left. There is dorsal subluxation of the seventh cervical vertebra. The synovial articulation between the sixth and seventh cervical vertebrae is enlarged and has focal radiolucent areas. The intervertebral foramina are narrowed caudally. The vertebral foramen of the seventh cervical vertebra is wedge-shaped, narrower cranially.

diameter of the vertebral canal is relatively wide, malalignment is often of no significance (Figure 10.14). The radiographs must be examined and interpreted in the light of the clinical signs, and if there is any doubt about the potential significance of a lesion it is helpful to obtain flexed lateral views, to measure intravertebral and intervertebral sagittal ratios (see pages 507–511) and possibly to perform myelography.

Caudal extension of the arch of the vertebral canal

In a normal vertebra the dorsal aspect of the arch of the vertebral canal (the dorsal lamina) reaches, but does not extend over, the cranial epiphysis of the next caudal vertebra. Caudal extension of the arch of the vertebral canal is identified by drawing a line perpendicular to the longitudinal aspect of the vertebral canal from the caudal tip of the vertebral arch (dorsal

[522]

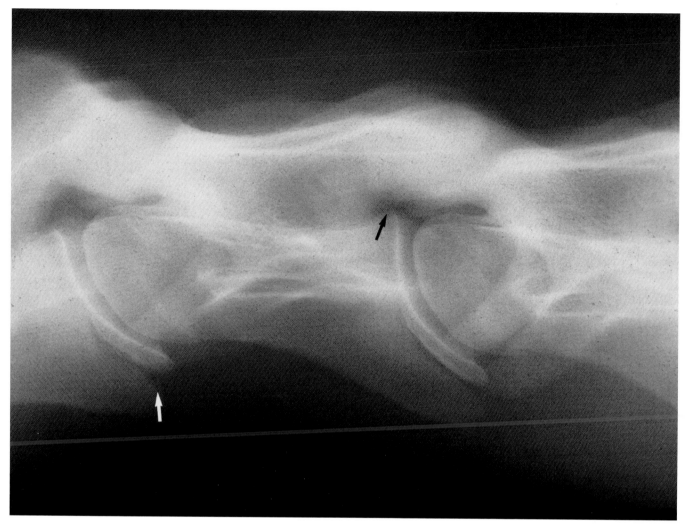

Figure 10.14 Lateral view of the second to fourth cervical vertebrae of an ataxic yearling Thoroughbred filly, obtained with the filly standing normally. There is apparent subluxation at C2–C3 (white arrow), but the dorsoventral diameter of the vertebral canal was not significantly narrowed. Spinal cord compression was confirmed at the C6–C7 level, in association with a severe arthropathy. Note the moderate enlargement of the caudal epiphysis of C3 (black arrow).

lamina) (Figure 10.13a). If this line extends on to the dorsal aspect of the cranial epiphysis of the next caudal vertebra, this is defined as mild caudal extension. Severe caudal extension is present if the line reaches the cranial physis of the vertebra.

Modelling of the cervical synovial articulations

Rooney (1963) described two distinct lesions of the synovial articulations (see 'Further reading'). Type 1 occurs at the C2–C3 articulation, associated with malalignment of the articular processes. It results in hyperflexion and stenosis of the vertebral foramen and usually causes ataxia. If the vertebrae are fused, however, it is possible for quite a marked stenosis to be present without signs of ataxia. In a Rooney type 2 lesion there is medial

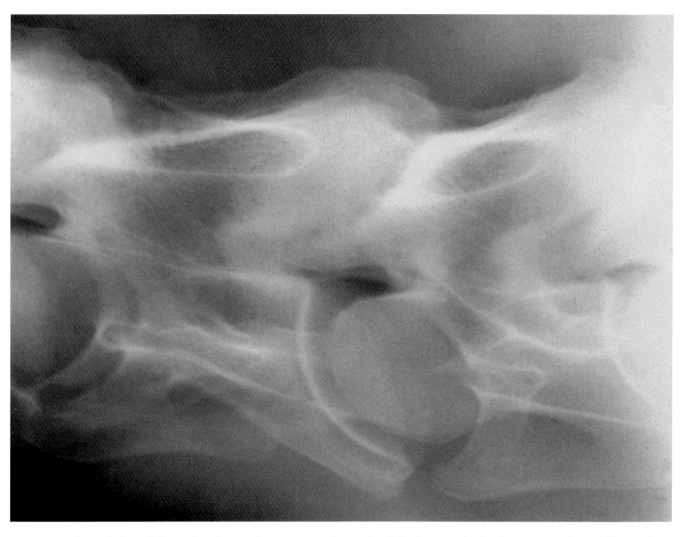

Figure 10.15 Lateral view of the sixth and seventh cervical vertebrae of a clinically normal adult horse. There is modelling and enlargement of the synovial articular facets, a common incidental finding. Note the absence of buttresses (compare with Figure 10.17). C6 is slightly rotated. There is transposition of one ventral process from C6 to C7.

enlargement of the articular processes of C4, or occasionally C5, and this may cause spinal compression, especially in foals. This lesion cannot be detected radiographically on a plain lateral view and is difficult to identify on a ventrodorsal view.

The articular facets of C5–C6 and C6–C7 are frequently enlarged and modelled in mature horses, resulting in blurring of the normally smooth contours of the articulations (Figure 10.15). This probably reflects the stresses placed on these highly mobile joints, but the comparatively wide spinal canal at this point means that stenosis of the vertebral canal usually does not occur, and so it is often of no clinical significance. These modelling changes, however, are the prerequisite for development of an epidural synovial bursa or 'cyst', which can intermittently or permanently compress the spinal cord and cause ataxia. Such modelling changes may also result in low-grade neck pain or stiffness.

[524]

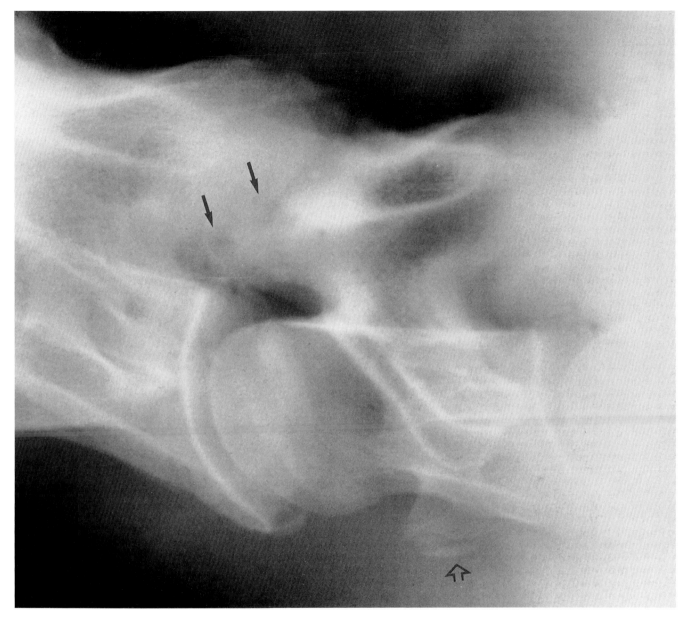

Figure 10.16 Lateral view of the caudal cervical vertebrae (C6 and C7) of an ataxic yearling Thoroughbred filly. There is extensive modelling of the articular facets of C6–C7 and an irregular joint contour. Radiolucent areas (solid arrows) represent pits in the vertebral pedicles. Spinal cord compression was confirmed at C6–C7, associated with a synovial cyst. One ventral process, with separate centre of ossification, was transposed from C6 to C7 (open arrow).

Periarticular new bone can be produced in association with articular cartilage lesions and this may be of clinical significance in a horse with neck stiffness or ataxia. Small lucent zones in the region of the articular processes represent deep pits in the vertebral pedicles (Figure 10.16). These are usually indicative of a clinically significant lesion.

A bony 'knob' may be seen on the ventral aspect of one or both cranial articular processes, in normal and ataxic horses. If well developed this 'buttress' impinges on to the body or arch of the more cranial vertebra and

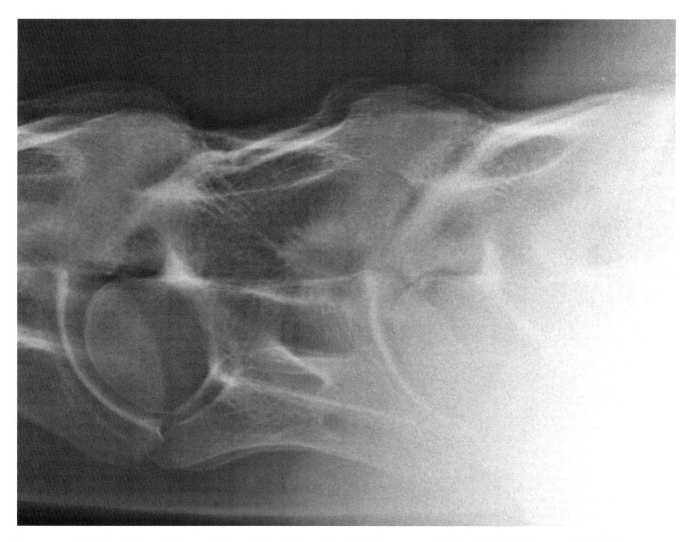

Figure 10.17(a) Lateral view of the caudal cervical vertebrae (C5–C7) of a 7-year-old Warmblood with generalized stiffness. Cranial is to the left. There is considerable enlargement of the synovial articular facet joints between the fifth and sixth and sixth and seventh cervical vertebrae, with almost complete obliteration of the intervertebral foramina.

forms a false joint. Radiographically the buttress partially obliterates the intervertebral foramen (Figure 10.17). This may be of no clinical significance unless the joint capsule balloons axially and compresses the spinal cord.

Massive enlargement of the synovial articular facet joints of C4–C5 and C6–C7 has been seen in association with unilateral forelimb lameness (Figures 10.18a and 10.18b). Nerve root impingement associated with atrophy of the caudal cervical musculature has been documented by contrast-enhanced computed tomography at C4–C5 and C5–C6, associated with severe degenerative joint disease of the synovial articular facet joints. In a horse with unilateral forelimb lameness of unknown cause, comparison of left to right and right to left lateral radiographs may be helpful.

A pathological fracture may develop secondarily to modelling of a cervical synovial articulation. There is usually minimal displacement of the fracture fragments, but a lucent line is detectable radiographically (Figure 10.19).

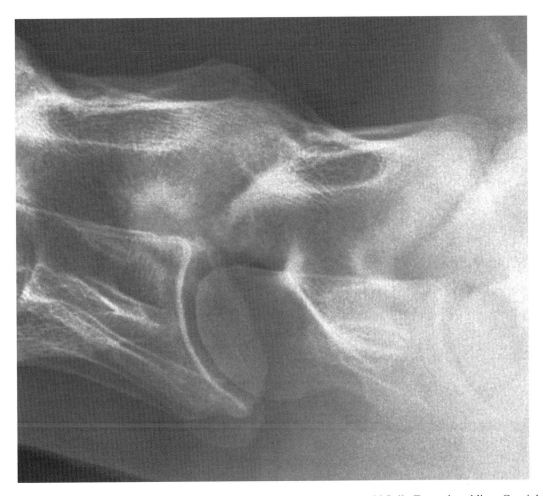

Figure 10.17(b) Lateral view of the caudal cervical vertebrae (C6–T1) of an 8-year-old Selle Français gelding. Cranial is to the left. The horse had a history of neck stiffness and poor performance and intermittently the neck locked in a low position with the horse unable to move. This usually resolved spontaneously. There is massive enlargement of the synovial articulations between the sixth and seventh cervical vertebrae; the ventral aspect of the articulation extends to the vertebral bodies. This is ventral buttressing. The intervertebral foramina are very small. The horse also had clinical evidence of back pain and sacroiliac joint region pain and had radiographic evidence of impinging dorsal spinous processes of the seventeenth and eighteenth thoracic vertebrae and osteoarthritis of the facet joints at the same level. Performance was markedly improved by analgesia of the impinging dorsal spinous processes and caudal thoracic facet joints together with the sacroiliac joint region. The radiographic abnormalities of the neck may result in episodic nerve root impingement and severe pain, causing the locking of the neck.

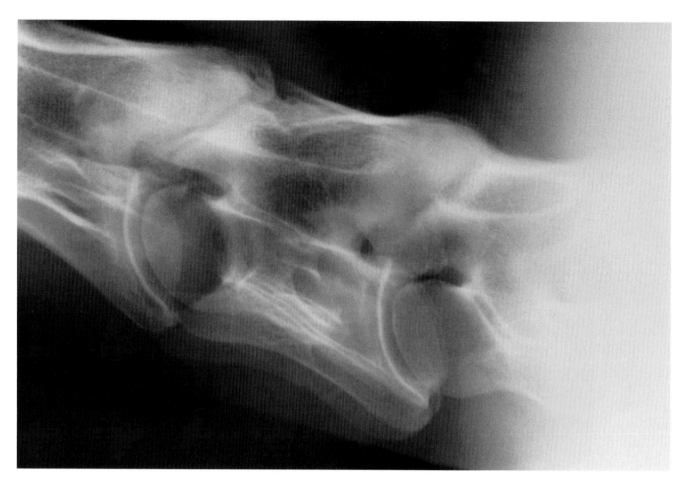

Figure 10.18(a) Lateral view of the caudal cervical region (C5–C7) of a 9-year-old riding horse, with right forelimb lameness and low-grade neck pain. The synovial articulations between the C5 and C6, and C6 and C7 are massively enlarged. There is obliteration of the intervertebral foramen between the fifth and sixth cervical vertebrae.

Fractures may occur unilaterally or bilaterally but this is difficult to assess on lateral radiographs. An associated ataxia warrants a poor prognosis.

Modelling of the caudal cervical synovial articular facet joints is common in mature horses and, unless radiographic abnormalities are dramatic, ascribing clinical significance to them can be difficult. Nuclear scintigraphy is often not helpful because there is frequently little change in the normal pattern of radiopharmaceutical uptake. Ultrasonography can be useful to identify joint capsule thickening and increased amounts of synovial fluid, but such abnormalities are not necessarily associated with pain. Ultrasound-guided local analgesia of the synovial articular facet joint is the most reliable method of confirming the presence of pain and the clinical significance of any radiological abnormality.

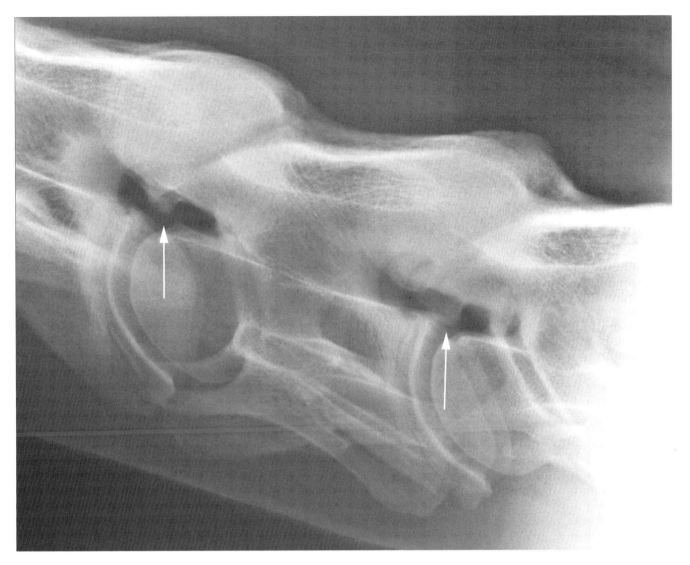

Figure 10.18(b) Lateral view of the caudal cervical vertebrae (C5–C7) of a 4-year-old Warmblood dressage horse, which was stiffer to the right and exhibited right forelimb lameness. Cranial is to the left. The sixth cervical vertebra appears slightly rotated because of asymmetrical enlargement of the synovial articulations between the sixth and seventh cervical vertebrae. Note also the large spurs (arrows) projecting from the ventral aspect of the articulations of both C5 and C6 and C6 and C7. Right forelimb lameness was abolished by intra-articular analgesia of the right C6–7 facet joint.

Subluxation

Subluxation of the atlanto-axial joint may occur in foals or less commonly in an adult horse, associated with damage of the ventral ligaments of the dens. It results in an abnormal neck posture, with or without ataxia. The abnormal position of the vertebra is easily seen on a lateral radiographic view (Figure 10.20), which should be scrutinized carefully for a concurrent fracture. The distance between the dorsal lamina of the first cervical vertebra and the dorsal aspect of the dens should be measured and compared with normal values. The prognosis is poor.

[529]

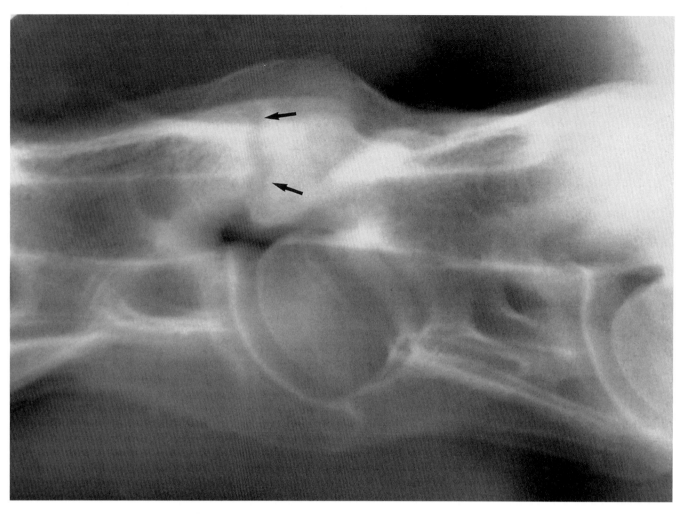

Figure 10.19 Slightly rotated lateral view of the fifth and sixth cervical vertebrae of an ataxic 2-year-old Thoroughbred colt. There is a fracture involving the articular process of C5–C6 (arrows). The cranial orifice of C6 was stenotic and this was considered to contribute to spinal cord compression.

Entheseophyte formation on the occiput associated with the nuchal ligament

New bone formation may occur in the region of insertion of the nuchal ligament on the occiput, also extending slightly dorsal and ventral to the site of insertion (Figure 9.8, page 429). It can be seen as an incidental finding, especially in Warmbloods. Clinically affected horses tend to resist the reins, find difficulty in flexion at the poll and may rear or head-shake. The significance of the bony abnormality may be determined by local infiltration of local anaesthetic solution. Treatment by osteopathic manipulation or local infiltration of corticosteroids and local anaesthetic solution, combined with modification of the training programme, has variable results.

Degenerative changes of the intercentral articulations

Narrowing of an intercentral articulation due to primary degeneration of an intervertebral fibrocartilage (disc) is rarely seen (see Discospondylitis,

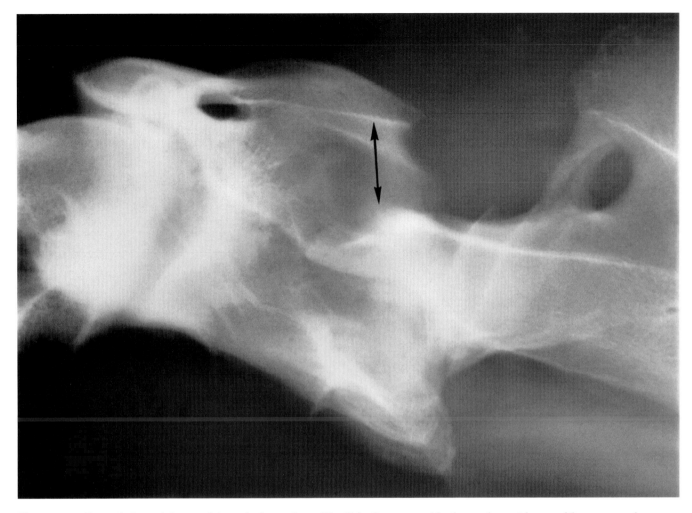

Figure 10.20 Lateral view of the cranial cervical vertebrae (C1–C2) of a 9-year-old advanced event horse with severe neck stiffness and an audible click associated with these vertebrae. There is subluxation of the atlantoaxial joint. Note the narrowed space between the dorsal aspect of the odontoid peg of the axis and the ventral aspect of the dorsal lamina of the atlas (arrowed). Compare with Figure 10.5.

page 533), but degenerative changes of the joint may occur secondary to trauma. Radiographic abnormalities include narrowing of the intercentral joint space, change in shape of the joint surfaces and change in the subchondral bone opacity (Figure 10.21).

Osteomyelitis

In foals, systemic infections may localize in cancellous bone, often in the vertebral bodies. This usually results in neck stiffness and recurrent pyrexia. Focal lucent areas are the first identifiable radiographic change, but if the foal survives, sclerotic bony changes may develop. In older horses local extension of a chronic soft-tissue infection (e.g. avian tuberculosis) can result in osteomyelitis and neck stiffness. Radiolucent areas, which are usually surrounded by more sclerotic margins, are seen within the vertebral bodies (Figure 10.22).

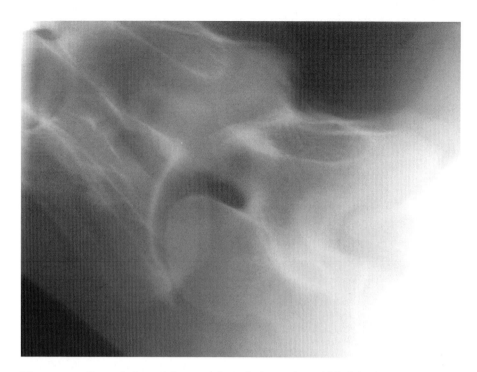

Figure 10.21 Lateral view of the caudal cervical vertebrae (C6–C7) of a 15-year-old Thoroughbred stallion with a history of difficulty in mounting mares and a non-specific hindlimb gait abnormality. Cranial is to the left. Clinical examination revealed mild hindlimb ataxia and weakness. There is ventral subluxation of the head of the seventh cervical vertebra. The intercentral joint space is narrowed ventrally. There is periarticular new bone on the caudoventral aspect of the sixth cervical vertebra and modelling of the dorsal articular margin consistent with degenerative joint disease. There is enlargement of the synovial articulation between the sixth and seventh cervical vertebrae.

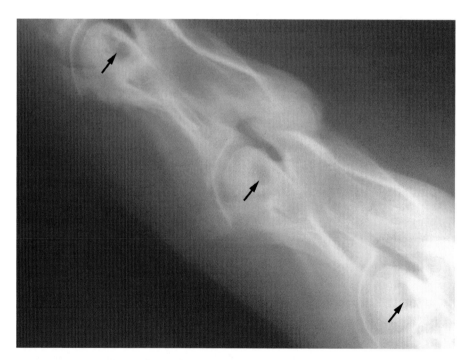

Figure 10.22 Lateral view of the fourth to sixth cervical vertebrae of a 5-year-old Thoroughbred mare with severe neck stiffness, persistent leucocytosis and neutrophilia, and an increase in β_2 globulins. There are irregular radiolucent areas in the vertebral bodies (arrowed) surrounded by sclerotic bone. Tuberculous osteomyelitis was confirmed post mortem.

Discospondylitis

Discospondylitis (inflammation of the vertebral body and associated intervertebral disc) is rare and is usually associated with infection. Clinical signs include neck pain, with or without ataxia or forelimb lameness, cervical hyperaesthesia or muscle twitching. At the time of onset of clinical signs radiography may be unrewarding, but follow-up radiographs usually reveal abnormalities. Focal or more diffuse radiolucent zones and some sclerosis are seen in the caudal end plate of one cervical vertebra and/or the cranial aspect of the adjacent vertebra, with or without alteration of the width of the disc space. Ultrasonographic examination may be useful to identify fluid accumulation typical of abscess formation. The prognosis with conservative management is poor, but successful surgical management has been recorded.

Neoplasia

Neoplastic invasion of cervical vertebrae is rare, but may present clinically as neck stiffness, neck pain or ataxia. Pressure caused by an expanding soft-tissue mass may cause smooth modelling of the bone. Neurofibromatosis can cause enlargement of the transverse and intervertebral foramina and cavitation of the vertebral arch, resulting in a large well defined radiolucent zone (Figure 10.23). A mottled opacity of the vertebral bodies may be suggestive of neoplastic invasion of the bone marrow (e.g. lymphosarcoma, plasma cell myeloma), which may result in osteomalacia and pathological fractures. It may be difficult to differentiate radiographically between the effects of neoplasia, infection and trauma.

Soft-tissue lesions

Mineralization in the soft tissues should not be confused with lesions involving the vertebrae. This may occur secondary to an intramuscular injection (Figure 10.24a) or as the result of previous trauma. A common site is in the ligamentum nuchae, caudal to the occiput. This dystrophic mineralization is readily identifiable radiographically (Figure 10.24b) but may not be of long-term clinical significance.

Tearing of muscle and ligamentous insertions on the ventral aspect of the vertebral bodies may result in entheseophyte formation, readily identifiable radiographically on a lateral projection. This may be of no long-term clinical significance.

Fractures

Fractures are usually the result of trauma (e.g. a fall) or occur secondarily to a pre-existing lesion (e.g. modelling of a cervical synovial articulation). They result in neck pain and stiffness, and may cause ataxia. In young horses, separation frequently occurs along unfused physes and this occurs most often in the axis. The prognosis depends on the site of the fracture,

[533]

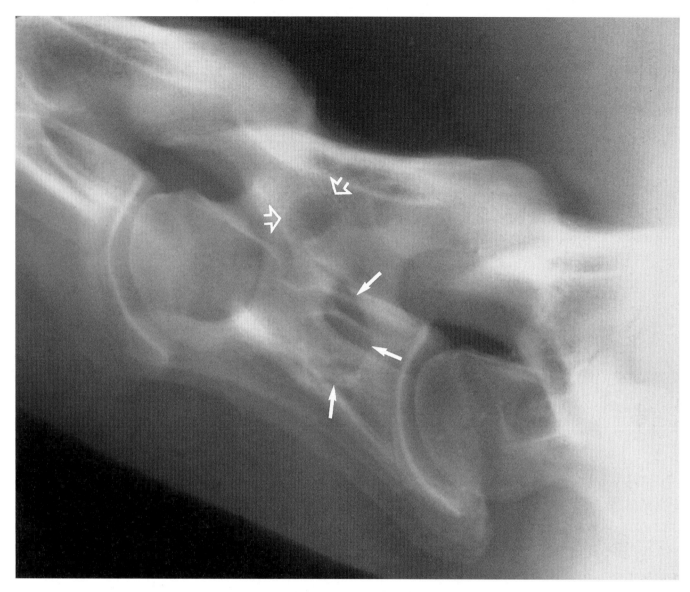

Figure 10.23 Lateral view of the fifth to seventh cervical vertebrae of a 2-year-old Thoroughbred colt with neck stiffness, patchy sweating on the left side of the neck, atrophy of the left supraspinatus and left forelimb lameness. There are radiolucent areas in the vertebral body (solid arrows) and in one of the pedicles of C6 (open arrows), secondary to invasion by neurofibromatous tissue. The horse died suddenly due to total collapse of the weakened C6 and laceration of the spinal cord.

particularly with reference to the vertebral foramen, the degree of fracture displacement and the amount of callus that develops subsequently.

In the acute stage it is often difficult to make an accurate prognosis based on the clinical signs or the radiographic appearance of the fracture (Figures 10.25 and 10.26). Initial ataxia may resolve, only to recur when callus impinges on the spinal cord. Fusion of adjacent vertebrae may develop and cause neck stiffness. Generally, fractures involving the bone surrounding the vertebral foramen or the articular process warrant a guarded prognosis.

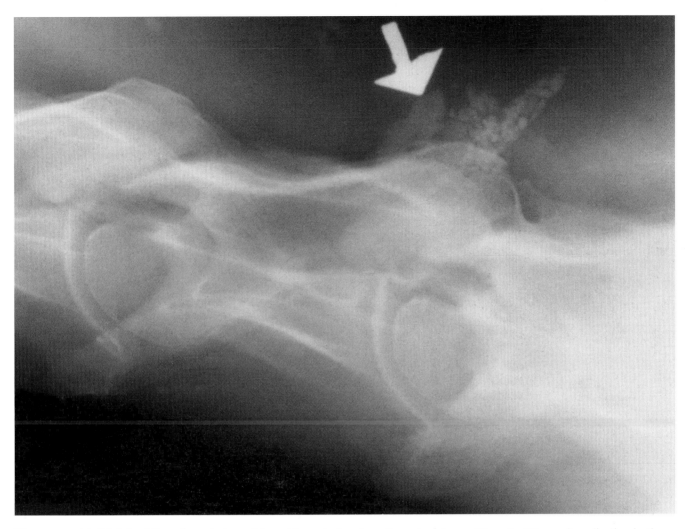

Figure 10.24(a) Slightly oblique lateral view of the mid-cervical region of a mature horse. There is diffuse mineralization in the soft tissues secondary to an intramuscular injection (arrow). This radiopacity is partially superimposed on the articulation between C4 and C5 and should not be confused with a lesion involving the vertebrae.

Occasionally a fracture of a caudal cervical vertebra may be associated with unilateral forelimb lameness.

Thoracolumbar spine

RADIOGRAPHIC TECHNIQUE

Equipment

Radiography of the thoracolumbar spine in adult horses poses a number of technical problems. The thickness of the back requires radiographic equipment with an output of 75–120 kV and 100–250 mAs, and the large mass of soft tissues causes considerable scattered radiation that must be controlled to obtain diagnostic radiographs.

[535]

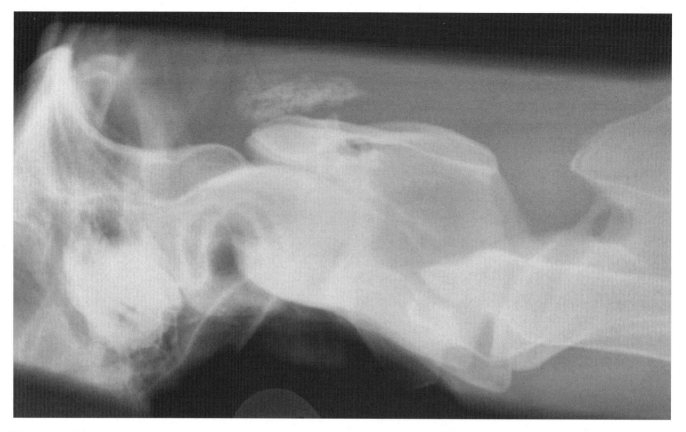

Figure 10.24(b) Lateral view of the cranial cervical vertebrae (C1–C2) of a 4-year-old Warmblood. There is a large focus of mineralization dorsal to the atlas, which was seen as an incidental abnormality.

Ideally the x-ray tube is mounted on an overhead gantry with a linked cassette holder to ensure alignment of the x-ray beam and the film. Diagnostic radiographs of limited areas of the spine can be obtained using a mobile unit, but care should be taken not to overdiagnose on the limited radiographs that are obtained. If a cassette holder is not linked to an overhead gantry, it is best mounted on the horizontal beam of a set of stocks, or directly on a wall. This improves safety and helps to reduce movement. Stocks are recommended not only to restrain the horse but also to ensure that it is standing straight, so that true lateral views are obtained.

Digital systems or rare earth screens and appropriate film are necessary. The effect of scattered radiation must be controlled and the use of a 10:1 ratio focused grid is recommended. In addition, a lead sheet (at least 0.01 mm lead equivalent) should be placed behind the cassette to prevent backscatter. These measures are particularly important for radiographs of the lumbar spine. To compensate for the differences in tissue density, an aluminium wedge filter is useful (see page 8) to prevent overexposure of the summits of the dorsal spinous processes. Alternatively an aluminium wedge can be placed on the horse's back, but some horses with back pain will not tolerate this.

With the above equipment, it is technically possible to obtain radiographs of the thoracolumbar spine from the first thoracic (T1) to approximately the third or fourth lumbar vertebrae (L3/L4), depending on the size and thickness of the horse. Further caudally, the lumbosacral spine and iliac wings are superimposed, making interpretation impossible (except in foals and small thin ponies). In the lumbar region, the mass of soft tissues results in a lot of scattered radiation, so that without the use of an appropriate grid, detail and contrast are lost.

To minimize movement of the patient, tranquillization is nearly always necessary. Radiographs are best obtained at the end of expiration. Only lateral and lateral oblique radiographs of the thoracolumbar spine can be obtained with the horse standing. Ventrodorsal radiographs of the caudal thoracic spine may be obtained under general anaesthesia. Ventrodorsal views of the lumbar region are discussed elsewhere (see Chapter 11, page 575).

To evaluate the thoracolumbar spine (T2–L3) adequately, it is necessary to use large cassettes (35 cm × 43 cm), and to obtain at least four to six radiographs. To help identify individual vertebrae on successive radiographs, it is helpful to tape small radiodense markers (e.g. lead arrows) to the skin on the midline of the back. Four or five of these should be evenly spaced between the withers and the croup.

Positioning

The horse should stand squarely taking weight evenly on all four limbs, with the head and neck straight. Resting a limb causes rotation of the vertebrae, resulting in radiographic images that are difficult to interpret. The first radiograph is normally obtained in the mid-thoracic region (approximately T9–T15). For routine radiographs, the x-ray beam is centred at the level of the vertebral canal (approximately 15–20 cm below the dorsal midline of the back in an adult Thoroughbred horse), and aligned at right angles to the long axis of the trunk. Successive radiographs are similarly aligned, centring cranial or caudal to the previous view. Adjacent radiographic images should overlap, as this greatly aids identification of vertebrae. At the withers, the x-ray beam needs to be centred so that the top of the cassette is just above the highest point of the withers.

For all areas of the thoracolumbar spine, at least two differently exposed films are needed, even when using digital systems: one to examine the dorsal spinous processes and a second to examine the vertebral bodies and their articulations. Visualization of the articular processes and their articulations (facet joints) requires high-quality, well collimated radiographs. Additional information about the left and right facet joints and the vertebral bodies can be obtained using oblique radiographic views. It is important to be able to assess the entire length of the dorsal spinous processes, the articular facet joints and the vertebral bodies for complete evaluation. Assessment of the summits of the dorsal spinous processes may be enhanced by the use of exposures at reduced kilovoltage, without a grid.

If linked equipment is not available, it is often helpful to mark the horse on each side with an adhesive label where each radiograph is centred, to aid alignment of the cassette.

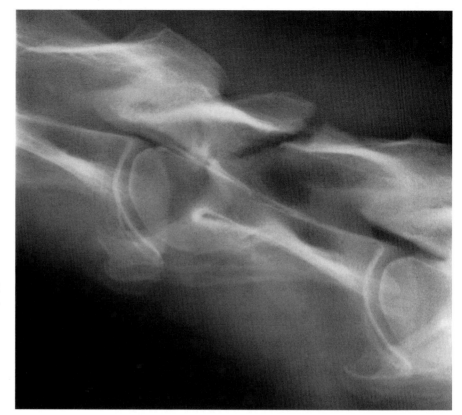

Figure 10.25(a) Lateral view of the third and fourth cervical vertebrae of a 9-year-old Dutch Warmblood dressage horse with severe neck pain and stiffness, and incoordination following a fall in a field 12 days previously. There is a comminuted, slightly displaced fracture of the dorsal arch of the fourth cervical vertebra.

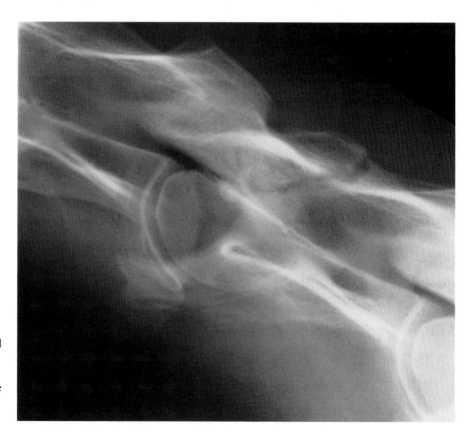

Figure 10.25(b) Lateral view of the third and fourth cervical vertebrae of the same horse as in Figure 10.25(a), obtained 6 weeks later. There is evidence of some bony union. The horse made a complete functional recovery.

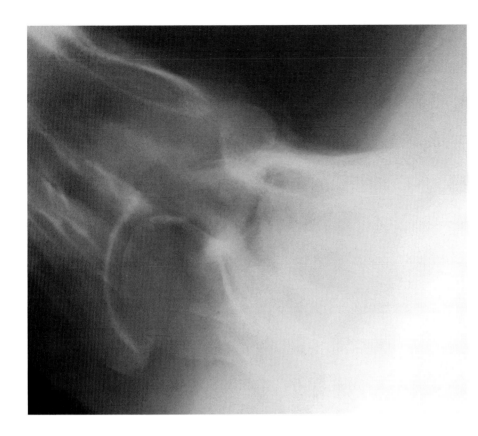

Figure 10.26(a) Lateral view of the cervicothoracic junction (C6–T1) of a 6-year-old Thoroughbred cross, which had fallen while jumping a hedge 10 days previously. There is a slightly displaced fracture through the dorsal arch and vertical pedicle of the seventh cervical vertebra. There is evidence of pre-existing enlargement of the synovial articulations between the sixth and seventh cervical vertebrae.

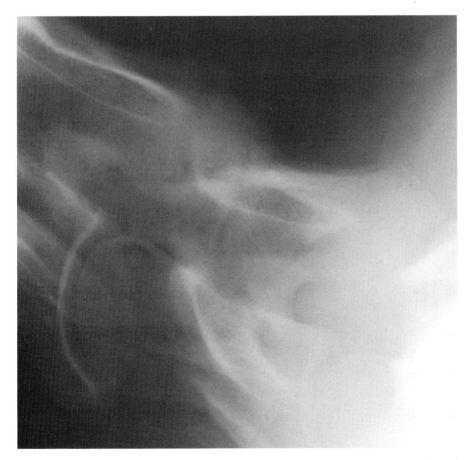

Figure 10.26(b) Lateral view of the cervicothoracic junction of the same horse as Figure 10.26(a) obtained 4 months later. There is some osseous union, but the fracture line is still evident. The horse had shown some clinical improvement but developed severe ataxia 1 month later.

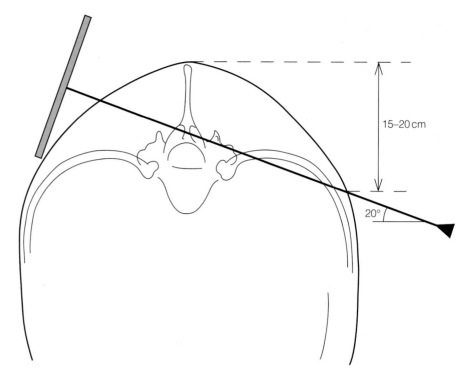

Figure 10.27 Positioning of the horse, imaging plate and x-ray beam to obtain a lateral 20° proximal oblique view of the thoracic facet joints. The x-ray beam, angled 20° proximal from horizontal, is centred at the level of the facet joints, 15–20 cm distal to the dorsal midline depending on the size of the horse. The imaging plate is aligned perpendicular to the x-ray beam and positioned as close to the horse as possible.

To obtain oblique radiographic views of the facet joints and vertebral bodies, the x-ray tube is aligned 20° proximal to the horizontal (Figure 10.27). The imaging plate is aligned perpendicular to the x-ray beam. The x-ray beam is centred at the approximate level of the facet joints. Radiographs are best obtained at the end of expiration to avoid the diaphragm being superimposed over the caudal thoracic facet joints. Radiographs should be obtained from left to right and right to left. However, such views are only useful in the thoracic region because caudal to the diaphragm abdominal structures are superimposed over the facet joints. Particular care with radiation safety should be taken whenever the x-ray beam is angled upwards, as most x-ray facilities are designed for vertical (down) or horizontal x-ray beams.

NORMAL ANATOMY, VARIATIONS AND INCIDENTAL FINDINGS

Immature horse

At birth the thoracolumbar spine is dorsally convex and remains so until it becomes straight at about 6 months of age. All the vertebral bodies have cranial and caudal physes, the cranial physes closing at about 6–12 months and the caudal physes between 2 and 4 years of age (Figure 10.28).

[540]

At approximately 12 months of age the cranial thoracic dorsal spinous processes (T2–T8) develop separate centres of ossification within their cartilaginous summits. This ossification is gradual. These centres of ossification have an irregular outline and mottled opacity, and usually remain separate from the parent bone and incompletely ossified throughout life (Figure 10.29).

Skeletally mature horse

The horse normally has 18 thoracic vertebrae. The number of lumbar and sacral vertebrae varies between horses. Most horses have six lumbar vertebrae and five sacral vertebrae, but a significant number of horses have only five lumbar vertebrae, or may have six sacral vertebrae. The donkey has only five lumbar vertebrae and four to six sacral vertebrae. The vertebral bodies are approximately rectangular in shape, cranially convex and caudally concave. They articulate at the intercentral joints which are uniform in width. Care should be taken not to interpret overlying lung opacities as modelling of the vertebral bodies. The vertebral canal is of similar height throughout the thoracolumbar spine. The synovial or facet joints are difficult to evaluate and higher exposures may be required (Figure 10.30). Large, well muscled horses are easier to examine than smaller, fatter horses. These articulations are identified as oblique radiolucent lines dorsal to the vertebral canal (Figure 10.31a). The articular facets in the lumbar region are larger than in the thoracic region; they appear more radiopaque and have a more irregular outline (see Figure 10.36, page 555). There are marked variations in shape of the articular facet joints from the cranial thoracic region to the caudal lumbar region (Figures 10.31b, 10.31c and 10.36), and comparison with articulated bone specimens is invaluable. The ribs articulate dorsal to the intercentral articulations and initially course dorsally and caudally, but then turn ventrally (Figure 10.30). If the ribs are 'highly sprung' they will be superimposed over the articular facet joints, prohibiting evaluation of the joints on lateral views.

The dorsal spinous process of T1 has a triangular shape and is considerably shorter than that of T2. The dorsal spinous process of T2 is noticeably shorter than T3 and more rectangular than T1. It shows marked variation in width between individuals. T1 has no separate dorsal ossification centre, but there are separate ossification centres from T2 to T7 or T8. These are usually single centres, but occasionally two are present. Further caudally the summit of each dorsal spinous process is smoothly rounded. Smoothly outlined, irregular new bone formation on the summit of a dorsal spinous process may reflect previous supraspinous enthesopathy. There is frequently rather irregular new bone on the cranial and caudal aspect of the body of one or more dorsal spinous processes, possibly reflecting entheseous reaction at the attachment of the interspinous ligament (Figure 10.32).

The dorsal spinous processes at the withers (approximately T2–T10) are long and slender and slope caudally (Figure 10.29, page 543). Their cranial aspects frequently have a smoothly outlined irregular border. Caudal to the seventh thoracic vertebra, the processes become shorter, more upright and

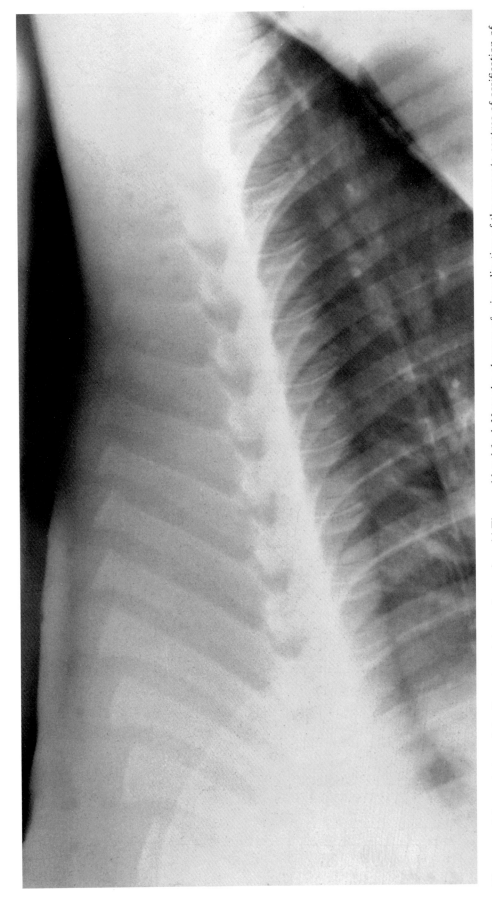

Figure 10.28 Lateral view of the thoracic vertebrae of a 10-day-old Thoroughbred foal. Note the absence of mineralization of the separate centres of ossification of the dorsal spinous processes of the more cranial vertebrae compared with an adult horse (Figure 10.29). The cranial and caudal physes of the vertebral bodies are clearly seen.

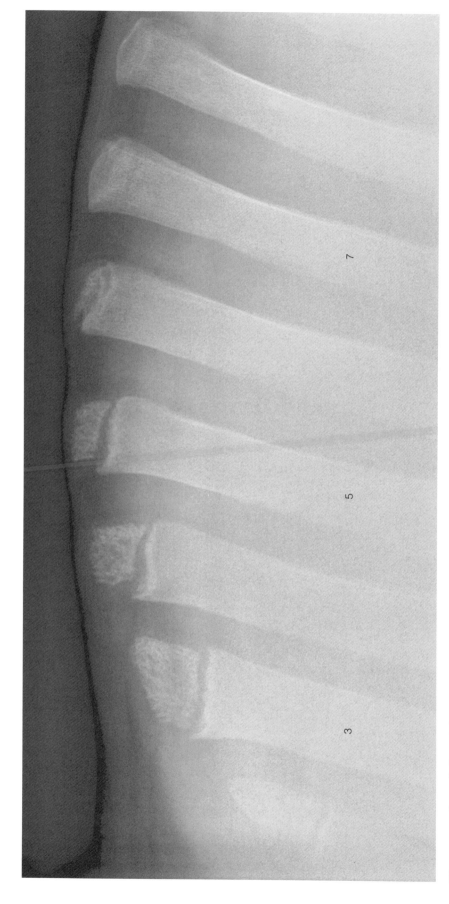

Figure 10.29 Lateral view of the cranial thoracic dorsal spinous processes of the withers region (T2–T8) of a normal adult horse. Note the uneven opacity of the separate centres of ossification of the summits of the dorsal spinous processes. This appearance persists throughout life. Note also the smooth contour of the cranial and caudal margins of each dorsal spinous process.

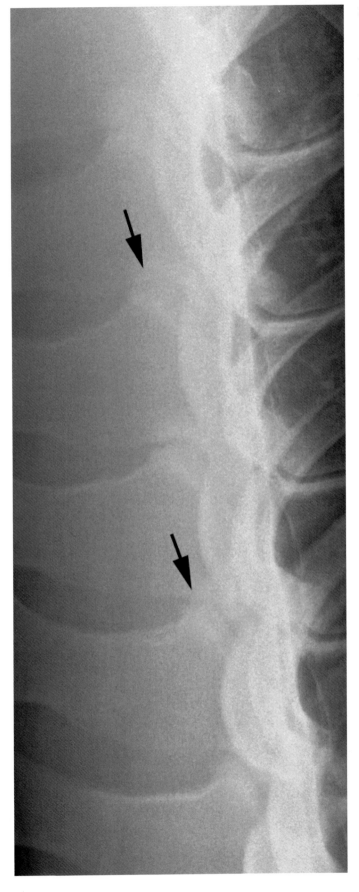

Figure 10.30 Lateral view of the facet joints in the mid to caudal thoracic region of a normal adult horse. Note the relatively opaque articular facets (arrows) crossed by a lucent line (the joints) coursing from caudodorsally to cranioventrally. The vertebral canal is obscured by superimposition of the ribs. In some horses with very highly curved ribs, the facet joints may also be obscured.

[544]

broader (Figure 10.33). The dorsal spinous processes are approximately parallel and any marked deviation from this indicates that the vertebral bodies and intervertebral facets should be examined carefully. The anticlinal vertebra (which has a vertical dorsal spinous process) is usually T15. Caudal to this the dorsal spinous processes slope cranially and the interspinous spaces are considerably narrowed. There is considerable variation between horses in the shape of the thoracic spinous processes and therefore in their spacing in the mid- to caudal thoracic region (Figures 10.34a and 10.34b). On either side of the anticlinal vertebra the dorsal spinous processes tend to be closer together (see Figure 10.39a, page 559). The dorsal spinous processes may be in apposition, especially in short-coupled horses. Normally they have a smooth, relatively straight cranial and caudal cortex, throughout their length. Smoothly irregular new bone is frequently seen on the cranial and caudal aspects of the dorsal spinous processes of the second to tenth thoracic vertebrae, unassociated with clinical signs. It is less common to see new bone formation on more caudal thoracic dorsal spinous processes in clinically normal horses. There is sometimes a cranially directed 'beak' on the summits of dorsal spinous processes in the caudal thoracic region. The spinous processes of the lumbar vertebrae resemble those of the caudal thoracic region (Figure 10.35); however, their orientation varies. In horses with five lumbar vertebrae, the dorsal spinous processes tend to be parallel, whereas in horses with six lumbar vertebrae there may be divergence of the two most caudal dorsal spinous processes.

The thoracic vertebrae have relatively small transverse processes compared with the lumbar vertebrae where the transverse processes are large and flattened, and can be identified on lateral radiographs (Figure 10.36).

Identification of individual vertebrae is most easily made by identifying the dorsal spinous processes of T1, and numbering caudally. As a rough guide, the following structures can be used:

1 The separate centre of ossification on the dorsal spinous process of T3 is broad and triangular shaped.
2 Separate centres of ossification are present on the dorsal spinous processes of T2–T7/T8.
3 The dorsal spinous process of T6 (or T7) normally forms the highest point of the withers.
4 T15 is normally the anticlinal vertebra.
5 Except in full inspiration, the image of the diaphragm usually lies over the vertebral body of T16 or T17.

SIGNIFICANT FINDINGS

It is important to recognize that several radiographic abnormalities of the thoracolumbar vertebrae may occur concurrently, which may influence treatment and prognosis. It is therefore important to evaluate the vertebrae in their entirety, not just for example the dorsal spinous processes. Radiographic abnormalities are not always of clinical significance and must be interpreted in the light of clinical findings and, where appropriate, the

[545]

response to local analgesia. Nuclear scintigraphic evaluation can be helpful in identifying which radiographic abnormalities are likely to be of clinical significance, although a negative result does not preclude the existence of back pain, nor does a positive result imply that the area is a source of pain. Ultrasonography may also be useful.

Sprain of the supraspinous ligament

The supraspinous ligament is a functional continuation of the nuchal ligament of the neck. It attaches to the periosteum of the summits of the dorsal spinous processes from T10/T11, caudally to the last lumbar vertebra. If these attachments are sprained following severe trauma such as a fall, there may be 'lifting' of the periosteum at the dorsal aspect of successive processes. This may be seen on softly exposed radiographs as a small radiopaque 'flake' dorsal to and in close proximity to the summit of the dorsal spinous process (Figure 10.37). Alternatively, entheseous new bone may develop on the summit of the dorsal spinous process. The condition is most frequently seen in the T10–T13 or L1–L3 regions. Ultrasonographic evaluation of the supraspinous ligament may be helpful, but architectural

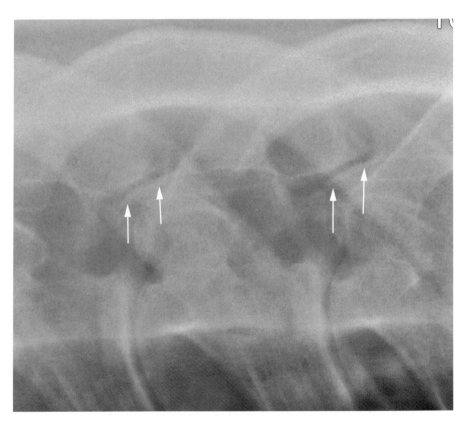

Figure 10.31(a) Close-up lateral 20° proximal view of the synovial intervertebral articulations (facet joints) between the thirteenth and fourteenth and fourteenth and fifteenth thoracic vertebrae (arrows) of a normal adult horse. Cranial is to the left. Note the oblique orientation of the joint spaces and the regularity of joint space width.

[546]

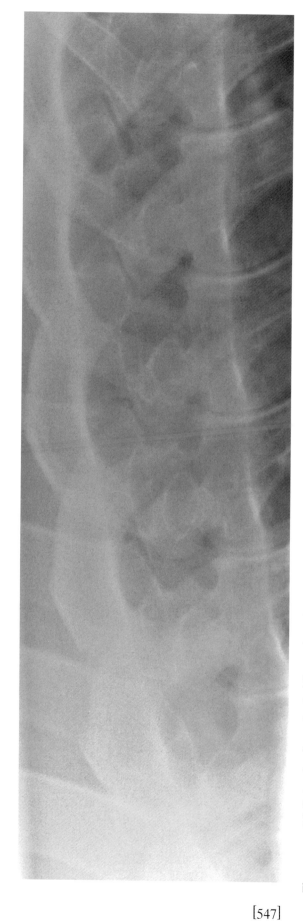

Figure 10.31(b) Lateral 20° proximal oblique view of the mid-thoracic region of a normal adult horse. Cranial is to the left. The facet joints all have similar opacity. Compare with Figure 10.31(c).

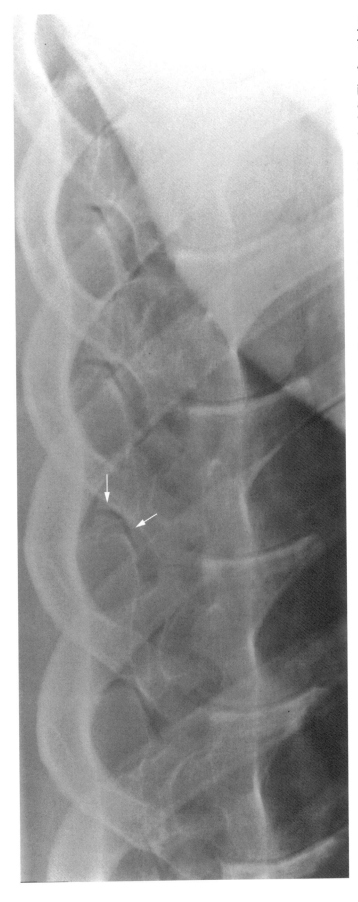

Figure 10.31(c) Lateral 20° proximal oblique view and diagram of the caudal thoracic region (T13–T18) of a normal adult horse. Cranial is to the left. The facet joints between T15–T16, T16–T17 and T17–T18 are approximately a rotated L-shape, with both oblique and vertical components (arrows).

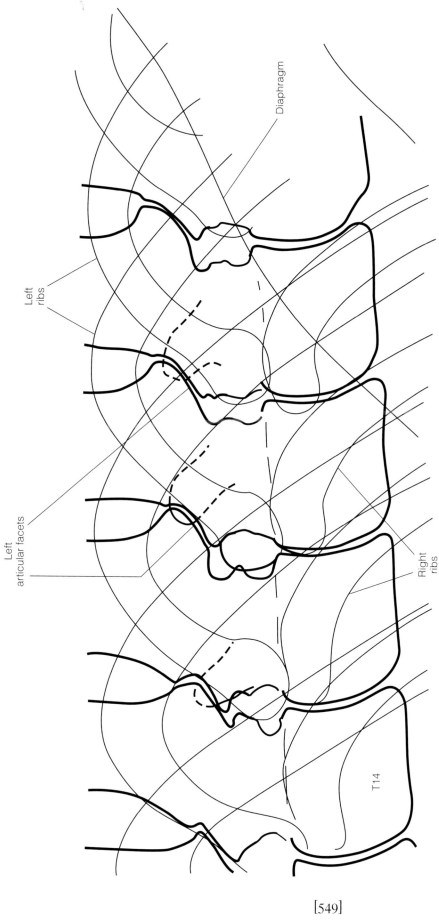

Left
ribs

Diaphragm

Left
articular facets

Right
ribs

T14

Figure 10.31(c) *Cont'd*

[549]

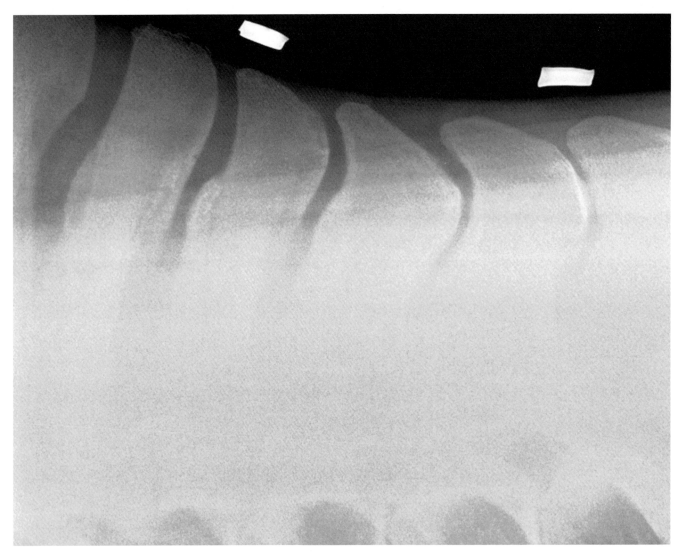

Figure 10.32 Lateral radiographic view of the dorsal spinous processes of the mid-thoracic region (T11–T15) of a 10-year-old Thoroughbred event horse with back stiffness and poor performance. Cranial is to the left. There is new bone on the cranial and caudal margins of the dorsal spinous processes of T11 and T12 and modelling of the cranial aspect of the dorsal spinous process of T13. The dorsal spinous processes of T13 and T14 are almost unseparable throughout their length. The summits of the dorsal spinous processes of T13–T15 are beak-shaped and overriding. The more caudal thoracic dorsal spinous processes were also overriding.

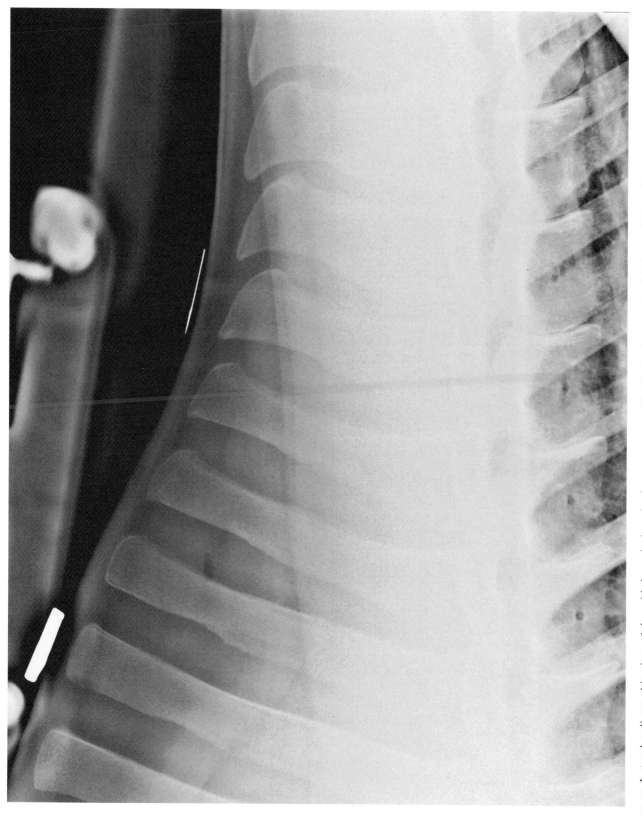

Figure 10.33 Lateral radiographic view of the mid-thoracic dorsal spinous processes (T7–T15) of a normal adult horse. The radiograph was obtained using an aluminium wedge filter and there are lead markers on the skin. The dorsal spinous processes in this region are completely ossified (compare with Figure 10.29). Note the rather irregular margin of the cranial and caudal aspects of the more cranial dorsal spinous processes. The facet joints are underexposed and cannot be evaluated.

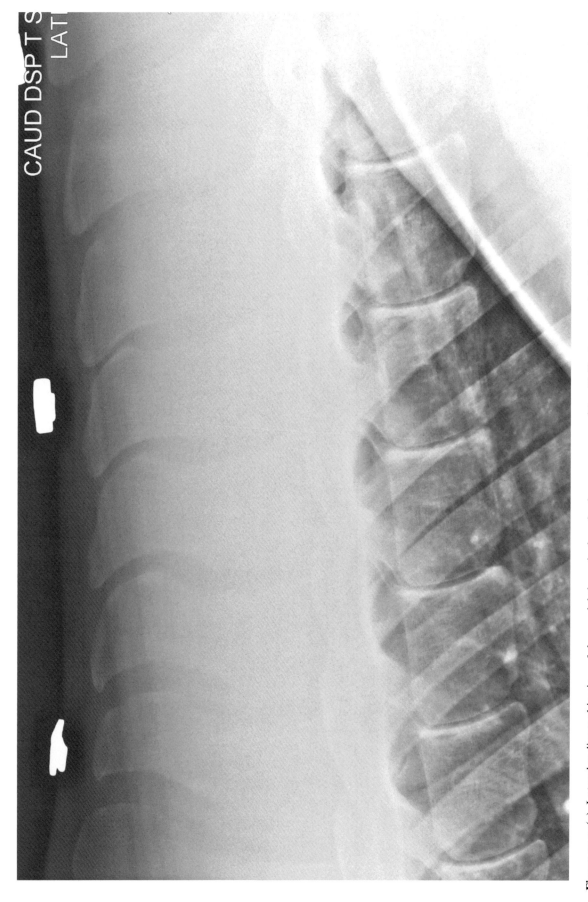

CAUD DSP T S
LAT

Figure 10.34(a) Lateral radiographic view of the caudal thoracic dorsal spinous processes (T12–T18) of a normal adult horse. Cranial is to the left. The dorsal spinous processes are well spaced; they are closer in some normal horses. The facet joints are obscured by the highly sprung ribs. The diaphragm crosses the vertebral bodies of T17 and T18.

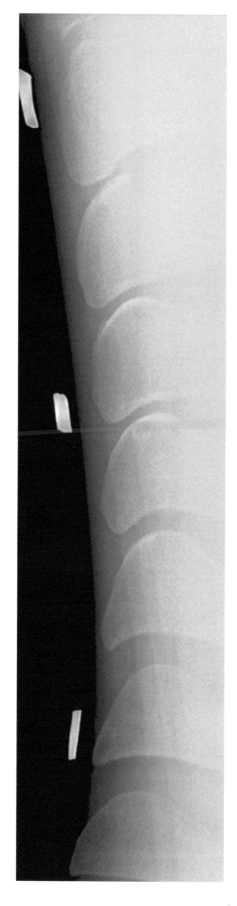

Figure 10.34(b) Lateral radiographic view of the proximal half of the dorsal spinous processes of the 11th to 17th thoracic vertebrae of a clinically normal horse. The dorsal spinous processes are well spaced, but there is a radiolucent zone in the subcortical bone on the caudal aspect of T14. There is mild cortical sclerosis of the caudal aspect of T14, 15 and 16. The cranial aspect of the dorsal spinous process of T17 is slightly beak-shaped.

[553]

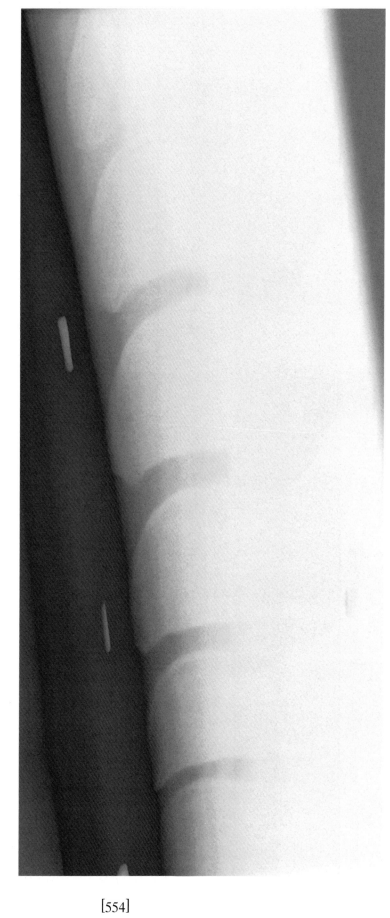

Figure 10.35 Lateral radiographic view of the dorsal spinous processes of the lumbar vertebrae of a normal adult horse. Cranial is to the left. The dorsal spinous processes are well spaced. Different exposures are required for assessment of the facet joints and vertebral bodies.

[554]

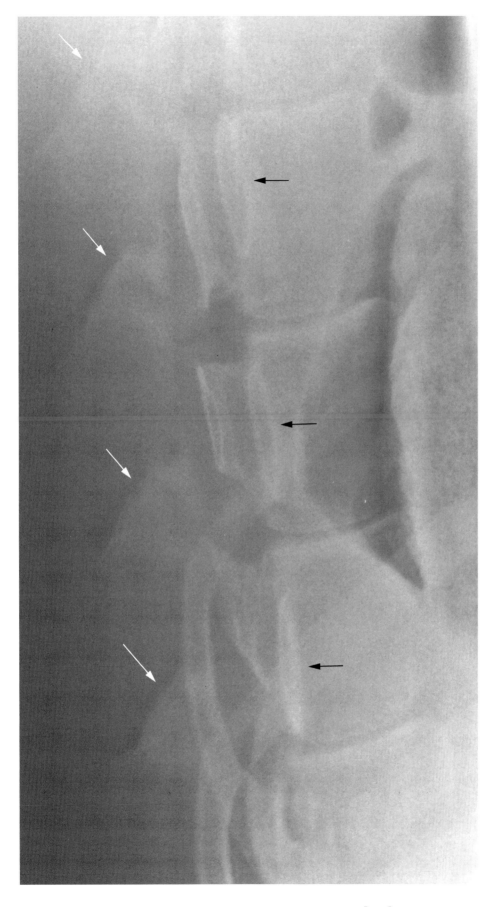

Figure 10.36 Lateral radiographic view of the articular facet joints and vertebral bodies of the cranial lumbar vertebrae. Superimposed over the more cranial vertebrae are the caudal ribs and abdominal viscera. Note the relatively sclerotic appearance of the facet joints (white arrows) through which a faint lucent line courses from caudodorsal to cranioventral. The oval-shaped sclerotic area (black arrows) on the dorsal aspect of each vertebral body represents a transverse process. Note the opaque caudal subchondral bone plate of each vertebral body.

[555]

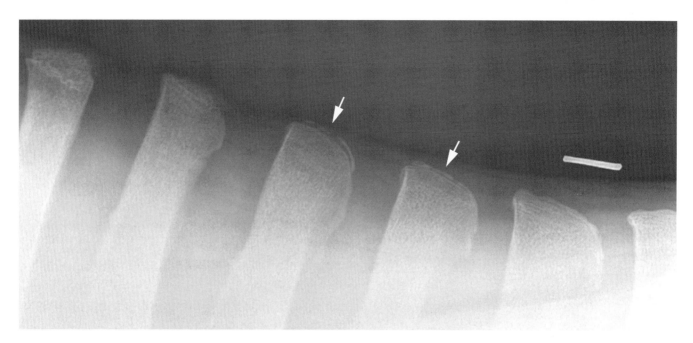

Figure 10.37 Lateral radiographic view of the summits of the dorsal spinous processes of the mid-thoracic region (T8–T13). Cranial is to the left. This 7-year-old Warmblood had chronic back pain. There is separation of a thin radiopaque flake on the dorsal aspect of two dorsal spinous processes (T10 and T11, arrows), which is believed to reflect elevation of the periosteum following damage to the supraspinous ligament.

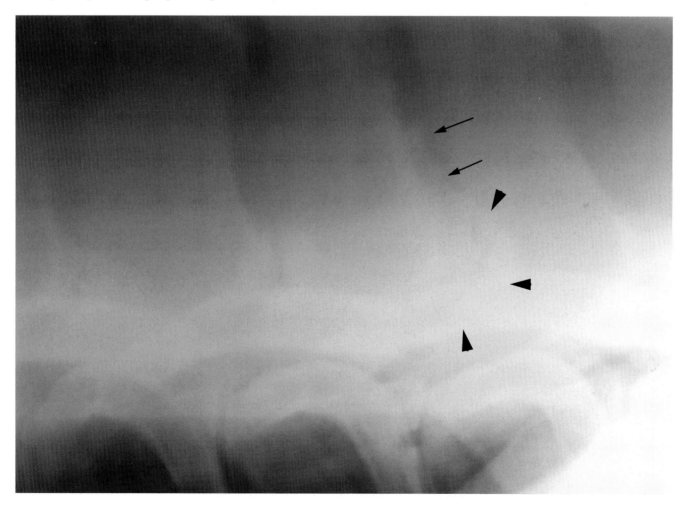

Figure 10.38(a) Lateral view of the dorsal spinous processes of the caudal thoracic vertebrae of a 4-year-old Hanoverian/Thoroughbred, which had become trapped under a horse box partition 10 weeks previously. There is extensive entheseous new bone on the caudal aspect of the dorsal spinous process of T15 (arrows), due to tearing of the interspinous ligament. The articular facet joint between T15 and T16 is also enlarged (arrowheads). The horse also damaged the supraspinous ligament and the summits of the dorsal spinous processes in the mid- to caudal thoracic regions.

variations and abnormalities can be seen in some asymptomatic horses. The condition may be accompanied by inflammation of other soft-tissue structures and can cause symptoms of back pain for several months. Satisfactory improvement normally occurs with rest, but the radiographic appearance does not necessarily alter, and these changes may therefore be an incidental radiographic finding. Nuclear scintigraphic evaluation may help to determine the presence of active bone modelling and thus the likely clinical significance; primary soft-tissue pain may be present in some horses.

Interspinous ligament enthesopathy

Smoothly irregular new bone formation on the cranial and caudal aspects of the dorsal spinous processes of the first 8–10 thoracic vertebrae is a common incidental finding (see Figure 10.29, page 543), but new bone formation on the dorsal spinous processes of more caudal vertebrae is more likely to be of clinical significance (Figures 10.38a and 10.38b), reflecting interspinous ligament enthesopathy. It may be seen alone or together with either impinging dorsal spinous processes or degenerative joint disease of the articular facet joints.

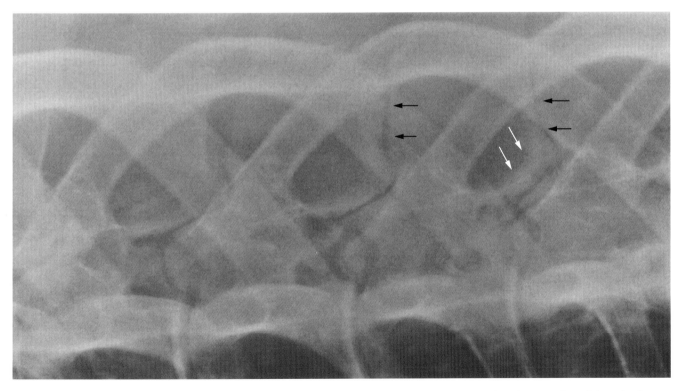

Figure 10.38(b) Lateral 20° proximal oblique radiographic view of the caudal thoracic facet joints (T13–T16) and dorsal spinous processes of a 16-year-old general purpose Cob with marked back stiffness. Cranial is to the left. The bases of the dorsal spinous processes of T14, T15 and T16 are very close, with subcortical sclerosis (black arrows). There is also thickening of the subchondral bone plate of the facet joint between T15 and T16 (white arrows). There was also bony bridging further proximally between the dorsal spinous processes of T13 and T14.

Impingement and overriding of the dorsal spinous processes

It is important to be aware that impingement and overriding of the summits of the thoracic dorsal spinous processes is a fairly common radiological observation, even in clinically normal horses (Figure 10.39a). Radiographic changes should be looked upon with some caution and must be interpreted in the light of a comprehensive clinical examination of the horse at rest and at work. It is not possible to relate the radiographic changes to the degree of clinical signs exhibited. Radiographic changes may simply be evidence of previous impingement and no longer of clinical significance. However, crowding of the dorsal spinous processes may reduce the patient's athletic potential and can alter the biomechanics of the thoracolumbar region and predispose to the development of other pathological lesions that may cause pain. A change in stance, with slight hollowing of the back, may also result in crowding of the dorsal spinous processes, which may therefore be secondary to some other cause of back pain. Clinical significance may also be influenced by the athletic demands placed on the horse.

Radiographic examination can be misleading if only a limited part of the thoracolumbar region is evaluated and the radiographic quality is not adequate. Clinically significant impingement or overriding dorsal spinous processes is usually restricted to the mid- and caudal thoracic regions. Abnormalities can extend throughout the lumbar region, or even occur exclusively in the lumbar region.

Impingement may result in discrete lucent zones in the subcortical bone and periosteal reaction with new bone formation. This may be followed by sclerosis and modelling of the opposing surfaces of the spinous processes (Figure 10.39b). The cranial aspect of the summit of one dorsal spinous process may model to envelop the caudal aspect of the adjacent cranial dorsal spinous process. Closeness or impingement of the summits of successive processes is frequently seen, but need not be of clinical significance. Active periosteal proliferative reactions are more likely to be of significance. Significance is best determined by infiltration of local anaesthetic solution, although both false-positive and false-negative results may occur.

Nuclear scintigraphic evaluation is helpful in some horses, but false-negative results occur and increased radiopharmaceutical uptake can be seen in the summits of one or more dorsal spinous processes in some horses without evidence of pain and no apparent impingement. In some cases where overt back pain is absent, 'overcrowding' of the processes (reduced interspinous spaces without marked reaction of the opposing bone surfaces) may reduce the flexibility of the back, and hence reduce performance at the highest levels of competition. The greater the number of dorsal spinous processes involved, the higher the likelihood of associated clinical signs.

Conservative management frequently results in clinical improvement, although there is generally little or no change in the radiographic appearance. Local infiltration with corticosteroids and/or pain-modifying drugs, shock wave treatment or osteopathic manipulation may help to control pain, but effects may be temporary in some horses. Surgical treatment by resection of the summits of one or more dorsal spinous processes should be

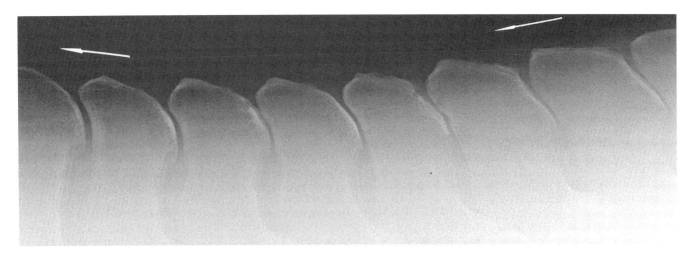

Figure 10.39(a) Lateral view of the dorsal spinous processes of the caudal thoracic and cranial lumbar region (T13–L2) of a 6-year-old Andalusian cross gelding with a stiff back, poor hindlimb impulsion and engagement and reluctance to canter. Cranial is to the left. The summits of the dorsal spinous processes are very close or impinging, with mild cortical sclerosis. There was intense increased radiopharmaceutical uptake associated with these dorsal spinous processes.

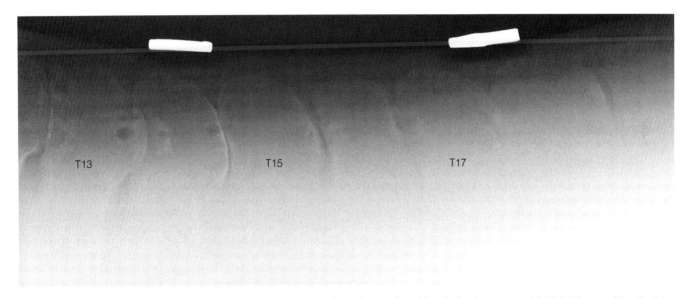

Figure 10.39(b) Lateral view of the caudal thoracic and cranial lumbar region (T12–L1) of a 9-year-old Irish Thoroughbred with stiffness, poor hindlimb impulsion, reluctance to go forwards and episodic explosions. The summits of the dorsal spinous processes are very variable in craniocaudal width. The dorsal spinous processes are impinging or overlapping. There is mild cortical sclerosis and extensive subcortical radiolucent areas.

contemplated in severe or intractable cases, but again results may only be temporary. It is important to evaluate the vertebrae in their entirety, to preclude other co-existing pathological changes of likely significance, which will adversely influence the prognosis.

Other abnormalities of the dorsal spinous processes

The alignment of the dorsal spinous process in the sagittal plane is best appreciated clinically and abnormalities can be verified using dorsal scintigraphic images. Deviation of a dorsal spinous process to the left or the right may result from uneven muscle tone between the two sides of the back, but is usually associated with other pathological abnormalities of the adjacent vertebrae. Radiographs of the entire group of vertebrae should be carefully inspected. The summits of the dorsal spinous processes generally follow a smooth curve; an abrupt change in height between two adjacent dorsal spinous processes is not normal and may be congenital or acquired. It is likely to be associated with other pathological abnormalities which compromise performance.

Bridges of bone between adjacent dorsal spinous processes are occasionally seen and are probably congenital in origin; if widespread they are likely to compromise movement of the thoracolumbar region and predispose to the development of other pathological changes. Huge variation in width of adjacent dorsal spinous processes is also a congenital abnormality which is usually associated with abnormalities of the vertebral bodies and the facet joints.

Vertebral fusion

Vertebral fusion may involve two or more vertebrae, but is rare in the thoracolumbar spine. The absence of irregular bony callus helps to distinguish a congenital abnormality from fusion following a recent fracture. A fracture that occurred a year or more previously may be indistinguishable from a congenital fusion, due to modelling of the callus.

Lordosis, kyphosis and scoliosis

Varying degrees of lordosis, kyphosis and, occasionally, scoliosis occur, although minor deviations may result from uneven muscle tone in the epaxial muscles.

Lordosis may be the result of congenital hypoplastic articular processes but may also be an acquired defect. Marked lordosis of the thoracolumbar spine is recognized radiographically as a ventral convexity (dipping) of the thoracolumbar spine, and may adversely affect performance, although it does not necessarily do so.

Kyphosis may also be congenital or acquired. It is recognized radiographically as a dorsal convexity (arching) of the thoracolumbar spine. A similar posture may be adopted by young horses with bilateral

[560]

osteochondrosis of the femoropatellar articulations, and this must be considered as a differential diagnosis.

Congenital scoliosis may occur (possibly due to uterine malpositioning). On lateral radiographs, twisting of the spine results in asymmetry of the positioning of the ribs and an apparent variation in the length of the vertebral bodies. Wedge-shaped vertebral bodies may be seen on lateral or dorsoventral radiographs.

Mild degrees of lordosis and kyphosis are frequently seen and are not necessarily associated with poor performance, although they may be of significance in horses undertaking particular athletic activities. Scoliosis is often of sufficient severity to interfere with any type of performance.

Degenerative joint disease

The articular processes (facet joints) in the thoracic region form simple arthrodial joints with small and flat articular surfaces which become angulated caudally (see Figure 10.30, page 544). In the lumbar region, the articular processes are hinge-like and have a slightly different radiographic appearance (see Figure 10.36, page 555). True lateral projections and oblique views that 'cut through' the joints (Figure 10.31a, page 546) are essential for assessment of any abnormality involving these structures. The joints under suspicion must be in the middle of the radiograph, and it may be helpful to compare the size and shape of the adjacent facet joints. Evaluation of the joints on lateral views can be extremely difficult if the ribs are 'highly sprung'.

Degenerative joint disease of the articulations of the articular processes (facet joints) (Figure 10.40a) is difficult to diagnose and requires high-quality radiographs, with good definition. Good collimation may markedly enhance radiographic quality. The condition was formerly thought to be a rare cause of back pain, but with improved radiographic technique, and also the use of nuclear scintigraphy, is now being recognized more frequently. Degenerative joint disease of the articular facet joints most often affects the caudal thoracic and cranial lumbar vertebrae.

Radiographic abnormalities include (Figure 10.40b):
- Asymmetry: no clear joint space is visible, or there is a double joint space
- Reduced joint space, with or without osteolysis
- Sclerosis: the subchondral bone plate is thickened and of increased opacity
- Osteolysis or subchondral bone stress fracture
- Dorsal periarticular proliferation, resulting in increased size of the joint. This is most easily recognized in the caudal thoracic and lumbar regions. There may be reduced space between the dorsal spinous processes, especially in the caudal thoracic region
- Ventral periarticular proliferation. This can only be recognized in the lumbar region, due to the superimposition of the ribs in the thoracic region

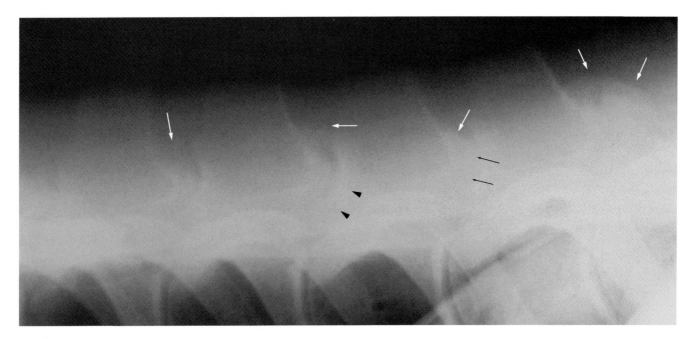

Figure 10.40(a) Lateral view of the caudal thoracic vertebrae of an 8-year-old horse with chronic back pain. Cranial is to the left. There is degenerative joint disease of the facet joints characterized by periarticular new bone formation (white arrows), thickening of the subchondral bone plate (arrowheads) and loss of joint space (black arrows). The changes are most advanced caudally.

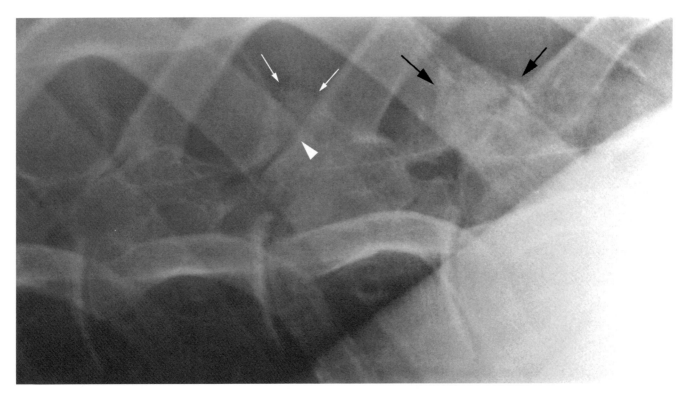

Figure 10.40(b) Lateral 20° proximal oblique view of the caudal thoracic vertebrae (T15–T18). There is degenerative joint disease characterized by narrowing of the facet joint between T16 and T17 proximally (white arrowhead) and periarticular new bone dorsally (white arrows). There is extensive subchondral bone sclerosis and periarticular new bone around the facet joints between the seventeenth and eighteenth thoracic vertebrae (black arrows) and complete loss of joint space.

Comparison of left and right oblique views helps to determine if the radiographic abnormalities are unilateral or bilateral. Ultrasonography may also be helpful. With low-grade radiographic abnormalities the results of nuclear scintigraphic examination may be normal in mature horses. In young Thoroughbreds there may be focal intensely increased radiopharmaceutical uptake associated with a stress fracture of the dorsal lamina in the cranial lumbar region. Severe degenerative changes are often associated with increased radiopharmaceutical uptake. Ultrasound-guided paravertebral local analgesia can be helpful to verify the significance of equivocal radiological abnormalities.

Occasionally concurrent abnormalities of the intercentral articulations are identified, which probably reflect previous trauma, or new bone may extend proximally between the dorsal spinous processes, reflecting interspinous enthesopathy.

Ossifying spondylosis (spondylosis deformans)

This is a relatively uncommon condition in the horse, the aetiology of which is not known. It is consistently found in the caudal half of the thoracic region (T10–T16). It may be multifocal and in some horses reflects ventral ligament enthesopathy.

Osteophytes (spondyles) arise from the ventral borders of the vertebral bodies near the intercentral articulations. The osteophytes usually extend across the intercentral joint towards similar osteophytes on adjacent vertebrae (Figure 10.41a). Frequently a slightly irregular radiolucent line of varying width remains between the opposing spondyles as an apparent continuation of the intercentral joint (Figures 10.41b and 10.41c), but complete bridging between adjacent vertebrae may occur (Figure 10.41d). There is considerable variation in the degree of spondylosis which develops, and the clinical significance of the changes has not yet been well established. Although spondylosis is usually seen in lateral radiographs, occasionally it can only be demonstrated on oblique radiographs.

Once spondylosis has started to form, it will frequently progress in caudal and cranial directions. Spondylosis may occur without obvious clinical signs. This may depend on the athletic demands placed on the horse. Some horses with associated back pain have been able to perform acceptably with controlled medication, although only limited athletic pursuits are possible.

Spondylosis has also been seen concurrent with other abnormalities, such as impinging dorsal spinous processes and degenerative joint disease of the caudal thoracic articular facet joints.

Osteomyelitis

Systemic infections may localize in the vertebral bodies, although this is a rare finding. This may result in some stiffness of the back and intermittent pyrexia. Radiographically, focal lucent areas, sometimes surrounded by a sclerotic rim, are seen. While a number of systemic infections may cause this

[563]

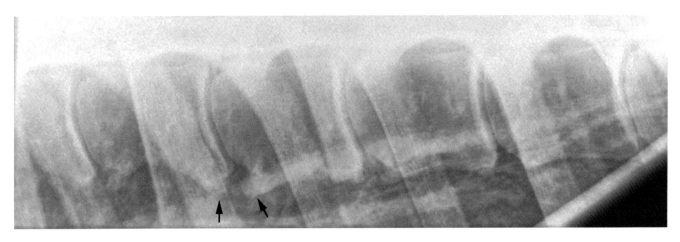

Figure 10.41(a) Lateral view of the vertebral bodies of the caudal thoracic region (T13–T18). Cranial is to the left. There is new bone reflecting early spondylosis involving the ventral aspect of the vertebral bodies of T14 and T15 (arrows). This 8-year-old Thoroughbred event horse had recently begun stopping and also had moderate impinging dorsal spinous processes in the same region. Care must always be taken to differentiate genuine new bone formation from superimposed lung opacities.

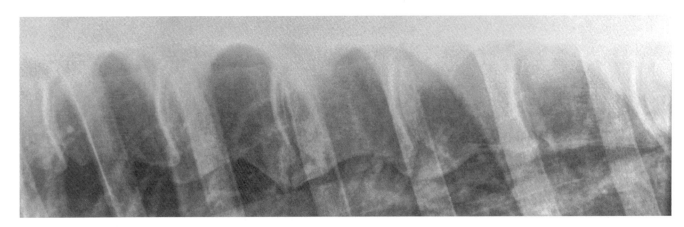

Figure 10.41(b) Lateral radiographic view of the vertebral bodies of the tenth to sixteenth thoracic vertebrae of an 8-year-old Irish Draught cross gelding with a history of an unspecified back injury 6 months previously, after which the horse had been reluctant to walk for several weeks. Currently the horse was stiff, short striding and reluctant to canter. Cranial is to the left. There is new bone on the cranial and caudal distal aspects of the vertebral body of T12 and the cranial distal aspect of T13. There is a large bridge of bone extending between the fourteenth and thirteenth thoracic vertebrae. There is slight modelling of the caudal distal aspect of the vertebral body of T14 and the cranial distal aspect of T15. This represents extensive spondylosis. The intercentral joints appear normal. Compare with Figure 10.41(c).

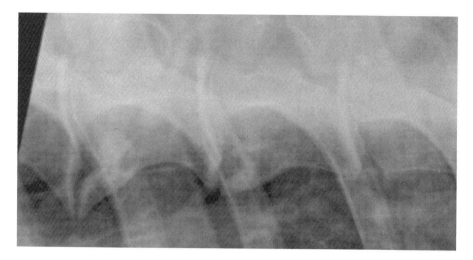

Figure 10.41(c) Oblique radiographic view of the vertebral bodies of the twelfth to fifteenth thoracic vertebrae of the same horse as in Figure 10.41(b). Cranial is to the left. Note the large spondyles which effectively extend the intercentral articulations.

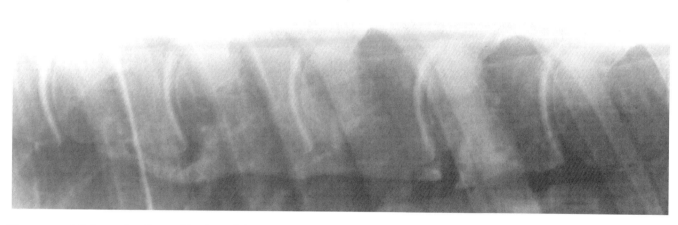

Figure 10.41(d) Lateral radiographic view of the vertebral bodies of the mid-thoracic vertebrae (T11–T16) of a 12-year-old Thoroughbred advanced event horse. The horse was stiff and evasive and short striding. There is advanced spondylosis with bone bridging between the twelfth to fourteenth thoracic vertebrae. The horse also had bilateral forelimb and hindlimb proximal suspensory desmitis and osteoarthritis of the centrodistal joint of the left hindlimb.

condition in foals, including *Rhodococcus equi*, the most common cause in the adult horse is tuberculosis. Neoplastic metastases may give a similar radiographic appearance. Negative radiographic findings do not preclude the possibility of vertebral infection. Nuclear scintigraphy may be more sensitive.

Infection in the withers region (fistulous withers) may involve the dorsal spinous processes. This may appear as lucency in the subcortical bone and periosteal new bone formation. It should not be confused with the normal radiographic appearance of the dorsal spinous processes in this region (see Figure 10.29, page 543). Positive contrast fistulograms and/or diagnostic ultrasonography may be helpful to determine if a draining tract is associated with osteomyelitis. This condition has become less common in the United Kingdom in recent years, probably due to the reduced incidence of brucellosis, with which it was commonly associated. Topical treatment with metronidazole has been found helpful in some cases. Surgery may be required, but some cases remain refractory to treatment.

Discospondylitis

Discospondylitis (inflammation of the vertebral body and associated intervertebral disc) has been seen rarely in association with infection, characterized by back stiffness and an abnormal stance and gait, with or without ataxia. Serum fibrinogen may be elevated. Radiographically there is alteration in the intervertebral joint space: either irregular widening with sclerosis and lysis of the vertebral endplates, or narrowing or obliteration of the intervertebral joint space, with new bone on the ventral and/or dorsal aspect of the vertebral bodies. There may be some malalignment of the vertebrae. Successful treatment with antimicrobial drugs has been reported.

Luxation

Subluxation or luxation of a vertebra in the thoracolumbar region is rare and is associated with severe pain, with or without ataxia. Luxation occurs most commonly in the lumbar region, where radiographic evaluation of the vertebral bodies is most difficult. The alignment of the vertebrae and the width of the intercentral articulations must be assessed carefully. The prognosis for athletic function is extremely poor.

Fractures

Fractures involving the bodies of the thoracolumbar vertebrae are relatively uncommon. They normally cause or are accompanied by damage to the spinal cord, which often results in immediate paraplegia.

Hairline fractures with minimal displacement may prove impossible to detect radiographically, but may be detected using nuclear scintigraphy. Stress fractures are now thought to occur more commonly in young Thoroughbreds in training than previously recognized, especially involving the

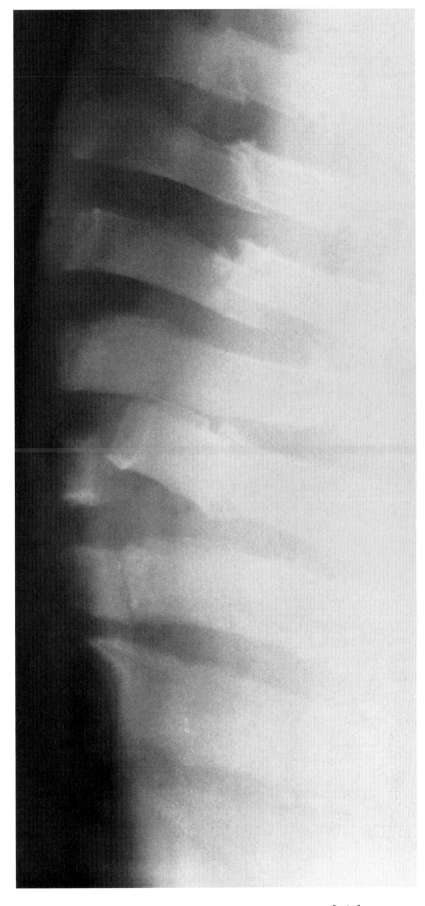

Figure 10.42 Lateral view of the dorsal spinous processes of the second to ninth thoracic vertebrae of an advanced event horse with acute onset of pain in the withers region following a fall in water, and subsequently becoming cast in a stable within 24 hours. There are displaced comminuted fractures of the dorsal spinous processes of T3–T9. The horse was treated conservatively and made a complete functional recovery, although slight malformation of the withers region persisted. The radiograph was obtained using an aluminium wedge filter.

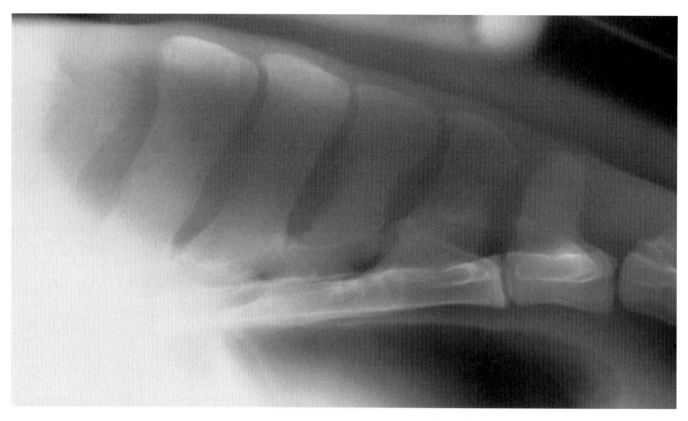

Figure 10.43 Lateral view of the sacrum and cranial coccygeal vertebrae of a normal adult horse. The horse was poorly muscled over its dorsal midline and the sacrum is defined better than in the majority of horses. The radiograph was obtained using an aluminium wedge filter.

facet joints in the lumbar region. Significant radiological signs of a vertebral fracture include: (a) apparent shortening of the length of the vertebral body; (b) a change in shape of the intercentral articulations, possibly with dorsal (upward) displacement of the vertebra; (c) callus formation.

In young animals, pathological fractures of vertebrae may occur secondarily to osteomyelitis following destructive and resorptive changes in the vertebral body.

Fracture of a vertebral body generally has a grave prognosis.

Fractures of the dorsal spinous processes usually occur at the withers as the result of a fall. Displacement of the fragments is often present (Figure 10.42). Complete osseous healing frequently does not occur and there is often deformation of the dorsal spinous processes. A good prognosis for future performance can be given, although a special saddle may be required.

Other fractures occur, but may be difficult to identify on radiographs.

Fracture of the ribs may present clinically as back pain. Fracture of the first rib may result in forelimb lameness or a neurological gait deficit (see Chapter 12, page 646).

[568]

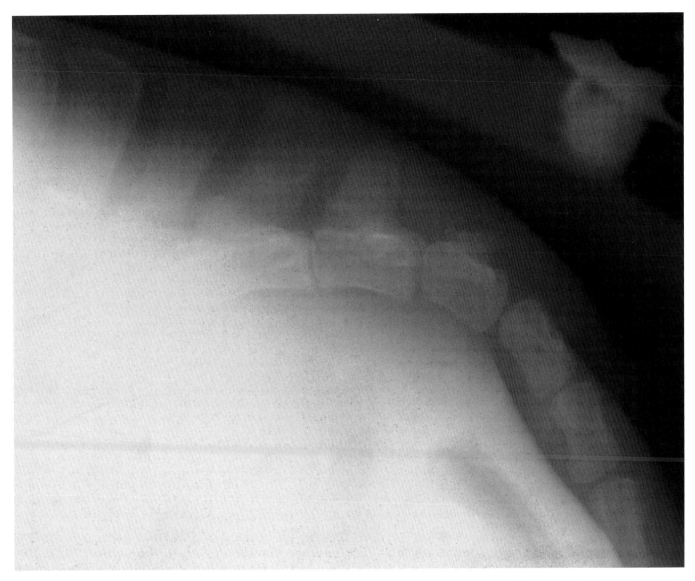

Figure 10.44 Lateral view of the caudal aspect of the sacrum and the cranial coccygeal vertebrae (CO1–CO5) of a normal adult horse. Note the different shape of each coccygeal vertebra. The radiograph was obtained using an aluminium wedge filter.

Sacrum and coccygeal vertebrae

Lateral radiographs of the sacrum and coccygeal vertebrae are obtained similarly to those of the thoracolumbar spine. Definition is often poor due to the overlying soft tissues and the resulting scattered radiation. Ventro-dorsal views can be obtained with the horse in dorsal recumbency under general anaesthesia (see Chapter 11, 'Pelvis', page 575).

On a lateral view of a normal horse, the sacrum is poorly defined, but its ventral border is seen as a linear opacity (Figure 10.43). The coccygeal vertebrae are aligned in a curvilinear manner (Figure 10.44).

Occasionally pain is associated with impinging dorsal spinous processes of the sacrum (Figure 10.45).

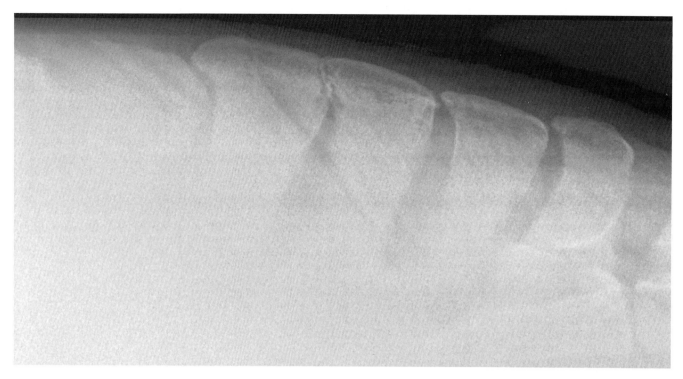

Figure 10.45 Lateral radiographic view of the dorsal spinous processes of the sacrum of a 14-year-old Arab endurance horse with poor performance and a reluctance to canter. The horse was painful to palpation throughout the thoracolumbar and sacral regions. There is overriding of three sacral dorsal spinous processes. There were also some architectural changes of the supraspinous ligament seen ultrasonographically.

Sacral fractures are often displaced in a dorsoventral direction, and thus are best identified in a lateral projection. Clinically these fractures may result in a change in conformation of the hindquarters and neurological abnormalities. Ultrasonographic examination both externally and per rectum may be useful for verifying the diagnosis.

FURTHER READING

Adams, A., Steckel, R. and Blevins, W. (1985) Diskospondylitis in five horses. *J. Am. Vet. Med. Ass.*, **186**, 270–272

Alitalio, I. and Karkkainen, M. (1983) Osteochondrotic changes in the vertebrae of four ataxic horses suffering from cervical vertebral malformation. *Nord. Vet. Med.*, **35**, 468–474

Alward, A., Pease, A. and Jones, S. (2007) Thoracic discospondylitis with associated epaxial muscle atrophy in a Quarter Horse gelding. *Equine vet. Educ.*, **19**, 67–71

Denoix, J.-M. (2005) Thoracolumbar malformations or injuries and neurological manifestations. *Equine vet. Educ.*, **17**, 191–194

Denoix, J.-M. (2007) Discovertebral pathology in horses. *Equine vet. Educ.*, **19**, 72–73

Erichsen, C., Eksell, P., Roethlisberger Hol, K. and Johnston, C. (2004) Relationship between scintigraphic and radiographic evaluation of spinous processes in the thoracolumbar spine in riding horses without clinical signs of back problems. *Equine vet. J.*, **36**, 458–465

Funk, K. and Erickson, E. (1968) A case of atlanto-axial subluxation in a horse. *Can. Vet. J.*, **9**, 120–123

Giguere, S. and Lavoie, J. (1994) *Rhodococcus equi* vertebral osteomyelitis in 3 Quarter Horses. *Equine vet. J.*, **26**, 74–78

Greet, T.R.C., Jeffcott, L.B., Whitwell, K.E. and Cook, W.R. (1980) The slap test for laryngeal adduction function in horses with suspected cervical spinal cord damage. *Equine vet. J.*, **12**, 127–131

Guffy, M., Coffman, J. and Strafuss, A. (1969) Atlantoaxial luxation in a foal. *J. Am. Vet. Med. Ass.*, **155**, 754–757

Haussler, K. and Stover, S. (1998) Stress fractures of the vertebral lamina and pelvis in Thoroughbred racehorses. *Equine vet. J.*, **30**, 374–383

Haussler, K., Stover, S. and Willits, N. (1997) Developmental variation in lumbosacropelvic anatomy of Thoroughbred horses. *Am. J. Vet. Res.*, **58**, 1083–1091

Hawkins, J. and Fessler, J. (2000) Treatment of supraspinous bursitis by use of debridement in standing horses: 10 cases (1968–1999). *J. Am. Vet. Med. Ass.*, **217**, 74–78

Hudson, N. and Mayhew, I. (2005) Radiographic and myelographic assessment of the equine cervical vertebral column and spinal cord. *Equine vet. Educ.*, **17**, 34–38

Jeffcott, L.B. (1975) The diagnosis of diseases of the horse's back. *Equine vet. J.*, **7**, 67–78

Jeffcott, L.B. (1979a) Radiographic examination of the equine vertebral column. *Vet. Radiol.*, **20**, 135–139

Jeffcott, L.B. (1979b) Radiographic features of the normal equine thoracolumbar spine. *Vet. Radiol.*, **20**, 140–147

Jeffcott, L.B. (1979c) Back problems in the horse – a look at past, present and future progress. *Equine vet. J.*, **11**, 129–136

Jeffcott, L.B. (1980) Disorders of the thoracolumbar spine of the horse – a survey of 443 cases. *Equine vet. J.*, **12**, 197–210

Jeffcott, L.B. and Dalin, G. (1980) Natural rigidity of the horse's backbone. *Equine vet. J.*, **12**, 101–108

Jeffcott, L.B. and Hickman, J. (1975) The treatment of horses with chronic back pain by resecting the summits of the impinging dorsal spinous processes. *Equine vet. J.*, **7**, 115–119

Kothstein, T., Eashmir-Raven, A., Thomas, M. and Brashier, M. (2000) Radiographic diagnosis: thoracic spinal fracture resulting in kyphosis in a horse. *Vet. Radiol. and Ultrasound*, **41**, 44–45

Leipold, H., Brandt, G., Guffy, M. and Blauch, B. (1974) Congenital atlanto-occipital fusion in a foal. *Vet. Med./Small Anim. Clin.*, **69**, 1312–1316

Mayhew, I. (1978) Congenital occipitoatlantoaxial malformations in the horse. *Equine vet. J.*, **10**, 103–113

Mayhew, I., Whitlock, R. and de Lahunta, A. (1978) Spinal cord disease in the horse. *Cornell Vet.*, **68**, Suppl. 6, 44–68

Mayhew, I., Donawick, W., Green, S. *et al.* (1993) Diagnosis and prediction of cervical vertebral malformation in Thoroughbred foals based on semi-quantitative radiographic indicators. *Equine vet. J.*, **25**, 435–440

McCoy, D., Shires, P. and Beadle, R. (1974) Ventral approach for stabilisation of atlantoaxial subluxation secondary to odontoid fracture in a foal. *J. Am. Vet. Med. Ass.*, **185**, 545–549

Moore, B., Holbrook, T., Stefanacci, J. *et al.* (1992) Contrast-enhanced computed tomography in six horses with cervical stenotic myelopathy. *Equine vet. J.*, **24**, 197–202

Moore, B., Reed, S., Biller, D. *et al.* (1994) Assessment of vertebral canal diameter and bony malformations of the spine in horses with cervical sclerotic myelopathy. *Am. J. Vet. Res.*, **55**, 5–13

Nout, Y. and Reed, S. (2003) Cervical vertebral stenotic myelopathy. *Equine vet. Educ.*, **15**, 212–223

Olchowy, T. (1994) Vertebral body osteomyelitis due to *Rhodococcus equi* in 2 Arabian foals. *Equine vet. J.*, **26**, 79–80

Owen, R. ap R. and Smith-Maxie, L. (1978) Repair of a dens of the axis in a foal. *J. Am. Vet. Med. Ass.*, **173**, 854–856

Perkins, J., Schumacher, J., Kelly, G., Pollock, P. and Harty, M. (2005) Subtotal ostectomy of dorsal spinous processes performed in nine standing horses. *Vet. Surg.*, **34**, 625–629

Pinchbeck, G. and Murphy, D. (2001) Cervical vertebral fracture in three foals. *Equine vet. Educ.*, **13**, 8–12

Randelhoff, A. (1997) Pathologische anatomische und histologische Untersuchungen zur Pathogenese von Wirbelsäulenveränderungen bei Pferden. Doctorate Thesis, Berlin

Rantanen, N., Gavin, P., Barbee, S. and Sande, R. (1981) Ataxia and paresis in horses, Part 2: Radiographic and myelographic examination of the cervical vertebral column. *Comp. Cont. Educ.*, **3**, 161–171

Rashmir-Raven, A., Thomas, M. and Brashier, M. (2000) Radiographic diagnosis: Thoracic spinal fracture resulting in kyphosis in a horse. *Vet. Radiol. and Ultrasound*, **41**, 44–45

Ricardi, G. and Dyson, S. (1993) Forelimb lameness associated with radiographic abnormalities of the cervical vertebrae. *Equine vet. J.*, **25**, 422–426

Richardson, D. (1986) *Eikenella corrodens* osteomyelitis of the axis in a foal. *J. Am. Vet. Med. Ass.*, **188**, 298–299

Rooney, J.R. (1963) Equine incoordination 1. Gross morphology. *Cornell Vet.*, **53**, 411–422

Rooney, J.R. and Prickett, M.E. (1966). Congenital lordosis of the horse. *Cornell Vet.*, **57**, 417–428

Smythe, R.H. (1962) Ankylosis of the equine spine; pathologic or biologic? *Mod. Vet. Pract.*, **43**, 50–51

Sweers, L. and Carstens, A. (2006) Imaging features of discospondylitis in two horses. *Vet. Radiol. and Ultrasound*, **47**, 159–164

Taylor, S., Murray, R., Donovan, T. and Scott, C. (2002) Conservative management of a sacrococcygeal fracture/luxation in a horse. *Equine vet. Educ.*, **14**, 63–70

Van Biervliet, J., de Lahunta, A., Ennulat, D., Oglesbee, M. and Summers, B. (2004) Acquired cervical scoliosis in six horses associated with dorsal grey column chronic myelitis. *Equine vet. J.*, **35**, 86–92

Vaughan, L. and Mason, B. (1975) *A Clinicopathological Study of Racing Accidents in Horses*, Adlard and Son, Bartholomew Press, Dorking, Surrey

Walmsley, J., Pettersson, H., Winberg, F. and McEvoy, F. (2002) Impingement of the dorsal spinous processes in two hundred and fifteen horses: case selection, surgical technique and results. *Equine vet. J.*, **34**, 23–28.

Whitwell, K. (1980) Causes of ataxia in horses. *In Practice*, **2**, 17–24

Whitwell, K. and Dyson, S. (1987) Interpreting radiographs 8: Equine cervical vertebrae. *Equine vet. J.*, **19**, 8–14

Wilson, W., Hughes, S., Ghoshal, N. and McNeel, S. (1985) Occipitoatlantoaxial malformation in two non Arabian horses. *J. Am. Vet. Med. Ass.*, **187**, 36–40

Witte, S., Alexander, K., Bucellato, M., Sofaly, C., Fife, W. and Hinchclife, K. (2005) Congenital atlantoaxial luxation associated with malformation of the dens in a Quarter horse foal. *Equine vet. Educ.*, **17**, 175–178

Wong, D., Scarratt, W. and Rohleder, J. (2005) Hindlimb paresis associated with kyphosis, hemivertebrae and multiple thoracic vertebral malformations in a Quarterhorse gelding. *Equine vet. Educ.*, **17**, 187–191

Chapter 11
The pelvis and femur

Pelvis

The primary indications for radiography of the pelvis are:

1 Asymmetry of the pelvis, assessed by comparison of the tubera coxae and sacrale

2 Hindlimb lameness in the absence of clinical and radiographic abnormalities of the lower limb

3 Audible or palpable crepitus in the pelvic region associated with hindlimb lameness (radiography performed with the horse under general anaesthesia should be postponed in these circumstances for at least 6 weeks – see 'Fractures', page 592). It should be noted that diagnostic ultrasonography can be useful to identify fractures, especially those of the ilial wing

4 Positive nuclear scintigraphic findings

RADIOGRAPHIC TECHNIQUE

Equipment

Radiographs of the pelvis require radiographic equipment with an output in excess of 100 kV and 200 mAs. Digital systems or rare earth screens and films are required. Large (35 cm × 43 cm) cassettes are recommended. Oblique lateral radiographic views of the pelvis in a standing horse can be obtained and yield adequate diagnostic information in foals, ponies and Thoroughbred-type horses, but their diagnostic value in large horses is more limited. Standing ventrodorsal oblique radiographs can be obtained and may be useful to diagnose obvious lesions of the coxofemoral joint and the ischium, particularly when general anaesthesia is clinically undesirable. Strict control of personnel is essential to minimize the radiation hazard. Standing radiographs may underestimate the degree of pathological abnormality. It is not possible to assess the ilial wings, tubera coxae and sacroiliac joints using this technique.

Much more detailed, high-quality radiographs of the entire pelvic region are obtained with the horse in dorsal recumbency under general anaesthesia. Because of the large exposures required, no personnel should be in the x-ray room during radiography. It is preferable to have an x-ray table that incorporates a cassette tunnel, since accurate positioning of the cassettes directly under a recumbent horse is difficult (Figure 11.1).

[573]

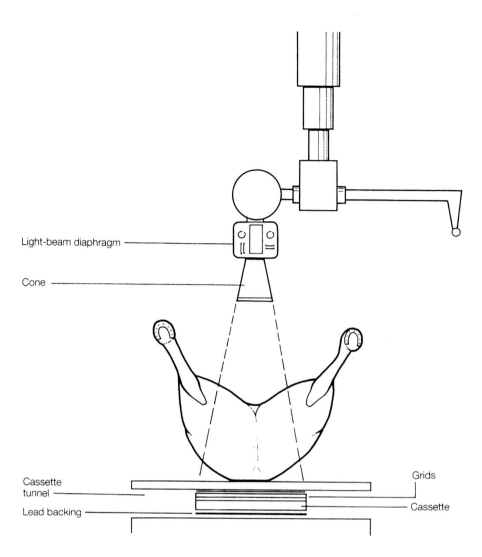

Light-beam diaphragm

Cone

Cassette tunnel

Lead backing

Grids

Cassette

Figure 11.1 Positioning of the x-ray machine, horse and cassette to obtain ventrodorsal radiographic views of the pelvis and lumbar vertebrae (not to scale).

Because of the large amount of soft tissue present, scattered radiation is a serious problem. It must be carefully controlled using one or more of the following:

- Precise collimation of the primary x-ray beam, using a light-beam diaphragm
- A focused grid (12:1 ratio), or ideally two focused grids with grid lines at right angles to each other (this will markedly increase the exposure required) (note, for computed or digital radiography, it may be necessary to experiment with grid types in order to eliminate moiré lines)
- A lead intensifying screen (lead equivalent 0.002 cm) placed in front of the grid(s) to absorb low-energy radiation
- A sheet of lead (0.01 mm lead equivalent) placed behind the cassette in order to reduce back-scatter
- A lead cone in addition to a light-beam diaphragm is helpful to collimate the primary beam fully

Ventrodorsal views of the pelvis with the horse in dorsal recumbency

For accurate assessment of pelvic radiographs it is important that the horse is positioned symmetrically in dorsal recumbency in the so-called 'frog-leg' position, i.e. with the caudal lumbar spine and the sacrum in a straight line, and the hindlimbs flexed and abducted. In horses with unilateral atrophy of the muscles of the hindquarters and/or severe asymmetry of the pelvis, positioning can be difficult. The best guide to ensure that positioning is correct is to assess the linea alba, which should be straight and lie vertically above the spine. Extra padding may need to be placed under the horse if there is pronounced uniaxial muscle atrophy of the hindquarters, to aid correct positioning. The position of the flexed hindlimbs, and in particular the points of the hocks, can be deceptive. All the radiographs are obtained with the x-ray beam aligned perpendicular to the table on which the horse is supported.

For complete assessment of the pelvis of an adult horse, at least seven standard overlapping radiographic views are recommended (using 35 cm × 43 cm cassettes) (Figure 11.2).

Three views are obtained along the midline of the pelvis. The x-ray beam in each case is centred on the linea alba.

1   To examine the tubera ischii, the caudal edge of the cassette is positioned immediately caudal to the tubera ischii.

2   To examine the region of the coxofemoral joints and obturator foramina, the cassette is moved cranially so that the two radiographic images overlap by about 5 cm. This also gives visualization of the caudal part of the sacrum.

3   To examine the sacroiliac and lumbosacral joints and the cranial part of the sacrum, the cassette is moved cranially, to overlap the previous position by about 5 cm.

Separate views are obtained of each tuber coxae. The cassette is positioned 5–10 cm cranial to the most cranial view of the pelvic canal, but is centred approximately 20 cm to the right or left of the midline. This view may aid definition of the individual sacroiliac joints.

For examination of the left and right coxofemoral joints, the horse should be rolled slightly so that the limb on the side to be radiographed is tilted nearer to the table, forming an angle of 10–15° with the horizontal. The cassette is positioned about 10 cm cranial to the position for the caudal pelvic view, and the x-ray beam is centred 5–10 cm lateral to the linea alba. This view also gives good visualization of the proximal femur.

Demonstration of specific lesions may require non-standard views. Subluxation of the coxofemoral joint may not be apparent in the frog-leg position and it may be necessary to extend the limb to demonstrate this abnormality. Oblique views are best obtained by rolling the horse, rather than angling the x-ray beam, in order to avoid grid cut-off.

Superimposition of gas- and ingesta-filled viscera over the pelvis is a problem. Routine starvation prior to general anaesthesia and radiography

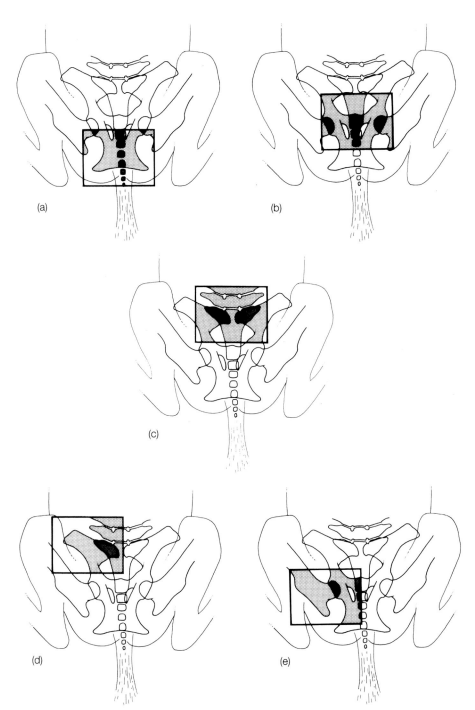

Figure 11.2 Positioning the cassette relative to the horse to obtain ventrodorsal views of (a) the tubera ischia, (b) the pelvic canal, (c) the sacroiliac joints, (d) an iliac wing and (e) a coxofemoral joint. The latter is obtained with the horse rocked towards the side to be examined.

unfortunately has little effect upon this. During radiography rectal manipulation of the viscera and manual emptying of the rectum can be tried, but tend to be ineffective in moving the intestinal contents significantly.

Lateral oblique views of the pelvis in the standing horse

Oblique lateral views of the pelvis can provide adequate diagnostic information in foals, ponies and Thoroughbred-type horses. Their diagnostic value in larger horses is limited. The horse should stand squarely on all four limbs,

[576]

however many horses with fractures of the pelvic region are not able to bear full weight on the lame limb. Rectal examination, including ultrasonographic examination, of the osseous structures of the pelvis is recommended to obtain further information about the possible site of fracture. Evacuation of faeces from the rectum helps avoid artefacts created by overlying faecal material. It is also beneficial to inject air into the rectum to provide better contrast for the visualization of overlying osseous structures.

A vertically positioned cassette supported by a cassette holder is positioned against the side of the pelvis to be examined (Figure 11.3). The x-ray machine is angled 30° distally from the horizontal, centring the x-ray beam between the level of the greater trochanter of the femur and the base of the tail, approximately two-thirds of the distance between the ipsilateral tuber sacrale and tuber ischii. If the horse is unable to bear weight on the limb to be examined the pelvis is tipped ventrally on that side, so the x-ray beam must be angled a further 5–10° distally and centred several centimetres further ventrally. The height of the cassette is adjusted accordingly. The precise craniocaudal position of the cassette and x-ray machine depends on the area of clinical interest.

Rare earth screens (or a digital system) and a stationary parallel grid aligned perpendicular to the x-ray beam give best results. This view permits evaluation of the caudal half of the ilial shaft, the ischium, the greater trochanter of the femur, the femoral head, the acetabulum and the coxofemoral joint. It permits the identification of displaced fractures, extensive periarticular new bone and lack of congruence of the coxofemoral joint. However it is not possible to detect more subtle radiographic abnormalities, such as periarticular osteophyte formation. Little information can be gained about the ilial wings and the tubera coxae.

This technique involves high exposure factors and the minimum number of personnel should be present.

Ventrodorsal views of the pelvis in the standing horse

It is essential that the horse is adequately sedated. It should stand with the hindlimbs abducted as far as is compatible with standing both comfortably and still. A cassette and cross-hatch grid are placed dorsal to the pelvic region, angled so that they will be perpendicular to the x-ray beam. The x-ray tube is then positioned ventral to the horse's abdomen, cranial to the hindlimbs, and the beam is angled dorsally 10–25° caudad. The cassette and cross-hatch grid are positioned over the hindquarter to be examined, or over the dorsal midline to examine both sides simultaneously (Figure 11.4). The cassette and the x-ray tube can be moved caudally, cranially or laterally to visualize the coxofemoral joints, the caudal pelvic canal and the tubera ischii. It is important to recognize the potential risk to personnel in the room, with the large exposure factors required (up to 150 kV, 400 mAs for a 500 kg horse). The use of a vertically mounted Bucky and cassette holder is highly recommended. The cassette should never be hand-held.

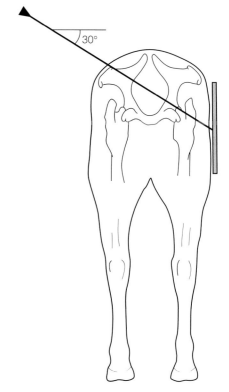

Figure 11.3 Positioning the x-ray beam and cassette to obtain a lateral oblique view of the coxofemoral joint in a standing horse. The cassette is positioned as close as possible to the horse, centred at the level of the coxofemoral joint. The x-ray beam is angled 30° ventrally and centred between the greater trochanter of the femur and the tail head, approximately two-thirds of the distance between the tuber sacrale and tuber ischii.

[577]

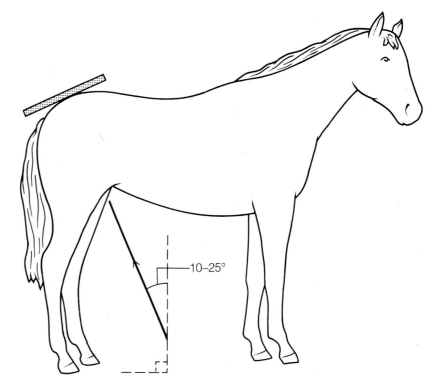

Figure 11.4 Positioning to obtain ventrodorsal views of the pelvis in the standing horse.

NORMAL ANATOMY, VARIATIONS AND INCIDENTAL FINDINGS

Immature horse

The pelvis consists of three paired bones (left and right): the ilium, pubis and ischium (Figure 11.5). At birth the symphyseal branches of the pubis and ischium are fused to each other, but ossification of their shafts, and fusion with the ilium to complete the acetabulum, does not occur until about 1 year of age (see page 713). In foals and yearlings the points of the tubera ischii are irregular and bluntly outlined due to incomplete ossification.

Separate ossification centres occur in each of the bones: ilium – iliac crest and tuber coxae; pubis – acetabular portion of the shaft; ischium – caudal portion of the bone and tubera ischii. The separate centres of ossification of the pelvis fuse by about 10–12 months, but the symphysis pubis remains unfused throughout life.

The proximal femur has separate centres of ossification for the femoral head, the trochanter major and the trochanter minor. The physis of the femoral head closes between 24 and 36 months, and the trochanter major fuses with the femoral shaft between 18 and 30 months. Fusion of the trochanter minor is less consistent, usually occurring at about 2 years.

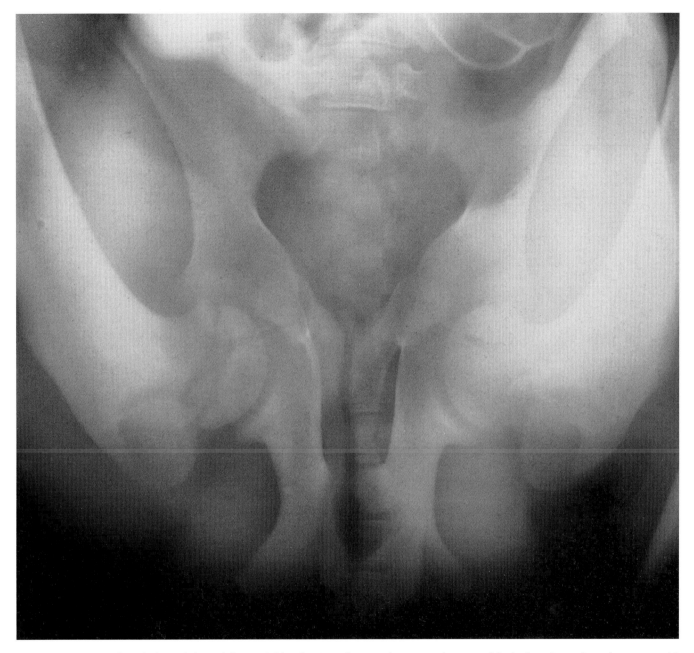

Figure 11.5 Ventrodorsal view of the pelvis, caudal lumbar vertebrae and sacrum of a normal foal of 11 days of age (compare with Figures 11.6a-c). Note the position of the symphyses between the ilium and pubis, and the ischium and the ilium, the wide pubic symphysis and the physis of the femoral head.

Skeletally mature horse: ventrodorsal views

When examining radiographs of the pelvis it is useful to start by assessing the obturator foramina (Figure 11.6b). If the horse is correctly positioned, these should appear symmetrical. If the foramina appear asymmetrical, this may be due to poor positioning or to traumatic damage to the pelvis. Asymmetry of the foramina is frequently seen in combination with pubic, ischial or acetabular fractures.

The symphysis pubis remains evident throughout life (Figure 11.6a). It is relatively straight. Occasionally a bony protuberance is evident at the cranial aspect of the pubic symphysis. The pubic bones should be aligned, with no step at the pelvic brim. Roughening on the cranial aspect of the pubis in the region of the pubic tubercle and iliopubic eminence may be seen.

The outline of the tubera ischii varies slightly between individuals, but should always be regular (Figure 11.6a).

The shaft of the ilium is smooth, with some roughening of the psoas tubercle. The ilium broadens cranially to form the body of the ilium and tuber coxae laterally, and the tuber sacrale medially (Figure 11.6d).

To compare the left and right coxofemoral joints, it is important that the pelvis is symmetrically positioned with similar rotation and abduction of the femurs. This can be evaluated on radiographs by comparing the angle formed between the trochanter major and the acetabular branch of the ischium.

The acetabulum is formed by fusion of the ilium, ischium and pubis. The dorsal rim has a smooth outline (Figure 11.6e). The ventral rim has, at its deepest point, a depression – the acetabular fossa – for attachment of the ligament of the femoral head (teres ligament). At the site of attachment of this ligament on the femoral head, a small focal lucent area – the fovea capitis – can sometimes be seen, opposite the acetabular fossa.

The sacroiliac joints (left and right) provide the only articulation between the pelvis and the spine, and have little movement (Figure 11.6c). They are diarthrodial joints with flattened joint surfaces which are angled at approximately 30° to the horizontal plane. The size and contour of the joints vary between individual animals. The joints are difficult to identify on a ventrodorsal projection, due to their angle and superimposition of abdominal viscera. It may be helpful to locate the narrowest (caudal) part of the sacrum between the shafts of the ilia and follow the diverging outlines of the sacrum cranially towards the external angle of the lumbosacral joint (Figure 11.6c). The sacroiliac joints are located where these lines are superimposed upon the wings of the ilia.

The five sacral vertebrae are fused, but have separate dorsal spinous processes which are seen as oval-shaped opacities in the midline, superimposed on the body of the sacrum (Figure 11.6c). The body of the sacrum broadens cranially. The first sacral vertebra has transverse processes which articulate with the transverse processes of the most caudal (the sixth) lumbar vertebra. The lumbosacral joints are easily recognized on dorsoventral radiographs (Figure 11.6c). The sacral body has intervertebral foramina between the adjacent vertebrae, but these can be difficult to identify radiographically. The intervertebral foramina between the sacrum and the most caudal lumbar vertebra and adjacent lumbar vertebrae are clearly seen as approximately circular lucent zones on the left and right sides of the intercentral articulations. The intercentral articulations are slightly variable in width and often appear wider in the sagittal midline than at the periphery of the joints, because the caudal articular surfaces are more curved than the cranial articular surface of the adjacent vertebra. The caudal subchondral bone plate of each lumbar vertebra is relatively sclerotic.

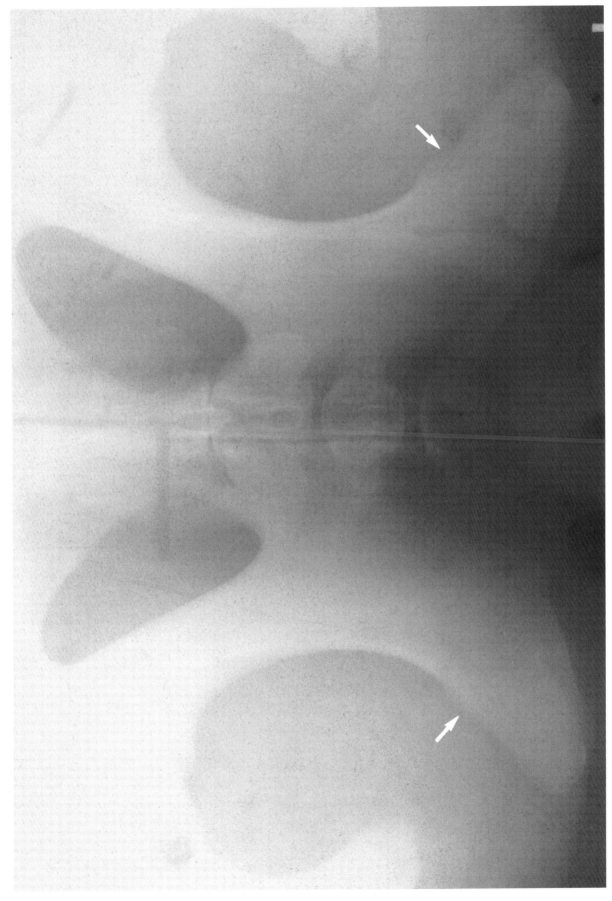

Figure 11.6(a) Ventrodorsal view of the caudal aspect of the pelvis of a normal adult horse. The cranial coccygeal vertebrae are superimposed over the pubic symphysis. Note the slight irregularity in outline of the cranial edge of each tuber ischium (arrows).

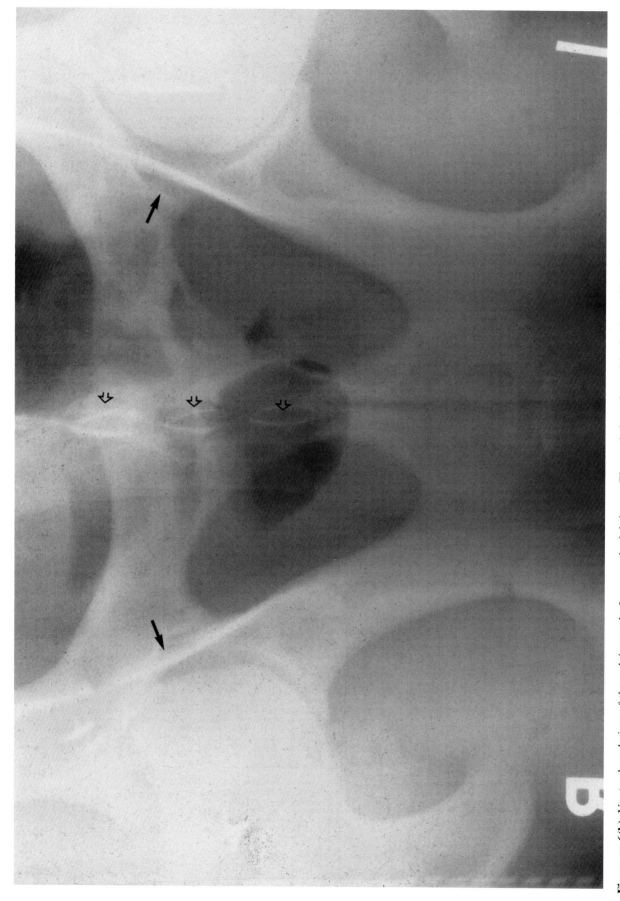

Figure 11.6(b) Ventrodorsal view of the pelvic canal of a normal adult horse. The oval-shaped opacities in the midline (open arrows) represent the dorsal spinous processes of the sacrum. Superimposed abdominal viscera cause the gas shadows. Note the symmetry of the obturator foramina, apparent widening of each coxofemoral joint in the region of the insertion of the teres ligament (closed arrows) and the flat appearance of the outline of the opposing femoral heads.

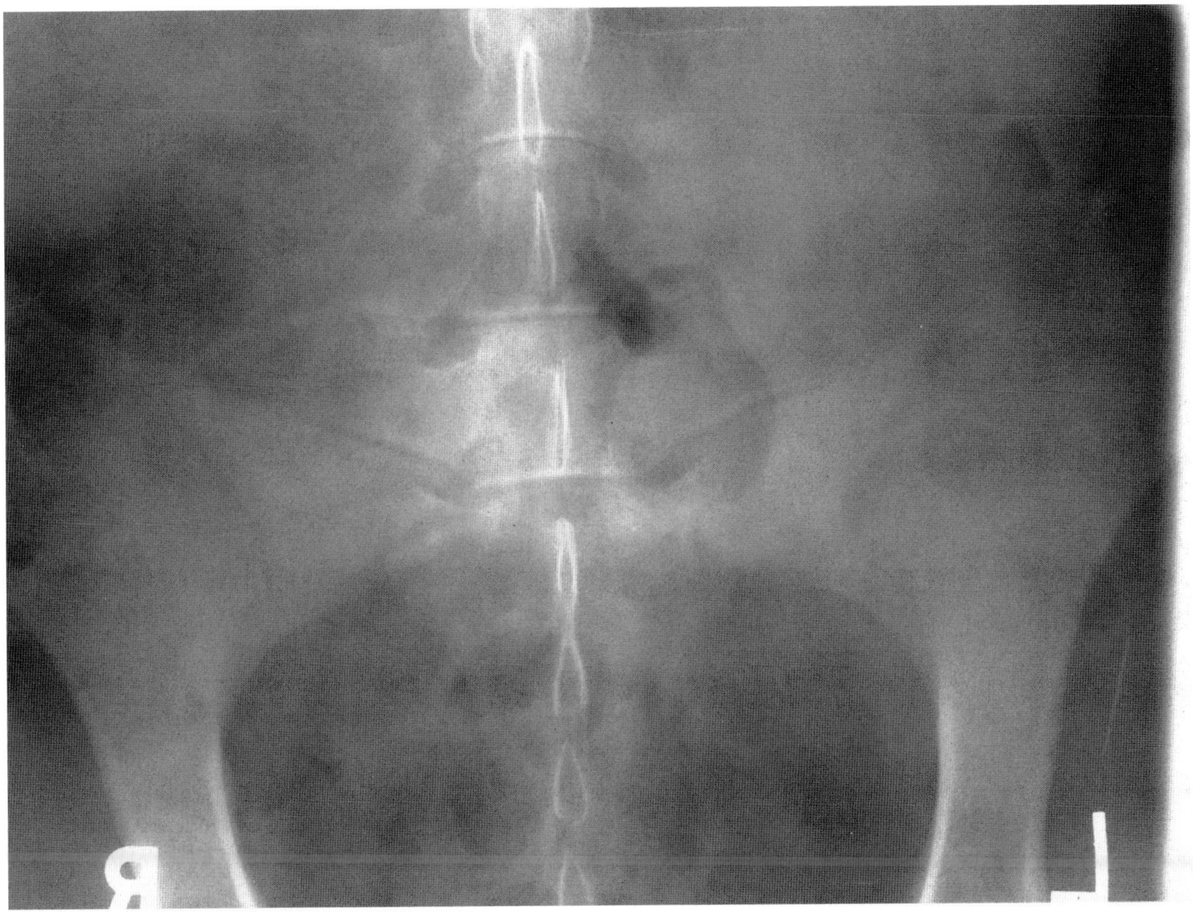
R
L

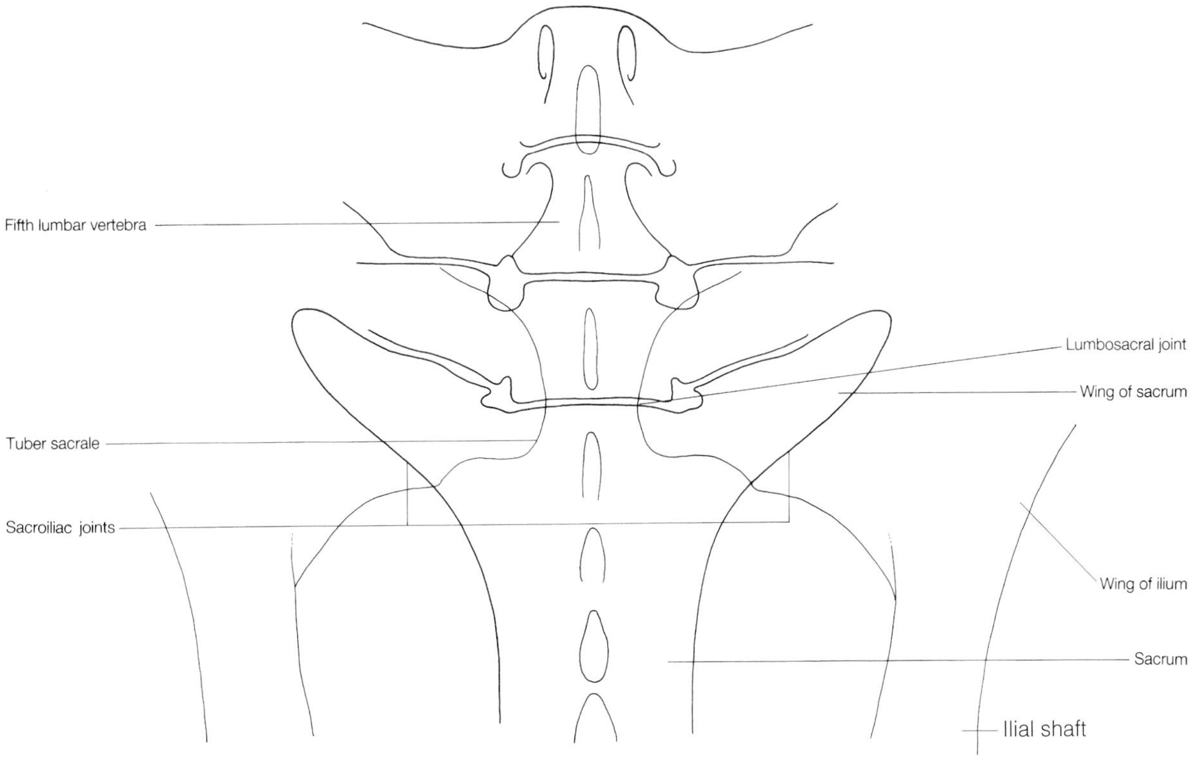
Fifth lumbar vertebra
Lumbosacral joint
Wing of sacrum
Tuber sacrale
Sacroiliac joints
Wing of ilium
Sacrum
Ilial shaft

Figure 11.6(c) Radiograph (above) and diagram of a ventrodorsal view of the lumbosacral region of a normal adult horse. Note the changing shape of the intercentral articulations of the lumbar vertebrae from cranially to caudally and the wider lumbosacral joint. The articulations between the transverse processes of the caudal lumbar vertebrae and the sacrum are well defined. The sacroiliac joint is less well defined on the left side due to superimposition of abdominal viscera.

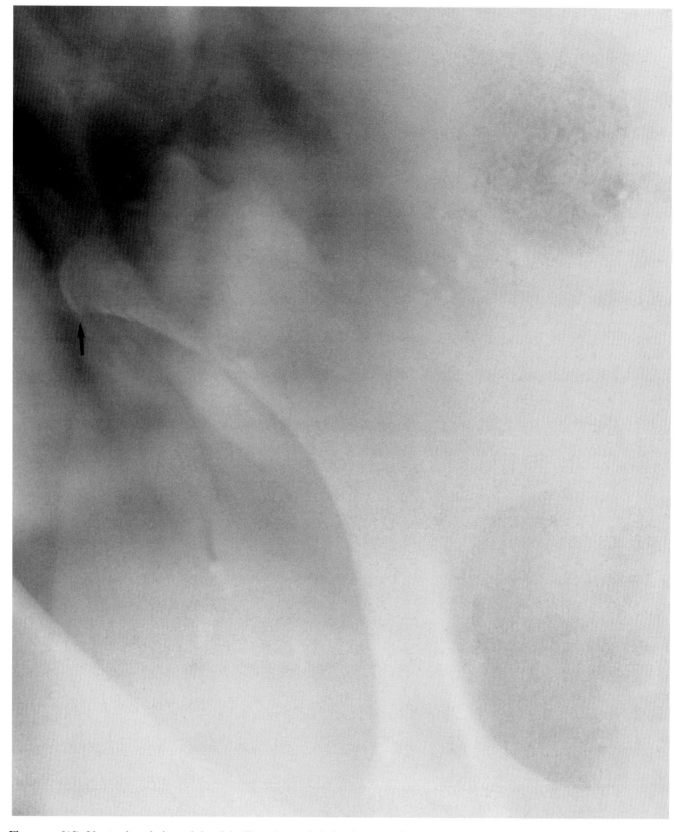

Figure 11.6(d) Ventrodorsal view of the right iliac wing and shaft of a normal 4-year-old horse. Note the incomplete fusion of the separate centre of ossification of the tuber coxae (arrow). The right sacroiliac joint is underexposed and therefore poorly defined.

[584]

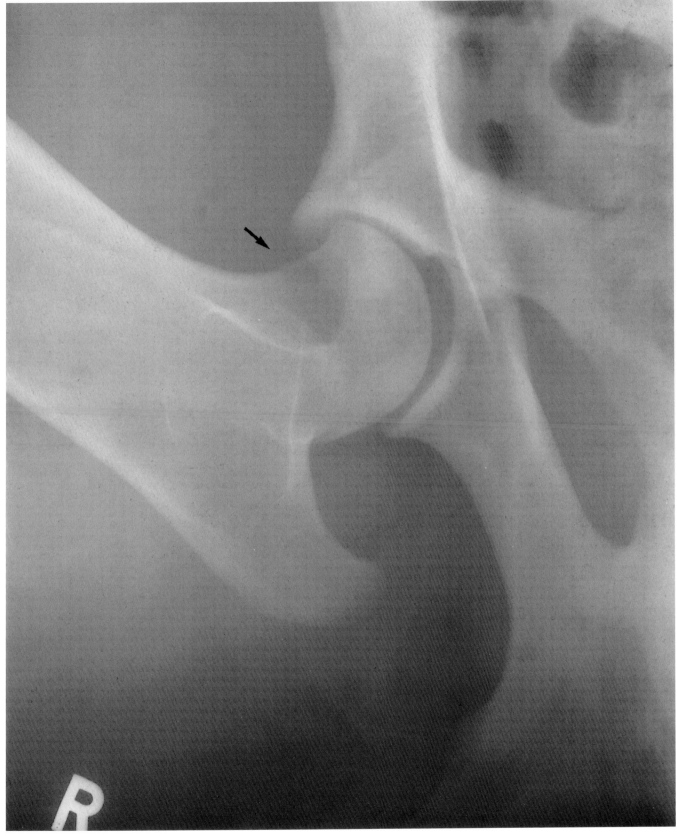

Figure 11.6(e) Ventrodorsal view of a coxofemoral joint of a normal adult horse. Note the slightly irregular margin of the cranial aspect of the proximal femur (arrow), which should not be confused with new bone formation.

Articulations between the transverse processes of the lumbar vertebrae are variable and may be asymmetrical. There is no relationship between age and the number of articulations, or the presence of ankylosis. The size and width of intertransverse articulations tends to be greatest at the lumbosacral joint and decreases craniad. The articulations between the transverse processes of adjacent lumbar vertebrae are often slightly irregular in outline. Occasionally irregular lucent zones and areas of sclerosis are seen in the cortical bone opposing the joints. The lumbosacral joint, and in some horses the intercentral joints between the fifth and sixth and fourth and fifth lumbar vertebrae and the intertransverse articulations, can also be assessed by per rectum ultrasonography.

Less commonly there may be fusion of the intercentral joints between the most caudal lumbar vertebrae and between the sixth lumbar vertebra and the sacrum, but this usually cannot be detected in a dorsoventral radiograph unless associated spondyles project laterally. The clinical significance of these changes is uncertain. Fusion may alter the biomechanical function of the back and predispose to other lesions of the thoracolumbar and sacroiliac regions.

In the standing horse acceptable images of the caudal ilium and ischium, the acetabulum and femoral head and neck can be obtained. Views of the obturator foramen are obliqued compared with views obtained with the horse under general anaesthesia, resulting in foreshortening. Caudal abdominal contents are superimposed over the pubis, making evaluation difficult. Evaluation of the ilia and sacroiliac joints is impossible.

Skeletally mature horse: oblique lateral views

In small standing horses, acceptable images of the ilial shaft, the coxofemoral joint, the greater trochanter of the femur, the femoral neck and the ischium can be obtained. Because of the obliquity of the x-ray beam they appear somewhat distorted (Figure 11.7). Knowledge of normal anatomy is essential, because in a horse that is unwilling to bear full weight on the lame limb, the radiographic images of the left and right sides will not be symmetrical. They are therefore not suitable for comparison to determine normality or abnormality.

SIGNIFICANT FINDINGS

Hip dysplasia

Hip dysplasia occurs very infrequently. Radiographic evidence includes flattening of the acetabulum, deformation of the femoral head and neck, subluxation and secondary degenerative changes in the joint. Such changes can only be appreciated on radiographs obtained with the horse under general anaesthesia. Even then care must be taken when evaluating radiographs, since relatively small changes in the position of the horse, or angle of the x-ray beam, can cause artefacts, especially in the region of attachment of the round ligament.

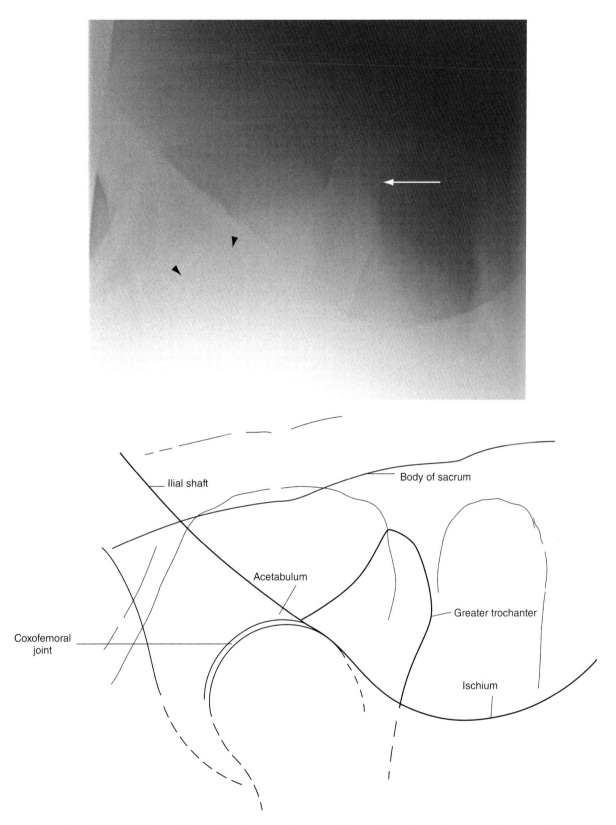

Figure 11.7 Lateral 30° distal oblique radiographic view and diagram of the pelvic region of a 3-year-old normal Thoroughbred. Cranial is to the left. The coxofemoral joint (arrowheads) and greater trochanter of the femur (arrow) can be identified. The ilial shaft extends to the left and the ischium to the right.

Subluxation of the coxofemoral joint

Subluxation of the coxofemoral joint has been described in association with malformation of the acetabulum and femoral head. Although the latter may be developmental in origin, it is also thought to occur secondarily to trauma and hip dysplasia (see above). The condition is characterized radiographically by flattening of the contour of the acetabulum and the femoral head, and an increase in the width of the joint space. These features can generally only be appreciated in radiographs obtained with the horse in dorsal recumbency under general anaesthesia.

Traumatically induced subluxation associated with partial tearing of the teres ligament can be a challenge to identify because, in the frog-leg position in dorsal recumbency, or in lateral oblique views obtained in a standing horse loading the limb, the joint may appear to be in normal alignment. Subluxation can be demonstrated in dorsal recumbency by extending the limb. If chronic there is usually also evidence of degenerative joint disease. There may be associated fracture(s). In a standing horse if the horse rests the limb then subluxation may be demonstrated. Transcutaneous ultrasonography is also useful for diagnosis.

Luxation of the coxofemoral joint

Luxation of the coxofemoral joint is rare and is usually the result of trauma with craniodorsal displacement of the femoral head. It can also be seen in association with multifocal stress fractures of the ilial shaft, pubis and ischium in young Thoroughbreds. It has been recognized in association with permanent upward fixation of the patella. Radiographically there is superimposition of the acetabulum and the femoral head. The radiographs should be inspected carefully for evidence of concurrent fractures of the femoral head and acetabulum. Luxation of the coxofemoral joint should be detectable on standing oblique views of the coxofemoral joint. The condition is characterized clinically by moderately severe to non-weight-bearing lameness, a tendency to abduct the stifle and foot, disparity in height of the hocks and dorsal displacement of the trochanter major of the femur. There is often audible and palpable crepitus. Ultrasonography may also be useful. Surgical treatment has been successful in some cases but the prognosis is generally poor.

Septic arthritis/osteomyelitis

Septic arthritis and osteomyelitis complex occurs occasionally in the coxofemoral joint of young horses. It is characterized radiographically by widening of the joint space, and productive and destructive bone changes involving both the acetabulum and the femoral head. The proximal femoral physis may also be involved in type P osteomyelitis (see Chapter 1, page 32).

Degenerative joint disease

Degenerative joint disease of the coxofemoral joint is an unusual cause of lameness in the horse. In some cases it is secondary to hip dysplasia, an acetabular fracture or damage to the teres ligament. Radiographic changes include: (a) modelling of the acetabulum, with osteophyte formation on the cranial and caudal margins (Figure 11.8); (b) flattening of the femoral head; (c) irregular width of joint space; (d) changes in subchondral bone opacity; (e) new bone formation on the neck of the femur.

Low-grade radiographic abnormalities are only detectable in radiographs obtained with the horse under general anaesthesia. More advanced radiographic abnormalities may be detectable in lateral oblique radiographs obtained in a standing horse. Ultrasonography may permit the identification of thickening of the joint capsule, presence of an abnormal amount of fluid and dorsal periarticular osteophytes. Nuclear scintigraphy may reveal increased radiopharmaceutical uptake, which may prompt more detailed radiographic examination.

The prognosis for future athletic function is hopeless in mature animals, but some horses may be sound enough to be retired for breeding purposes.

Sacroiliac joint disease

The radiographic features associated with a chronic sacroiliac lesion are usually minimal or absent. Occasionally there may be increase of the width of the joint space, or asymmetry of the two joints. The relative positions of the tubera sacrale and the summits of the sacral dorsal spinous processes may be altered. In a few advanced cases, peripheral osteophytes near the most caudal margin of the joint can be seen, disrupting the relatively smooth caudal outline of the medial aspect of the wing of the ilium (Figure 11.9). It is not possible to demonstrate radiographic abnormalities in the majority of cases where clinical signs are suggestive of lameness associated with the sacroiliac joints.

Linear tomography has shown potential for examining the lumbosacral region, including abnormalities of the sacroiliac joint. This equipment is only available at a very small number of clinics and therefore is not discussed further.

Nuclear scintigraphic examination may also be valuable; asymmetry of radiopharmaceutical uptake in the sacroiliac joint regions is not normal. Transrectal ultrasonography can give limited information about the caudal aspect of the joint space and reveal alteration in joint space width and bone contour.

The tubera sacrale are not easily examined radiographically, but ultrasonography may reveal altered bone contour reflecting enthesopathy and structural abnormalities of the dorsal sacroiliac ligament.

Osseous cyst-like lesions

Osseous cyst-like lesions have been recorded in the femoral head and the acetabulum. There is insufficient information for any prognosis or treatment to be recommended.

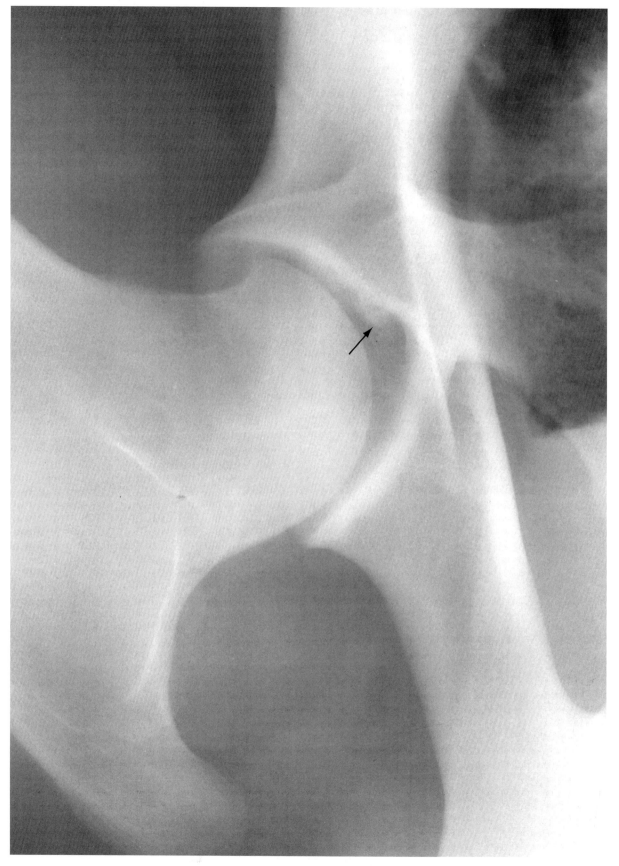

Figure 11.8 Ventrodorsal view of the right coxofemoral joint of a 14-year-old part Thoroughbred with evidence of degenerative joint disease. The cranial half of the acetabulum is poorly defined due to osteophyte formation (arrow) (compare with Figure 11.6e); there is also slight loss of definition of the caudal half of the acetabulum.

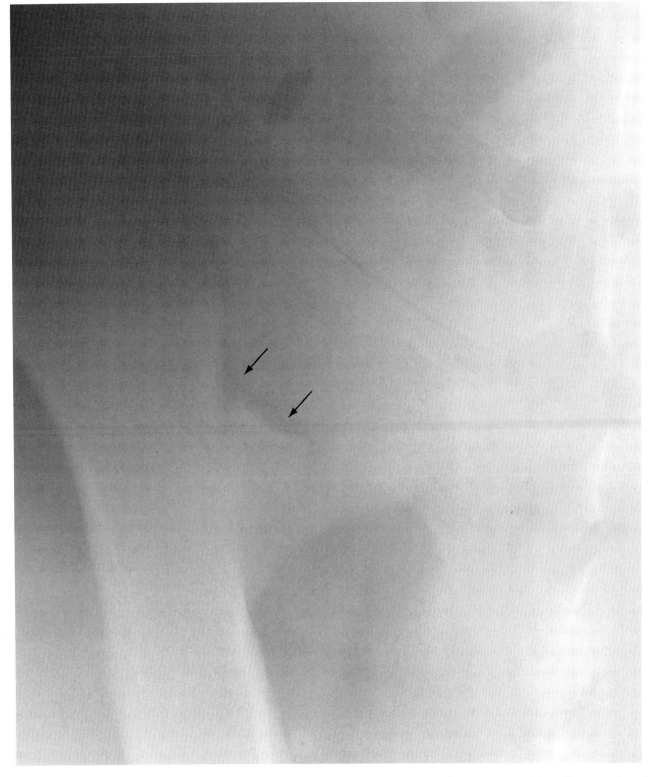

Figure 11.9 Ventrodorsal view of the sacrum and right iliac wing of a 5-year-old Arab with asymmetry of the tubera sacrale and right hindlimb lameness. The right sacroiliac joint is abnormal in shape and widened irregularly (arrows). There is no evidence of new bone formation on the caudal aspect of the joint.

Osteochondrosis

The coxofemoral joint is an unusual site for osteochondrosis. Radiographic abnormalities have been described in both the acetabulum and the femoral head, and include poorly defined lucent zones in the subchondral bone, with or without a surrounding sclerotic rim. Circular lucent zones in the subchondral bone have been referred to as subchondral bone cysts, but there is little evidence to show whether these are true subchondral bone cysts. Modelling of the caudal aspect of the acetabulum without associated lucent zones in the subchondral bone has also been described. The prognosis for further athletic soundness is generally considered to be poor.

Fractures

If a fracture of the pelvis is suspected, standing radiography may be useful in some cases. Percutaneous and transrectal ultrasonography may yield diagnostic information. If radiographs are to be obtained with the horse in dorsal recumbency, it is recommended that anaesthesia should be delayed for at least 6 weeks in order to avoid further displacement of the fracture during induction and recovery.

Although severe direct trauma is normally required to fracture the pelvis, 'spontaneous' fracture (often of the wing or shaft of the ilium) does occasionally occur during exercise in young Thoroughbreds in training. Spontaneous fractures are more common in females. These fractures initiate as incomplete stress fractures. With the more routine use of nuclear scintigraphic evaluation combined with diagnostic ultrasonography, fatigue fractures have been detected earlier and the incidence of complete fractures has decreased.

The most common sites of fractures are the ilium (including the tuber coxae), acetabulum and ischium (Figure 11.10). As a general rule the prognosis is considerably worse if there is an articular component to the fracture (coxofemoral or sacroiliac), due to subsequent secondary degenerative joint disease.

Fractures of the ilium

Fractures of the tuber coxae alone are recognized by a slight palpable irregularity of the external angle of the ilium, and seldom require radiography for diagnosis. On radiographs the tuber coxae appears blunted but the displaced fragment may not be visible. These fractures carry a good prognosis. Oblique radiographic views of the affected tuber coxae can be obtained in a standing horse, but ultrasonography is generally easier and equally informative.

Complete fractures of the ilial wing frequently extend obliquely in a craniocaudal direction. There is often displacement due to the action of the muscle masses that attach to the tuber coxae. Large fissures which frequently ramify towards the centre of the wing (Figure 11.11) can occur with minimal displacement of the ilium. These may extend towards and some-

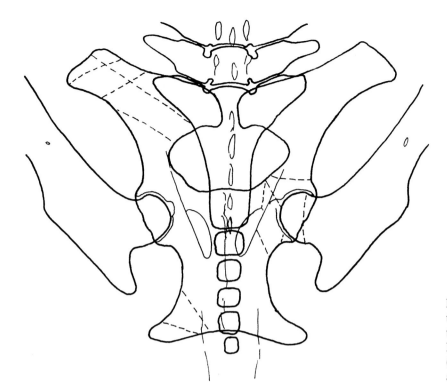

Figure 11.10 Common fracture sites of the pelvis. Compare with the position of the symphyses of the immature horse in Figure 11.5. See also Little and Hilbert (1987), Rutowski and Richardson (1989) and Pilsworth *et al.* (1994).

times involve the sacroiliac joint. Such fractures can usually be demonstrated using diagnostic ultrasonography.

Fractures of the ilial wing alone carry a fair prognosis if there is osseous union, but fibrous union accompanied by continual lameness may occur. If the fractures involve either the sacroiliac or (less frequently) the lumbosacral joints, the prognosis is guarded to poor.

Stress fractures of the ilial shaft in young Thoroughbreds are less common than ilial wing stress fractures and are sometimes scintigraphically silent or associated with only mildly increased radiopharmaceutical uptake. If a fracture becomes complete then diagnosis may be possible using lateral oblique radiographic views obtained in a standing horse. Fractures of the shaft of the ilium may be articular (see below). The prognosis is poor.

Fractures involving the coxofemoral joint

Fractures of the bones comprising the acetabulum are frequently accompanied by deformation of the ipsilateral side of the pelvis due to the severity of the initiating trauma. It must be borne in mind that the large forces required to create a fracture may result in multifocal fractures and identification of all the fractures may be important for prognosis. The most common site is at or close to the symphysis between the ilium and pubis. Such fractures are difficult to detect in lateral oblique radiographs in a standing horse, but may be detectable by transrectal ultrasonography, or in ventrodorsal radiographs obtained under general anaesthesia. If the fracture involves

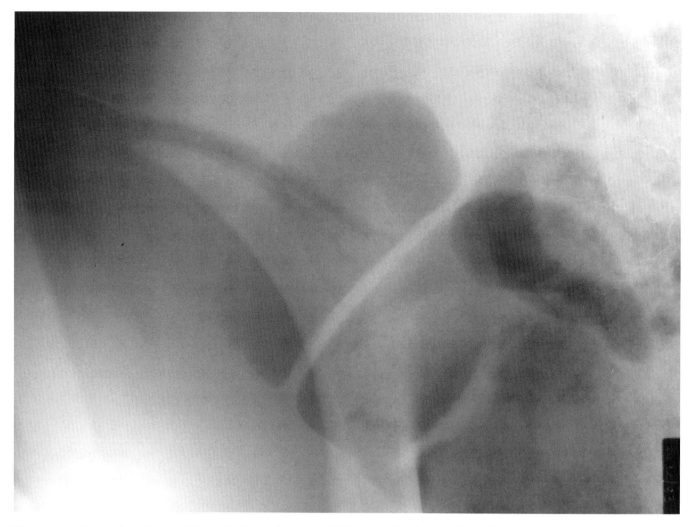

Figure 11.11 Ventrodorsal view of the right ilium of a 2-year-old Thoroughbred mare with a history of acute onset severe right hindlimb lameness after work 6 weeks previously. There is a displaced fracture of the right iliac wing, ramifying towards the iliac shaft. There is no bony union. The right sacroiliac joint is obscured by superimposed abdominal viscera. The radiograph was obtained using an aluminium wedge filter.

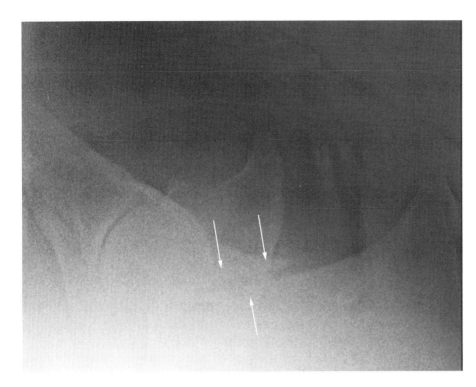

Figure 11.12(a) Lateral 30° distal oblique radiographic view of a 2-year-old Thoroughbred flat racehorse with acute onset of right hindlimb lameness. Cranial is to the left. There is a displaced fracture of the cranial aspect of the ischium (arrows).

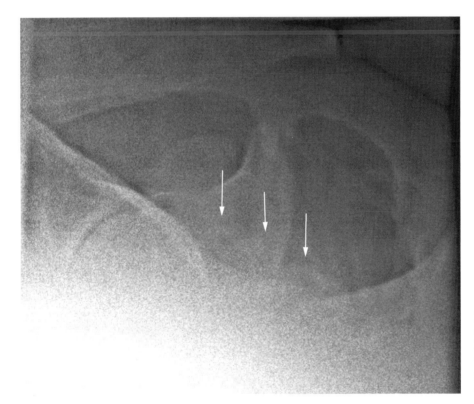

Figure 11.12(b) Lateral 30° distal oblique radiographic view of the same horse as in Figure 11.12(a), obtained 6 weeks later. Cranial is to the left. There is extensive callus bridging the fracture site (arrows).

only a small part of the acetabulum in a skeletally immature horse, satisfactory modelling of the joint may occur without radiographic evidence of degenerative joint disease. Such an animal may be capable of an athletic career. If large parts of the acetabular surface are involved, particularly in a skeletally mature animal, and/or articular incongruity exists, secondary degenerative joint disease is inevitable. This may be recognized radiographically within 4–5 weeks.

Fractures of the proximal femoral physis occasionally occur in foals. If a complete Salter-Harris type 1 fracture occurs, this may result in displacement of the femoral head (Figure 11.13). Internal fixation may be attempted, but with a very guarded prognosis. Secondary degenerative changes may ensue. Fracture of the femoral head may follow severe trauma in an adult. The prognosis is hopeless. Fracture of the greater trochanter of the femur is a rare injury and diagnosis is usually made using nuclear scintigraphy and ultrasonography.

If there is marked deformation of the pelvis, even without articular involvement, changes in apposition of the joint surfaces of the coxofemoral or sacroiliac joints may result in a change in gait or lameness.

Fracture of the ischium

The acetabular branch of the ischium is frequently involved in fractures of the acetabulum (see above). Fractures of the tuber ischii occur separately and are often related either to direct trauma or to the distracting effect of the semitendinosus and semimembranosus muscles, which originate on the ventral surface of this bone. There is often slight displacement of the most peripheral 5–7 cm of the tuber ischii. The prognosis for this fracture is usually good, the majority responding satisfactorily to 3–6 months of rest. Osseous healing with slight deformation of the tuber usually occurs, although occasionally lameness resolves despite lack of bony union. Non-union fractures with continual lameness rarely occur. Sequestration with sinus discharge occasionally occurs. A fracture of the tuber ischii is usually detectable using nuclear scintigraphy and ultrasonography, but can be confirmed radiographically.

Less commonly, a fracture of the body of the ischium occurs, usually the result of a fall when jumping at speed. Such fractures are usually complete and displaced and can be detected in lateral oblique radiographs of the ischium obtained in a standing horse (Figures 11.12a and 11.12b).

Femur

RADIOGRAPHIC TECHNIQUE

Equipment

The proximal two-thirds of the femur are best radiographed with the horse under general anaesthesia. It is not easy to obtain more than one view with the horse in a single position. High-output x-ray equipment and digital

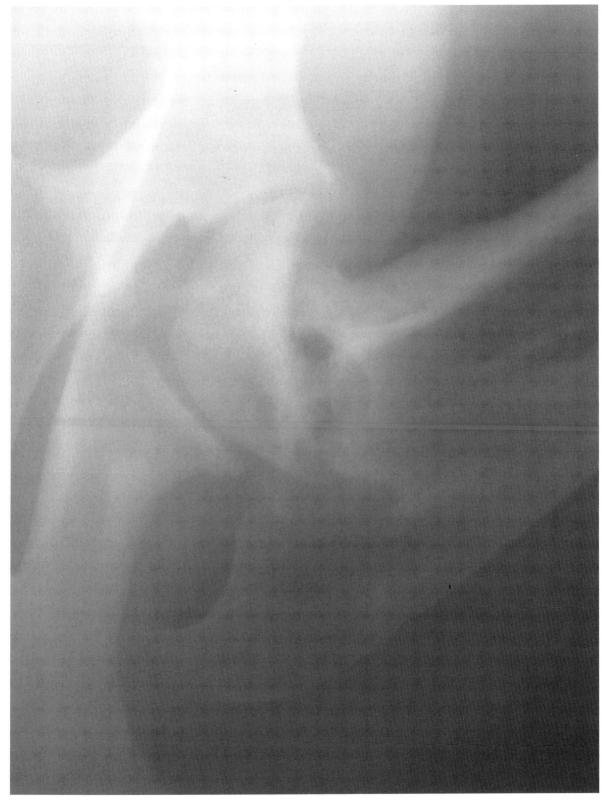

Figure 11.13 Ventrodorsal view of a coxofemoral joint of a yearling Thoroughbred with lameness of approximately 2½ months' duration. There is a displaced fracture of the femoral head through the physis (Salter-Harris type 1) with secondary changes in the femoral head and degenerative joint disease. Note the sclerosis of the femoral head adjacent to the physis.

systems or fast rare earth screens are essential, and a grid is beneficial, because of the large muscle mass which must be penetrated.

Positioning

A craniolateral-caudomedial oblique view is the easiest to obtain. The horse is positioned in dorsal recumbency, tipped towards the limb to be examined, as described for radiography of the coxofemoral joint (see page 575). It is usually necessary in an adult horse to obtain more than one radiograph in order to assess the entire length of the femur. It is difficult to obtain other projections, but this can be done by adjusting the position of the horse and limb.

An alternative technique is to place the horse in lateral recumbency, lying on the limb to be examined. This limb is then extended caudally and the contralateral limb extended cranially. This technique does not give such good results for the most proximal aspect of the femur.

The distal one-third of the femur may be radiographed using the same techniques as for the stifle joint (see page 364) and caudocranial, lateromedial and oblique views are readily obtained either with the horse standing or under general anaesthesia.

RADIOGRAPHIC ANATOMY

For details of the anatomy of the proximal and distal aspects of the femur, the reader is referred to the coxofemoral joint (pages 579–586) and the stifle joint (pages 366–379).

The proximal femur has separate centres of ossification for the femoral head, the trochanter major and the trochanter minor. The physis of the femoral head closes between 24 and 36 months, and the trochanter major fuses with the femoral shaft between 18 and 30 months. Fusion of the trochanter minor is less consistent, usually occurring at about 2 years of age.

The distal femoral physis is wavy and irregular in outline, closing at 24–30 months of age.

The greater and lesser trochanters and the third trochanter of the femur are readily seen in a craniolateral-caudomedial oblique view.

RADIOGRAPHIC ABNORMALITIES

Fractures of the femur

Fractures involving the proximal and distal epiphyses are discussed in conjunction with the coxofemoral joint (page 592) and the stifle joint (page 402).

Diaphyseal fractures of the femur

Diaphyseal fractures are relatively uncommon and result in a non-weight-bearing lameness. In immature or small horses it may be possible to detect crepitus, but in adult horses this may be concealed by the large muscle mass and soft-tissue swelling. In young horses the fractures are usually simple and oblique, but in adults the fractures are generally comminuted. There is often considerable overriding of the fracture fragments. Surgical repair of simple diaphyseal fractures may be attempted in foals, provided that the nutrient foramen is not involved. In older horses the prognosis is extremely bad.

Fracture of the third trochanter

Fracture of the third trochanter of the femur occasionally occurs (Figure 11.14). The horse shows moderate lameness and there may be palpable

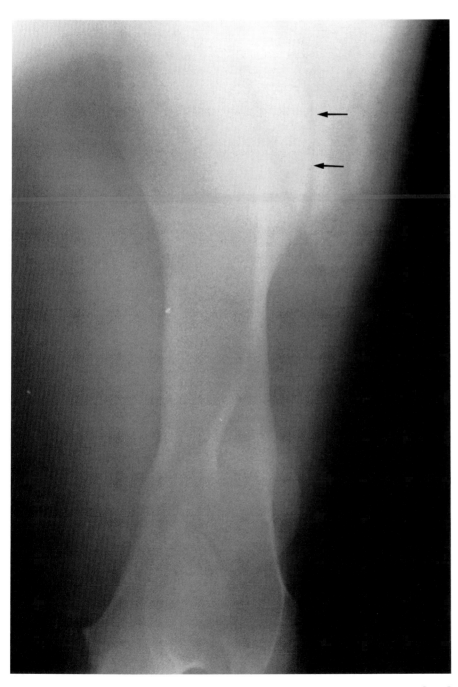

Figure 11.14 Caudocranial view of a femur of an 8-year-old advanced event horse, with acute onset hindlimb lameness of 2 weeks' duration, after being cast. There is a fracture of the third trochanter of the femur (arrows). The horse made a complete recovery.

crepitus, although this may be difficult to detect in a well muscled horse. Nuclear scintigraphic examination may help to identify such fractures. Although the fracture may heal only by fibrous union, the horse may return to full athletic function. Increased radiopharmaceutical uptake in the third trochanter of the femur could also be the result of entheseous trauma. Differentiation may be possible in some horses using ultrasonography.

FURTHER READING

Barrett, E., Talbot, A., Driver, A. *et al.* (2006) A technique for pelvic radiography in the standing horse. *Equine vet. J.*, **38**, 266–270

Bennet, D., Campbell, J. and Rawlinson, J. (1977) Coxofemoral luxation complicated by upward fixation of the patella in the pony. *Equine vet. J.*, **9**, 192–194

Brenner, S. and Whitcomb, M. (2007) How to diagnose equine coxofemoral subluxation with dynamic ultrasonography. *Proc. Amer. Assoc. Equine Pract.*, **53**, 433–437

Dalin, G. and Jeffcott, J. (1986a) Sacroiliac joint of the horse: 1. Gross morphology *Anat. Histol. Embryol.*, **15**, 80–94

Dalin, G. and Jeffcott, J. (1986b) Sacroiliac joint of the horse: 2. Morphometric features *Anat. Histol. Embryol.*, **15**, 97–107

Davenport-Goodall, C. and Ross, M. (2004) Scintigraphic abnormalities of the pelvic region in horses examined because of lameness or poor performance : 128 cases (1993–2000). *J. Am. Vet. Med. Ass.*, **224**, 88–95

Davison, P. (1967) A case of coxofemoral subluxation in a Welsh pony. *Vet. Rec.*, **80**, 441–443

Dyson, S., Murray, R., Branch, M., Whitton, C. *et al.* (2003a) The sacroiliac joints: evaluation using nuclear scintigraphy. Part 1: The normal horse. *Equine vet. J.*, **35**, 226–232

Dyson, S., Murray, R., Branch, M. and Harding, E. (2003b) The sacroiliac joints: evaluation using nuclear scintigraphy. Part 2: lame horses. *Equine vet. J.*, **35**, 233–239

Garcia-Lopez, J., Boudrieau, R. and Provost, P. (2001) Surgical repair of coxofemoral joint luxation in a horse. *J. Am. Vet. Med. Ass.*, **219**, 1254–1258

Hance, S.R., Bramlage, L.R., Schneider, R.K. and Embertson, R.M. (1992) Retrospective study of 38 cases of femur fractures in horses less than one year of age. *Equine vet. J.*, **24**, 357–363

Haussler, K., Stover, S. and Willits, N. (1997) Developmental variation in lumbosacropelvic anatomy of Thoroughbred horses. *Am. J. Vet. Res.*, **58**, 1083–1091

Haussler, K. and Stover, S. (1998) Stress fractures of the vertebral lamina and pelvis in Thoroughbred racehorses. *Equine vet. J.*, **30**, 374–383

Jeffcott, L.B. (1979a) Radiographic examination of the equine vertebral column. *Vet. Radiol.*, **20**, 135–139

Jeffcott, L.B. (1979b) Radiographic features of the normal equine thoracolumbar spine. *Vet. Radiol.*, **20**, 140–147

Jeffcott, L.B. (1982) Pelvic lameness in the horse. *Equine Pract.*, **4**, 21–47

Jeffcott, L.B. (1983a) Technique of linear tomography for the pelvic region of the horse. *Vet. Radiol.*, **24**, 194–200

Jeffcott, L.B. (1983b) Radiographic appearance of equine lumbosacral and pelvic abnormalities by linear tomography. *Vet. Radiol.*, **24**, 201–213

Little, C. and Hilbert, B. (1987) Pelvic fractures in horses: 19 cases. *J. Am. Vet. Med. Ass.*, **190**, 1203–1205

May, S., Patterson, J., Peacock, J. and Edwards, G. (1991) Radiographic technique for the pelvis in the standing horse. *Equine vet. J.*, **23**, 312–314

Miller, C. and Todhunter, R. (1987) Acetabular osteochondrosis dissecans in a foal. *Cornell Vet.*, **77**, 75–83

Nixon, A., Adams, R. and Teigland, M. (1988) Subchondral cystic lesions (osteochondrosis) of the femoral heads in a horse. *J. Am. Vet. Med. Ass.*, **192**, 360–362

Pilsworth, R.C., Shepherd, M.C., Herinckx, B.M.B. and Holmes, M.A. (1994) Fracture of the wing of the ilium, adjacent to the sacroiliac joint in Thoroughbred racehorses. *Equine vet. J.*, **26**, 94–99

Roneus, B., Svanholm, R. and Carlson, J. (1987) Diagnostik, etiologi och prognos vid skadar i backenregionen hos häster. *Svensk Veterinärtidning*, **39**, 315–323

Rose, J., Rose, E. and Smylie, D. (1981) Case history: acetabular osteochondrosis in a yearling thoroughbred. *Equine Vet. Surg.*, **1**, 173–174

Rutowski, J. and Richardson, D. (1989) A retrospective study of 100 pelvic fractures in horses. *Equine vet. J.*, **21**, 256–259

Skidell, J. (1987) Backenfractur hos häst – en litteratursammanstallning och beskrivning av 33 fall. *Svensk Veterinärtidning*, **39**, 326–333

Smyth, G. and Taylor, G. (1992) Stabilization of a proximal femoral physeal fracture in a filly by use of cancellous bone screws. *J. Am. Vet. Med. Ass.*, **210**, 895–898

Speitz, V.C. and Wrigley, R. (1979) A case of bilateral hip dysplasia in a foal. *Equine vet. J.*, **11**, 202–204

Stecher, R. and Goss, L. (1961) Ankylosing lesions of the spine of the horse. *J. Am. Vet. Med. Ass.*, **138**, 248–255

Swor, T., Schneider, R., Ross, M., Hammer, E. and Tucker, R. (2001) Injury to the origin of the gastrocnemius muscle as a possible cause of lameness in four horses. *J. Am. Vet. Med. Ass.* **219**, 215–219

Turner, A., Milne, D., Hohn, R. and Rouse, G. (1979) Surgical repair of fractured capital epiphysis in three foals. *J. Am. Vet. Med. Ass.*, **175**, 1198–1202

Chapter 12
The thorax

RADIOGRAPHIC TECHNIQUE

Equipment

Complete radiographic examination of the thorax of adult horses is only possible with large stationary x-ray units and a grid (10:1 ratio, or suitable equivalent for digital systems) or moveable Bucky. If a grid is not available the effects of scattered radiation can be reduced by leaving an air gap between the patient and the cassette. This technique should be avoided whenever possible because of the increased parallax and magnification that occurs.

A short exposure time is required to eliminate motion unsharpness; therefore it is best to use fast rare earth screens and compatible film, or digital equivalents. Large cassettes (35 cm × 43 cm) are recommended. Foals can occasionally be radiographed in lateral and ventrodorsal recumbency by placing the cassette and grid on the floor or by using a machine with an x-ray table incorporating a Bucky grid. The use of digital radiography can make assessment of lung density more difficult to assess than when using conventional film, and extra care needs to be taken to ensure that increased density is not overlooked.

Positioning

The adult or standing horse should be positioned with the forelimbs slightly forward in order to decrease the amount of muscle mass over the cranial thorax. The radiographs should be obtained at full inspiration (see pages 614 and 615). Expiratory radiographs are of value for comparison with inspiratory radiographs in two instances: to evaluate the effect of respiration on tracheal diameter or for evaluation of restrictive lung disease (see 'Chronic obstructive pulmonary disease', page 626). It is recommended that four 35 cm × 43 cm radiographs of the thorax be obtained with overlap of the fields (Figure 12.1): (a) dorsocaudal, (b) ventrocaudal, (c) dorsocranial and (d) ventrocranial (Figures 12.1a–d). Fields (a) and (b) are possible to radiograph with large mobile units, but fields (c) and (d) usually require larger equipment in order to penetrate the greater muscle mass in this area. The entire thorax can often be evaluated on one or two radiographs in foals (Figure 12.2), ponies and small horses (Figures 12.3a and 12.3b).

In order to compensate for parallax and magnification, views (a) and (b) should be obtained with the right side (right lateral projection) and then the left side (left lateral projection) of the thorax next to the cassette.

[603]

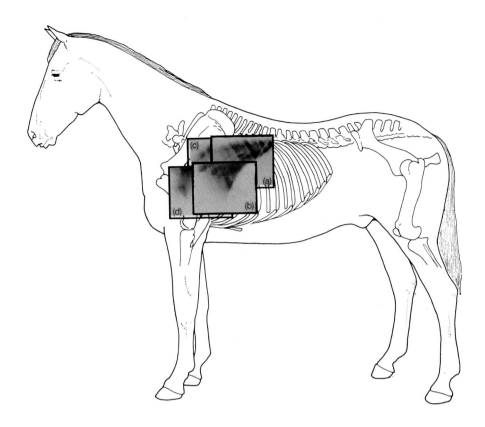

Figure 12.1 Placement of cassettes for the four overlapping views of the thorax.

Parallax and magnification are major problems in evaluation of the equine thorax, but they can be used to advantage by utilizing the changes in position, size and image sharpness to determine the location of the lesion (left side versus right side). Structures close to the cassette will be well visualized and have sharp margins, whereas those away from the cassette will be magnified and less distinct due to the large object–film distance (Figures 12.4a and 12.4b).

Examination of neonates or miniature horses in lateral recumbency should include both right and left lateral recumbent views. Ventrodorsal views should be obtained when possible. When obtaining recumbent lateral radiographs, care must be exercised not to extend the forelimbs excessively as this will cause the chest to rotate and a true lateral radiograph will not be obtained.

It is recommended that thoracic radiographs be obtained using a film–focal distance of 100–120 cm.

Other imaging techniques

Nuclear scintigraphy

Nuclear scintigraphy, when coupled with radiography, offers advantages in evaluation of intrathoracic disease and is particularly helpful in the investi-

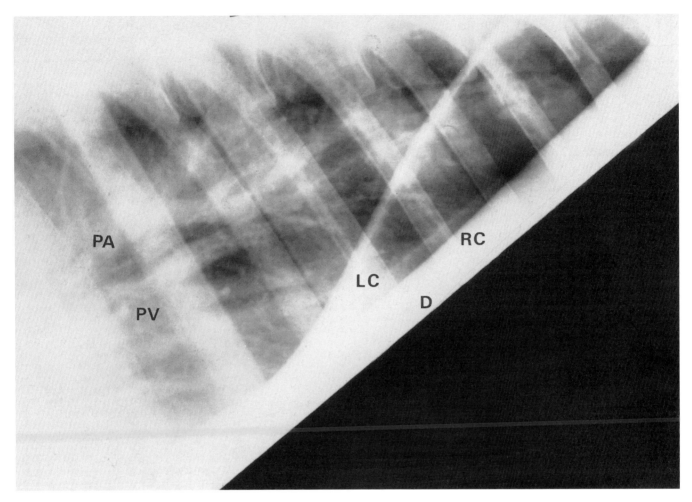

Figure 12.1(a) Dorsocaudal portion of the thorax of a normal adult horse. The branching pulmonary arteries (PA) and pulmonary veins (PV) pass dorsocaudad. The diaphragm (D) is separated into the left crus (LC) which overlies the major portion of the gastric gas cap which is also partially seen below the right crus (RC).

gation of chronic obstructive pulmonary disease (COPD) and exercise-induced pulmonary haemorrhage (EIPH) (see pages 626 and 641).

Ultrasonography

The greater availability, economy and safety of ultrasonography make it more desirable for the evaluation of cardiac and pleural disease than radiography.

Diagnostic ultrasonography is more reliable than survey radiography for the documentation of heart chamber enlargement, for the evaluation of the contractility of the myocardium and for the diagnosis of pericardial disease, pericardial effusion and valvular disease. Diagnostic ultrasonography is the most valuable imaging modality for evaluation of intrathoracic disease in the presence of pleural fluid, and is an invaluable adjunct to the evaluation and differentiation of pulmonary abscesses, granulomas and tumour masses provided that these masses are in contact with the pleural surface. Masses

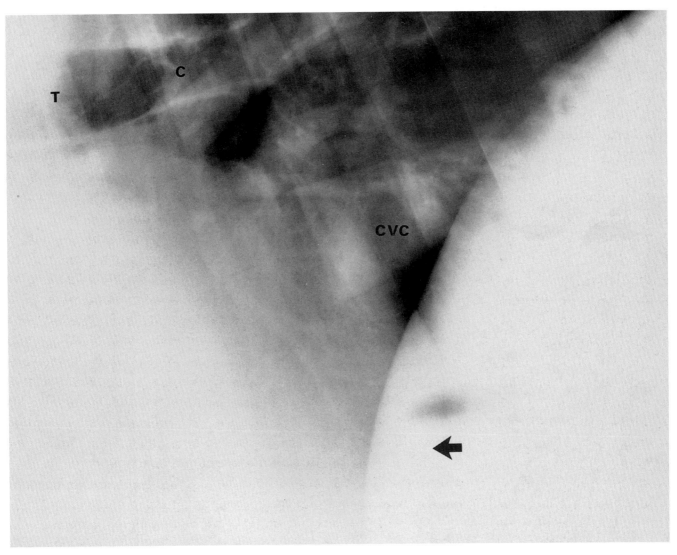

Figure 12.1(b) Ventrocaudal portion of the thorax of a normal adult horse. The caudal border of the heart overlaps the right diaphragmatic crus and is marked by the large black arrow. The pulmonary vessels overlie the caudal margin of the cardiac silhouette. The cranial portion of the cardiac silhouette is obscured by muscle mass which is not penetrated on this film. The caudal vena cava (CVC) is clearly delineated below the pulmonary arteries and veins as they exit and enter the heart, respectively. The trachea (T) passes caudally over the base of the heart and bifurcates at the carina (C). There is a lucent gas shadow in the cranial ventral abdomen adjacent to the diaphragm and the cardiac silhouette.

within the lung and surrounded by air are not adequately visualized because of attenuation of the ultrasound beam by air.

Monitoring pulmonary and/or pleural disease

It should be borne in mind that radiography may be much more informative than auscultation of the thorax. For example, a neonatal foal may have minimal or no abnormalities detectable by auscultation, but there may be significant abnormalities detectable radiographically. In the adult, however, development of radiographic abnormalities may lag behind clinical signs. It

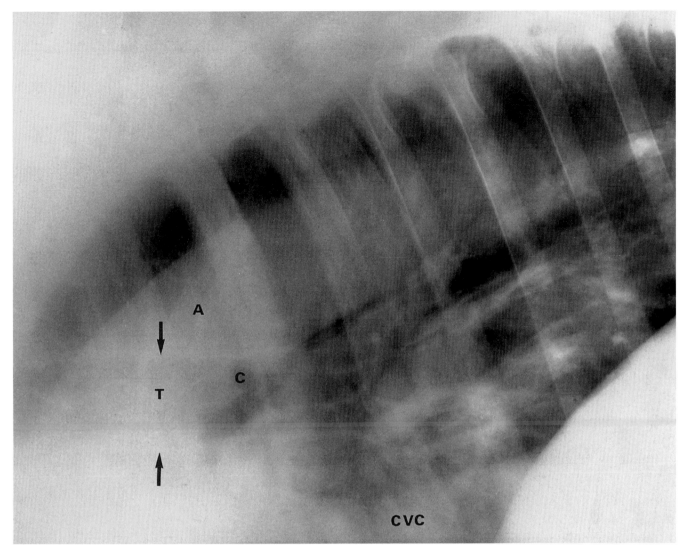

Figure 12.1(c) Dorsocranial portion of the thorax of a normal adult horse. The aorta (A) arises from the base of the heart and passes dorsocaudad, where it is lost from view due to over-penetration of the radiograph. The great pulmonary vessels arise from and enter the heart between the aorta and the caudal vena cava (CVC). The trachea (T) lies between the black arrows as it passes caudad and ends at the carina (C), where the mainstem bronchi branch.

should also be recognized that radiographic signs of improvement may lag behind clinical improvement in both the immature and mature horse.

NORMAL ANATOMY

It should be noted that the age of the horse, its size, the width of the thorax, the phase of respiration at which exposures are made, and the exposure factors will all influence the radiographic appearance of the lungs. High-speed film–screen combinations are required, but this means some loss of resolution. Scattered radiation also reduces contrast and resolution,

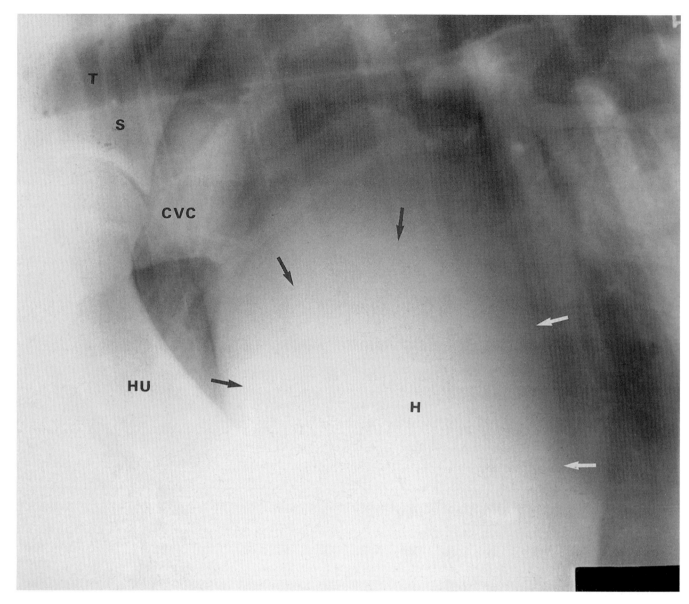

Figure 12.1(d) Ventrocranial portion of the thorax of a normal adult horse. High exposure factors are required to penetrate the muscle mass, humerus (HU) and scapula (S). The cranial vena cava (CVC) lies between the trachea (T) and the oesophagus in the cranial mediastinum. The cranial and caudal margins of the heart (H) are clearly visible and vessels arch over the top of the cardiac silhouette. The approximate border of the cardiac notch of the lungs is indicated by arrows (black and white).

especially in the ventral lung fields. Thoracic wall, visceral and parietal pleura and mediastinal structures all contribute to the overall radiographic density. Interpretation of pulmonary patterns is therefore not easy. Underexposure may create artefactual lung opacities, whereas overexposure may mask lesions. It is therefore not surprising that even experienced radiologists may interpret radiographs of the thorax differently. Using a high kV, low mA technique helps to reduce artefacts created by exposure factors. For comparison of radiographs between horses, or for serial examinations of the same horse, it can be helpful to try to achieve a constant radiopacity of the vertebral bodies as a guide to exposure.

[608]

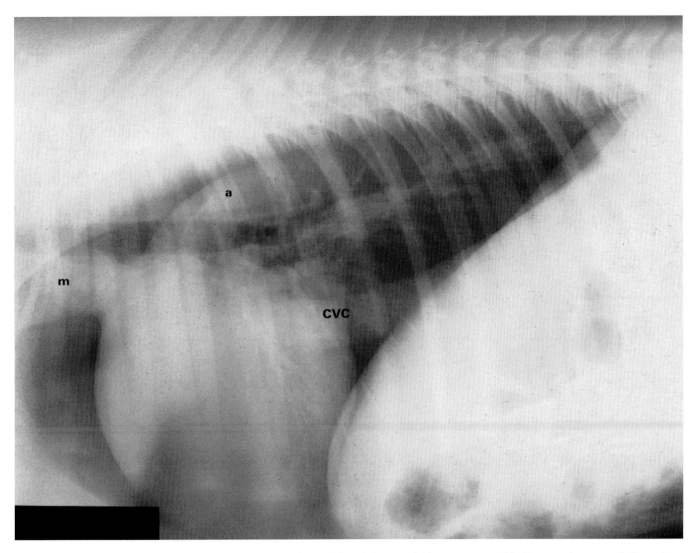

Figure 12.2 A normal 1-day-old Arabian colt. The portions of the abdomen which are seen on this film are also normal. Note the position of the trachea and its slightly ventral course, and the inability to visualize the margins of the aorta (a) beyond the caudal cardiac margin. The caudal vena cava (CVC) is well visualized. The great vessels in the cranial mediastinum are masked by other soft tissues in the mediastinum (m). Note how the fine vascular structures can be seen over the cardiac silhouette and extending to the periphery.

Immature horse

The cardiac silhouette occupies a greater proportion of the thoracic cavity in the neonate than in the adult (compare Figures 12.1, 12.2 and 12.3). In the normal foal the craniocaudal dimension should be between 5.6 and 6.3 times the length of a mid-thoracic vertebra, and the apicobasilar dimension should be 6.7–7.8 times the length of a mid-thoracic vertebra. Radiographs of the thorax of foals obtained within the first few hours of birth usually have a generalized interstitial opacity due to incomplete inflation. Within 12 hours the lungs become more lucent as the foal becomes active and the lungs are more completely inflated. The initial increased opacity leads to some diagnostic challenges during the first few days of life, as premature

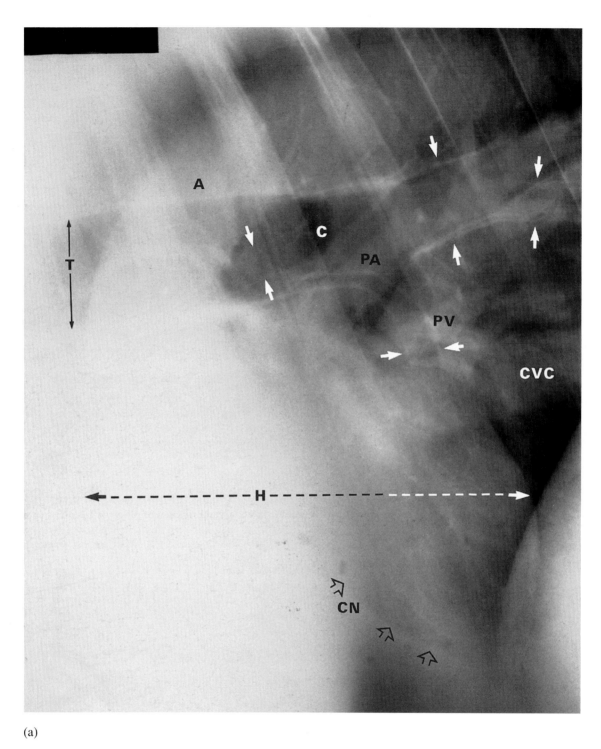

(a)

Figure 12.3 Normal adult thorax. Due to the small size of the patient, the entire thorax was obtained on two radiographs, both right lateral projections. Portions of the dorsocranial and ventrocranial thorax as well as a portion of the ventrocaudal thorax are demonstrated in (a), whereas (b) demonstrates the normal dorsocaudal thorax and a portion of the ventrocaudal thorax. (a) The tracheal diameter (T) is marked by solid arrows. The trachea bifurcates at the carina (C). Some of the major bronchi are marked between short white arrows. The cranial to caudal dimension of the cardiac silhouette is defined by (H) and arrows. Major pulmonary vessels can be seen and include the aorta (A), pulmonary arteries (PA), pulmonary vein (PV) and the caudal vena cava (CVC). The caudal ventral lung margin can be seen over the cardiac notch (CN) and is marked by open arrows. Fine vascular structures are readily identified over the caudal margin of the heart, aorta and vertebral bodies.

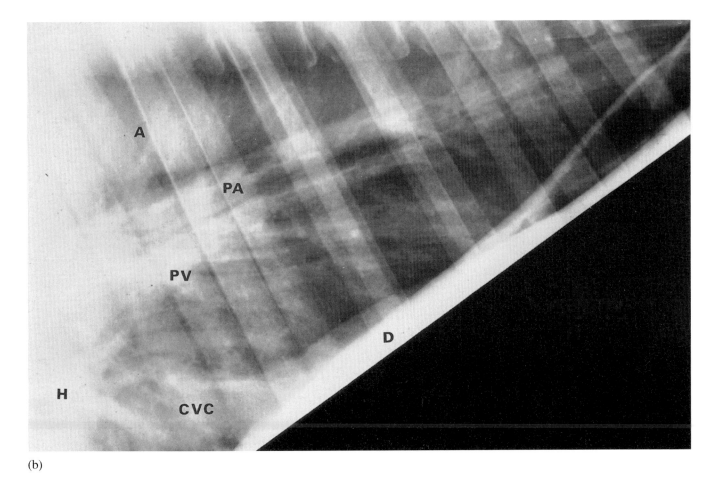

(b)

Figure 12.3 *Cont'd* (b) The caudodorsal lung fields are clear, and close inspection allows visualization of fine bronchial structures with parallel walls. Fine vascular structures can be seen over the vertebral bodies and ribs where the x-ray beam is attenuated. The margins of the aorta (A) are no longer visualized caudally. The pulmonary arteries (PA) and pulmonary veins (PV) can be seen exiting and entering the heart (H) above the caudal vena cava (CVC), which can be seen passing from the heart to the diaphragm (D). Dorsocaudally the gas in the stomach can be seen against the left diaphragmatic crus, while the right crus is flatter and lies over the hepatic shadow. Many pulmonary vascular structures can be seen centrally, but are lost caudodorsally due to beam penetration. The lungs are clear and normal.

(see Figure 12.18, page 636) and septicaemic foals will also have increased interstitial opacity. Foals with questionable abnormalities should therefore be re-evaluated in 24 and 48 hours.

Mature horse

Normal lung should appear lucent with well defined vascular structures that are largest at the heart base and taper gradually to the periphery of the lungs. These vessels should be most opaque over their greatest dimension and gradually decrease in opacity as they progress peripherally. The trachea enters the thoracic inlet as a lucent tubular structure that has well defined tracheal cartilages within the wall. The outer wall cannot be differentiated from other mediastinal soft tissues. The tracheal cartilages are not usually

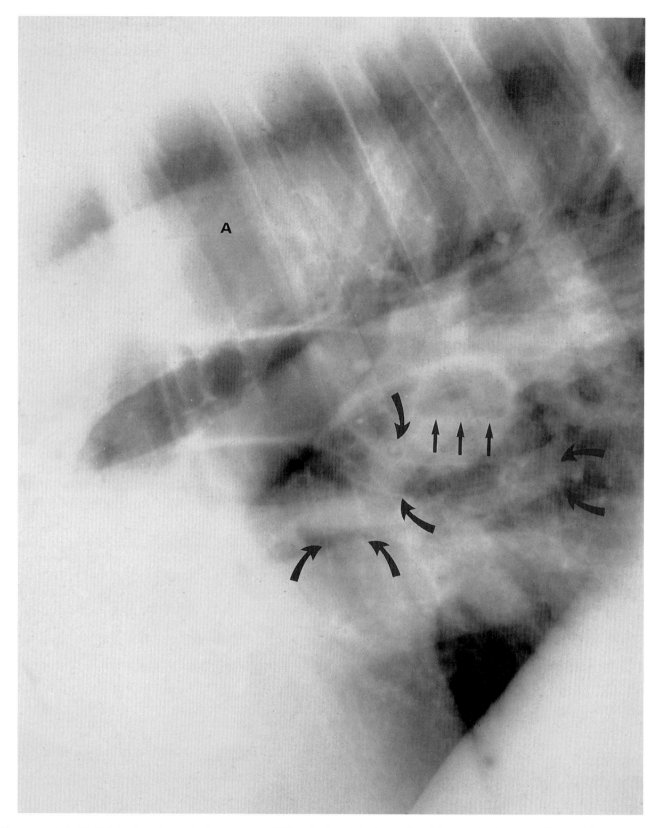

Figure 12.4(a) Right lateral radiograph of a 10-year-old Standardbred stallion with a history of pulmonary disease. There was mucus and pus in the trachea. This figure demonstrates a solitary cavitary pulmonary lesion. There is a well circumscribed mass containing both air and fluid. The air–fluid interface (straight arrows) is demonstrated on both views. The lungs are normal and fine vascular structures can be seen in the dorsal lung fields and over the aorta (A). Bronchial walls and end-on bronchi (curved arrows) are also seen.

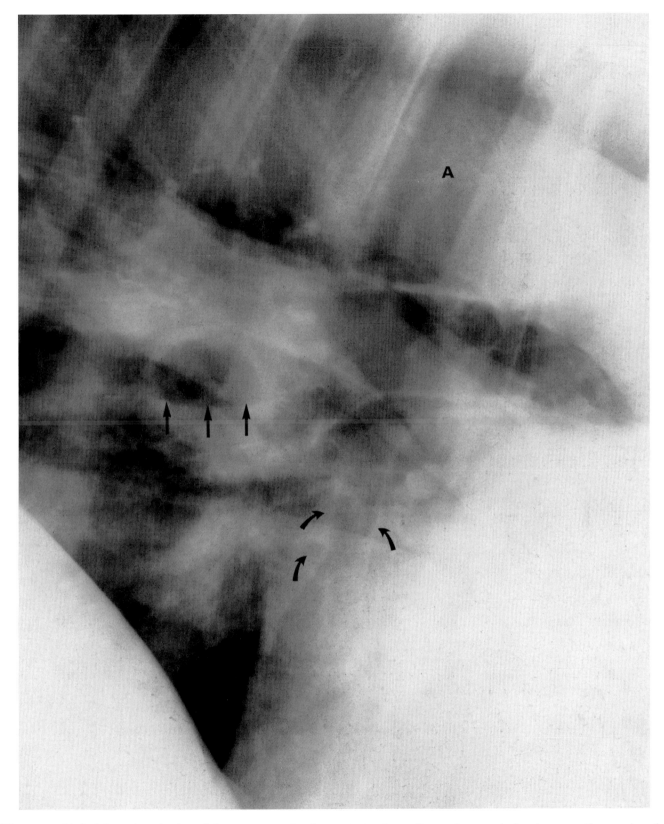

Figure 12.4(b) Left lateral projection of the same area also demonstrates the cavitary pulmonary lesion; however, the margins of the fluid line and mass are less well defined and slightly magnified, indicating that the lesion is in the right hemithorax. On both views, bronchial walls and end-on bronchi are also identifiable (curved arrows).

seen in young animals because they lack mineral content, which develops with age. The trachea terminates at the carina (point of bifurcation) at the base of the heart (Figure 12.1b, page 606) where it becomes the right and left mainstem bronchi. The mainstem bronchi if seen end-on are round, well demarcated structures at the base of the heart; in longitudinal plane their linear, opaque, well defined walls are seen. Bronchi are not normally seen much beyond the bifurcation (carina) (Figures 12.1c, page 607 and 12.3a, page 610). The left mainstem bronchus is more dorsal than the right because of the close association of the left bronchus with the left atrium.

A lucent triangle of normal lung tissue is usually identifiable caudoventrally in radiographs obtained at full inspiration. The sides of the triangle are made up of the caudal vena cava dorsally, the cardiac silhouette cranially and the diaphragm caudally. This triangle should be evaluated to determine the degree of inspiration. At peak inspiration, the apex of the triangle may be slightly blunted as the diaphragm and the cardiac silhouette separate, and the apex is formed by the sternum.

The cardiac notch in both the right and left lung leaves an area overlying the mid-ventral heart that is not covered by lung tissue; thus this area over the cardiac silhouette is devoid of pulmonary vessels. Care must be taken not to confuse the lack of vessels in this area with consolidated lung which might, in another location, have a similar appearance.

Dorsocaudal lung field

A portion of the aorta is usually observed just below or slightly overlapping the bodies of the thoracic vertebrae. The caudal portion of the aortic silhouette is only seen when the radiograph is obtained at peak inspiration. This is because the aortic silhouette becomes incorporated in the increasing lung opacity in the dorsocaudal lung, when the lungs contain less air (expiration). The pulmonary artery and vein extend from the base of the heart towards the vertebral bodies. Small pulmonary vessels are seen at the periphery of the lungs and can best be evaluated over the vertebral bodies, the cardiac silhouette and the diaphragm (see Figure 12.1a, page 605).

Ventrocaudal lung field

The dorsal portion of this radiographic view should overlap field (a). The caudal edge is defined by the silhouette of the diaphragm while the ventral side is defined by the diaphragm, sternum and the caudal aspect of the heart. The caudal vena cava is best evaluated in the right lateral projection as it lies on the right side of the thorax (see Figure 12.1b, page 606).

Dorsocranial lung field

The dorsocranial region overlaps portions of fields (a) and (b) but extends craniad. The aortic arch is the most prominent structure in this view and only a small amount of lung tissue, which is not obscured by the base of the heart and the muscle mass over the shoulders, is seen. A part of the trachea and the carina can be seen just above the cardiac silhouette. The great vessels can be evaluated as they leave the base of the heart (see Figure 12.1c, page 607).

Ventrocranial lung field

In this view the ventrocranial thorax can be evaluated, but the lungs are often obscured by the forelimbs cranially and by the cardiac silhouette caudally. This can be improved by extending and pulling forward the limb that is closest to the x-ray tube. There is some overlap with the other three fields at the dorsocaudal portion of this view. This is usually the least useful of the four views (see Figure 12.1d, page 608).

NORMAL VARIATIONS AND INCIDENTAL FINDINGS

An increase in lung opacity (interstitial density) may be noted as horses age, resulting in an inability to visualize the fine vascular structures and in loss of structural detail. This change in appearance is due to chronic pulmonary fibrosis. With age, the mainstem bronchi and tracheal rings may be more prominent due to cartilage mineralization.

Factors influencing interpretation

A single set of radiographs of the equine thorax represents the status at the time the radiographs are obtained. Many diseases will pass through similar stages during progression or regression, and radiographic findings will often, but not always, lag behind the clinical signs. Underexposed thoracic radiographs give the appearance of increased lung opacity while overexposure results in apparent decreased opacity. If an error is to be made, overexposure is preferable because information can be retrieved by the use of high-intensity illumination. Digital systems can make assessment of opacity more difficult, because of the ease of manipulation of the image. It is important to achieve consistent image opacity, and this may be best controlled by reference to some structure not significantly affected by lung density, e.g. a rib. Expiratory radiographs (radiographs obtained at end expiration) give the appearance of increased lung opacity because the air to tissue ratio is decreased; thus the soft tissues summate and result in a false interstitial pattern. The same phenomenon occurs when there is a large amount of intra-abdominal fluid or an abdominal mass, both of which interfere with normal diaphragmatic excursion and thus prevent peak inspiration.

Interpretation of thoracic radiographs is based on a thorough understanding of the patterns that make up the various thoracic diseases as well as their pathophysiology and the effect of positioning.

When evaluating lateral recumbent thoracic radiographs of young or small horses, it is important to understand that the image and its interpretation have been slightly altered by position. The sharpest image will be in the upper lung because the dependent lung will partially collapse. This partial collapse obscures opacities within the lung because of the lack of adjacent air to contrast with them. Concurrently the well aerated upper lung will allow for better definition of structures despite parallax and magnification artefacts. Therefore, both lateral projections should be obtained in the recumbent as well as standing patients.

SIGNIFICANT FINDINGS

Patterns of lung disease

Interstitial

Within the connective tissue framework of the lungs are the arteries, veins, lymphatics, nerves and the bronchi. The walls of the bronchi and the alveoli separate the interstitium from the air space. Thus, any inflammatory or infiltrative disease that affects any of these structures will result in what is referred to as an interstitial pattern (Figures 12.5 and 12.6). Although the pattern may vary to some degree depending upon the pathogenesis of the disease process, its hallmark is an increase in background opacity that results in the loss of visualization of the fine vascular structure that typifies a normal, well inflated (aerated) lung. Because of the varied tissues involved, this is the predominant pattern noted in the early stages of most pulmonary disease, including: viral, bacterial, mycotic, parasitic, hypersensitive, haemorrhagic, neoplastic and cardiogenic. In the foal an interstitial pattern is seen in both septicaemic and immature patients, and has recently been described in proliferative interstitial lung disease.

A generalized interstitial pattern may indicate the presence of pulmonary interstitial oedema from cardiac origin, an early phase of viral or bacterial pneumonia, or chronic pulmonary fibrosis due to age and chronic irritation. Expiration also decreases the proportion of air to tissue density and can thus create the impression of an interstitial opacity; this is undoubtedly the most common cause of misdiagnosis of pathology in normal lung. A granular or fine nodular interstitial pattern suggests a cellular infiltrate in the interstitium. This would lead to consideration of metastatic or mycotic disease in the differential diagnosis, as well as other causes of cellular infiltrates.

Vessels are within the interstitium and as such can only be differentiated prior to the accumulation of interstitial fluid (oedema) or infiltrate. These mask the underlying fine vascular structures or give them an indistinct outline. An increase in pulmonary vasculature may be associated with congenital or acquired heart disease or early stages of inflammatory lung disease. Radiographically there appears to be an increase in the number and size of vessels. These are most easily recognized as round to ovoid fluid densities of varying size that lie over the other vessels as they are seen end-on in the peripheral lung tissue. Many pulmonary diseases start within the interstitium, before involving the air spaces, so the presence of this pattern alone is not pathognomonic for any disease. Follow-up radiographs are always advisable.

[616]

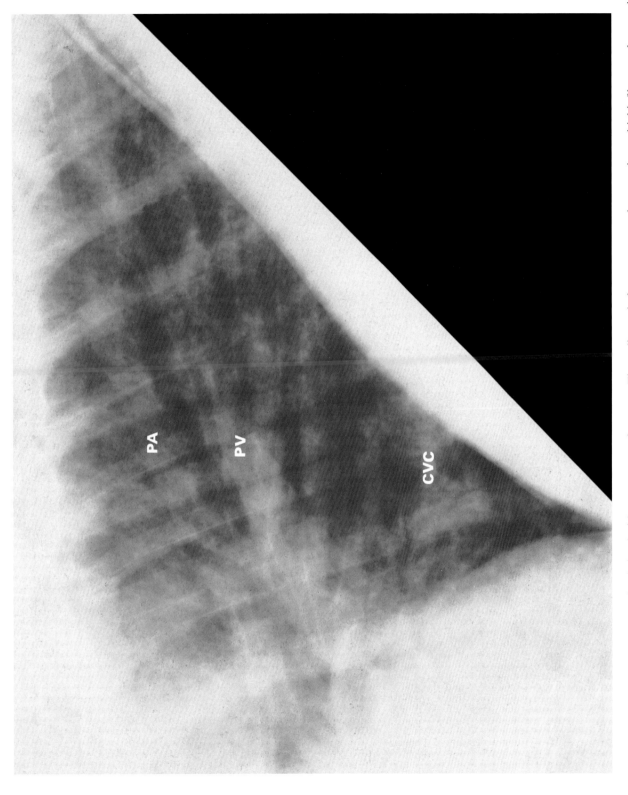

Figure 12.5 Five-month-old Thoroughbred colt admitted with severe acute dyspnoea. The radiograph demonstrates pulmonary interstitial infiltrates, characterized by a generalized increased lung opacity and the inability to visualize the fine vascular markings. The right pulmonary artery (PA) and the right pulmonary vein (PV) are still visible but poorly marginated, as is the caudal vena cava (CVC) and other vessels.

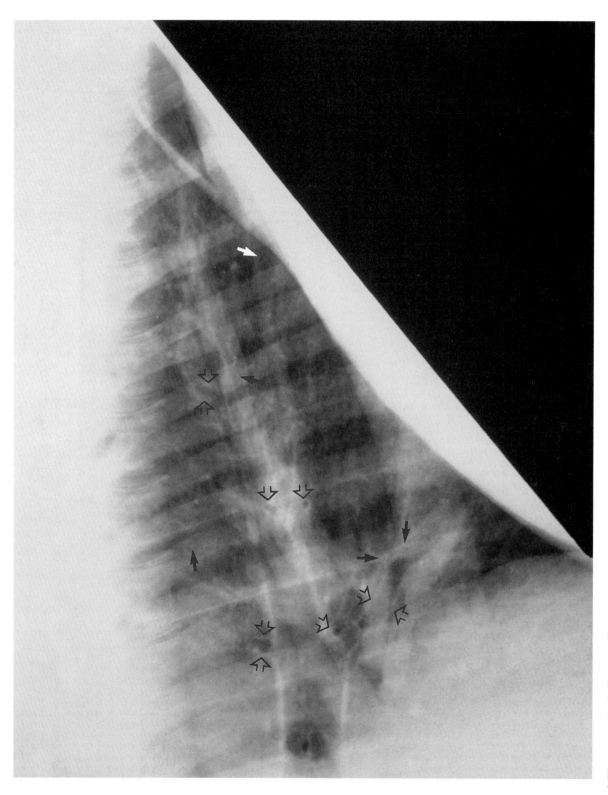

Figure 12.6 Three-month-old Thoroughbred colt which had previously had guttural pouch empyema with a recent 2-week history of pneumonia and nasal discharge. The nasal discharge had improved within the previous 3–4 days. The radiograph demonstrates interstitial and bronchial pattern due to bacterial pneumonia. There is a generalized increase in interstitial density of which a major component is a bronchial pattern, increased visualization of bronchial markings and well circumscribed end-on bronchial are marked with open arrows. Some of the larger bronchi are marked with open arrows. Note the width of the bronchus and prominent bronchial walls. Solid arrows mark small bronchi in the periphery.

Bronchial

Although the bronchi are part of the interstitial complex, diseases of the conducting system are often considered separately. The linear pattern can be differentiated on the basis of whether the bronchi appear sharply defined (bronchial pattern, Figure 12.6), or ill defined with apparently thickened walls (peribronchial pattern). A bronchial pattern is more indicative of chronic disease with changes in the bronchi themselves, such as mineralization or bronchiectasis (see Figure 12.14, page 629). A peribronchial pattern is indicative of an infiltrate around the bronchi and therefore of acute or chronic inflammatory disease such as allergic pneumonitis or early bronchopneumonia.

The radiographic signs of bronchial disease include:

1 Increased thickness of bronchial structures due to peribronchial infiltrates; this is often referred to as peribronchial cuffing. Apparent thickening of the bronchi by material which lines the inside of the airways, such as a diphtheritic membrane, may cause the bronchial walls to appear thicker than normal and also to have a decreased luminal clarity. This aids differentiation of these two causes of apparent wall thickening.

2 Increased diameter or change in shape of bronchi as seen in tubular or saccular bronchiectasis.

3 Apparent increased numbers because previously invisible bronchi are now more easily seen due to changes in opacity of the bronchi themselves or due to the enhanced lucency of surrounding air spaces.

Alveolar

When the terminal air spaces become involved in any disease process, the alveoli begin to fill with fluid (transudate, exudate or blood) or tissue and thus assume a soft-tissue opacity rather than normal lucency of air. In the early stages when few alveoli are involved, the structures that are normally visualized will be obscured by fluffy or cloudy fluid opacities. With the involvement of more and more alveoli there is a progressive coalescence and summation of these opacities, which eventually results in the formation of air bronchograms. These appear as lucent branching structures within an opaque lung field (Figure 12.7; see also Figure 12.16, page 633). The finding of air bronchograms is an indication of nearly complete alveolar filling; thus the only remaining air space is the bronchi, which are then visible as dark branching structures in a background of grey. At this stage the distribution of the air bronchograms will aid in the differentiation between various causes of alveolar filling. The differential diagnosis includes: bacterial, mycotic and aspiration pneumonia, and pulmonary oedema of both cardiogenic and non-cardiogenic origin (see 'Diseases of the lung', page 626).

Diseases of the pleural space and mediastinum

Hydrothorax (pleural effusion, free pleural fluid)

Radiography should be used in conjunction with ultrasonography as complementary tools for the evaluation of the presence of pleural fluid and any

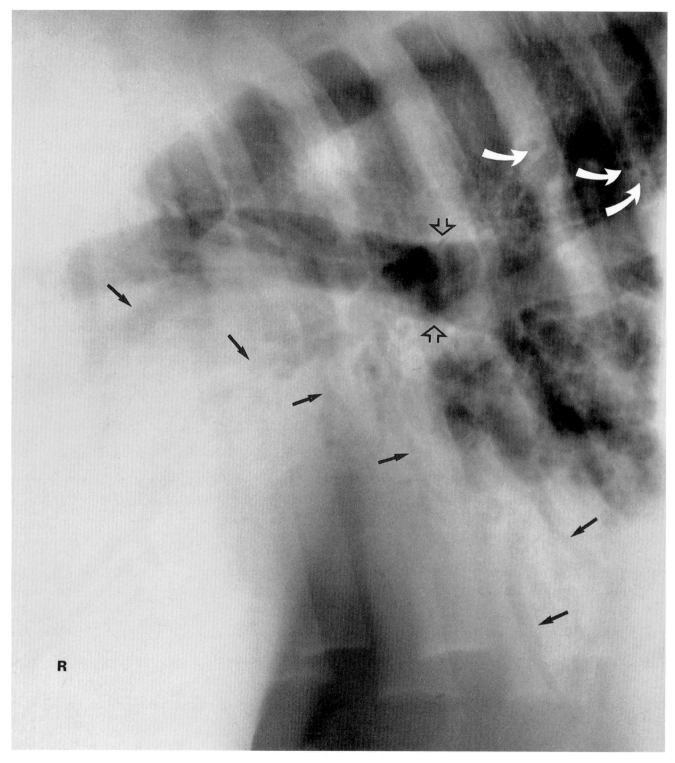

Figure 12.7 Three-month-old Thoroughbred filly with a history of acute onset of respiratory distress. There is an irregular fluid opacity which involves the entire ventrocaudal thorax and obscures the cardiac silhouette. Air bronchograms (black solid arrows) are readily visible. Dilatation of the caudal trachea at the carina (open arrows) is indicative of maximal inspiratory effort and dyspnoea. Peribronchial changes are noted dorsal to the carina (white curved arrows). These changes are typical of either severe aspiration or bacterial pneumonia. The air bronchograms branch as they extend towards the periphery and are indicative of alveolar infiltrate and consolidation. Diagnosis: bacterial and aspiration pneumonia.

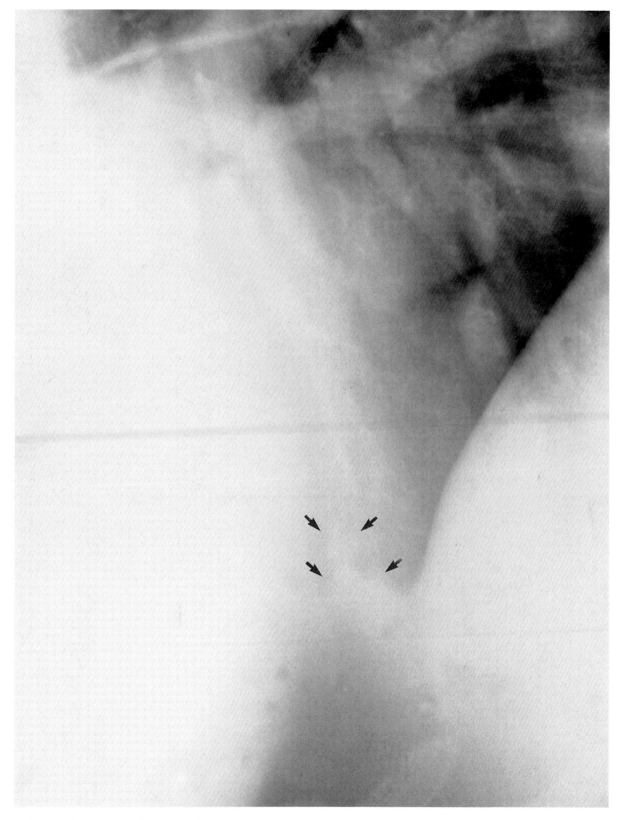

Figure 12.8 Yearling Thoroughbred colt with a history of thoracic disease. There is a small irregular fluid opacity in the ventrocaudal thorax over the cardiac silhouette (arrows). The remainder of the thorax is normal. This opacity represents a small amount of free pleural fluid at the base of the ventrocaudal lung adjacent to the cardiac notch.

concurrent lung disease. Small amounts of fluid in the pleural space may be seen as fluid opacities, which occupy the pleural fissures (Figure 12.8). With increased amounts of fluid there is a diffuse fluid opacity in the ventrocaudal thorax of the standing patient. The presence of large amounts of fluid results in a loss of definition between the heart and the diaphragm (Figure 12.9). This fluid line is poorly demarcated because of the capillary action of the pleural space and is only sharply delineated when there is concurrent pneumothorax. The loss of definition progresses dorsally with increasing amounts of fluid, which may at times be defined by the lung margins as they begin

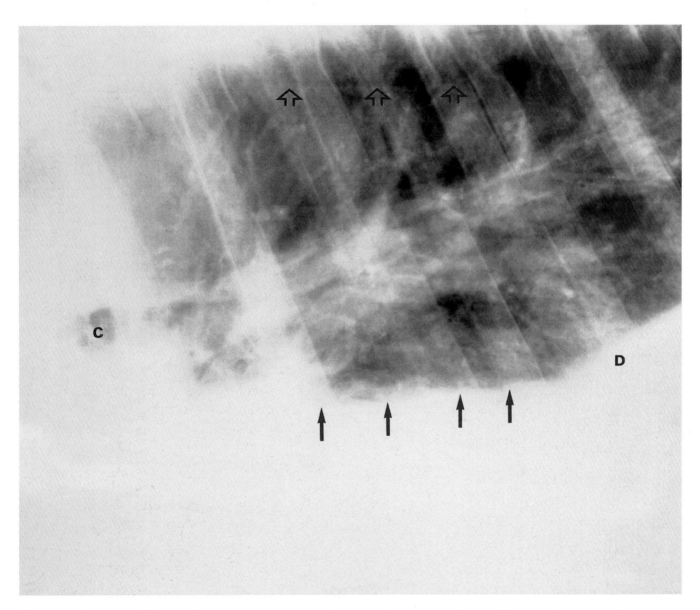

Figure 12.9 Six-year-old Thoroughbred stallion with an 8-week history of respiratory distress. Thirty-two litres of fluid were removed the day prior to radiographic evaluation. There is an irregular fluid level (black solid arrows) ventral to the carina (C) and extending to the diaphragm (D). The cardiac silhouette and ventral thorax are completely obscured by the fluid opacity. The lung cannot expand normally, which has resulted in increased interstitial pattern in all lung lobes. The margin of one lung is just visible dorsally (open arrows), indicating a small amount of pneumothorax which probably resulted from the drainage procedure on the previous day.

to retract dorsally. This results in an undulating fluid–lung interface, which indicates that the lungs are near normal. Abnormal (pneumonic) tissue tends to remain more ventral and summate with the fluid.

All fluids appear similar and cannot be differentiated radiographically as either transudate, modified transudate, exudate, haemorrhage and lymph (chyle). They have a uniform ground-glass appearance similar to the cardiac silhouette or the diaphragm and underlying liver. Malignant mesothelioma must be considered in the differential diagnosis when pleural fluid is present. In these cases the pericardial sac may also be involved and result in pericardial effusion. A final diagnosis must rely on additional techniques such as ultrasonography and pleurocentesis. Diagnostic ultrasound adds to the study of pleural disease by occasionally defining the character of the fluid and often allowing identification of fibrin, adhesions or concurrent cardiac disease, pericardial disease, pericardial effusion, lung consolidation and occasionally masses or abscesses within the consolidated lung.

It is advisable to re-radiograph the thorax after the removal of pleural fluid in order to evaluate the lungs both for possible causes and for involvement of areas that could not be evaluated in the presence of the fluid.

Pneumothorax

Free air in the pleural space rapidly collects dorsally, in the paraspinal recess and the dorsal caudal reflection of the pleura adjacent to the diaphragm at the highest portion of the paraspinal recess. The dorsocaudal area of the thorax is, therefore, the most important area to evaluate when small amounts of gas are expected. Radiographically the lung margins are retracted both from the diaphragm caudally and the vertebral bodies dorsally, thus allowing the pleural surface of the lung to be visualized (Figure 12.10). Unilateral pneumothorax may occur, and in these cases it is possible to see one lung margin retracted and to visualize the vessels in the contralateral lung. In cases of bilateral pneumothorax, both lung lobes are retracted.

Pneumothorax can arise as a result of a penetrating wound, which allows air to enter the pleural space either from the lung itself or from the outside, or from the rupture of a bulla, bleb or abscess. Pneumothorax secondary to trauma is often bilateral, but not always, and when associated with pleuropneumonia is usually unilateral. Pneumothorax can also arise secondary to pneumomediastinum, or tearing of a pleural adhesion. The entire thorax should be scrutinized for signs of concurrent pathology such as rib fractures and foreign bodies.

Pneumomediastinum

Radiographically, pneumomediastinum is seen as air outlining mediastinal structures. Both sides of the trachea are clearly defined together with other structures that cannot normally be seen within the mediastinum, such as the oesophagus and the great vessels at the base of the heart (Figure 12.11).

Pneumomediastinum may be progressive, extending into the pleural space and resulting in a pneumothorax. The converse is never true; an

[623]

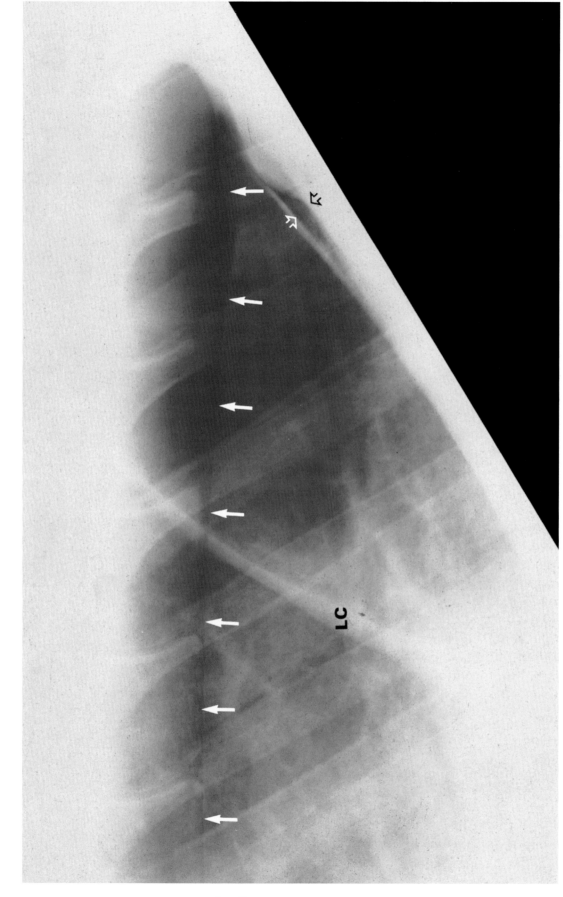

Figure 12.10 Eight-year-old Thoroughbred gelding with a 10-day history of lower respiratory tract disease. The right lung is retracted ventrally and cranially from the thoracic margins and the diaphragm, respectively. Free air is seen between the right diaphragmatic crus and the lung margin (open arrows). The dorsum of the right lung is identified by solid arrows. The left diaphragmatic crus (LC) is cranial to the gas-distended stomach which is displacing the left lung lobe cranially. Note that vessels can be seen over the three more cranial vertebral bodies and not over the caudal three. Diagnosis: pneumothorax.

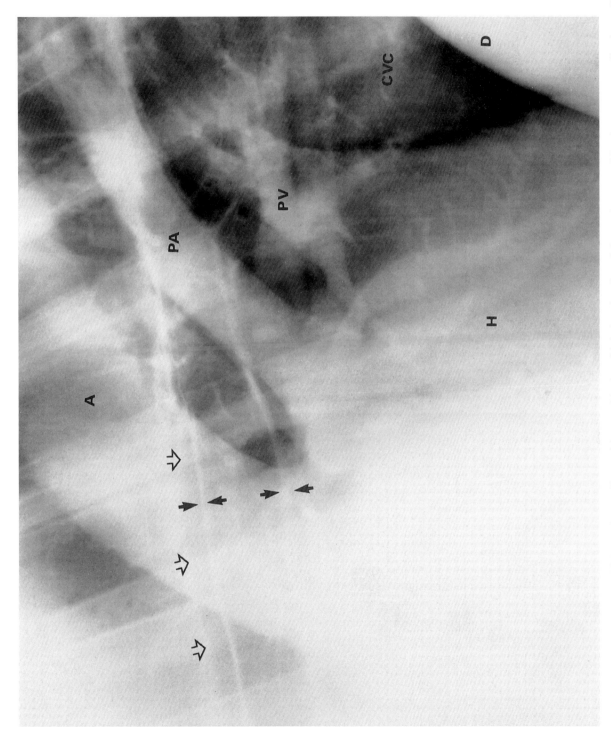

Figure 12.11 Yearling female Quarterhorse which was in a trailer accident and had multiple head and neck lacerations, resulting in pneumomediastinum. There is free air in the mediastinum which outlines both sides of the tracheal wall (between solid black arrows). Air in the mediastinum is seen between the dorsal tracheal wall and the open black arrows. Air in the mediastinum also allows for visualization of the major pulmonary vascular structures. The aorta (A), pulmonary arteries (PA) and the pulmonary veins (PV) are easily visualized. The pulmonary arteries and veins to the caudal ventral lung lobes are visualized over the heart (H). The diaphragm is identified (D). The caudal vena cava (CVC) is poorly visualized.

[625]

increase in intrathoracic pressure compresses the mediastinum, thus preventing the entrance of air into the potential mediastinal space. Pneumothorax and pneumomediastinum can exist concurrently, usually as the result of trauma.

Free air in the mediastinum may result from rupture of a tracheal ring, a penetrating wound or an abscess, or may be iatrogenic following techniques such as a transtracheal wash or intravenous fluid administration.

Mediastinal masses

Mediastinal masses may be seen as areas of increased soft-tissue opacity that summate with or displace other structures in the mediastinum such as the trachea, great vessels or the heart. Although rare they are often associated with free pleural fluid and are therefore obscured by the fluid that has the same opacity as the mass. The most common mediastinal disease in the horse is lymphosarcoma. Diagnosis and differentiation are aided by diagnostic ultrasound and/or drainage of the pleural fluid, followed by radiographic re-evaluation.

Tracheal collapse and stenosis

When tracheal collapse or tracheal stenosis is suspected, comparison of inspiratory and expiratory films may show a change in tracheal dimension, which aids in the interpretation.

Congenital abnormalities of the trachea such as hypoplastic trachea are occasionally seen and are most common in miniature horses (Figure 12.12). Occasionally focal narrowing of the tracheal lumen is seen. True tracheal masses must be differentiated from material being expectorated. With the latter there is usually an associated pneumonia and the mass will move with continued coughing (Figure 12.13).

Diseases of the lung

Bronchitis and bronchiolitis

These diseases may result in only minor increases in lung opacity associated with the bronchial walls and therefore do not have pathognomonic radiographic signs. Bronchiectasis due to chronic bronchitis has the pathognomonic changes of large well delineated and/or irregularly shaped bronchi (Figure 12.14).

Chronic obstructive pulmonary disease (COPD)

Radiographic abnormalities are only detectable in relatively advanced cases of COPD. In the case of emphysema there is air trapping, the lung is more lucent than normal and local contrast is improved. The lung parenchyma will have the same appearance on both inspiratory and expiratory radiographs, and although the lungs appear well aerated they may have a slightly

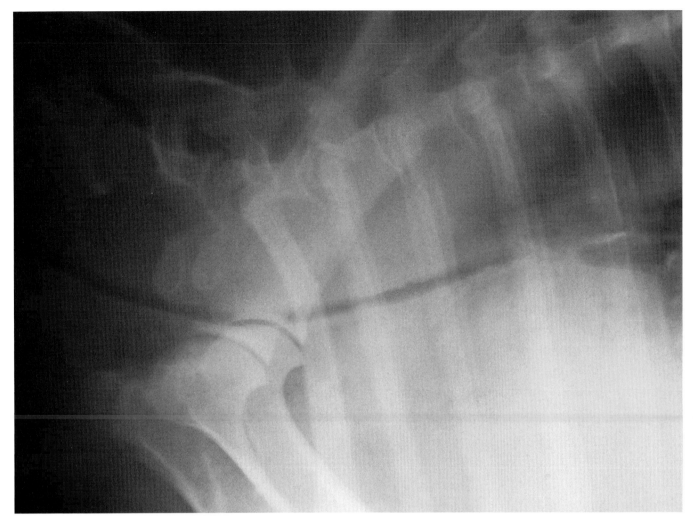

Figure 12.12 Fourteen-year-old miniature horse with a history of chronic inspiratory stridor and, when exercised, a 'honking' sound on expiration. There is severe collapse of the cervical and thoracic trachea. The cardiac silhouette appears to be slightly enlarged. Diagnosis: hypoplastic trachea.

reticulated interstitial pattern. This is often referred to as a honeycomb appearance and results from over-expanded terminal airways and consolidation of tissue and/or interstitial fibrosis. Redistribution of vascular flow has also been shown to contribute to this pattern. Late in the disease, bronchiectasis may be seen (Figure 12.14).

Bacterial pneumonia

This disease is usually bilateral and often associated with abscess or granuloma formation (see pages 635–637 and Figure 12.4a–b, pages 612–613). Although bacterial pneumonia may be generalized it often has a ventral distribution (see Figures 12.7, page 620 and 12.16, page 633). With abscessation there is often cavitation (see Cavitary pulmonary lesion(s), page 632) and evidence of an air–fluid interface with a 'fluid line' in the cavity. With

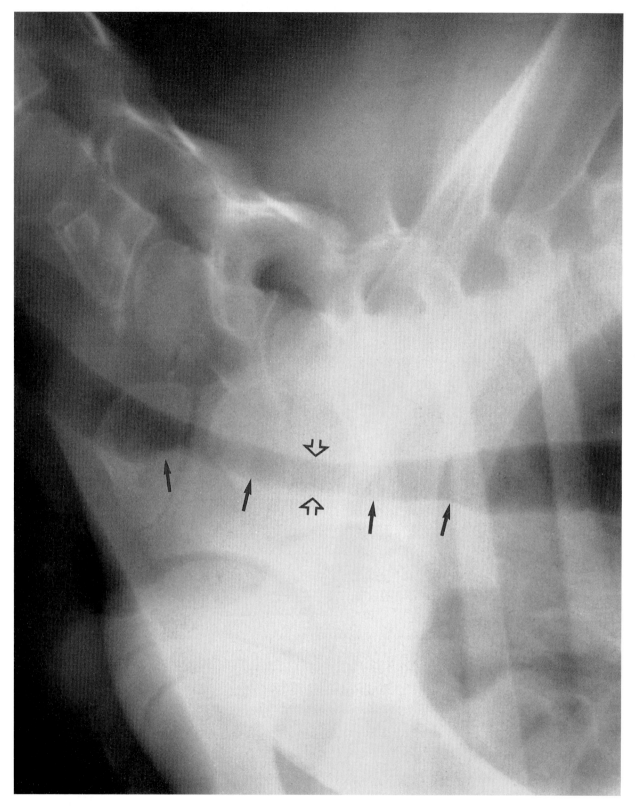

Figure 12.13 Three-month-old Arab colt with chronic pneumonia. There is narrowing of the trachea to approximately 50% of its diameter (open arrows). A tracheal mass is demonstrated on the ventral tracheal wall (solid arrows). This mass may represent either a true intraluminal mass or material that is being expectorated. Note the open physes of the scapulae and humeri. Diagnosis: material in the trachea that is being expectorated from the lungs.

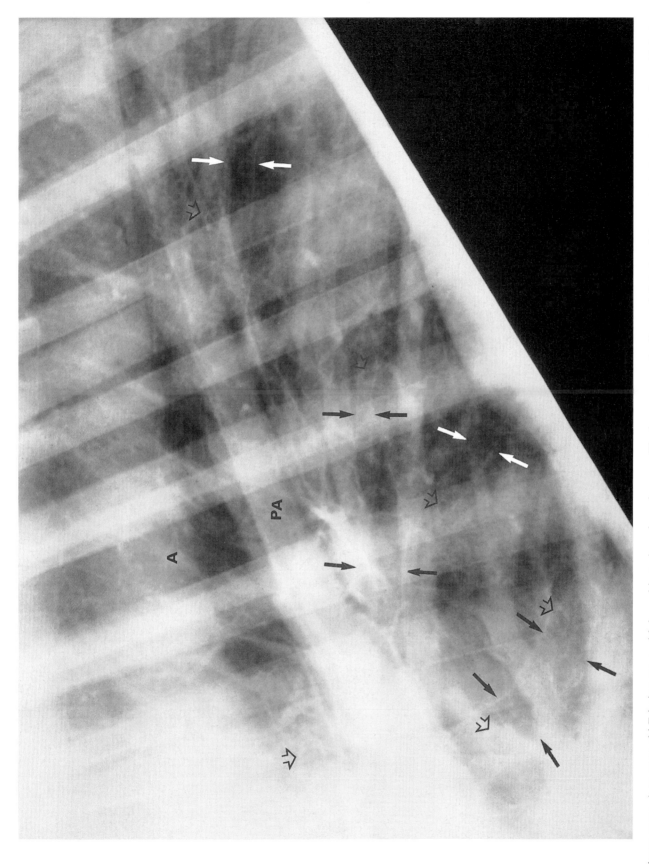

Figure 12.14 A 23-year-old Friesian mare with bronchiectasis and emphysema. The lungs are markedly overinflated and demonstrate large tortuous bronchi, between solid arrows (black and white). Thin-walled end-on bronchial structures are marked with open arrows. Only a few of the bronchi are marked. The aorta (A) and the pulmonary arteries (PA) are readily visualized extending caudal to the periphery.

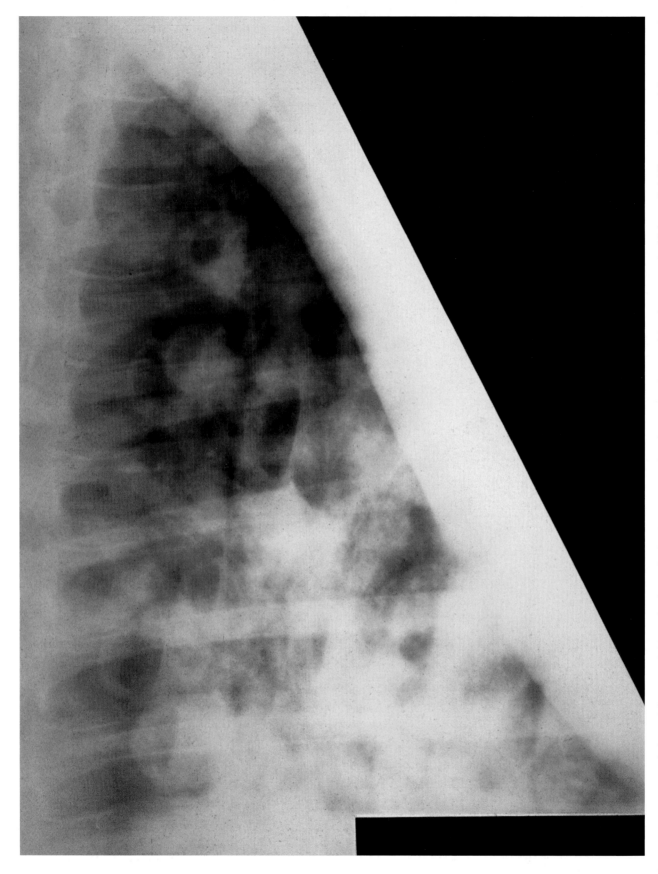

Figure 12.15(a) Lateral view of dorsocaudal lung field of a foal. There are multiple large circular opacities, in many of which are fluid lines. The caudal vena cava is obscured by 'cottonball' opacities. This is typical of the radiographic appearance of *Rhodococcus equi* pneumonia.

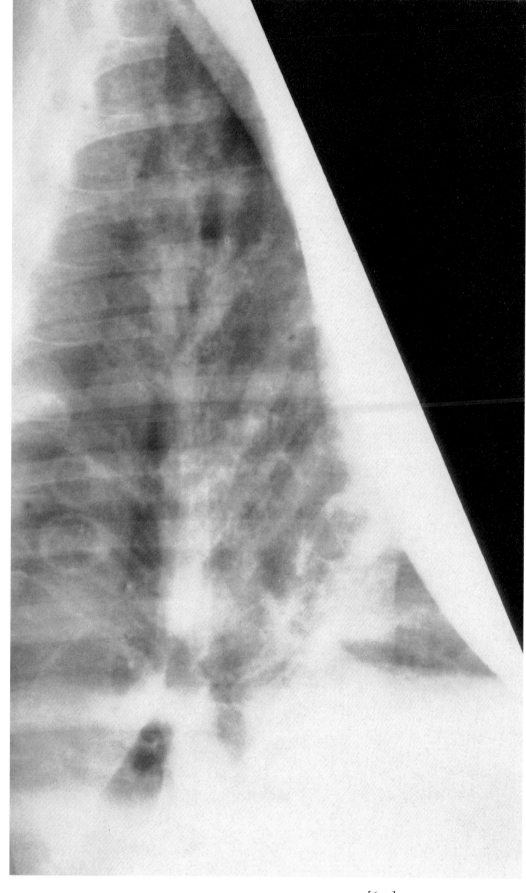

Figure 12.15(b) The same foal as in Figure 12.15(a), 19 days later, following treatment with erythromycin and rifampin. Although several round cavitated abscesses persist, many of the 'cottonball' opacities are no longer detectable and the caudal vena cava is now visible. An increase in interstitial density persists.

thick material in the abscess the dorsal margins may curve upwards, forming a meniscus. Although most bacterial pneumonias cannot be differentiated on the basis of radiographic signs, chronic *Rhodococcus* pneumonia of young horses usually has a cottonball appearance (Figures 12.15a and 12.15b), which may later cavitate or consolidate.

Aspiration pneumonia

This disease is almost always ventral in distribution due to the aspiration of particulate matter, and is often associated with severe consolidation. This results in a generalized increase in lung opacity and loss of all lung detail except for air bronchogram formation (Figure 12.16; see also Figure 12.7, page 620). If aspiration occurs when the patient is in dorsal or lateral recumbency the distribution will be dorsal or to the downside lung, depending upon the position of the patient at the time of aspiration.

Inhalation pneumonia

This disease usually has a more dorsocaudal distribution due to the non-particulate nature of the inhalant. In general, inhalation pneumonia is less consolidative than aspiration pneumonia and results in a more generalized interstitial pattern. If the inhalant is very irritating (smoke or toxic fumes), the lining of the air spaces may become so damaged that it results in oedema and alveolar flooding. Air bronchograms may then be seen in the consolidated lung.

Cavitary pulmonary lesion(s) (CPL)

This term is used to describe a cavity that occurs in the lung. In the horse the most common form is the result of abscess formation, liquefaction and loss of the fluid centre through a communicating bronchus (Figure 12.17; see also Figure 12.4a–b, pages 612–613). These are usually seen in young horses and have a thick opaque wall. Other abscesses or granulomas may also be seen. An air–fluid interface is often present. The lesions usually resolve with the associated pneumonia, but may be the last radiographic sign to disappear. The effect of geometric distortion is substantial and therefore positioning, phase of respiration and change due to growth of the patient must be taken into consideration when evaluating the size, progression and resolution of a CPL.

Other forms of CPL exist, but are rare in the horse. They include neoplastic, traumatic and congenital cavitary lesions (Figures 12.18 and 12.19). Neoplastic cavitary lesions have not been described in the horse, but might be difficult to distinguish from infective CPLs because both infectious and neoplastic CPLs have thick walls. Traumatic cavitary lesions (in other species) have walls that vary in thickness and usually resolve spontaneously. They may remain as thin-walled ring shadows, which in the horse might be hard to distinguish from an end-on bronchus, without a history of known thoracic trauma. Congenital CPLs in other species are usually thin walled

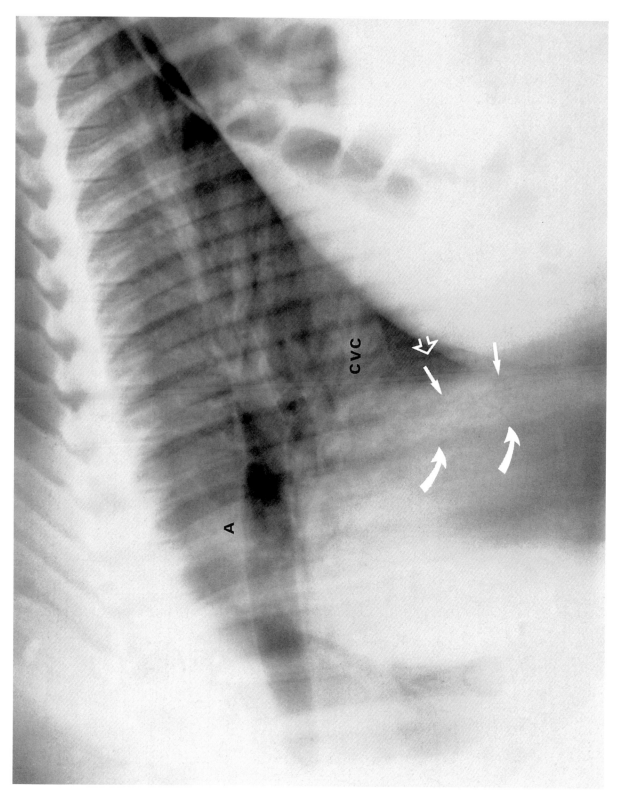

Figure 12.16 Right lateral recumbent view of the thorax of a newborn foal. There is an interstitial pattern in all lung lobes and an alveolar pattern over the cardiac silhouette extending from the curved white arrows to the caudal aspect of the heart (open arrow), below the caudal vena cava (CVC). Straight white arrows demonstrate air bronchograms. The interstitial density obscures the aortic root (A). The bowel pattern is normal. Because of the ventral distribution and the air bronchogram formation, both aspiration and bacterial pneumonia should be considered.

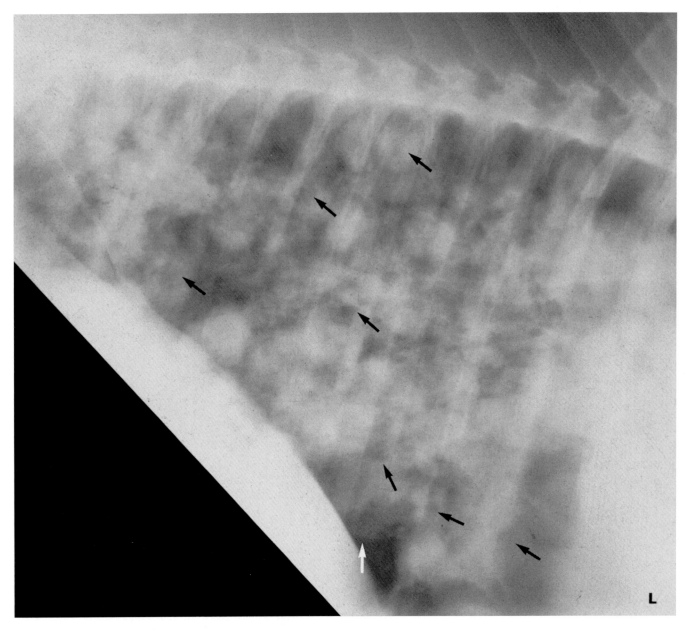

Figure 12.17 Six-week-old colt with a 2-week history of coughing. Left (this page) and right (opposite) lateral thoracic films are characterized by generalized nodular opacities through all lung lobes. The cardiac silhouette is obscured by the coalescing opacities. Some of the opacities have lucent centres indicating cavitation (white and black arrows). Cavitation is more obvious in the left (L) lateral radiograph, indicating that most of the cavitation is on that side. Diagnosis: granulomatous pneumonia with cavitation. Compare with Figures 12.4a, 12.4b, 12.18 and 12.19.

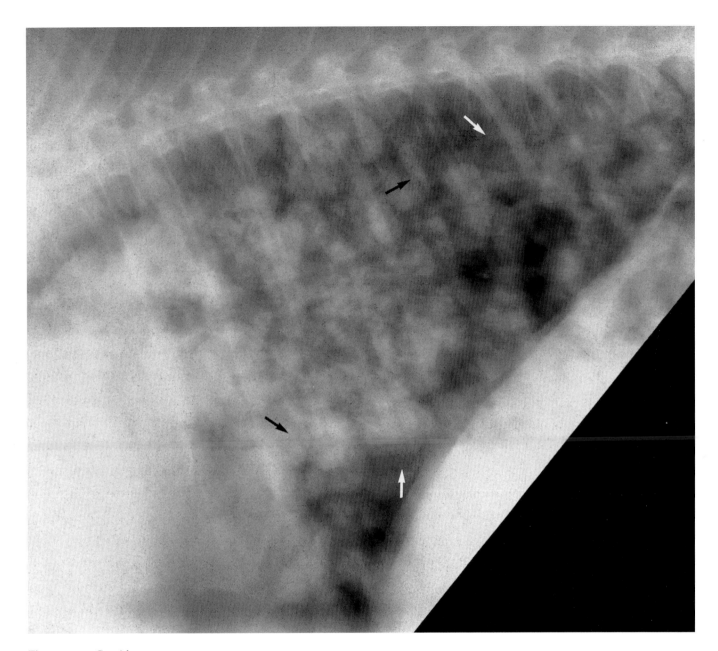

Figure 12.17 *Cont'd*

and may contain some fluid. Any cavitary lesion may rupture and result in pneumothorax (see page 623), pneumomediastinum (see page 623) or other complications, depending on their content.

Pulmonary masses

ABSCESSES

In the horse the most common form of pulmonary masses are abscesses, which appear as opaque masses with or without a lucent gas cap dorsally (see Figure 12.4, page 612). Solitary abscesses may be quite large

[635]

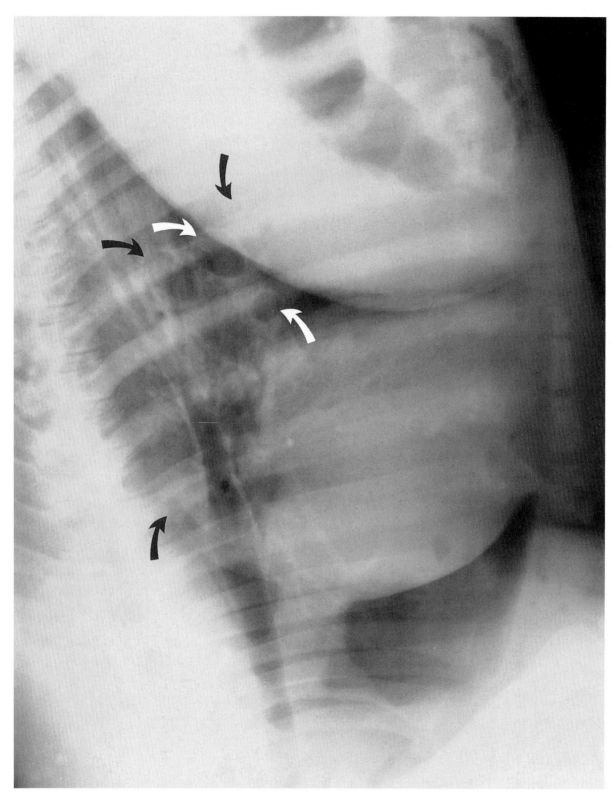

Figure 12.18 A foal 2 weeks premature, with a profuse watery diarrhoea. There are multiple, various-sized, thin-walled cavitary pulmonary lesions (white and black arrows). The cranial lung lobes are normal. The caudal lung lobes have an increase in both interstitial and bronchial markings which are felt to be age related. Diagnosis: multiple cavitary pulmonary lesions. The cavitary pulmonary lesions may represent a congenital cyst, resolving haematomas from a difficult parturition or, less likely, abscessation. Compare with Figures 12.4a, 12.4b, 12.17 and 12.19.

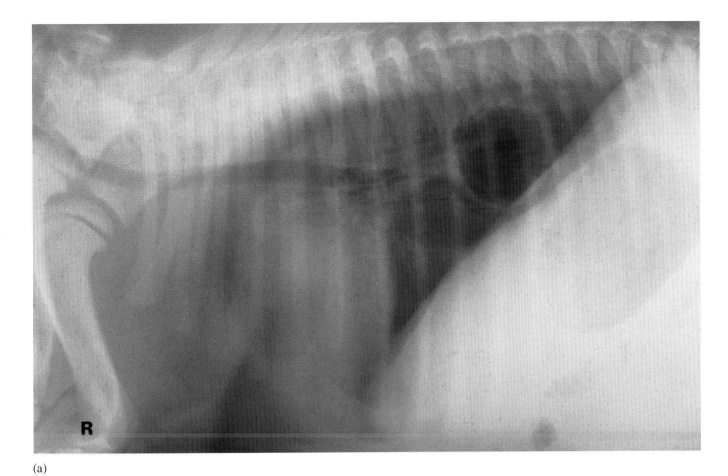

(a)

Figure 12.19 Six-day-old miniature horse born prematurely, with *Salmonella* diarrhoea but no clinical signs of respiratory disease. A lateral radiograph (a) shows a large, thick-walled air-filled bulla which can be seen in the caudal right lung lobe. The inner wall of the bulla is irregular. The remainder of the thorax is normal. A dorsoventral radiograph (b) also demonstrates the lesion. Differential diagnosis should include a congenital bulla or a pneumatocoele secondary to haematoma or infarct. Abscessation is felt to be less likely because of the lack of associated pulmonary disease. Compare this case with Figures 12.4a, 12.4b, 12.17 and 12.18. Diagnosis: congenital cavitary pulmonary lesion.

(Figure 12.20) and if cavitated may be confused with a hollow viscus from a diaphragmatic hernia (see Figure 12.23, page 644). Abscesses are always associated with other signs of infection including interstitial and usually alveolar infiltrates. In general they have irregular indistinct margins and may form CPLs (see page 632).

GRANULOMAS

Like abscesses, granulomas may be associated with other intrapulmonary disease, but may also be the only remnants of a previous more active disease. Granulomas are opaque and their margins may be more distinct than abscesses. Mycetomas have a tendency to have indistinct margins and are multi-compartmented.

[637]

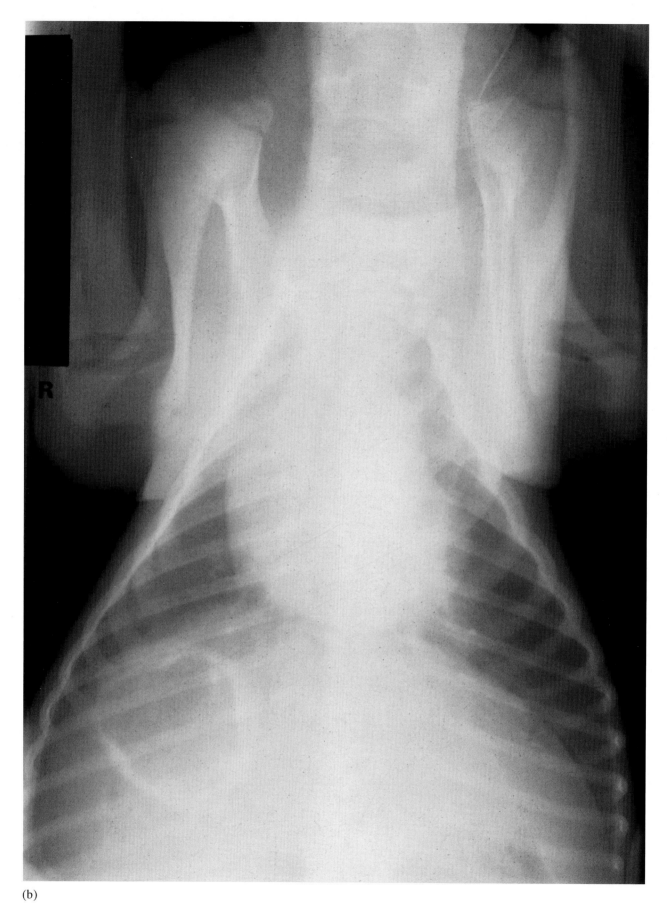

R

(b)

Figure 12.19 *Cont'd*

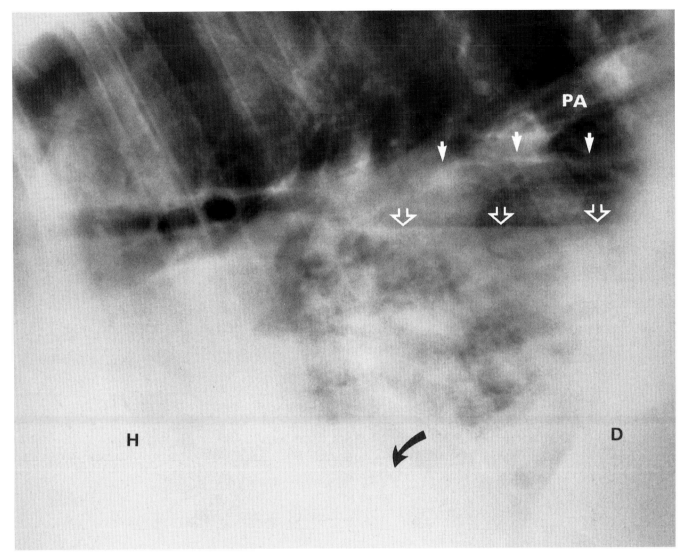

Figure 12.20 Two-year-old Thoroughbred stallion with a 3-week history of pleuropneumonia. Twenty-two litres of fluid were drained from the left hemithorax the day before these radiographs were obtained. There is a large pulmonary abscess in the caudal ventral thorax between the heart (H) and the diaphragm (D), ventral to the solid white arrows. There is a fluid line below the open arrows and an air space between the open arrows and the wall of the abscess (solid white arrows). The pulmonary arteries (PA) are marked. There is a generalized interstitial and bronchial pattern in the remainder of the thorax. Other smaller and less well defined abscesses can be seen above the heart. They are poorly defined because they are in the right hemithorax and this radiograph is a left lateral projection in order to demonstrate the size and character of the larger abscess. A chest tube is in place in the thoracic cavity: the curved black arrow denotes the position of a metallic marker on the chest drain. Diagnosis: multiple pulmonary abscesses with a large cavitating abscess in the left hemithorax; hydrothorax.

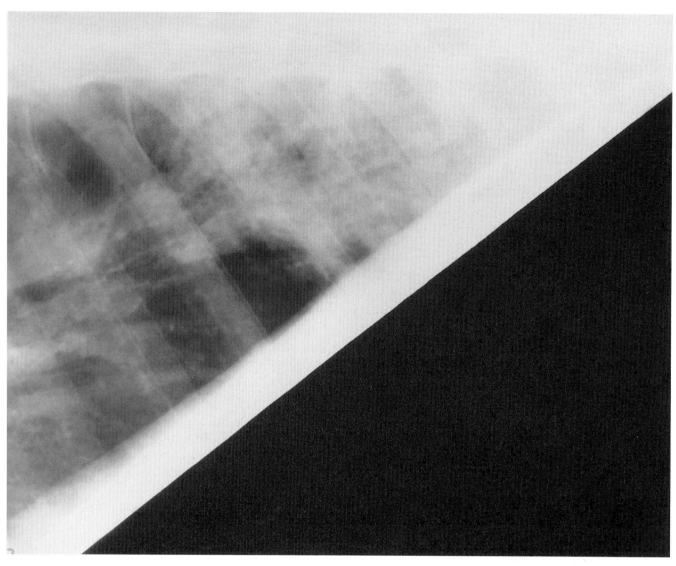

Figure 12.21 Three-year-old Thoroughbred filly with a history of chronic pleuritis and weight loss. There is a caudodorsal lung mass of mixed interstitial and alveolar infiltrates. The cranial margins of the mass are well circumscribed. The findings are suggestive of infarct or pulmonary haemorrhage. The possibility of bacterial pneumonia cannot be ruled out. The smooth margins cranially, the triangular shape and less distinct peripheral margins are more characteristic of infarct. Diagnosis: caudal thoracic mass, probably an infarct.

INFARCTS AND EMBOLISM

These occur occasionally, especially in the caudal dorsal lung lobes. They usually have a somewhat triangular shape with a sharply defined cranial margin and an indistinct periphery (Figure 12.21). Infarcts and exercise-induced pulmonary haemorrhage (EIPH) appear similar radiographically, but may be differentiated by obtaining serial radiographs. Infarcts persist, whereas EIPH resolves rapidly.

This is occasionally seen as multiple circular opacities that vary in size and in the sharpness of their margins. The appearance of the metastatic lesion will depend on the cell type of the original tumour, the tumour-doubling time, the location of the nodule in the lung and whether there have been single or multiple showers of neoplastic cells. Solitary masses of 0.5 cm or less in diameter will usually be missed, and masses as large as 2 cm in diameter may be overlooked. However, superimposition of multiple nodules of 1 cm or larger will usually be identified after careful examination.

PRIMARY LUNG TUMOURS

These are rare but, when they occur, tend to be well circumscribed and solitary. The most common lung tumour in the horse is adenocarcinoma. When present a tumour usually appears as a singular mass; these vary in size depending on the tumour-doubling rate and the length of time that they have been present. They are usually quite large when found and may be seen as incidental findings when examining the lung for other diseases. They must be differentiated from abscesses, granulomas and resolving EIPH.

Exercise-induced pulmonary haemorrhage (EIPH)

The diagnosis of EIPH is usually based on the presence of haemorrhage from the nostrils and in the bronchi on endoscopic examination immediately following strenuous exercise. Radiographic findings when present are limited to the caudodorsal lungs and consist of interstitial opacities with a wispy appearance that often obliterate the thoracophrenic angle and summate with the diaphragmatic shadow. The opacities are usually more circumscribed toward the hilus and less well defined toward the periphery. Resolution of the opacity has been reported as early as 10 days, but it may last for several months with a gradual decrease in size and increase in margination. Cavitation and pleural fluid accumulation have both been reported as sequelae to this condition. A pre-existing abscess may predispose to haemorrhage.

Collapsed lung

Collapse of a lung results in loss of normal lung tissue dorsally. Ventrally there is a more consolidated appearance, with loss of normal lung pattern. If it occurs unilaterally the dorsal aspect of the collapsed lung appears as an oblique radiopaque line superimposed on the normally aerated contralateral lung (Figure 12.22). See also Pneumothorax (page 623 and Figure 12.10). A collapsed lung resulting from previous pleural disease may have increased opacity of the lung margins, because of fibrin on the pleural surface of the lung.

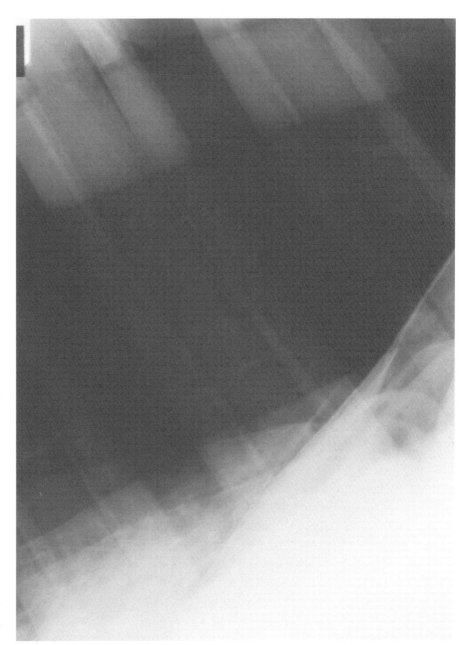

Figure 12.22 Lateral radiographic view of the caudal aspect of the thorax of a polo pony which had sustained a stake wound in the pectoral region 24 days previously. Cranial is to the left. The left and right lungs have collapsed so there is no lung pattern in the proximal half of the lung field, which appears radiolucent. The aorta is seen proximally.

Diaphragmatic hernia

Diaphragmatic hernias may be either congenital or acquired. Congenital diaphragmatic hernias may occur dorsally, in the mid-diaphragm on the left side, or ventrally, where they are usually larger. Although congenital hernias are reported to have smooth, well rounded margins, this change is not seen radiographically. Large defects have been reported in foals with arthrogryphosis and scoliosis.

Acquired diaphragmatic hernias are usually associated with trauma or violent exercise (jumping) or increased intra-abdominal pressure (parturition, a fall or colic). When signs of trauma are absent consideration must be

[642]

given to the existence of a congenital defect that has been exacerbated by exercise or increased intra-abdominal pressure.

There may be no clinical signs that relate to the diaphragmatic rupture immediately after the initial trauma. However, acute signs of abdominal distress (colic) or respiratory distress may be noted later on.

The radiographic signs of diaphragmatic rupture include gas-capped fluid levels and bowel patterns in the ventral thorax with or without free fluid (Figure 12.23). Fluid opacities may be present when liver, spleen or omentum are in the thoracic cavity without accompanying bowel structures. Striations or crescent-shaped lines through gas-containing structures may indicate haustra of the large bowel. Normal structures such as the pulmonary vessels and the heart may be displaced by the presence of abdominal viscera in the thoracic cavity.

Laterality may be determined by obtaining both right and left lateral projections of the thorax and comparing the image sharpness and magnification. Lesions or structures will be on the side in which they appear small and sharply delineated. If laterality cannot be determined by this method, the defect may be near the midline.

Ultrasonographic evaluation can aid in differentiating diaphragmatic hernias from other disease, as well as defining the structures that have been displaced.

Cardiac diseases

In general, cardiac disease in the large equine patient does not lend itself to radiographic diagnosis, but congenital cardiac disease may occasionally be diagnosed in the foal (Figure 12.24). The use of diagnostic ultrasonography is usually much more valuable in the diagnosis of cardiac disease in the horse. Occasionally other radiographic signs may lead to the inclusion of cardiac disease in the differential diagnosis. Decreased number and diminished size of pulmonary vessels, although quite subjective, should lead to the consideration of diseases that cause hypoperfusion. Increasing size of these structures should lead to the consideration of overperfusion, which might lead to other signs such as progression from interstitial to alveolar oedema. Marked enlargement of the cardiac silhouette may be indicated by dorsal displacement of the carina or a rounded appearance, and points to cardiac or pericardial disease.

Rib lesions

TUMOURS

When productive lesions are noted on the ribs or when a pleural mass appears to be associated with a rib, chondrosarcoma must be considered. These tumours may appear as a mass lesion and it may be difficult to define either bone destruction or production, although both components are usually present.

[643]

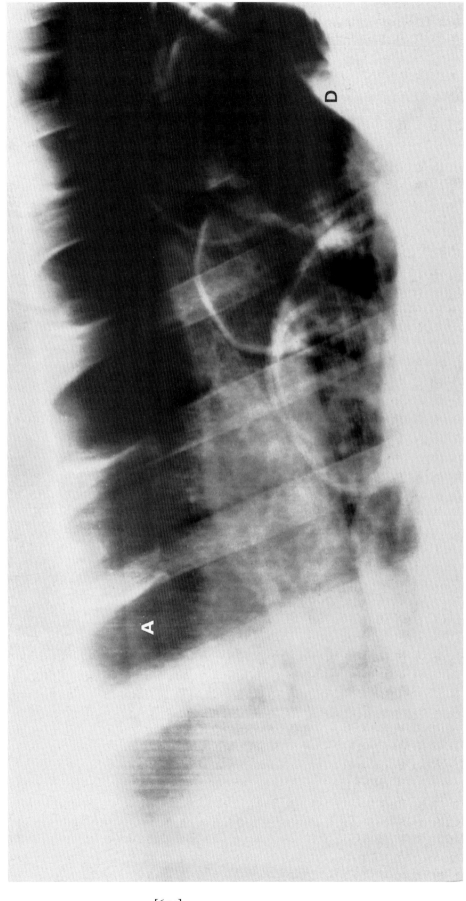

Figure 12.23 Radiographic abnormalities characteristic of a diaphragmatic hernia. There is fluid obscuring the ventral thorax. There are gas-filled bowel loops cranial to the diaphragm (D), containing gas and fluid at various levels. The dorsal margin of the aorta (A) passes over the vertebral bodies. The lungs are displaced ventrally from the paraspinal gutter by pneumothorax. The lungs appear opaque due to the atelectasis caused by the fluid and pneumothorax.

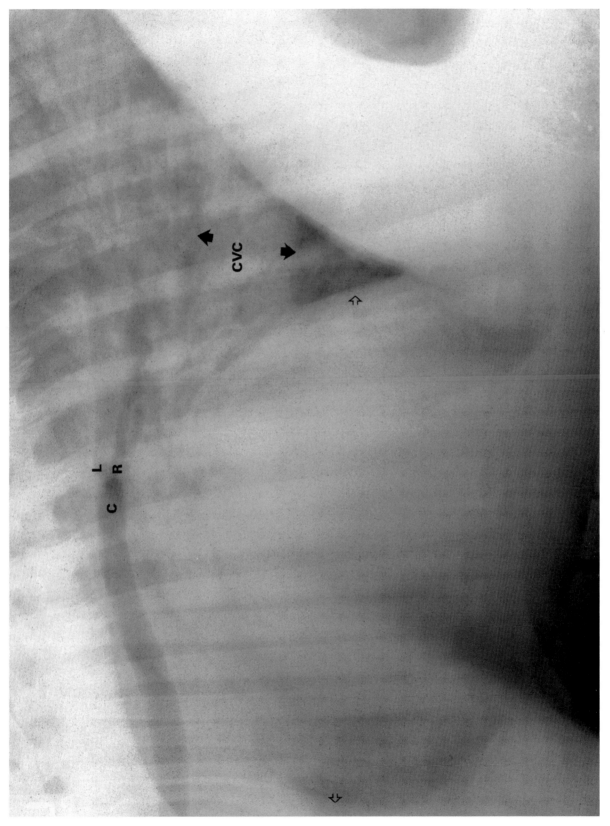

Figure 12.24 A 45-day-old Thoroughbred colt with harsh lung sounds and poor growth. There is cardiac enlargement with dorsal displacement of the trachea just cranial to the carina (C). The left mainstem bronchus (L) is slightly elevated over the right (R). The caudal vena cava (CVC) is markedly dilated (solid arrows). There is a generalized increase in pulmonary interstitial infiltrates in all lung lobes. This results in an overall opacification of the lungs. The cranial and caudal margins of the cardiac silhouette are marked with an open arrow. Diagnosis: congenital right and left heart enlargement with congestive heart failure.

RIB FRACTURES

Rib fractures may lead to pneumothorax, lung contusion or pleural haemorrhage. A fracture of a more cranial rib may result in abnormal behaviour when the horse is tacked-up or mounted. Rib fractures are often hard to find radiographically and may be defined by centring the x-ray beam over an area of suspected trauma. Ultrasonography is also useful for the identification of rib fractures. Fractures may persist as chronic non-union fractures due to motion. The ends of the opposing ribs may appear slightly flared adjacent to the lucent fibrous union. A fracture of the first rib may result in forelimb lameness and muscle atrophy; the fracture may best be identified by using the technique described for radiography of the shoulder (see page 273).

MULTIPLE OSTEOCHONDROMAS

Multiple hereditary osteochondromatosis has been reported in the horse and should be suspected when smoothly marginated bone protrusions are noted on flat bones. Other osteochondromas may be found on long bones (see pages 257 and 315). Osteochondromas are not usually of any clinical significance, but they may be considered to be potentially pre-cancerous growths.

Abnormalities of the oesophagus are dealt with in Chapter 13 (page 659).

Also see 'Hypertrophic osteopathy', Chapter 1, page 22.

Sternum

Lateral views of the sternum can be obtained using portable x-ray equipment. Digital systems or rare earth screens and appropriate film are recommended. The sternum is best radiographed with one forelimb protracted to minimize the amount of soft tissues that the x-ray beam has to penetrate. An aluminium wedge filter can be useful. The x-ray beam is centred caudal to the elbow approximately 10 cm proximal to the ventral aspect of the thorax.

At birth the sternum consists of seven bony segments, sternebrae, which are united by intersternebral cartilages. The two most caudal sternebrae fuse by approximately 3 months of age, but the remainder only partially fuse. Only the caudal one-third to one-half of the sternum can easily be seen radiographically because of the overlying structures of the forelimb cranially. The sternum inclines ventrally from cranial to caudal (Figure 12.25a). The dorsal border is straight, whereas the ventral border is smoothly curved with indentations at the site of the intersternebral articulations. The most caudal aspect of the sternum is rather variable in shape between horses, being either pointed, or slightly rounded. The so-called costal cartilages are mineralized and are seen radiographically. They articulate with the ribs dorsally.

Radiographic abnormalities of the sternum, costal cartilages or ribs are not common, but have been identified in horses demonstrating abnormal

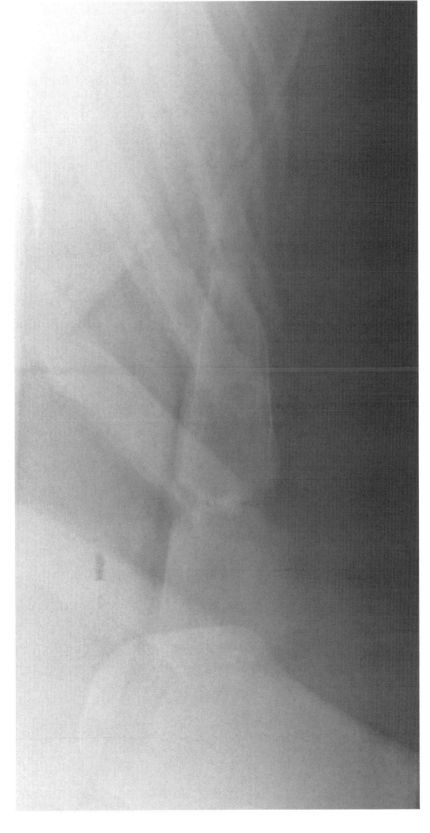

Figure 12.25(a) Lateral view of the caudal one-third of the sternum and the costal cartilages of a normal adult horse. Note the indentations ventrally at the intersternebral articulations.

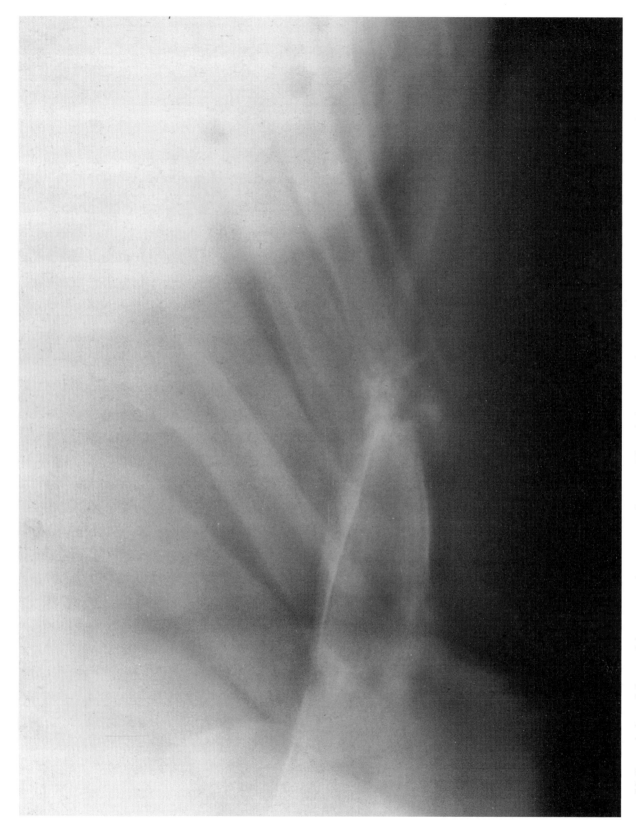

Figure 12.25(b) Lateral view of the caudal sternum of a mature polo pony. There is fragmentation at the most caudal aspect of the sternum (compare with Figure 12.25a). The pony had shown a sudden onset of violent bucking behaviour when tacked-up or when mounted. When re-examined 6 weeks later, the sternum had modelled considerably; the pony resumed full work without recurrence of abnormal behaviour.

behaviour when tacked up or mounted. Abnormalities include a fracture of a costal cartilage and fragmentation of the most caudal aspect of the sternum (Figure 12.25b).

FURTHER READING

Ainsworth, D., Eicker, S., Yeagar, A., Sweeney, C. *et al.* (1998) Associations between physical examination, laboratory and radiographic findings and outcome and subsequent racing performance of foals with *Rhodococcus equi* infection: 115 cases (1984–1992). *J. Am. Vet. Med. Ass.*, **213**, 510–515

Ainsworth, D., Erb, H., Eicker, S., Yeagar, A. *et al.* (2000) Effects of pulmonary abscesses on racing performance of horses treated at referral Veterinary medical teaching hospitals: 45 cases (1985–1997). *J. Am. Vet. Med. Ass.*, **216**, 1282–1287

Boy, M. and Sweeney, C. (2000) Pneumothorax in 40 cases (1980–1997). *J. Am. Vet. Med. Ass.*, **216**, 1965–1967

Buergelt, C.D., Hines, S.A., Cantor, G., Stirk, A. and Wilson, J.H. (1986) A retrospective study of proliferative interstitial lung disease of horses in Florida. *Vet. Pathol.*, **23**, 750–756

Carlsten, J. (1986) Imaging of the equine heart. An angiographic and echocardiographic investigation. *Thesis*, Uppsala, Sweden, Merkantil-Tryckeriet AB, Uppsala

Carlsten, J., Kvart, C. and Jeffcott, L.B. (1984) Method of selective and non-selective angiocardiography for the horse. *Equine vet. J.*, **12**, 47–52

Carr, E., Carlsen, G., Wilson, D. and Reed, D. (1997) Acute haemorrhagic pulmonary infarction and necrotizing pneumonia in horses: 21 cases (1967–1993). *J. Am. Vet. Med. Ass.*, **210**, 1774–1778

Cook, G., Divers, T. and Rowland, P. (1995) Hypercalcaemia and erythrocytosis in a mare with associated metastatic carcinoma. *Equine vet. J.*, **27**, 316–318

Farrow, C.S. (1981a) Equine thoracic radiology. *J. Am. Vet. Med. Ass.*, **179**, 776–781

Farrow, C.S. (1981b) Radiography of the equine thorax: anatomy and technique. *Vet. Radiol.*, **22**, 62–78

Farrow, C.S. (1981) Radiographic aspects of inflammatory lung disease in the horse. *Vet. Radiol.*, **22**, 107–114

Farrow, C.S. (1976) Pneumomediastinum in the horse: a complication of transtracheal aspiration. *Vet. Radiol.*, **17**, 192–195

Farrow, C.S. (1982) Inhalation pneumonia in a horse. *Can. Vet. J.*, **23**, 340–341

Gehlen, H., Stadler, P. and Ohnesorge, B. (2005) Tracheal obstruction in a horse with oesophageal stenosis and diverticulum. *Equine vet. Educ.*, **17**, 132–134

Gronvold, A., Ihler, C. and Hanche-Olsen, S. (2005) Conservative treatment of tracheal perforation in a 13 year old hunter stallion. *Equine vet. Educ.*, **17**, 142–145

Hillidge, C.J. (1986) Review of *Corynebacterium* (*Rhodococcus*) *equi* lung abscess in foals: pathogenesis, diagnosis and treatment. *Vet. Rec.*, **119**, 261–264; *Vet. Radiol.*, **9**, 80–88

Jean, D., Lavoie, J.-P., Nunez, L. and Lagace, A. (1994) Cutaneous haemangiosarcoma with pulmonary metastasis in a horse. *J. Am. Vet. Med. Ass.*, **204**, 776–778

Jorgensen, J., Geoly, F., Berry, C. and Breuhaus, B. (1992) Lameness and pleural effusion associated with an aggressive fibrosarcoma in a horse. *J. Am. Vet. Med. Ass.*, **210**, 1328–1331

Kangstrom, L.E. (1968) The radiological diagnosis of equine pneumonia. *Vet. Radiol.*, **9**, 80–88

Kohn, C.W. (1981) Recognition and management of equine viral respiratory disease. *Compend. Contin. Educ.*, **3**(3), 73–81

Kosch, P.C., Koterba, A.M., Coons, T.J. and Webb, A.I. (1984) Developments in management of the newborn foal in respiratory distress 1: Evaluation. *Equine vet. J.*, **16**, 312–318

Koterba, A.M., Brewer, B.D. and Tarplee, F.A. (1984) Clinical and clinicopathological characteristics of the septicaemic neonatal foal: review of 38 cases. *Equine vet. J.*, **16**, 376–383

Kvart, C., Carlsten, J., Jeffcott, L.B. and Nilsfors, L. (1985) Diagnostic value of contrast echocardiography in the horse. *Equine vet. J.*, **17**, 357–360

Lamb, C.R., O'Callaghan, M.W. and Pradis, M.R. (1990) Thoracic radiography in the neonatal foal: a preliminary report. *Vet. Radiol.*, **31**, 11–16

Lavoie, J., Fiset, L. and Laverty, S. (1994) Review of 40 cases of lung abscesses in foals and adult horses. *Equine vet. J.* **26**, 348–352

Mair, T. (1991) Treatment and complications of pleuropneumonia. *Equine vet. J.*, **23**, 5

Mair, T., Hillyer, M. and Brown, P. (1992) Mesothelioma of the pleural cavity in a horse. *Equine vet. Educ.*, **4**, 59–61

Mair, T., Rush, B. and Tucker, R. (2004) Clinical and diagnostic features of thoracic neoplasia in the horse. *Equine vet. Educ.*, **16**, 30–36

Martens, R.J., Martens, J.G. and Fiske, R.A. (1989) *Rhodococcus equi* foal pneumonia: pathogenesis and immunoprophylaxis. *Proc. Am. Ass. Equine Prac.*, **35**, 199–213

Martens, R.J. and Renshaw, H.W. (1982) Foal pneumonia. A practical approach to diagnosis and therapy. *Compend. Contin. Educ.*, **4**(9), 217–228

Mazan, M., Vin, R. and Hoffman, A. (2005) Radiographic scoring lacks predictive value in inflammatory airway disease. *Equine vet. J.*, **37**, 541–545

Morris, D.D. and Beech, J. (1983) Disseminated intravascular coagulation in six horses. *J. Am. Vet. Med. Ass.*, **183**, 1067–1072

Nout, Y., Hinchcliffe, K., Smaii, V., Kohn C. *et al.* (2002) Chronic pulmonary disease with radiographic interstitial opacity (interstitial pneumonia) in foals. *Equine vet. J.*, **34**, 542–549

O'Callaghan, M.W. and Seehermans, H.J. (1989) New ways of looking at lung disease in the horse using radiography and scintigraphy. *Proc. Am. Ass. Equine Prac.*, **35**, 221–232

Pascoe, J.R., O'Brien, T.R., Wheat, J.D. and Meagher, D.M. (1983) Radiographic aspects of exercise-induced pulmonary hemorrhage in racing horses. *Vet. Radiol.*, **24**, 85–92

Pusterla, N., Pesavento, P., Leutenegger, C., Hay, J. *et al.* (2002) Disseminated pulmonary adiaspiromycosis caused by *Emmonscia crescens* in a horse. *Equine vet. J.*, **34**, 749–752

Rantanen, N.W. (1986) Diagnostic ultrasound. *Vet. Clin. N. Amer.: Equine Practice* 2, No. 1, W.B. Saunders, Philadelphia

Rantanen N. and McKinnon, A. (1998) *Equine Diagnostic Ultrasonography*, 1st edn, Williams and Wilkins, Baltimore

Reef, V. (1998) *Equine Diagnostic Ultrasound*, 1st edn, W.B. Saunders, Philadelphia

Rossdale, P., Greet, T., McGladdery, A., Ricketts, S. and Aqel, N. (2004) Pulmonary leiomyosarcoma in a 13 year old Thoroughbred stallion presenting as a differential diagnosis to recurrent airway obstruction. *Equine vet Educ.*, **16**, 21–28

Schwarzwald, C., Stewart, A., Morrison, C. and Bonagura, J. (2006) Cor pulmonale in a horse with granulomatous pneumonia. *Equine vet. Educ.*, **18**, 182–187

Seltzer, K. and Byars, T.D. (1996) Prognosis for return to racing after recovery from pleuropneumonia in Thoroughbred racehorses: 70 cases (1984–1989). *J. Am. Vet. Med. Ass.*, **208**, 1300–1301

Shively, J.F., Dellers, R.W., Buergelt, C.D. *et al.* (1973) *Pneumocystis carinii* pneumonia in two foals. *J. Am. Vet. Med. Ass.*, **162**, 648–652

Silverman, S., Poulos, P.W. and Suter, P.F. (1976) Cavitary pulmonary lesions in animals. *J. Am. Vet. Radiol. Soc.*, **17**, 134–146

Sweeney, C. and Gillette, D. (1989) Thoracic neoplasia in equids: 35 cases (1967–1987). *J. Am. Vet. Med. Ass.*, **195**, 374–377

Toal, R.L. and Cudd, T. (1986) Equine neonatal thoracic radiography: a radiographic-pathologic correlation. *Proc. Am. Ass. Equine Pract.*, **32**, 117–128

Uhlorn, M., Hurst, M. and Demmers, S. (2006) Disseminated eosinophilic pulmonary granulomas in a pony. *Equine vet. Educ.*, **18**, 178–181

Verschooten, F., Oyaert, W., Muylle, E., DeMoor, A., Steenhaut, M. and Moens, Y. (1977) Diaphragmatic hernia in the horse: four case reports. *J. Vet. Radiol.*, **18**(2), 45–50

Walker, M. and Goble, D. (1980) Barium sulphate bronchography in horses. *Vet. Radiol.*, **21**, 85–90

Wisner, E., O'Brien, T., Lakritz, J. *et al.* (1993) Radiographic and microscopic correlation of diffuse interstitial and broncho-interstitial pulmonary patterns in the caudodorsal lung of adult Thoroughbred horses in race training. *Equine vet. J.*, **25**, 293–298

Chapter 13
The alimentary and urinary systems

Although the oesophagus could be discussed in a regional manner, we have chosen to include it in its entirety with the alimentary system. Diseases of the diaphragm are discussed with the thorax (see Chapter 12, page 642). Abdominal radiography in an adult horse is difficult and only limited information can be obtained. In many instances ultrasonography has the potential to yield more information. Therefore emphasis is placed on those conditions in which abdominal radiography is of real value: abdominal radiography of foals and on the use of contrast studies for the diagnosis of abdominal diseases.

RADIOGRAPHIC TECHNIQUE

Equipment

With the exception of the cervical oesophagus, the radiographic evaluation of the alimentary system of adult horses cannot be accomplished with portable equipment. High-output portable units can be used in small horses and foals, and small-animal x-ray units can be used for young foals and miniature horses. Radiography of the abdomen of adult horses is of little value except for the diagnosis of enterolithiasis, diaphragmatic hernia (see page 642), bowel obstruction, sand impaction in the large colon and urinary calculi. These studies in adult horses can only be performed with large stationary equipment and exposures in the range 90–120 kVp and 180–600 mAs. It is difficult, if not impossible, to obtain diagnostic radiographs from horses with an abdominal width greater than 70 cm. Digital systems or conventional radiography using fast rare earth screens are recommended and a focused grid is essential. A grid with a 140 cm focus, 103 lines per cm and a 10:1 ratio is recommended for use with film. Grids used for digital systems must be chosen by trial and error, to avoid the production of moiré lines.

Abdominal radiography in an adult horse is usually performed standing, using four views with overlapping fields: (a) cranioventral, (b) mid-ventral, (c) mid-dorsal and (d) dorsocaudal. In young foals and miniature horses one or two views are usually sufficient to evaluate the entire abdomen (Figures 13.1, 13.2a and 13.2b). Recumbent radiographs may be obtained, but standing lateral films are preferred (Figures 13.3a and 13.3b). The radiographs should be obtained with the side with the area of interest next to the cassette. Regardless of positioning for the initial radiograph, a second one should be obtained in the opposite lateral position, centred over the area of concern. Evaluation of the stomach should always be performed

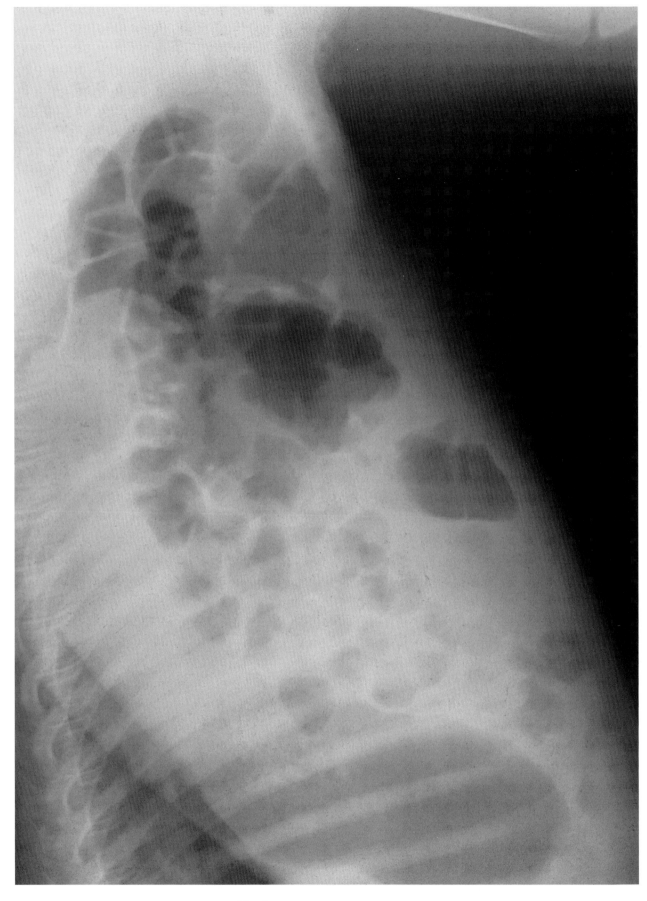

Figure 13.1 Lateral radiograph of a normal abdomen of a 6-day-old Thoroughbred filly, obtained with the foal recumbent. There is gas, fluid and food material within the stomach. The lack of abdominal visceral detail is due to the age of the patient. There is gas in the large and small bowel.

with the left side against the cassette. In a recumbent foal both lateral and ventrodorsal views are recommended, especially when contrast material is used.

Positioning

The oesophagus

Examination of the oesophagus of adult horses should be performed with the patient standing with its left side next to the cassette. If recumbent radiographs are obtained, the patient should be in left lateral recumbency. If contrast material is to be used in a conscious recumbent animal, it should be limited to barium paste which is easier to swallow and less likely to be aspirated than barium suspension.

The abdomen

Abdominal radiography in young and adult horses is always performed in the standing position, whereas abdominal radiography of the neonatal equine patient or a miniature horse may be carried out either standing or in lateral recumbency, with the cassette placed on the floor or using a standard x-ray table. Standing and recumbent abdominal radiographs differ in the distribution of gas and fluid. Gas-capped fluid levels can only be evaluated on radiographs obtained in the upright (standing) position (Figure 13.3b). Ventrodorsal radiographs of adult horses are seldom used because of the need for general anaesthesia and the paucity of information gained; however, they can be obtained in neonates and miniature horses using minimal chemical restraint.

Contrast examinations

Contrast examinations are covered in detail with each specific area to be examined, but the clinician must be aware of the basic principle that proper evaluation of a hollow viscus requires that the viscus must be distended. The distension can be obtained with positive contrast (barium- or iodine-containing compounds), negative contrast (air) or a combination of the two. In general, micropulverized barium sulphate should be administered as a 30% (weight per volume) suspension. In foals and young horses, a dosage of 5 ml/kg body weight may be used, whereas in adult horses a dosage of 3 ml/kg body weight is recommended. When a barium paste is used the dosage is quite variable, depending on the tolerance of the patient; usually half a tube of esophotrast is adequate. The paste is placed in the mouth and the patient is allowed to swallow in a normal manner. For contrast studies of the abdomen the patient should be starved for 12 hours prior to the examination to enhance detail.

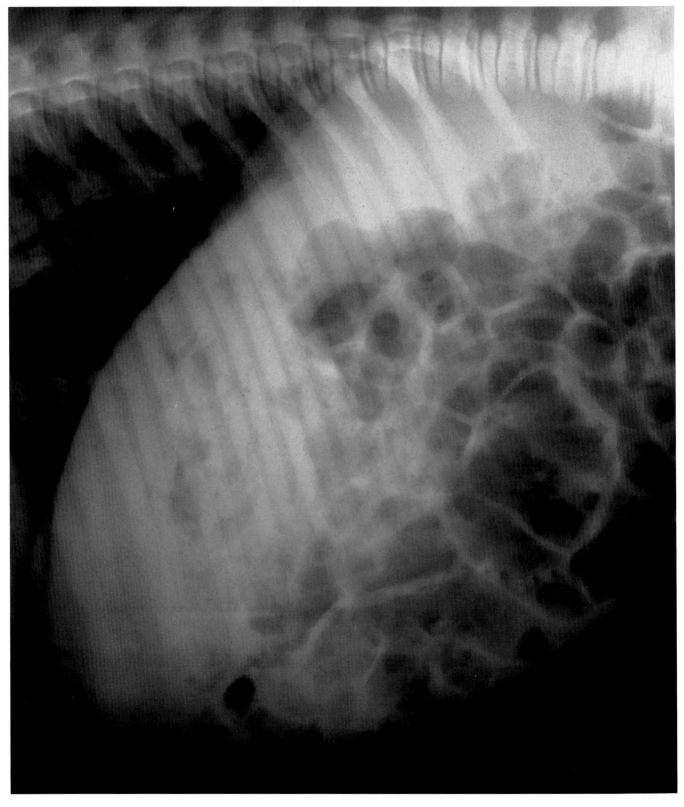

Figure 13.2(a) Lateral recumbent radiograph of the normal cranial abdomen of a 3-day-old foal. There is food and gas within the stomach. The large and small bowel are mostly gas-filled loops without evidence of overdistension.

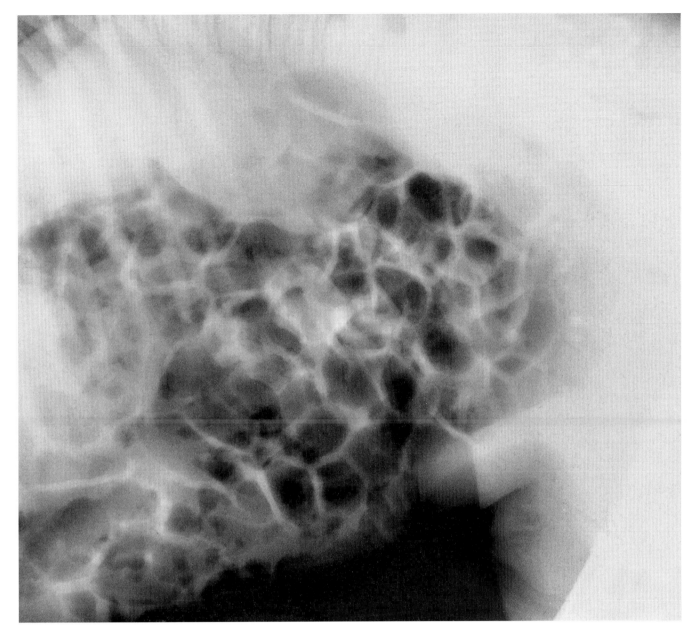

Figure 13.2(b) Lateral recumbent radiograph of the normal caudal abdomen of a 3-day-old foal, demonstrating gas- and fluid-filled large and small bowel loops. The urinary bladder can be seen adjacent to the caudoventral abdominal wall.

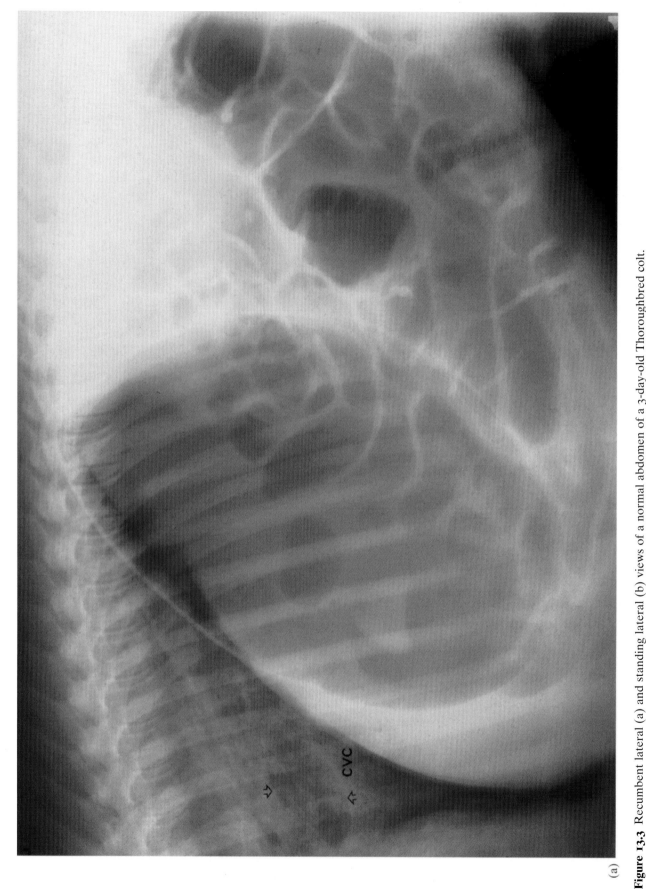

(a)

Figure 13.3 Recumbent lateral (a) and standing lateral (b) views of a normal abdomen of a 3-day-old Thoroughbred colt. (a) There is a well circumscribed gas lucency noted in the caudal oesophagus (arrows) overlying the caudal vena cava (CVC). There is gas and fluid distension of the stomach. The large and small bowel contain both gas and fluid, but there is no indication of overdistension or obstruction. There is a generalized increase in interstitial markings in the portions of the lung that are visible. This is probably due to age and pressure from the distended stomach, preventing complete inflation.

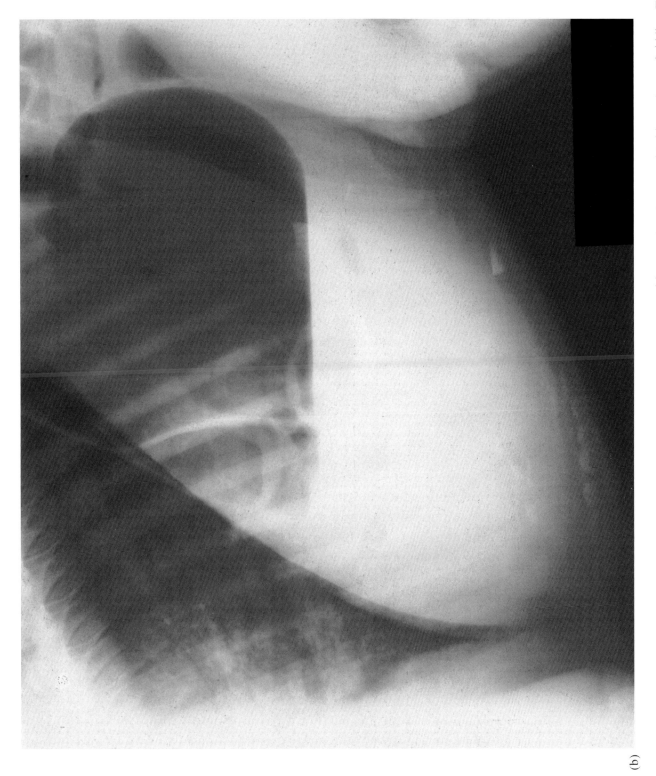

(b)

Figure 13.3 *Cont'd* (b) This standing lateral projection of the abdomen was obtained several hours after (a). Note that the gas and fluid now form a fluid line. The caudal abdomen cannot be as well visualized in the standing lateral film due to the position of the limbs which cover the caudal abdomen. Gas and fluid can be seen in both the large and small bowel. Opaque material in the ventral colon is sand.

Oesophagus

RADIOGRAPHIC TECHNIQUE

The appropriate technique is discussed on page 651, and contrast studies on page 653.

NORMAL ANATOMY AND ACTION OF THE OESOPHAGUS

In the normal horse there is no air in the oesophagus. As the oesophagus passes through the thoracic inlet it may drape over, and partially obscure, the dorsum of the trachea. The oesophagus then elevates slightly as it passes over the heart and caudally through the cardia into the stomach.

When eating, a bolus of food (or contrast material) gradually collects rostral to the epiglottis at the base of the tongue. When the horse swallows, the bolus passes into the retropharyngeal area and on into the oesophagus. It is carried rapidly down the oesophagus by the stripping motion of the oesophageal contractions. The passage of a bolus takes between 4 and 10 seconds. Although the act of deglutition can only be followed with fluoroscopy, the results can often be noted on serial radiographs obtained after the administration of contrast material.

Contrast examination of the oesophagus

When there is a history of dysphagia, oesophageal obstruction or recurrent oesophageal disease, and survey radiographs are normal, a contrast examination of the oesophagus should be performed. Barium paste is used to evaluate the oesophageal mucosa. The paste coats the mucosa and has the advantage of outlining structures for several minutes. In the normal oesophagus the contrast medium is seen as fine radiopaque linear streaking outlining the longitudinal oesophageal mucosal folds after the passage of the bolus. A bolus may be seen on a single radiograph, but will normally pass on gradually, or be carried away with the next bolus. The bolus should not be in the same location in subsequent radiographs.

Barium suspension is the contrast medium of choice when diverticuli or mega-oesophagus are suspected, because of the greater volume of contrast material required to demonstrate such changes. Liquid barium given per os or by stomach tube into the cranial oesophagus is passed in a similar manner to barium paste, but does not coat the oesophageal mucosa as well. Occasionally a small amount of contrast material is held momentarily at the thoracic inlet or just cranial to the cardiac silhouette. Contrast medium may also remain momentarily at the cardia, but will pass gradually into the stomach. Barium-coated food such as pellets or hay can also be used to demonstrate strictures which may not be demonstrated by the use of liquid barium alone.

Delayed oesophageal emptying and distension with air and contrast material have been reported as a sequel to recent passage of a nasogastric tube and have been associated with the use of tranquillizers.

If liquid barium is administered by mouth, in some cases traces will be seen dorsal to the soft palate, or in the larynx or trachea. This is abnormal and indicative of abnormal pharyngeal function. A clinical evaluation of the nasopharynx and larynx should be performed to differentiate conditions such as cleft palate, a foreign body and Eustachian tube diverticulum mycosis from primary oesophageal diseases.

DISEASES OF THE OESOPHAGUS

Diseases of the oesophagus can be divided into three main categories.

Diseases that decrease the diameter

Stricture from scar tissue

Scar tissue results from damage due to previous trauma such as choke, a foreign body, a penetrating wound, previous surgery or overzealous attempts to relieve a choke. The stricture can usually be demonstrated with barium paste, but may require a mixture of food and barium. The wall is normally smooth at the point of stricture and barium and/or food will be retained cranial to the stricture (Figure 13.4).

Abscessation

Abscessation of the oesophageal wall may result from penetration from inside or outside. Soft-tissue swelling and irregularity of the mucosal surface may be noted when an abscess originates from internal trauma. The mucosal surface may be smooth if the abscessed wall has not yet ruptured into the lumen. Wounds to the oesophagus may result in fistula formation as well as scarring and abscessation as noted above. Following rupture of the oesophagus, food and gas may be seen in the perioesophageal tissues (Figure 13.5).

Spasm

Spasm is usually a temporary condition and may not be found on subsequent radiographs. The mucosal surface is smooth and a second examination is often necessary to differentiate spasm from stricture.

External masses

Pressure from adjacent tissue such as a tumour, goitre or external abscess may be identified by noting that the oesophagus, dilated by contrast material, appears to deviate around a soft-tissue mass rather than being

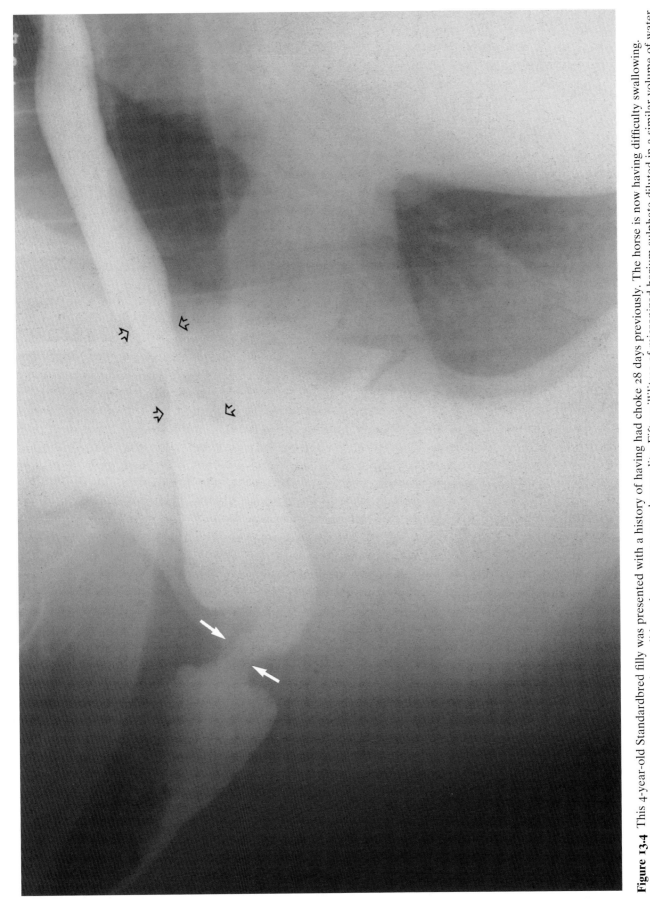

Figure 13.4 This 4-year-old Standardbred filly was presented with a history of having had choke 28 days previously. The horse is now having difficulty swallowing. Survey radiographs of the cervical oesophagus did not demonstrate any abnormality. Fifty millilitres of micronized barium sulphate diluted in a similar volume of water was administered via stomach tube in the cranial oesophagus. There is a stricture of the oesophagus at the thoracic inlet (solid arrows), with pre- and post-stenotic dilatation. A second area of stenosis is noted caudal to the first (open arrows). The remainder of the oesophagus is normal. Diagnosis: oesophageal stricture at two locations.

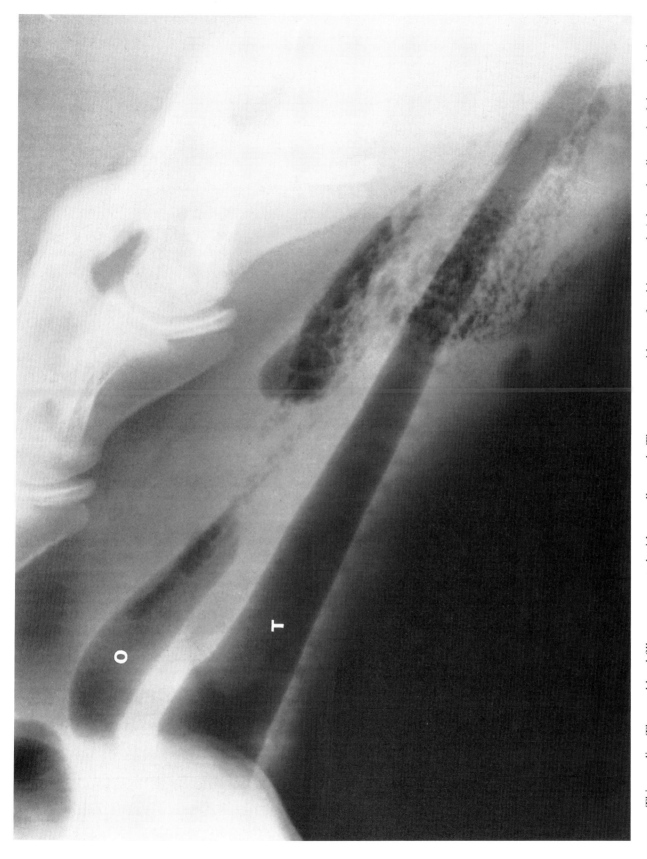

Figure 13·5 This yearling Thoroughbred filly was presented with a swollen neck. There was no evidence of a skin wound. A lateral radiograph of the cervical area demonstrates the soft-tissue swelling which appears to compress the trachea (T) and narrow the tracheal lumen. There is gas in the cranial oesophagus (O) and a mottled irregular appearance representing both gas and food material in the soft tissues. Diagnosis: ruptured oesophagus with food and gas in the peri-oesophageal soft tissues.

completely encircled by the mass. Ultrasonographic examination may be very helpful in these cases.

Neoplasia

Oesophageal neoplasia is extremely rare in the horse, but must be considered in cases where there is a mass and irregularity of the mucosal surface of the oesophagus. The differential diagnosis includes abscessation.

Diseases that increase the diameter

Mega-oesophagus – dilatation of the oesophagus

The affected segment of the oesophagus may be dilated with gas (Figure 13.6), fluid or food, either alone or in combination (Figure 13.7).

Mega-oesophagus may be focal, resulting from a stricture, a foreign body or an annular ring anomaly, or may involve the entire oesophagus due to neuromuscular dysfunction or abnormality of the cardiac sphincter. Generalized mega-oesophagus has been reported in chronic grass sickness in the United Kingdom. In foals, generalized mega-oesophagus may be seen in gastroduodenal ulcer disease (Figure 13.7) (see page 665). Focal mega-oesophagus with accumulation of food is usually considered to be the result of oesophageal obstruction (see below). Lack of oesophageal motility can be demonstrated using liquid barium and obtaining several exposures without moving the patient. If oesophageal motility is present, the contrast column or contrast–air interface will change. A common sequel to mega-oesophagus is aspiration pneumonia (see page 632).

Diverticuli

Horses with a diverticulum may have either a history of spontaneous occurrence or of previous injury or choke. Diverticula may be classified as either pulsion or traction. A pulsion diverticulum is the result of mucosal herniation through an acquired defect in the muscularis, due to overdilatation at an impaction site which caused separation of the muscularis. These diverticuli may be large. Regardless of size or cause, a diverticulum appears as a rounded out-pouching of the oesophagus rather than the linear appearance of the normal oesophagus cranial and caudal to the diverticulum (Figures 13.8a-c and 13.9a-c). A traction diverticulum is usually small and of little significance. It may have a pointed rather than rounded appearance because it results from perioesophageal scarring which exerts traction on a segment of the wall.

Oesophageal dysfunction and obstruction (choke)

Choke

Although oesophageal obstruction is often related to the rapid ingestion of food, it may also occur secondarily to scar formation or diverticula (Figures 13.8 and 13.9) within the oesophagus or as a result of impingement upon the oesophagus from masses or annular ring anomalies, or for no discernible reason.

The radiographic appearance varies depending upon the cause of the obstruction, but most often has a mottled gas and soft-tissue opacity resulting from the mixture of gas and food material (Figures 13.8 and 13.9). The mass is most commonly oval in shape. Air may be seen at one or both ends of the mass and conforms to the shape of the mass and then tapers sharply to a point. The obstruction may occur at any location within the oesophagus, but the thoracic inlet, base of the heart and the cardia are the most common sites when there is no underlying pathology as the cause of the obstruction.

Contrast material will aid in the definition of the obstruction, but care must be taken that reflux of the contrast into the trachea does not occur. Aspiration pneumonia may be seen as a sequel to oesophageal obstruction (see page 632). A post-treatment control study, using barium sulphate paste, is helpful in the evaluation of the oesophagus after the obstruction has been relieved (Figure 13.9).

Grass sickness

In some cases of grass sickness (in the United Kingdom) a bolus of food (or contrast medium) passes down the oesophagus more slowly than normal and may oscillate to and fro, particularly at the thoracic inlet or at the diaphragm. A bolus may remain stationary at the diaphragm for several minutes before passing into the stomach.

Abdomen and gastrointestinal tract

RADIOGRAPHIC ANATOMY

Foal abdomen

The most common reason for abdominal radiography in a foal is acute abdominal discomfort. In young foals, abdominal structures may be poorly visualized due to the lack of abdominal fat that usually helps differentiation of structures (Figure 13.10). A normal standing lateral abdominal radiograph has the appearance of a mixture of gas, fluid and ingesta, with occasional bowel loops showing gas-capped fluid levels. There is often a large amount of gas in the terminal bowel. Distension of small bowel loops is considered to be present when their diameter is slightly greater than the length of the body of the first lumbar vertebra. This measurement can only be made when there is enough gas distension for the small bowel loops to be identified.

Right lateral standing position

The fundus of the stomach is located adjacent to the left crus of the diaphragm, with the body of the stomach inclining slightly forward against the

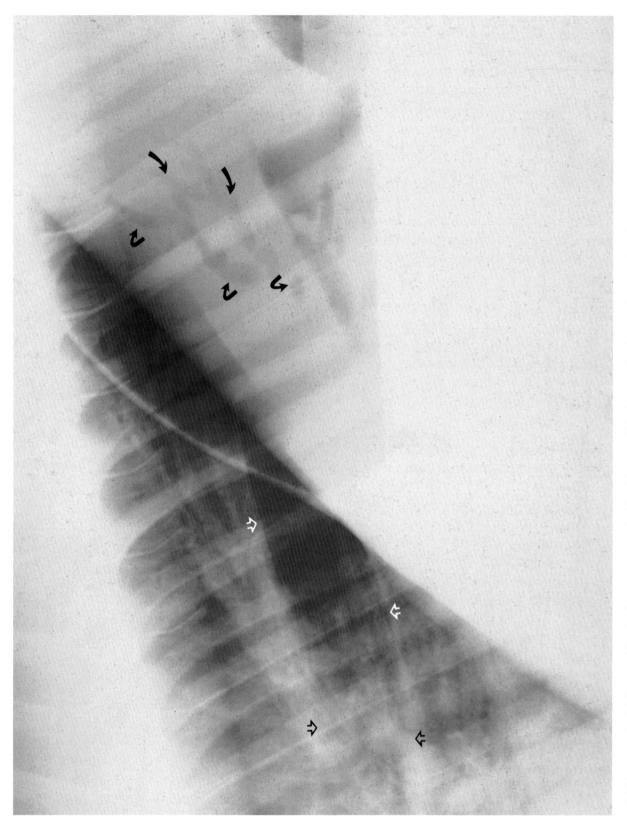

Figure 13.6 This 4-month-old Thoroughbred colt was presented with a history of black tarry diarrhoea. The tentative diagnosis was gastroduodenal ulcer disease. The gas-distended oesophagus is seen in the caudal dorsal thorax, between open arrows. The increased opacity in the caudal dorsal lung lobes is due to pulmonary interstitial infiltrates. A fluid line can be seen in the gas- and fluid-distended stomach. Gas is seen in the biliary tree (curved arrows). Radiographic diagnosis: gastric dilatation with air and fluid, mega-oesophagus, pulmonary interstitial infiltrates and gas in the biliary tree. These findings are indicative of gastroduodenal ulcer disease of the foal.

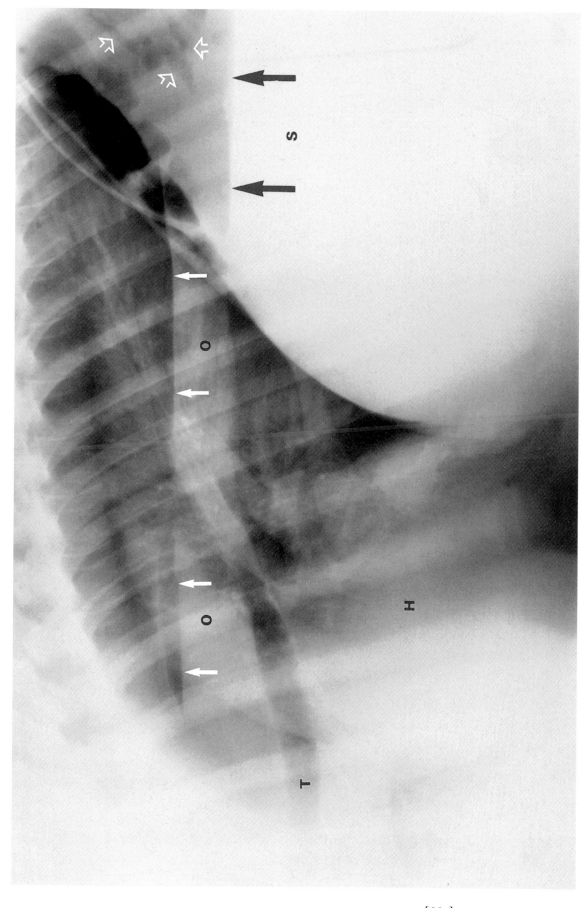

Figure 13-7 This 1-month old Thoroughbred colt was presented depressed and with a painful abdomen, with a 3-week history of signs compatible with gastric ulcer disease. The lateral radiograph demonstrates mega-oesophagus with fluid and air resulting in a gas-capped fluid line (solid white arrows) in the dilated oesophagus (O). The oesophagus is depressing the trachea (T) over the base of the heart (H). There is a mixed alveolar and interstitial pattern in the caudal ventral lungs which is best seen over the caudal margin of the cardiac silhouette. The stomach (S) is distended with fluid and air, resulting in a gas-capped fluid level (large black arrows). Gas can also be seen in the biliary tree as branching lucencies (open white arrows) over the opaque liver. Diagnosis: gastroduodenal ulcer disease with mega-oesophagus, aspiration pneumonia and gas in the biliary tree.

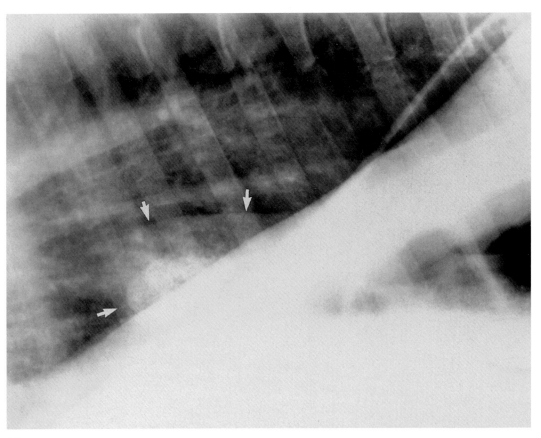

(a)

Figure 13.8 This 14-year-old Quarterhorse mare had a history of four episodes of nasal regurgitation in the previous 6 months.

(a) Survey radiograph of the caudal thorax demonstrates focal dilatation of the caudal oesophageal hiatus (arrows). There is dense granular food material within the mass. Tentative diagnosis: oesophageal diverticulum or gastro-oesophageal invagination.

(b) Approximately 50 ml of micropulverized barium sulphate was administered via stomach tube and a radiograph of the suspected diverticulum was obtained immediately. Contrast material is seen in the normal oesophagus to the level of the mass, where it passes over the mass and delineates the dorsal border. Increased interstitial markings in the lungs probably represent chronic fibrosis secondary to regurgitation.

(c) Administration of additional barium sulphate and air dilates the oesophagus and demonstrates the extent of the diverticulum (curved white and black arrows). A fluid line can be seen in the oesophagus due to the air–fluid interface. The dorsal oesophageal margins are marked (open white and black arrows). Diagnosis: oesophageal diverticulum and secondary pulmonary fibrosis.

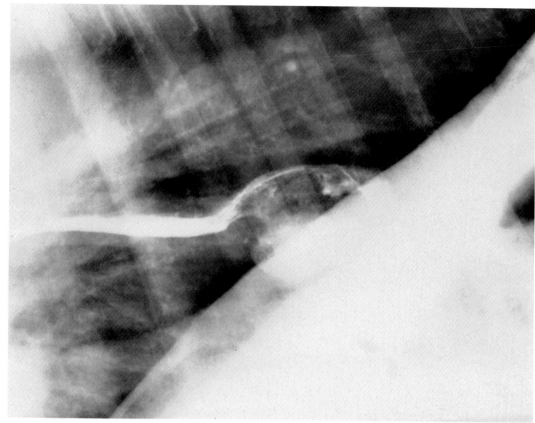

(b)

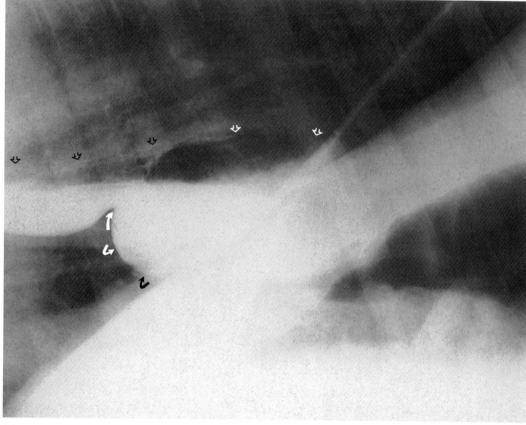

(c)

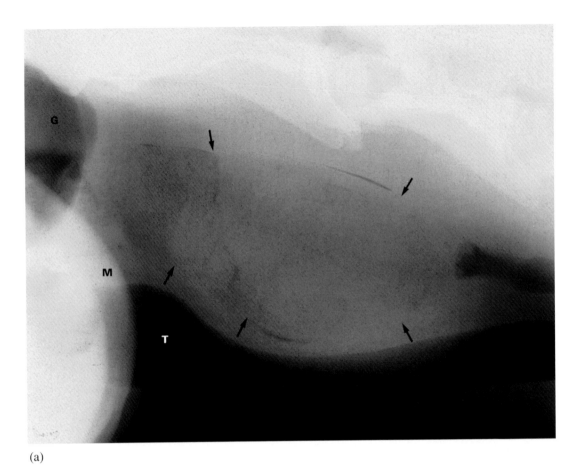

(a)

Figure 13.9(a) A lateral radiograph of the cranial cervical oesophagus demonstrating a large granular gas- and fluid-containing mass within the oesophagus (arrows), compressing the trachea ventrally. There is gas caudal to the mass within the oesophageal lumen. The guttural pouches are identified (G). The right and left rami of the mandible (M) can be seen over the guttural pouches, a portion of the oesophagus and the trachea (T). Diagnosis: oesophageal obstruction, 'choke' of the cervical oesophagus.

Figure 13.9(b) Six days after relief of the 'choke' the oesophagus remains dilated and somewhat irregular. There appears to be mucosal folding at several locations (curved arrows). The trachea remains compressed beneath the gas-containing mass. Gas can also be noted in the lateral ventricle (L).

Figure 13.9(c) Barium sulphate paste was administered immediately following the survey radiographs (b). The contrast examination demonstrates mucosal irregularity and contrast material in the wall of the oesophagus. The thickened oesophageal wall can be seen between the contrast column and the trachea. The trachea is depressed by the mass. Aspirated contrast material lines the tracheal wall. The oesophagus is normal beyond the developing diverticulum. Diagnosis: oesophageal obstruction due to chronic oesophageal wall disease and developing diverticulum.

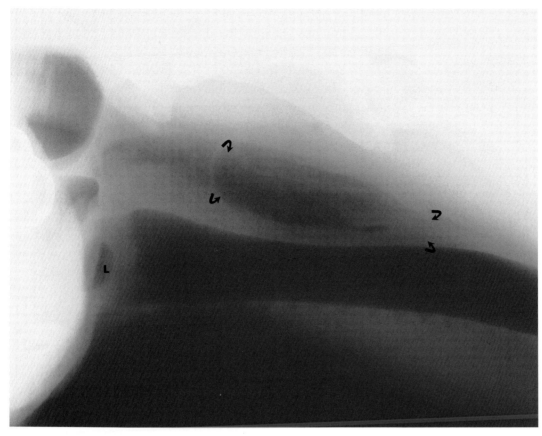

(b)

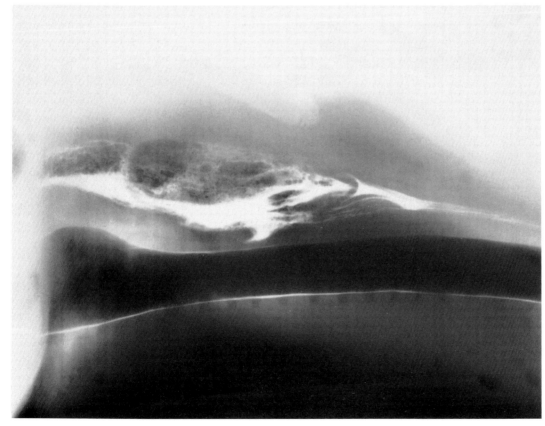

(c)

[669]

liver. When both air and fluid are present in the stomach, there is a gas cap dorsally in the fundus and against the diaphragm. Fluid and/or food are located ventrally in the pyloric area. Gastric size is considered normal when the width is approximately half the length. The duodenum exits the pylorus near the mid- to ventral third of the abdomen. The diaphragmatic flexure of the colon is found ventral to the stomach and in contact with the liver. The ventral colon is just caudal to the diaphragmatic flexure against the ventral abdominal wall. Crescent-shaped folds may be identified between the haustra of the ventral colon when the content is more or less dense than soft tissue. The caecum is located in the mid-abdomen and often has a gas cap. The colon lies ventrally with the sternal flexure, beneath the diaphragmatic flexure. The dorsal and ventral flexures of the colon cannot usually be separated. The pelvic flexure is found ventrally adjacent to the urinary bladder. The small colon and rectum are located dorsocaudally. The kidneys are rarely seen radiographically.

Right and left lateral recumbent positions

There is little change in the anatomical location of structures, but they may become more or less visible due to the shifting of air and fluid contents or, in the case of contrast examination, the passage of contrast material silhouetted against soft tissue or a gas-filled viscus.

Ventrodorsal position

The stomach is located to the left of the midline, with the diaphragmatic flexure of the colon crossing over against the liver and occupying the right cranial abdomen. The duodenum exits the pyloric antrum caudal to the main body of the stomach and the sigmoid loop extends approximately two-thirds of the way to the right body wall, just caudal to the ventral colon, before passing caudally as the descending loop. The descending loop passes caudally to about the level of the last rib before changing course medially and cranially to form the caudal flexure. The jejunum is caudal to the stomach and lies mostly on the left side. The base of the caecum is located in the right caudal abdomen, with the apex near the xiphoid cartilage. The small colon is located on the left side. The right and left ventral and dorsal large colon lie on both sides ventrally.

Adult abdomen

The liver lies adjacent to the diaphragm and separates the stomach from the sternum in the cranioventral abdomen. The stomach is craniodorsal on the left side, but is not fixed in position.

ANATOMICAL VARIATIONS

The main difference in the anatomy of the foal and the adult horse is the relative change in size of the stomach, the caecum and large colon. In the foal the stomach is larger in proportion, but this decreases with age as the caecum and colon increase in size.

Contrast studies in the foal

Survey radiographs should always be obtained before the administration of contrast material in order to have baseline information regarding the size, shape and position of organs prior to contrast administration.

A foal cannot be fasted for the same time interval as an adult because fluid and electrolyte balance must be maintained. Therefore, fasting should not be more than 4 hours in foals that are still on fluid diet and 12 hours for foals that are eating solid food. Fasting should be limited to solid matter and not fluids. Contrast material should be administered by nasogastric tube at the rate of 5 ml of barium sulphate suspension (30%w/v) per kilogram. Radiographs should be obtained immediately and at 30 minutes, 1 hour and then at hourly intervals thereafter until the contrast reaches the small colon. Additional radiographs can be obtained as required. When possible, standing right lateral and ventrodorsal radiographs should be obtained. Normal transit time is approximately 8 hours.

The stomach is best evaluated using a double-contrast technique following a 4–12-hour fast (see above). Barium sulphate suspension 30%w/v is then administered via stomach tube at a rate of 5 ml/kg. Normally there is adequate air in the stomach, but if not it should be slightly distended by administration of air. Care must be taken not to overdistend the stomach. The standing patient is placed with the left side to the cassette and radiographed. In a recumbent foal, right and left lateral recumbent and ventrodorsal radiographs should be obtained immediately following administration of the contrast and air. These radiographs should be repeated at 30 minutes, 1 hour and 2 hours post-administration. Contrast material may begin to exit the stomach as early as 10 minutes after administration, but emptying may vary greatly depending on the gastric content. The pylorus and the duodenum may not be recognized as distinct features, but contrast material may be defined in the descending duodenum within the first 10 minutes as it exits the pylorus in the mid- to lower third of the abdomen and passes over the gas-filled stomach. The remainder of the small bowel then fills and contrast usually reaches the caecum in 4–5 hours.

DISEASES OF THE GASTROINTESTINAL TRACT

Small intestinal obstruction

Multiple small intestinal loops are distended with gas and fluid (Figures 13.10, 13.11; see also Figure 13.13a, page 676). Hairpin curves are often noted, as well as many gas-capped fluid levels. The stomach may also be gas distended. Mechanical or functional obstruction cannot be differentiated.

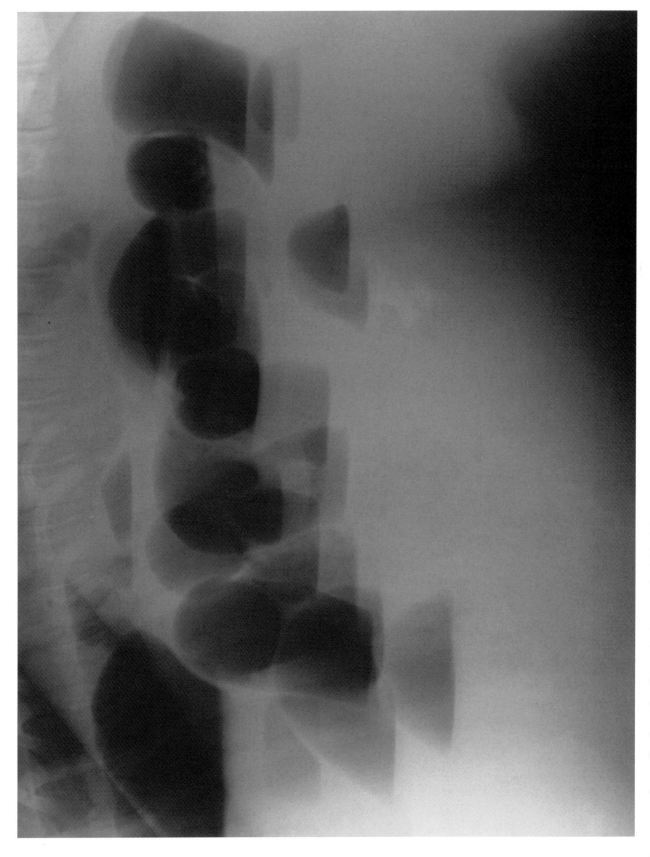

Figure 13.10 A standing lateral radiograph of a 3-week-old foal demonstrates lack of abdominal visceral detail which is apparently within the large intestinal structures. The very opaque material is sand within a bowel segment. The moderately dilated small intestinal loops with unequal fluid levels (inverted Us) are suggestive of mechanical ileus.

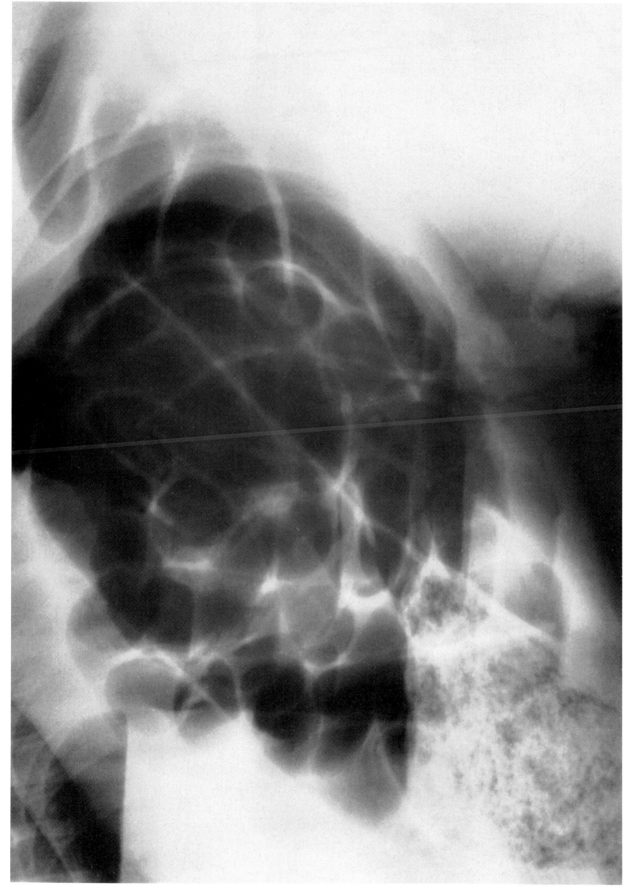

Figure 13.11 Thoroughbred foal with suspected meconium impaction. There are gas-distended large and small intestines. Cranioventrally there is granular-appearing material in the large bowel which probably represents retained meconium. Gas in the rectum is thought to be secondary to enemas. Radiographic diagnosis: obstructive ileus, probably due to meconium in the mid-large bowel.

Large intestinal obstruction

Meconium retention or large intestinal obstruction may be visualized on lateral standing or recumbent radiographs as an ileus (Figures 13.11 and 13.12). Gas-distended bowel may outline the meconium retention. If the meconium is not visualized on a survey radiograph, barium or air may be placed in the rectum with the aid of either a stomach tube and gravity flow or a rubber syringe, thus demonstrating the area of blockage. With a barium or air enema care must be exercised. Stop immediately if pressure is encountered.

Atresia coli

Atresia coli has been reported in foals and must be differentiated from other causes of ileus and colic. The lesion can be demonstrated by injection of contrast into the rectum, showing a lack of communication with the remainder of the large intestine (Figure 13.13b).

Ileocolonic aganglionosis

Ileocolonic aganglionosis occurs in white progeny of Overo Spotted Horses: 'lethal white foal'. These foals are normal at birth but do not defaecate. They develop signs of colic in the first day of life and this must be differentiated from meconium retention, atresia coli (which may also occur in these foals) and atresia ani, as well as other causes of colic. Radiographic diagnosis in these cases is based on ruling out other causes of colic and on the presence of distension of the stomach, small intestines and large bowel. A barium enema will not be expelled due to lack of contractility.

Gastroenteritis

There is a decrease in the granular appearance of the bowel content, which appears to be more uniformly fluid filled than normal. Gas-capped fluid levels may be common, but there is no distension and hairpin loops are seldom seen. The gas caps do not stay in the same location on subsequent films, indicating that there is intestinal motility. Transit time is usually much shorter than the expected 8 hours.

Gastroduodenal ulcer disease in foals

Standing lateral radiographs demonstrate gastric distension that does not diminish with fasting. A gas cap is usually noted and air is often seen in the hepatic ducts (see Figures 13.6, page 664 and 13.7, page 665). Double-contrast gastrography, performed with the foal in right lateral recumbency, demonstrates delayed gastric emptying for up to 4 hours and the contrast fills the pylorus and duodenal ampulla. Ulcers in the non-glandular portion of the stomach may be demonstrated as round to elliptically shaped lucent (black) filling defects with well marginated walls of increased opacity (white).

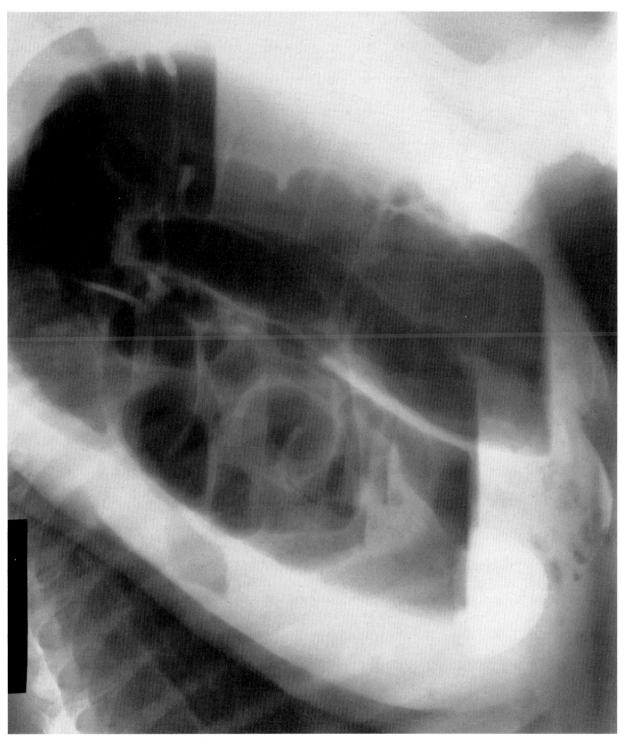

Figure 13.12 This 1-week-old Quarterhorse filly was presented because of recurrent colic. Meconium has passed normally, but there had been no faecal matter noted since then. Radiographs of the abdomen demonstrated markedly dilated large bowel structures with variable fluid lines. The small bowel appears normal. There is sand in the stomach. Radiographic diagnosis: large bowel obstruction.

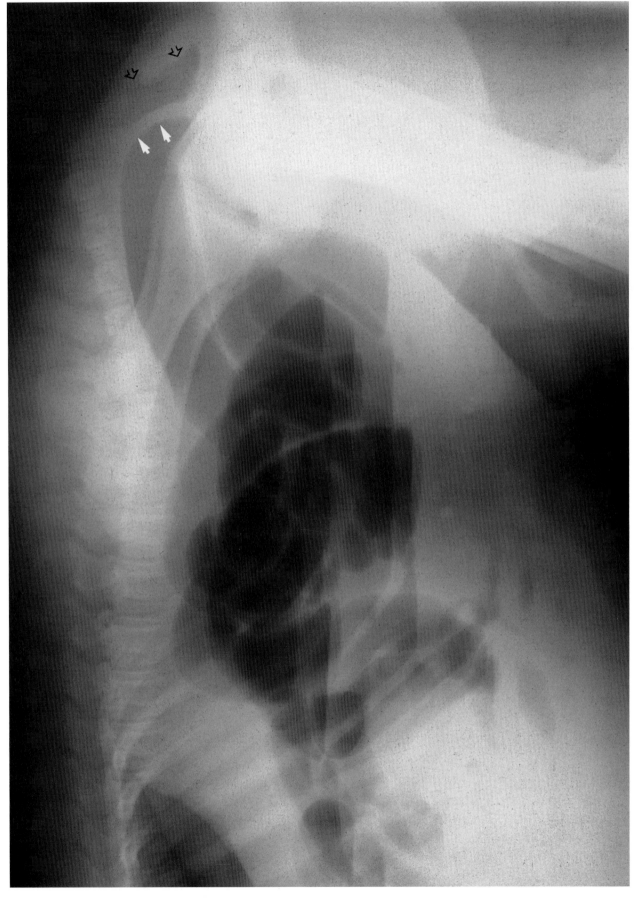

Figure 13.13 This 12-hour-old Arabian foal was born 3 weeks prematurely and had not passed meconium. (a) A survey radiograph shows fluid- and gas-distended bowel loops with varying fluid levels indicative of obstructive ileus. The large bowel appears to terminate at a soft-tissue wall (solid white arrows). Gas in the rectum (open arrows) does not appear to communicate with the remainder of the bowel.

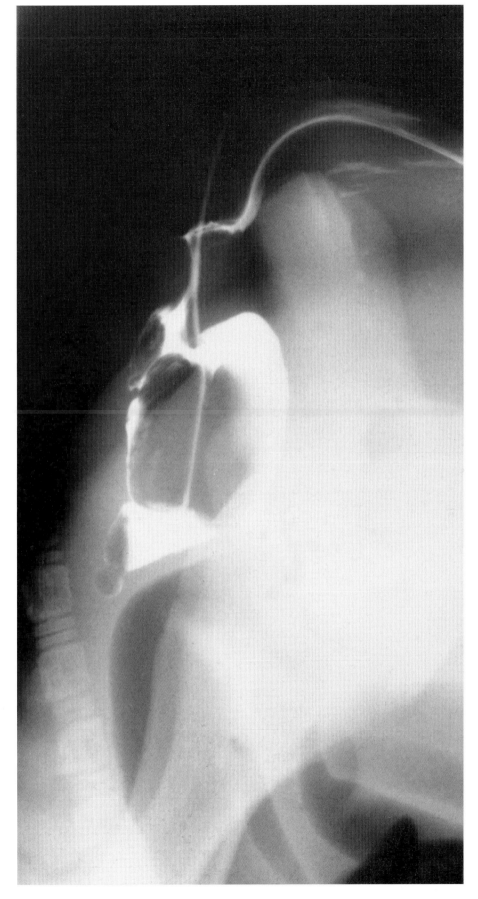

Figure 13.13 *Cont'd* (b) Barium sulphate injected into the rectum does not communicate with the terminal large bowel. The soft-tissue wall is again noted. Radiographic diagnosis: atresia coli.

Ulcers can best be demonstrated by obtaining both right and left lateral recumbent and ventrodorsal radiographs, which allow for double-contrast coating of the mucosal surfaces. Standing thoracic radiographs may demonstrate mega-oesophagus with fluid and/or air. Contrast studies may demonstrate gastro-oesophageal reflux or retention of contrast in the oesophagus. These foals often have increased interstitial lung markings which are in part due to an inability to make a maximal inspiratory effort due to the abdominal distension. Inhalation pneumonia may be a complication of this disease (see Chapter 12, page 632).

Rupture of a hollow viscus

A hallmark of rupture of a hollow viscus is free abdominal gas (Figure 13.14), which allows for visualization of the poles of the kidneys and is often seen between the stomach and the diaphragm. Gas-filled bowel loops appear to be elevated in the abdomen or to float due to free abdominal fluid, which also causes loss of abdominal visceral detail. The abdomen may appear pendulous and there may be a generalized increase in opacity of the abdomen.

Enterolithiasis of adult horses

Enterolithiasis should be suspected in patients with moderate, recurrent abdominal pain which is refractory to conservative therapy and when there is evidence of bowel obstruction. Enterolithiasis has been described in both the small intestine and the rectum, but the majority of cases occur in the colon.

When enteroliths are suspected, radiographs should be obtained with the right side of the horse against the cassette. Left lateral radiographs should be obtained if further information is needed. Radiographic diagnosis is made by defining single or multiple opaque enteroliths. The diagnosis is sometimes aided by the presence of air adjacent to an enterolith. Absence of radiographic findings does not preclude the presence of enteroliths, nor does the presence of an enterolith alone signify the presence of obstructive bowel disease.

Sand impaction

Sand impaction occurs most often in the ventral colon and results in occlusion of the lumen by an opaque mass.

Urinary system

In an adult horse, abdominal radiography for the diagnosis of urinary tract disease is primarily of use for identification of calculi. The use of ultrasound is generally superior for the evaluation of the kidneys.

[678]

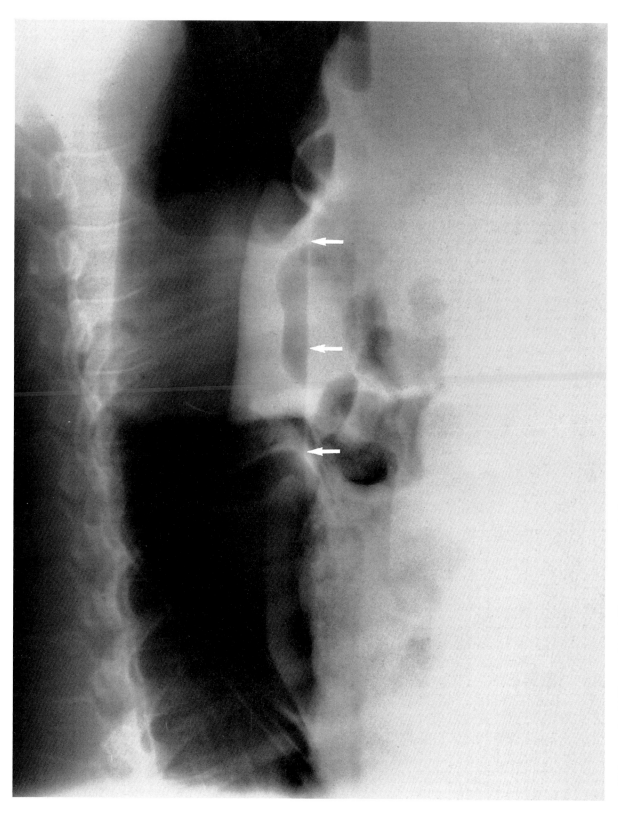

Figure 13.14 This 5-week-old Thoroughbred filly was presented with a history of prolonged diarrhoea. The patient had acute abdominal pain. The standing lateral radiograph reveals a lack of abdominal visceral detail ventrally. In the mid-portion of the radiograph, gas can be seen in bowel loops and multiple fluid levels are noted. Centrally in the mid-abdominal area there is a fluid line (arrows) which is not within a hollow viscus. This finding is indicative of free peritoneal air. Radiographic diagnosis: lack of abdominal visceral detail with free peritoneal air indicative of peritonitis and ruptured hollow viscus.

CONTRAST EXAMINATION

Intravenous pyelography is of limited value, but can be used to visualize the kidneys and ureters (see page 705). Cystography (positive or double contrast) is useful for evaluating the bladder of a foal (see below and page 704).

Positive contrast cystography should be preceded by survey radiography of the caudal abdomen to assess bladder size and position. A flexible catheter is then placed in the urinary bladder and urine withdrawn. This allows for evaluation of the urine as well as giving some idea of the volume of urine present. Since the catheter is now filled with fluid, air will not be injected into the bladder, causing artefacts at the beginning of the examination. Between 2 and 5 ml of local anaesthetic solution is injected through the catheter into the urinary bladder so that the bladder may be distended without causing discomfort. A solution of equal volumes of any water-soluble contrast material, which is recommended for intravenous use, and sterile saline is then injected. The total volume of contrast mixture required to distend the urinary bladder adequately can be calculated, at the rate of 12 ml/kg of body weight.

If no urine is retrieved after catheterization, half of the calculated amount of contrast can be infused and a radiograph obtained to evaluate the urinary bladder for content and placement. Additional contrast material, over the amount of urine withdrawn, or 50% of the calculated dose should be given slowly by syringe or by gravity flow. When resistance is noted, the filling should stop. Lateral and two ventrodorsal oblique radiographs are then obtained. These three views allow for visualization of the entire urinary bladder and assessment of the bladder wall. The positive contrast is then removed and an equal volume of air placed in the urinary bladder and the three radiographic views are repeated.

DISEASES OF THE URINARY BLADDER OF THE FOAL

Patent urachus

Although the diagnosis of congenital patent urachus does not require radiography, cystography and/or catheterization of the urachal remnant, these techniques may be of value in assessing the degree of the defect and the condition of the urinary bladder. Ultrasonographic examination of the urachus is often helpful in defining associated abscesses, free fluid and to monitor patency. A patent urachus (Figure 13.15) or urachal remnant (Figure 13.16) often result in cystitis (see below) and may be the nidus for recurrent cystitis as well as for the development of polyarthritis/polyosteomyelitis (see page 32). Patency may be demonstrated radiographically either by placing contrast material in the urinary bladder or by injection of the urachal remnant. Umbilical cord infection is often present without the presence of a patent urachus. Acquired patent urachus is caused by extension of inflammation and necrosis from the umbilical artery, vein or urachal remnant causing the urachus to reopen.

[680]

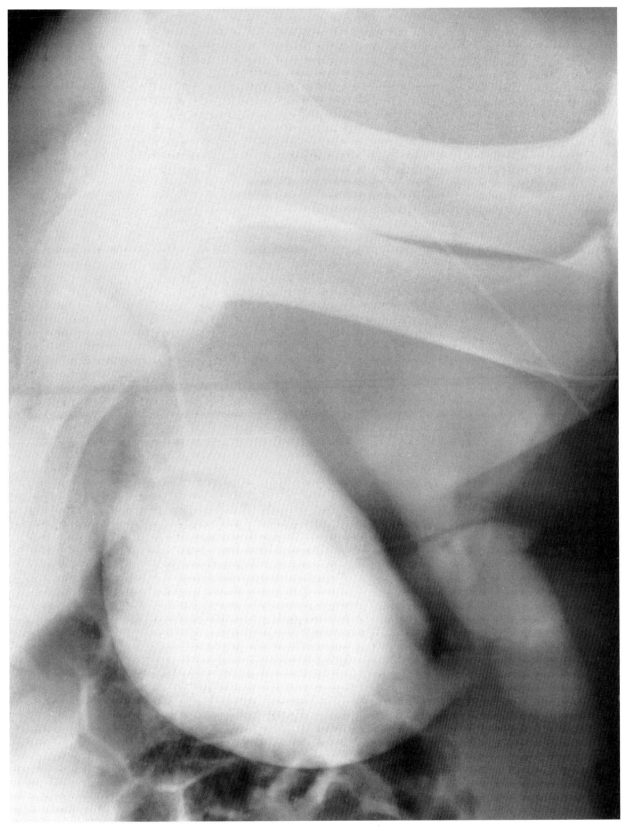

Figure 13.15 This 1-day-old Thoroughbred colt was presented because of a swollen prepuce and umbilicus. A patent urachus was suspected and a cystogram was performed by the placement of a catheter into the urinary bladder. Distension of the urinary bladder with contrast material demonstrates a patent urachus in the cranial ventral bladder wall and accumulation of contrast material in the subcutaneous tissues of the abdominal wall.

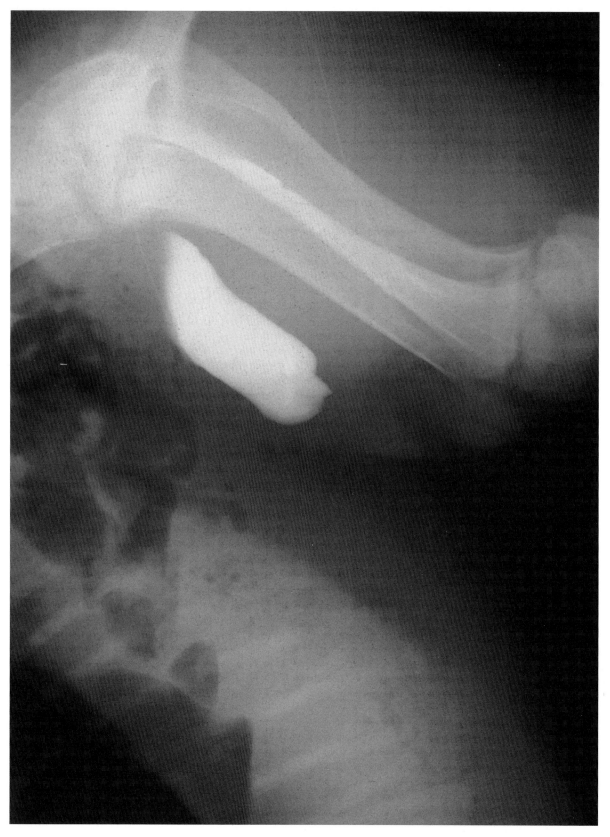

Figure 13.16 This 10-day-old Arabian colt presented because he did not exteriorize his penis and had urine scalds. Cystitis was suspected and a cystogram was performed by injection of contrast material through a urethral catheter. The standing lateral radiograph demonstrates a normal foal abdomen. The urinary bladder is in a normal position, but there is a urachal remnant noted in the mid-ventral portion of the urinary bladder. The bladder wall is thickened adjacent to the diverticulum. Radiographic diagnosis: urachal diverticulum with concurrent cystitis.

Cystitis

Cystitis, regardless of cause, is evident radiographically by the appearance of a thickened and irregular bladder wall. The cranial ventral portion of the bladder is often more severely affected. In severe cases the entire bladder wall may be involved. Thickness and irregularity of the bladder wall can only be assessed when the urinary bladder has been adequately distended.

Rupture

Rupture of the urinary bladder is most common in the foal. The most consistent radiographic sign is the presence of free abdominal fluid, but an ileus may result and signs of ileus as well as the presence of fluid may be noted (see page 678).

The area of rupture may be demonstrated by cystography but demonstration may require that radiographs are obtained while contrast material is being instilled into the urinary bladder. Free contrast material in the abdominal cavity does not present a problem so long as a sterile solution of water-soluble contrast is used and the patient is well hydrated. Barium should never be placed in the urinary bladder.

Ultrasonographic examination can demonstrate free fluid in the abdomen but will not demonstrate a tear.

FURTHER READING

Aanes, W.A. (1975) The diagnosis and surgical repair of a diverticulum of the oesophagus. *Proc. Am. Ass. Equine Pract.*, **21**, 211–222

Adams, S.B. and Fessler, J.F. (1987) Umbilical cord remnant infections in foals: 16 cases (1975–1985). *J. Am. Vet. Med. Ass.*, **190**, 316–318

Bowman, K.F., Vaughan, J., Quick, C., Hankes, G., Redding, R., Purohit, R., Rumph, P., Powers, R. and Harper, N. (1978) Mega-oesophagus in a colt. *J. Am. Vet. Med. Ass.*, **172**, 334–337

Campbell, M.L., Ackerman, N. and Peyton, L.C. (1984) Radiographic gastrointestinal anatomy of the foal. *Vet. Radiol.*, **25**, 194–204

Campbell-Thompson, M.L., Brown, M., Slone, D., Merritt, M., Moll, H. and Levy, M. (1986) Gastroenterostomy for treatment of gastroduodenal ulcer disease in 14 foals. *J. Am. Vet. Med. Ass.*, **188**, 840–844

Dik, K.J. and Kalsbeek, H.C. (1985) Radiography of the equine stomach. *Vet. Radiol.*, **26**, 48–52

Fischer, A.T., Kerr, L.Y. and O'Brien, T.R. (1987) Radiographic diagnosis of gastrointestinal disorders in the foal. *Vet. Radiol.*, **28**, 42–48

Fischer, A. and Yarbrough, T. (1995) Retrograde contrast radiography of the distal portions of the intestinal tract in foals. *J. Am. Vet. Med. Ass.*, **207**, 734–737

Gehlen, H., Stadler, P. and Ohnesorge, B. (2005) Tracheal obstruction in a horse with oesophageal stenosis and diverticulum. *Equine vet. Educ.*, **17**, 132–134

Greet, T.R.C. (1982) Observations on the potential role of oesophageal radiography in the horse. *Equine vet. J.*, **14**, 73–79

Greet, T.R.C. and Whitwell, K.E. (1986) Barium swallow as an aid to the diagnosis of grass sickness. *Equine vet. J.*, **18**, 294–297

Hultgren, B.D. (1982) Ileocolonic aganglionosis in white progeny of Overo Spotted Horses. *J. Am. Vet. Med. Ass.*, **180**, 289–292

Korolainen, R. and Ruohoniemi, M. (2002) Reliability of ultrasonography compared to radiography in revealing intestinal sand accumulation in horses. *Equine vet. J.*, **34**, 499–504

Pankowski, R.L. and Fubini, S.L. (1987) Urinary bladder rupture in a two-year-old horse: Sequel to a surgically repaired neonatal injury. *J. Am. Vet. Med. Ass.*, **191**, 560–562

Pearson, H., Pinsent, P.J.N., Polley, L.R. and Waterman, A. (1977) Rupture of the diaphragm in the horse. *Equine vet. J.*, **9**, 32–36

Peterson, F.B., Donawick, W., Merritt, A., Raker, C., Reid, C. and Rooney, J. (1972) Gastric stenosis in a horse. *J. Am. Vet. Med. Ass.*, **160**, 328–332

Rantanen N. and McKinnon, A. (1998) *Equine Diagnostic Ultrasonography*, 1st edn, Williams and Wilkins, Baltimore

Reef, V. (1998) *Equine Diagnostic Ultrasound*, 1st edn, W.B. Saunders, Philadelphia

Rose, J.A., Rose, E.M. and Sande, R.D. (1980) Radiography in the diagnosis of equine enterolithiasis. *Proc. Am. Ass. Equine Pract.*, **26**, 211–220

Ruohoniemi, M., Kaikkonen, R., Raekallio, M. and Luukkanen, L. (2001) Abdominal radiography in monitoring the resolution of sand accumulation from the large colon of horses treated medically. *Equine vet. J.*, **33**, 59–64

Schleining, J. and Voss, E. (2004) Hypertrophic osteopathy secondary to gastric squamous cell carcinoma in a horse. *Equine vet. Educ.*, **16**, 304–307

Schneider, J.E. and Leipold, H.W. (1978) Recessive lethal white in two foals. *J. Equine Med. Surg.*, **2**, 479–482

Swain, J., McGorum, B., Scudamore, C. and Pirie, R. (2004) Persistent oesophageal obstruction (choke) associated with diverticulum of the terminal oesophagus in a pony. *Equine vet. Educ.*, **16**, 195–200

Traub, J.L., Gallina, A., Grant. B., Reed S., Gavin, P. and Paulsen, L. (1983) Phenylbutazone toxicosis in the foal. *Am. J. Vet. Res.*, **44**, 1410–1418

Verschooten, F., Oyaert, W., Muylle, E., De Moor, A., Steenhaut, M. and Moens, Y. (1977) Diaphragmatic hernia in the horse: four case reports. *Vet. Rec.*, **18**, 45–50

West, H.J. and Kelly, D.F. (1987) Renal carcinomatosis in a horse. *Equine vet. J.*, **19**, 548–551

Wimberly, H.C., Andrews, E.J. and Haschek, W.M. (1977) Diaphragmatic hernias in the horse: a review of the literature and analysis of six additional cases. *J. Am. Vet. Med. Ass.*, **170**, 1404–1407

Yarsborough, T., Langer, D., Snyder, J. *et al.* (1994) Abdominal radiography for diagnosis of enterolithiasis: 141 cases (1990–1992). *J. Am. Vet. Med. Ass.*, **205**, 592–595

Chapter 14
Miscellaneous techniques

ARTHROGRAPHY AND BURSOGRAPHY

Arthrography is the technique of introducing a contrast medium into a joint prior to obtaining radiographs. It has been used to aid evaluation of articular cartilage, meniscal damage, subchondral bone and synovial membrane. It may be indicated in cases showing chronic joint distension, without apparent radiological abnormality on plain radiographs, radiographic findings incompatible with the clinical signs, or suspected joint capsule or articular cartilage damage. More specific indications include: evaluation of joint capsule ruptures or penetration; evaluation of cartilage flaps in osteochondrosis; to look for a cartilaginous joint fragment; and to differentiate between intra-articular and extra-articular bone fragments. It can also be used to determine whether an osseous cyst-like lesion communicates with a joint. Bursography is the technique of introduction of a contrast medium into a bursa. It can be used to assess the integrity of the bursal wall, to identify filling defects due to a space-occupying lesion and, for example, to facilitate identification of a fibrocartilage defect of the navicular bone. Diagnostic ultrasonography can also be useful in assessment of some of these problems. Contraindications for arthrography may include infections of the joint or adjacent tissues, inflammation and patients known to be allergic to contrast media.

For positive (or radiopaque) contrast studies, any media approved for intravenous use may be used. Concentrated contrast media may obscure the joint surface, and thus obscure the lesions they are intended to outline, so dilution of the media may be required. Approximately 25% triiodinated water-soluble contrast material is recommended. Some radiologists recommend the use of negative (or radiolucent) contrast (air, nitrogen or carbon dioxide), or double contrast, i.e. the use of negative and positive agents together. Negative-contrast techniques may cause artefacts, due to gas bubbles forming in the synovial fluid during injection, and for this reason negative and double-contrast studies are not often carried out. The formation of bubbles can be reduced by injecting the gas prior to the positive medium, and by using a positive medium with a low viscosity.

Technique

The patient may require sedation or general anaesthesia. The skin overlying the joint is prepared aseptically. Plain survey radiographs should be obtained immediately prior to the contrast study in order to re-evaluate the joint, as the contrast agent may remain in the joint or adjacent tissues for some time, making subsequent plain radiography impracticable.

A needle is introduced into the joint using aseptic technique. A volume of synovial fluid is then withdrawn and the equivalent volume of contrast agent introduced. The volumes will vary from 2 to 20 ml, depending on the size of the joint concerned. For double-contrast studies, as much fluid as possible is withdrawn initially, and after injection of positive contrast as much fluid as possible is again withdrawn. The joint is then distended with gas in order to outline the structures of the joint. (Although this is the normal technique, allowing radiographs to be made with positive contrast only if desired, it has been suggested that introduction of the gas first results in fewer artefacts from the formation of bubbles.)

After the injection of contrast agents, the joint should be extended and flexed, in order to spread the agents evenly throughout the joint. The study should be completed as soon as possible, and certainly within 20 minutes, or the contrast material will begin to be absorbed through the synovial membrane and the sharp appearance of the structures will be lost (see Figure 3.80b, page 165, and Figure 6.10, page 286).

Diagnostic criteria

Positive contrast medium will fill the joint, mixing with the synovial fluid. It will thus outline the joint pouches and will lie as a thin layer over the cartilage surfaces. The radiograph should be carefully examined, initially to ensure that areas of contrast conform with the normal anatomical shape of the joint. Subsequently the areas of contrast should be searched for any lucent areas (filling defects). These may represent radiolucent tissue masses (e.g. in chronic proliferative synovitis, see Figure 3.80b, page 165), or simply be areas of the joint to which contrast has failed to be dispersed for some other reason. The differentiation between the two may be difficult, but further passive movement of the joint may help ensure even filling. The cartilage surfaces should be carefully examined for irregularity of the contrast film adherent to the cartilage surface. This may be particularly useful for detection of cartilage flaps, where contrast medium will be seen between the flap and the underlying bone, resulting in a visible cartilage irregularity and a lucent area in the contrast medium overlying the defect.

Positive contrast arthrography is frequently used to determine if a wound has penetrated a synovial cavity. The joint capsule must be adequately distended with the contrast medium to determine if there is any leakage.

If double contrast studies are used, care must be taken that bubbles of gas are not misdiagnosed as tissue masses.

TENDONOGRAPHY

The term 'tendonography' includes any radiographic study of tendons. However, plain radiography of tendons is generally not very rewarding and so this section only describes studies involving the use of contrast agents. The tendons and ligaments on the palmar and plantar aspects of the third metacarpal and metatarsal bones may be visualized using contrast agents. This can be useful in the diagnosis of tendonitis, tendovaginitis and contracture of the palmar/plantar annular ligaments of the metacarpophalangeal and metatarsophalangeal joints. *The techniques have been largely superseded by the use of the diagnostic ultrasonography.*

Technique

Radiological examination of the tendon sheaths and bursae can be made in a manner similar to that described above for arthrography, using similar techniques and concentrations of contrast medium. For evaluation of soft-tissue structures, however, the use of air as the contrast agent is often preferable.

Air tendograms can be made of the tendons between the tendon sheaths. The technique is normally carried out under mild sedation with the horse standing, although general anaesthesia may improve the results. An area of skin is clipped over the centre of the flexor tendons of the metacarpus/metatarsus, on the palmar or plantar surface. The skin is then prepared aseptically. Local anaesthetic is infiltrated at the site where the contrast is to be injected, to desensitize the area of injection. A needle is passed through the skin and air injected subcutaneously and between the flexor tendons and ligaments. One hundred millilitres of air is usually sufficient. In order to separate the tendons and peritendonous tissues, considerable pressure may be required. Most of the air will be resorbed in 24 hours, and no adverse reactions have been reported. Standard radiographic views are made, using approximately half the mAs normally required.

Diagnostic criteria

The radiographic anatomy of the tendon sheaths is relatively complex, and the reader is referred to specific papers in the 'Further reading' list if they wish to embark upon this technique. Contrast studies permit the assessment of sheath or dorsal wall thickness, integrity of the synovial wall and adhesion formation.

Air tendograms of the flexor structures of the limb aid assessment of the thickness of the flexor tendons, and allow accurate measurement and comparison. Enlargements are normally indicative of tendon strain. If peritendonous swelling is present, the outlines of the tendons lose sharpness. Adhesions will result in failure of the structures to separate. Rupture of ligaments and tendons can also be confirmed. *However, ultrasonography has largely superseded this technique.*

ANGIOGRAPHY

Angiography is the technique whereby blood vessels are visualized by the injection of a positive-contrast agent at the time of radiography. It is used to gain information about the anatomical position of blood vessels, to gain evidence of vascular disease and, in some circumstances, to study the flow of blood through the vessels. Although it has been largely used for experimental purposes in equine veterinary medicine, it has an important role to play in the investigation and treatment of certain diseases, such as auditory tube diverticulum mycosis (see page 492) and suspected vascular abnormalities. It has also been used extensively in studies of the distal limb of the horse.

The technique is normally (but not invariably) carried out under general anaesthesia. For examination of the arteries, a positive contrast agent is injected into a major artery supplying the area. For venous studies, however, contrast may be injected via a major artery, allowing normal flow to carry it into the veins, or it may be injected directly into a suspected venous abnormality. It is also possible to stop venous outflow from an area with a tourniquet, and inject contrast into a vein, filling the veins 'against the flow', i.e. a retrograde injection. Although it is advantageous to obtain a series of radiographs after injection in order to visualize flow through the blood vessels, it may be adequate for many clinical cases to obtain a single radiograph, the timing depending on the area to be examined, but generally being about 2–5 seconds after the end of the injection.

Technique

The skin over the vessel to be injected is prepared as for surgery. Subcutaneous vessels may be injected directly with a percutaneous injection, but deeper vessels such as the carotid or common digital arteries are best approached surgically. It is important that arteries are handled with care, as trauma may cause spasm and give false results. It is recommended that the Seldinger technique be used to catheterize arteries, as this permits the introduction of a catheter of relatively large diameter with the minimum of trauma. After the study is completed, the catheter may be withdrawn and haemorrhage controlled by applying finger pressure to the vessel for at least 2 minutes. For deeper injection sites, it is recommended that the tissues should be sutured and the incision closed prior to the withdrawal of the catheter, unless the patient is suspected to have clotting defects. Subsequent to withdrawal, pressure applied to the area with fingers or a pressure pad and bandage is normally adequate to stem haemorrhage. If a very large-diameter catheter is used, then a purse-string suture should be placed in the vessel wall prior to removal of the catheter, and pulled tight and tied after catheter withdrawal. Once a catheter has been introduced into a blood vessel, it may be passed on through the vessel, and manipulated to follow branches of the vessel (e.g. the internal carotid artery may be catheterized by passing a catheter with a curved tip along the common carotid artery). When injections of contrast are made, the tip of the catheter should be positioned at least 5 cm to the cardiac side of any branches of the vessel that are to be examined as part of the study.

A pressure injector is recommended if flow studies are required, or for adequate visualization of large vessels where a large volume of contrast is required. Hand injections are adequate in many practice situations, although they may require the use of a larger-diameter catheter to allow injection of adequate volumes of contrast medium. There are many contrast media available for use in angiography and there are no special requirements for

[688]

the horse. The volume of contrast agent required should be just sufficient so that when the injection is completed, it fills the arterial vessels only, with no contrast evident in the capillary bed or veins. This varies with the area involved and the size of patient (approximately 5 ml for an injection into the common digital artery or 20 ml for injection into the common carotid).

Diagnostic criteria

Figures 14.1, 14.3(a), page 692, and 14.3(b), page 693, show normal angiograms of the head and distal limb of a horse. A detailed description is not given, since reference to the figures will give adequate information on the normal. More detailed information on the techniques and results can be obtained from the 'Further reading' list given at the end of the chapter. The information that follows gives a general outline of the changes that can be anticipated to be found on angiograms of any area.

Clinically significant lesions found will vary with the site radiographed, but may include those given below.

Irregular arterial wall

1 There may be an irregular 'roughened' appearance to the arterial wall. There may be little overall change in diameter of the arterial lumen, or there may be obvious narrowing of a section or all of the artery. This may indicate arterial disease, e.g. thrombosis. This is seen in the internal carotid in some cases of auditory tube diverticulum mycosis, where it may indicate the initial stages of the artery thrombosing. It also occurs in the digital arteries of many horses, both 'normal' and with conditions such as navicular disease.

2 A condition known as 'beading' may occur, when the arterial wall goes into spasm. This gives regular narrowed bands along the length of the vessel, although the wall appears to have a generally smooth internal surface. This can occur in normal vessels, and is probably triggered by the pressure of the injection. It is most common in vessels that are already sensitive, either from rough handling when being catheterized or if suffering from arterial disease.

Distension of a vessel

1 A vessel may become enlarged because of an increased peripheral resistance or increased flow to an inflamed area, and does not necessarily indicate arterial disease.

2 Outpouchings of a vessel are abnormal. The most common cause is an aneurysm (Figure 14.2). This results from a weakness of the arterial wall, which allows the arterial lining to be forced through a defect in the wall. They are seen on angiograms as an outpouching, with a slight narrowing on the cardiac side of the defect. They may be congenital or acquired. Frequently they will give rise to spontaneous haemorrhage.

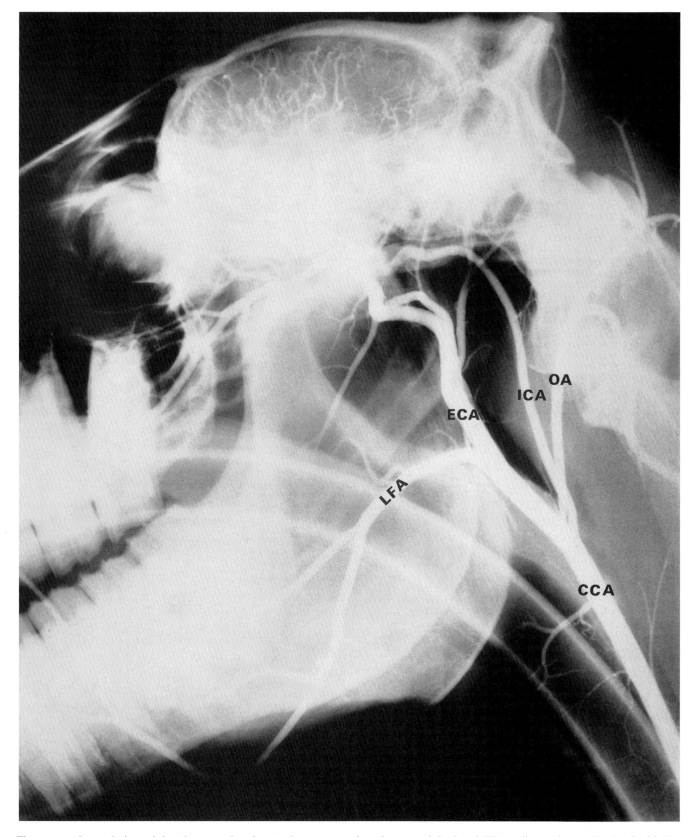

Figure 14.1 Lateral view of the pharyngeal region to show a normal angiogram of the head. The radiograph was obtained with the horse under general anaesthesia. Note the endotracheal tube, common carotid artery (CCA), occipital artery (OA), internal carotid artery (ICA), external carotid artery (ECA) and linguofacial artery (LFA).

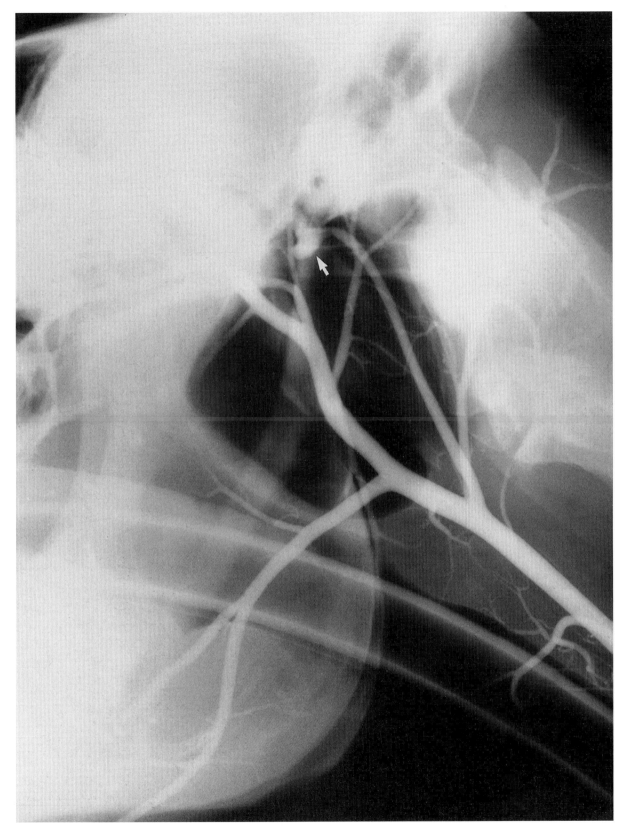

Figure 14.2 Lateral view of the pharyngeal region of a 7-year-old Thoroughbred with a recent history of epistaxis and dysphagia. Endoscopic examination confirmed the presence of auditory tube diverticulum mycosis. This angiogram demonstrates an aneurysm of the internal carotid artery (arrow).

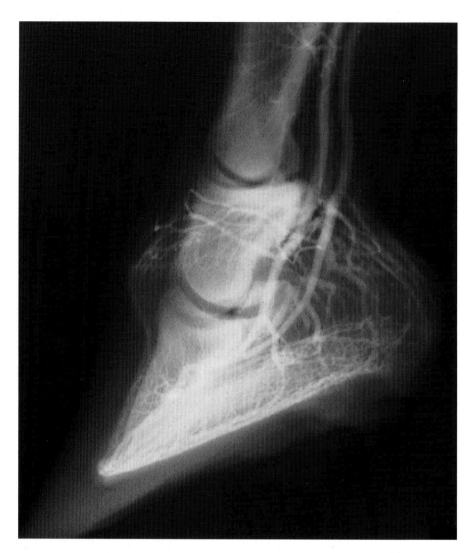

Figure 14.3(a) Lateral view of the foot of a normal pony. This angiogram was obtained 2.5 seconds after injection of the contrast medium into the common digital artery approximately 5 cm distal to the carpus (the pony was under general anaesthesia).

Narrowing of a vessel and failure to fill

Narrowing of a vessel and failure to fill have many common causes, which must be determined in the light of the available clinical information:

1 Arterial spasm may prevent a vessel filling or may cause partial filling or beading (see above). If serial radiographs are obtained using a rapid automatic serial plate changer, the vessel may be visible for part of the time, being occluded usually at the start of the injection. Repeat injections may be needed, but may result in repeat occlusion or narrowing of the vessel.

2 Another common cause of failure of an artery to fill is external pressure on the vessel. This may be caused by a haematoma, abscessation, neoplasia or incorrect positioning of the patient.

3 Arterial thrombosis may cause partial or complete occlusion of vessels (see also 'Distension of a vessel', above).

[692]

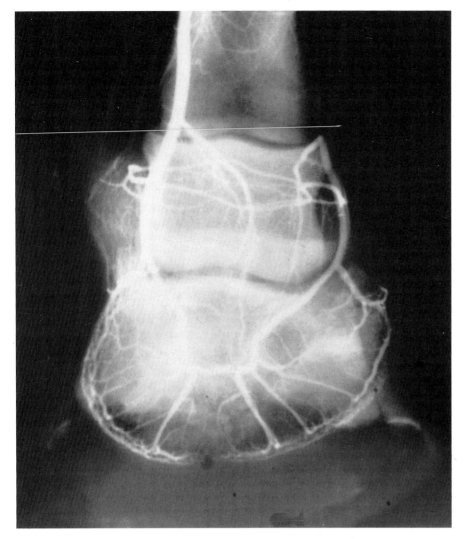

Figure 14.3(b) Dorsoproximal-palmarodistal oblique view of the foot of a normal pony. The angiogram was obtained 2.5 seconds after injection of the contrast medium into the common digital artery approximately 5 cm distal to the carpus (the pony was under general anaesthesia).

4 Inadequate concentration, volume or rate of injection of contrast medium may result in inadequate contrast for visualization of a vessel, or in vessels showing poor contrast.

VENOGRAPHY

Digital venograms are used to obtain information about the functional integrity of the venous blood flow within the digit, usually in cases of laminitis. The technique can be performed in a standing sedated horse, but requires a team of well prepared people. The pastern region in the region of the lateral palmar digital vein should be clipped. Perineural analgesia of the palmar nerves at the level of the proximal sesamoid bones is performed. A radiopaque marker is placed on the dorsal aspect of the hoof wall. The horse is positioned with the foot on a low wooden block. A tourniquet is fixed around the fetlock. The veterinarian positions himself in front of the limb so that shoulder pressure can be applied against the horse's carpus if it tries to move. A 21 gauge, 1.9 cm butterfly catheter with 30.5 cm tubing is placed in the lateral digital vein in the mid-pastern. Blood should flow freely. An assistant attaches a 12 ml luer lock syringe filled with 10 ml of diatrizoate sodium and the veterinarian injects the contrast agent; the first syringe is replaced by a second preloaded syringe. During injection of the second syringe the carpus is flexed and then extended to unload and reload the heel. When the injection is complete the catheter is clamped using mosquito forceps and lateromedial and dorsoproximal-palmarodistal oblique views are obtained, followed immediately by second lateromedial views. All radiographic views need to be acquired within 45 seconds of injection.

The lateral and medial digital veins, capillaries and arteries are filled retrograde, permitting visualization of the terminal arch, coronary plexus, dorsal lamellar vessels, circumflex vessels and vessels of the heel region (see Figure 3.34a, page 98). The second lateromedial view can demonstrate the contrast agent diffusing into the soft tissues, and may delineate an abnormality. In chronic laminitis, displacement of the distal phalanx, morphological changes in the laminae and compression of vessels can all contribute to alterations of the vasculature, notably in the coronary plexus, dorsal lamellar vessels and circumflex vessels (see Figure 3.34b, page 98). Such abnormalities may have some influence on treatment and prognosis.

MYELOGRAPHY

Myelography is the technique of introducing contrast agent into the spinal canal for radiography. It is usually performed to define the site or sites of cervical spinal cord compression in an ataxic horse, when a detailed clinical examination has suggested a lesion involving the cervical spinal cord. It is essential if surgical treatment is being considered. Survey radiographs should be obtained prior to myelography and are often suggestive of the site of a lesion. Recent evidence suggests that the technique can be unreliable and that semiquantitative evaluation of plain radiographs may be more accurate.

Technique

Myelography is best performed under general anaesthesia, since it results in fewer untoward side-effects, and the neck can be examined radiographically in the normal, flexed and extended positions. This is essential for identification of dynamic compressive lesions. Ventrodorsal views can also be obtained (see Chapter 10, page 507 for details of the radiographic technique). Myelography has been performed in the standing horse, but is not recommended.

At present, the following anaesthetic regimen is recommended for myelography, since it has been associated with minimal side-effects: premedication with acepromazine, detomidine or xylazine, followed by induction of anaesthesia using guianfenesin and thiopentone or ketamine, and maintenance using isoflurane or halothane in oxygen. Pretreatment with phenylbutazone is recommended.

The horse is positioned in lateral recumbency and plain lateral survey radiographs are obtained. It is important to support the neck with radiolucent cushions in order to obtain true lateral projections, which are essential for correct interpretation.

The skin over the poll is clipped and prepared as for surgery. The head is elevated approximately 30° and positioned so that the long axis of the head is perpendicular to the long axis of the neck. This prevents cranial passage of contrast material. An 18 gauge 86 mm spinal needle is inserted at the intersection of a line joining the cranial borders of the wings of the atlas and the dorsal midline. It is directed perpendicularly to the skin, aiming for the lower incisor teeth. A change of resistance can usually be appreciated as the needle penetrates the dorsal atlanto-occipital membrane and the cervical dura mater. The needle's stilette is withdrawn, and cerebrospinal fluid (CSF) will appear at the hub if the needle is correctly positioned. It is important not to insert the needle too deeply, since spinal cord puncture may result, with severe adverse consequences.

Approximately 40 ml of CSF is slowly withdrawn before injecting a similar volume of contrast agent over 3–5 minutes. Once injection is complete the needle is removed.

A superior technique involves the insertion of needles at both the cisterna magna and the lumbosacral subarachnoid cistern. A spinal needle is inserted on the dorsal midline approximately level with the cranial edge of the tubera sacrale and the caudal border of each tuber coxae, between the caudal edge of the dorsal spinous process of the sixth lumbar vertebra and the cranial edge of the second sacral dorsal spinous process. The latter landmarks can be difficult to palpate in a well muscled horse. Care should be taken to advance the needle in the sagittal plane. The needle is advanced into the ventral subarachnoid space, through the interarcuate ligament, dorsal dura mater and arachnoid and the conus medullaris. Forty to sixty millilitres of contrast are injected slowly via the cisterna magna, and CSF is allowed to flow from the lumbosacral site. The stilette should be replaced in the needle at the lumbosacral site while images are obtained. This method, although technically more difficult, encourages contrast agent to flow in a caudal direction.

Metrizamide has been successfully used in the horse, although there have been a number of side-effects, including delayed recovery from anaesthesia, muscle fasciculations, depression, pyrexia and deterioration of ataxia (it is not clear whether this last is due to the contrast agent or the affects of manipulating the neck during myelography and recovery from anaesthesia). Other, less irritant, non-ionic, water-soluble contrast agents have been introduced, and the use of either iopamidol (370 mg iodine/ml) or iohexol (350 mg iodine/ml) is strongly recommended. An iodine concentration of 300 mg/ml will give an adequate density in a small horse, but contrast may be poor in larger horses.

Approximately 5 minutes after completion of the injection (or 1–2 minutes if the double-needle technique is used), the horse's head may be

[695]

repositioned level with the rest of the body, and radiography can be repeated. Cranial, mid-neck and caudal neck views should be obtained routinely, with the neck in the neutral position. With the neck in flexion, at least cranial and mid-neck views should be repeated, and with the neck in extension, at least a caudal neck view should be repeated. Flexion and extension of the neck should be performed carefully to obtain radiographs in these 'stressed' positions, which will help to define any dynamic component to compression. If necessary, the horse may then be positioned in dorsal recumbency in order to obtain ventrodorsal radiographic views and identify sites of lateral compression. These views are difficult to obtain and are limited to the cranial two-thirds of the neck. The myelographic study should be performed quickly, since radiographic contrast may be reduced with time by dilution and resorption of the contrast agent.

Occasionally the contrast medium 'fails to flow' and accumulates in the region of the most cranial cervical vertebrae. It usually does eventually mix with cerebrospinal fluid, although resultant image quality may be poor. This is thought to be characteristic of subdural injection.

Interpretation of the myelogram

The myelogram should be evaluated with the neck in normal, flexed and extended positions in order to identify both static and dynamic lesions. Using 40 ml of contrast agent there should be complete filling of the subarachnoid space to the cervicothoracic junction. With the neck in the neutral position, the dorsal column of contrast agent is usually of more uniform width, and is wider than the ventral column (Figures 14.4a and 14.5). There is slight widening of the dorsal contrast column at the caudal aspect of each vertebral foramen, and slight narrowing at the cranial aspect of each vertebral foramen. The ventral contrast column usually narrows slightly and is slightly elevated at the intervertebral spaces.

If the neck is flexed, the width of the dorsal contrast column remains uniform (Figure 14.4b), whereas the ventral column becomes narrower at the intervertebral spaces due to pressure from the intervertebral disc. This is most marked at the articulations between the third and fourth, and fourth and fifth cervical vertebrae. Extension of the neck results in slight widening of the ventral column in the fifth, sixth and seventh cervical vertebrae, with no change in the dorsal column.

Diagnostic criteria

The aim is to determine if there is compression of the spinal cord. Focal narrowing of the dorsal contrast column when the neck is extended or flexed (Figures 14.6a, 14.6b and 14.7), together with narrowing of the ventral contrast column at similar sites, or occlusion of the passage of contrast agent, may be indicative of a site of spinal cord compression. Several different criteria have been used for determination of likely spinal cord compression using myelography, including a dorsal contrast column of <2 mm, narrowing of the dorsal contrast column by more than 50% and reduction of the dural diameter by more than 20%. However, a recent study that compared subjective assessment of plain radiographs, semiquantitative scoring of plain radiographs and myelography (positive results defined as ≥50% reduction in dorsal contrast column) in a group of horses with histologically confirmed spinal cord disease due to cervical vertebral malformation and a second group with other causes of spinal cord disease found that the semiquantitative method was most accurate. Semiquantitative measurements resulted in a higher sensitivity (87%) and specificity (94%) and more powerful positive predictive value (95%) and negative predictive value (84%) than either of the other techniques for identification of horses with spinal cord compression due to cervical vertebral malformation.

Narrowing of the dorsal column by more than 50% was generally considered to be significant, but should be interpreted with care and in the light of other findings. It is reasonably sensitive, but not very specific. False-positive results can occur. Focal narrowing of the ventral contrast column alone, when the neck is in the normal position or flexed, or of the dorsal column alone when the neck is extended, must be interpreted with extreme care, since these are normal findings. If a horse has either a narrow vertebral foramen or a small subarachnoid space, stress radiography is more likely to narrow the dural sac or obliterate the subarachnoid space. Overflexion can result in obliteration of both contrast columns in the mid-neck region, especially in small horses, and may potentially accentuate spinal cord damage. However, dorsal displacement of the spinal cord, so-called 'lifting', does usually reflect significant vertebral malalignment. The shape and angulation of the spinal cord should be assessed carefully. The myelogram should be carefully inspected for evidence of more than one site of potential narrowing of the vertebral canal, since this will influence surgical treatment and prognosis. In some instances, interpretation of the myelogram by subjective evaluation of the width of the contrast columns is equivocal. In these cases, measurements of the minimum dural sagittal diameter (Figure 14.8) may be useful, provided that a standardized radiographic technique is employed to allow for magnification, and comparison is made with horses of similar size. Alternatively the maximum and minimum dural sagittal diameters can be compared within a horse, with a 20% reduction in dural diameter being considered significant. In the caudal neck region (C6–C7) this technique has high sensitivity and specificity for detection of cervical stenotic myelopathy in both neutral and flexed positions, but in the mid-neck region this test has low sensitivity and high specificity in the neutral position. Flexion of the neck increases the frequency of false-positive diagnoses.

Separation of the dorsal or ventral contrast column from the wall of the vertebral foramen is suggestive of an epidural or extradural space-occupying lesion, e.g. epidural haemorrhage or a prolapsed intervertebral disc. False-negative results may occur due to failure to identify a laterally compressive lesion. With a laterally compressive lesion associated with cervical vertebral malformation the minimum sagittal diameter of the vertebra is often quite small, resulting in a low minimum sagittal dural diameter but within the normal range. There may be a blanching of the overall contrast column, widening of the sagittal shadow of the spinal cord and sometimes

[697]

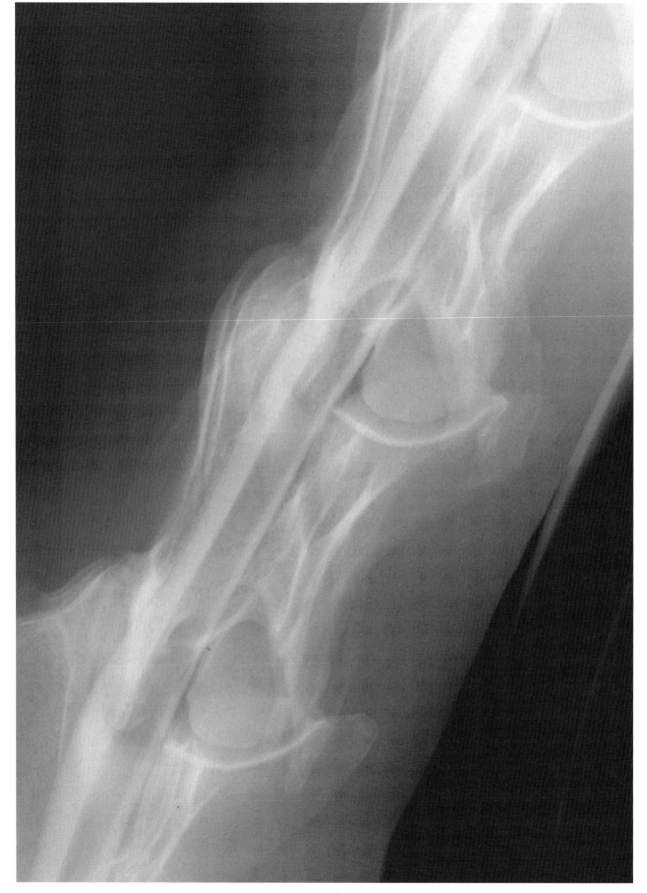

Figure 14.4(a) Lateral view of the second to fifth cervical vertebrae to show a normal myelogram of a mature Thoroughbred. Note that the dorsal contrast column is much wider than the ventral column. The ventral column narrows slightly at the intervertebral articulations, but the dorsal column remains of uniform width.

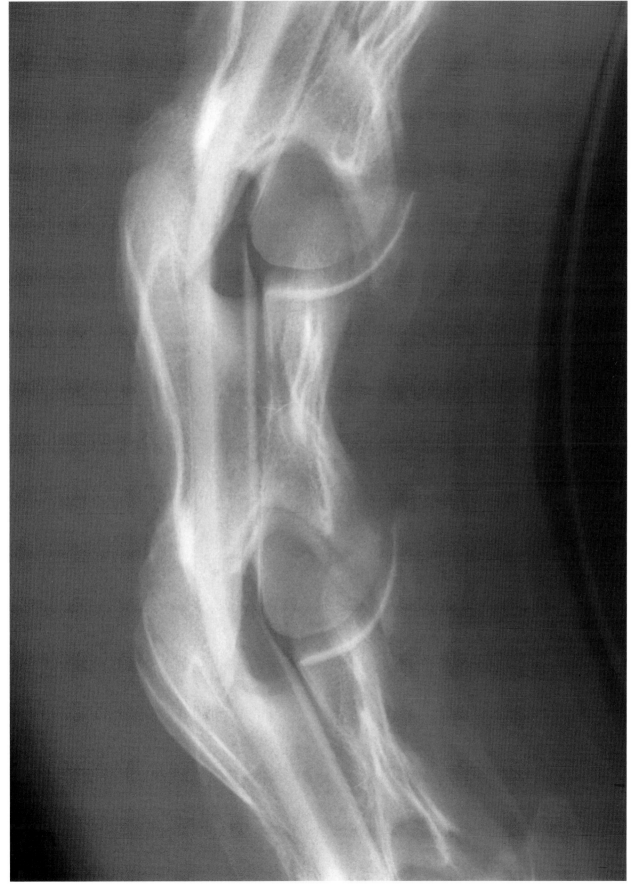

Figure 14.4(b) Flexed lateral view of the third to fifth cervical vertebrae to show a normal myelogram (the same horse as in Figure 14.4a). Narrowing of the ventral contrast column is accentuated at the intervertebral articulations, but the dorsal column remains a uniform width.

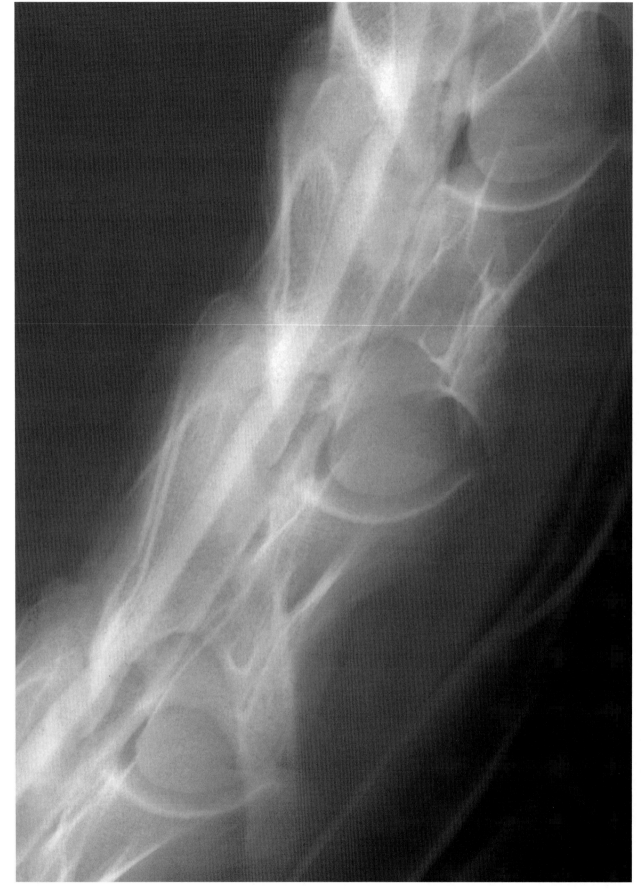

Figure 14.5 Lateral view of the fourth to seventh cervical vertebrae to show a normal myelogram (same horse as in Figures 14.4a and 14.4b).

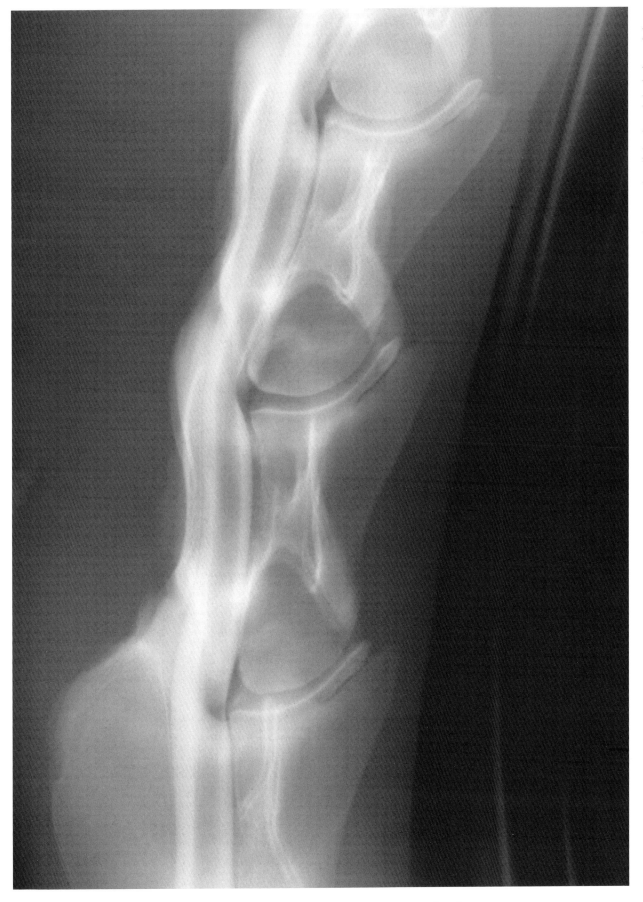

Figure 14.6(a) Lateral view of the second to fifth cervical vertebrae of a yearling Thoroughbred colt with mild hindlimb ataxia. Note the slight dorsal deviation of the fourth cervical vertebra, the suggestion of slight stenosis at its cranial orifice and the prominent caudal epiphysis of the third cervical vertebra. The myelogram was obtained with the neck in a normal (neutral) position. There is subtle narrowing of the dorsal contrast column at the articulation between the third and fourth cervical vertebrae. The ventral contrast column is narrower at each of the intervertebral articulations – a normal feature.

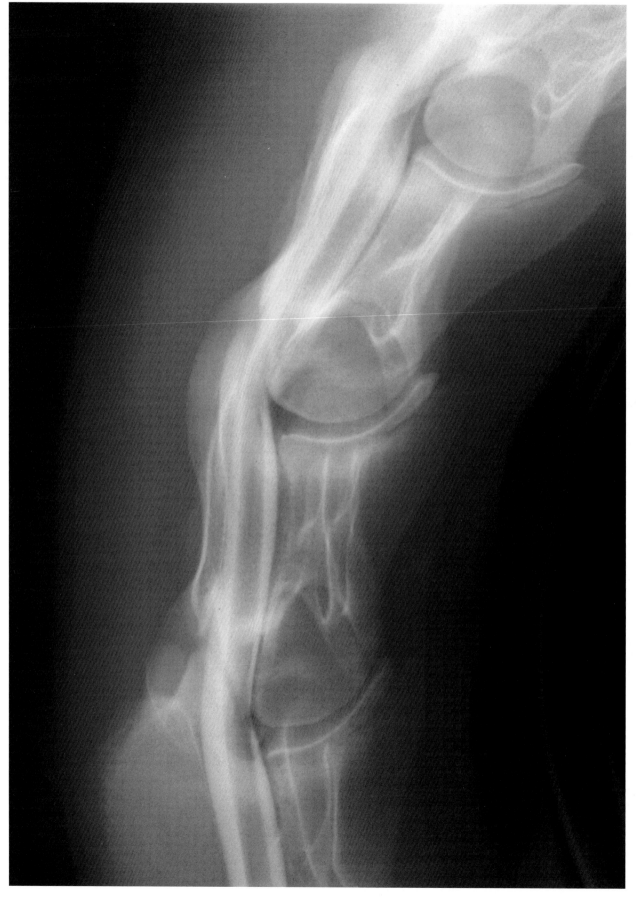

Figure 14.6(b) Flexed lateral view of the second to fifth cervical vertebrae (the same colt as in Figure 14.6a). Dorsal displacement of the head of the fourth cervical vertebra is accentuated and there is more obvious narrowing of the dorsal contrast column at this level, confirming a site of spinal cord compression. This was verified at post-mortem examination.

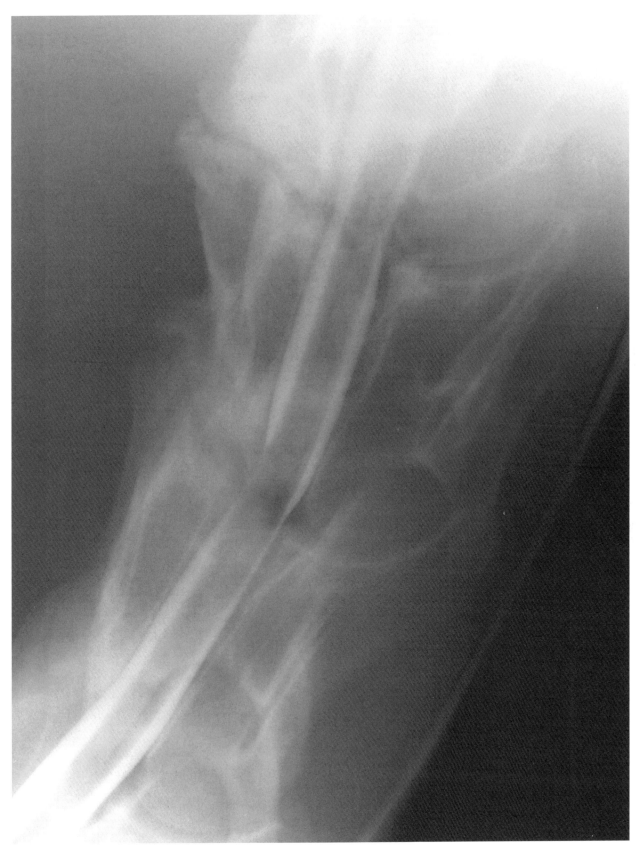

Figure 14-7 Lateral view of the fifth to seventh cervical vertebrae of a 3-year-old Thoroughbred filly with severe hindlimb and forelimb ataxia. There is tremendous enlargement of the articular facets of the synovial articulations between the fifth and sixth and sixth and seventh cervical vertebrae, with marked irregularity of the joint spaces. These changes are compatible with severe degenerative joint disease. There is marked narrowing of the dorsal and ventral contrast columns at the articulations between the fifth and sixth cervical vertebrae and to a lesser extent between the sixth and seventh. This is indicative of two sites of spinal cord compression. The filly was treated by fusion of the fifth, sixth and seventh cervical vertebrae and showed marked clinical improvement associated with some remodelling of the synovial articulation.

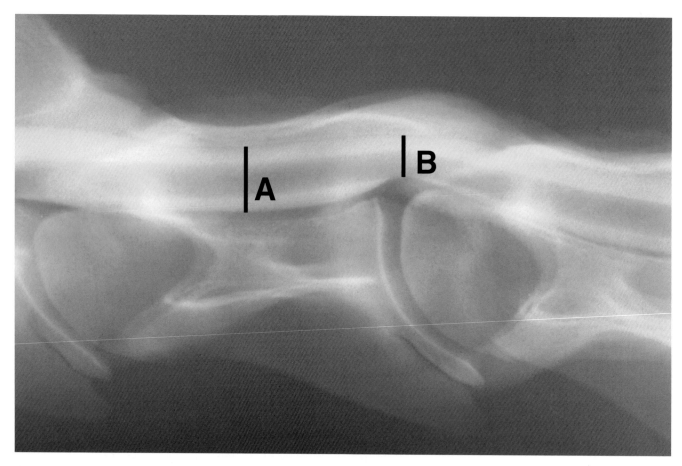

Figure 14.8 Lateral myelogram of the cranial cervical vertebrae (C2–C4). Cranial is to the left. Measurement of the minimum dural sagittal diameter. 'A' denotes the minimum dural sagittal diameter in the middle of C3; 'B' denotes the minimum dural sagittal diameter at the intervertebral articulation between C3 and C4. Note that the ventral contrast column is markedly narrowed as this site, but the dorsal contrast column is only slightly changed. Note also the 'ski jump' appearance of the proximocaudal aspect of the vertebral body of C3 and the slight malalignment between C3 and C4.

two dorsal borders of the contrast column caused by asymmetrical dorsolateral compression. A ventrodorsal myelogram may confirm transverse compression, although diagnostic-quality ventrodorsal radiographs of the caudal cervical vertebrae are difficult to acquire.

PNEUMOCYSTOGRAPHY

Chapter 13, page 680, describes the use of positive contrast cystography. Pneumocystography involves the introduction of air into the bladder, prior to radiographs being obtained. This provides negative (radiolucent) contrast within the bladder, allowing radiographic visualization of the internal surface of the bladder wall. While this can be carried out with the horse standing, the bladder can only be visualized on lateral radiographs of small horses. It is therefore normally necessary to carry out the technique under general anaesthesia, so that the bladder can be radiographed using the standard ventrodorsal views used for the pelvis (see Chapter 11, page 575).

Technique

This technique can be used in conscious foals or, if necessary, under mild sedation. The horse is positioned in dorsal recumbency as for pelvic radiography (see Chapter 11, page 575). A urinary catheter is then introduced into the bladder (a standard equine urinary catheter of approximately 7 mm diameter is adequate for this purpose in either sex). Any urine present should be withdrawn, and air is then introduced into the bladder and a radiograph obtained. The urethra in mares and geldings is sufficiently narrow for little air to escape around the catheter, but some device must be used to prevent egress of air through the catheter during the exposure. In adult Thoroughbreds, up to 5 l of air may be used.

Diagnostic criteria

In the normal horse, the bladder is seen as a roughly pear-shaped lucent shadow lying in the abdomen and pelvic canal, the broader part being within the abdomen. It is important to realize that the outline of the cranial portion of the bladder may be modified by pressure on the bladder from the intestines. In some horses, there is a tendency for a mineralized 'sandy' deposit to collect in the bladder. Normally this is voided in part or in total with the urine, but if a portion is left in the bladder, it will be evident on radiographs as a rather amorphous radiopacity lying in the dependent part of the bladder.

This technique is particularly useful in foals with suspected rupture of the bladder, where it can be carried out in the standing foal. It is important to look for air escaping from the bladder into the abdominal cavity, and not just to assess the outline of the bladder.

Positive (opaque) and double-contrast studies can also be made, either introducing opaque contrast medium into the bladder via a catheter as above, or as a result of intravenous pyelography (see below). Interpretation is similar to that outlined above, but is generally more difficult than with pneumocystography.

INTRAVENOUS PYELOGRAPHY

This technique is of limited value, but can be used to assess the outline of the kidneys, ureters and bladder. It is normally performed under general anaesthesia with the horse in dorsal recumbency. Ventrodorsal views of the pelvic and abdominal areas are required (see Chapters 11 and 13), but lateral views of the abdominal region may also be helpful in thinner horses. Ultrasonography is often helpful for evaluation of the kidneys.

Technique

There is little information available on the use of this technique in the horse, but it can be successfully performed as follows. The horse is placed in dorsal recumbency, and the bladder catheterized. Any urine present is withdrawn.

The jugular vein is catheterized, and 100 ml of Urografin (Schering Chemicals) is injected over 30 seconds. Radiographs are taken at five 5-minute intervals, centring over the kidneys. Good visualization of the kidneys and ureters can be obtained using ventrodorsal views. The exact entrance of the ureters to the bladder is difficult to see on ventrodorsal or lateral views, as it tends to be superimposed upon the pelvis or abdominal viscera. This makes this technique of limited value in cases of suspected ectopic ureter. Within 15–20 minutes, the contrast medium collects in the bladder, and good positive-contrast films of the bladder can be obtained.

OTHER TECHNIQUES

Contrast agents can be used to outline sinus tracts (so-called *sinography or fistulography*), and to determine whether they extend to other pathological lesions (Figures 14.9a and 14.9b). They may also outline foreign bodies lying

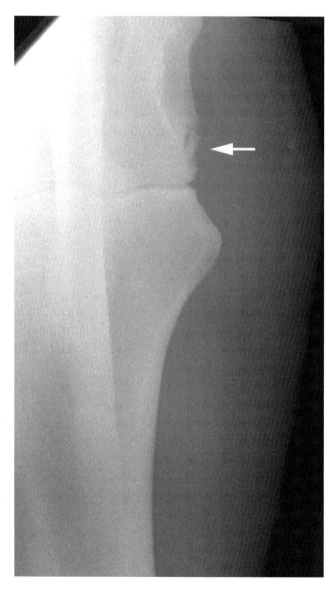

Figure 14.9(a) Craniocaudal radiographic view of the right elbow of an 11-year-old Irish Draught horse that had sustained a kick injury 3 weeks previously. Lateral is to the right. There was soft tissue swelling and a discharging sinus on the lateral aspect of the elbow. There is diffuse soft-tissue swelling and a small displaced chip fracture on the distal lateral aspect of the humerus (arrow).

[706]

within sinuses. The technique varies, depending on the position and size of the sinus. If possible, a Foley catheter should be used, to limit leakage and allow injection under pressure if necessary. In smaller tracts, it may be sufficient to introduce the contrast agent through a flexible catheter of 2–3 mm external diameter, introduced no more than 1 cm into the sinus. In other situations, contrast agent may be introduced by passing a flexible catheter as far into the sinus as possible. Sedation of the patient may be necessary, and the infusion of local anaesthetic solution into the sinus may also be beneficial. Diagnostic ultrasonography may also be useful.

Water-soluble, positive intravenous agents may be used, although contrast agents are manufactured specifically for fistulography. Contrast medium is likely to 'leak' from the sinus during injection, and should be cleaned from the skin surface prior to radiography. As always, more than one view of the area should be obtained. Interpretation of the results should be guarded. Sinuses frequently do not fill fully and artefactual filling defects are quite common.

The nasolacrimal duct can also be visualized using intravenous contrast agents (*dacryocystorhinography*). The contrast medium is introduced

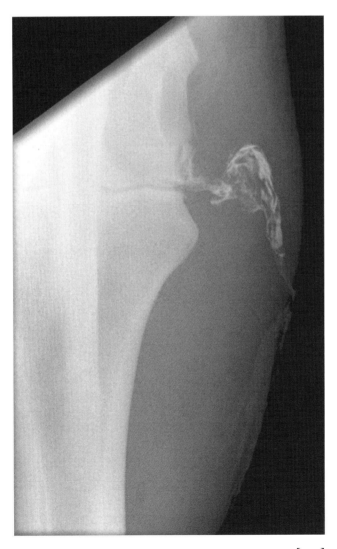

Figure 14.9(b) Craniocaudal radiographic view of the right elbow of the same horse as in Figure 14.9(a). A radiopaque contrast medium has been injected into the sinus, which communicates with the site of the chip fracture.

through a flexible catheter most easily via the puncta lacrimalia, but can be retrograde through the nasal ostium. If the duct is blocked, it is important to take care that it is not ruptured, as contrast media may cause a marked soft-tissue reaction.

The duct commences as two separate branches about 1 cm from the medial canthus of the eye. They join at the medial canthus, the duct then passing forward over the outer wall of the frontal sinus to open at the lower commissure of the nostril. The duct generally has a consistent diameter throughout its length, and runs a relatively straight course. There may be several openings into the nostril.

FURTHER READING

Arthrography

Arnbjerg, J. (1969) Contrast studies of joints and tendon sheaths in the horse. *Nord. Vet. Med.*, **21**, 318

Dik, K.J. (1984) Equine arthrography. *Vet. Radiol.*, **25**, 93–96

Meredith, W.J. and Massey, J.B. (1971) *Fundamental Physics of Radiology*, 2nd edn, Wright and Sons, Bristol

Nichols, F. and Sande, R. (1989) Radiographic and arthroscopic findings in the equine stifle. *J. Am. Vet. Med. Ass.*, **181**, 918–924

Nixon, A. and Spencer, C. (1990) Arthrography of the equine shoulder. *Equine vet. J.*, **22**, 107–113

Stashak, T.S. (1987) *Adams' Lameness in Horses*, 4th edn, Lea and Febiger, Philadelphia, pp. 171–172

Swanstorm, O. and Lewis, R. (1969) Arthrography of the equine fetlock. *Proc. Am. Ass. Equine Pract.*, **15**, 221–225

Tendonography

Hago, B.E.D. and Vaughan, L.C. (1986) Radiographic anatomy of tendon sheaths and bursae in the horse. *Equine vet. J.*, **18**, 102–106

Stashak, T.S. (1987) *Adams' Lameness in Horses*, 4th edn, Lea and Febiger, Philadelphia, pp. 172–174

Verschooten, F. and De Moor, A. (1978) Tendinitis in the horse: radiographic diagnosis with air tendograms. *J. Am. Vet. Radiol. Soc.*, **19**, 23–30

Angiography

Colles, C.M. and Cook, W.R. (1983) Carotid and cerebral angiography in the horse. *Vet. Rec.*, **113**, 483–489

Colles, C.M., Garner, H.E. and Coffman, J.R. (1979) The blood supply of the horse's foot. *Proc. 25th Am. Ass. Equine Pract.*, pp. 385–398

Herbert, W.W. (1964) Angiographic artefacts which simulate or mask abnormality. *Am. J. Roentgenol.*, **92**, 907–917

Hertsh, B-W. (1983) *Arteriographische Untersuchungen an den Extremitäten beim Pferd*, Habilitationsschrift, Hanover

Lindbom, A. (1957) Arterial spasm caused by puncture and catheterisation. *Acta Radiol.*, **47**, 449–459

Seldinger, S.I. (1953) Catheter replacement of the needle in percutaneous arteriography. *Acta Radiol.*, **39**, 368

Wickbom, I. and Bartley, O. (1957) Arterial spasm in peripheral arteriography. *Acta Radiol.*, **47**, 433–448

Venography

Redden, R. (2001) A technique for performing digital venography in the standing horse. *Equine vet. Educ.* **5**, 172–178

Rucker, A., Redden, R., Arthur, E. *et al.* (2006) How to perform the digital venogram. *Proc. Am. Ass. Equine Pract.*, **52**, 526–530

Myelography

Beech, J. (1979) Metrizamide myelography in the horse. *J. Am. Vet. Radiol. Soc.*, **20**, 22–31

Burbidge, H., Kannegieter, N., Dickson, L. and Goulden, B. (1988) Iohexol myelography in the horse. *Equine vet. J.*, **21**, 347–350

Conrad, R. (1984) Metrizamide myelography of the equine cervical spine: 14 case histories. *J. Am. Vet. Radiol. Soc.*, **25**, 73–77

Foley, J., Gatlin, S. and Selcer, B. (1986) Standing myelography in 6 adult horses. *J. Am. Vet. Radiol. Soc.*, **27**, 54–57

Hubbell, J., Reed, S., Myer, C. and Muir, W. (1988) Sequelae of myelography in the horse. *Equine vet. J.*, **20**, 438–440

Hudson, N. and Mayhew, I. (2005) Radiographic and myelographic assessment of the equine cervical vertebral column and spinal cord. *Equine vet. Educ.*, **17**, 34–38

May, S., Wyn-Jones, G., Church, S., Brouwer, G. and Jones, R. (1986) Iopamidol myelography in the horse. *Equine vet. J.*, **18**, 199–202

Nyland, T., Blythe, L., Pool, R., Helphrey, M. and O'Brien, T. (1980) Metrizamide myelography in the horse: clinical, radiographic and pathological changes. *Am. J. Vet. Res.*, **41**, 204–211

Papageorges, M., Gavin, P., Sande, R., Barbee, D. and Grant, B. (1987) Radiographic and myelographic examination of the cervical vertebral column in 306 ataxic horses. *Vet. Radiol.*, **28**, 53–59

Rantanen, N., Gavin, P., Barbee, D. and Sande, R. (1981) Ataxia and paresis in horses, part ii: radiographic and myelographic examination of the cervical vertebral column. *Comp. Cont. Educ.*, **4**, 161–171

Schwarz, T., Edwards, G. and Sullivan, M. (2002) Subdural injection of myelographic contrast in two horses. *Equine vet. Educ.*, **14**, 179–181

Van Biervliet, J., Scrivani, P., Divers, T., Erb, H., de la Hunta, A. and Nixon, A. (2004) Evaluation of decision criteria for detection of spinal cord compression based on cervical myelography. *Equine vet. J.*, **35**, 14–20

Widmer, W., Blevins, W., Jakovljevic, S. *et al.* (1998) A prospective clinical trial comparing metrizamide and iohexol for equine myelography. *Vet. Radiol. Ultrasound.*, **39**, 106–109

Other techniques

Crispin, S. (1988) Nasolacrimal duct cannulation in the horse. *In Practice*, **10**, 154–156

Lundin, C., Clem, M., DeBowes, R. and Bertone, A. (1988) Diagnostic fistulography in horses. *Comp. Cont. Educ.*, **10**, 639–645

Appendix A
Fusion times of physes and suture lines

HEAD AND VERTEBRAL COLUMN

Area	Centres	Notes	Closure	
HEAD				
Occipital	Squamous Lateral Basilar		Lateral-basilar Squamous to lateral-basilar Parieto-occipital Spheno-occipital Occipitomastoid	By 4 months 12–24 months 5 years* 5 years* Aged*
Sphenoid	Pre-sphenoid Post-sphenoid		Spheno-occipital	Uncertain, but in first year 5 years*
Ethmoid	Perpendicular Cribriform			Uncertain, but soon after birth
Parietal	One centre		Parietal suture Parieto-occipital	4 years* 5 years*
Premaxilla	One centre		Left and right	During 4th year*
Nasal	One centre		Left and right Naso-frontal	Do not fuse 1 year*
Mandible	Two halves		Left and right	3 months*
CERVICAL SPINE				

Atlas	Two halves	Faint longitudinal line
		  evident in
		  ventrodorsal view in
		  neonate		

Axis	Dens, head, body, caudal epiphysis		Dens to head Caudal epiphysis	About 7 months Complete 4–5 years
C3–C7	Cranial vertebral physis Caudal vertebral physis			Complete by 2 years Complete by 4–5 years
THORACOLUMBAR SPINE				
T1–L6	Cranial vertebral physis Caudal vertebral physis			6–12 months 2–4 years

T2–T8	Separate centres of ossification in
	  cartilaginous summits
		Develop at about 12
		  months
		Gradual ossification
				Remain separate throughout
				  life

*Obliteration of suture; all others are fusion of suture.

[711]

Area	Centres	Notes	Closure	
SCAPULA	Scapular cartilage Body of scapula Cranial glenoid cavity of scapula	Cranial glenoid cavity of scapula and supraglenoid tubercle incompletely ossified at birth	Cranial glenoid cavity with body	About 5 months
	Supraglenoid tubercle		Supraglenoid tubercle	By 12–24 months
HUMERUS Proximal	Diaphysis Humeral head Greater tubercle	Lesser tubercle develops from same ossification centre as humeral head – incompletely ossified at birth	Centres of proximal epiphysis	Merge about 3–4 months
			Proximal physis	24–36 months
Distal	Diaphysis Distal epiphysis Epiphysis of medial epicondyle			11–24 months
RADIUS Proximal	Single epiphysis			11–24 months
Distal	Diaphysis Epiphysis Lateral styloid process		Lateral styloid process with epiphysis	Within 1 year
			Physis	20–24 months
ULNA	Single proximal epiphysis	Incompletely ossified at birth Occasionally a separate centre for anconeal process	Physis	24–36 months
METACARPUS Third metacarpus	Proximal physis Distal physis		Physis Physis	Fused at birth About 6 months
Second and fourth		Distal epiphysis cartilaginous at birth, gradually ossifies	Fuses with shaft	1–9 months
PROXIMAL PHALANX	Proximal epiphysis Diaphysis Distal epiphysis		Proximal physis Distal physis	About 1 year Fused at birth
MIDDLE PHALANX	Proximal epiphysis Diaphysis Distal epiphysis		Proximal physis Distal physis	8–12 months Fused at birth
DISTAL PHALANX	Single centre	Models until about 18 months Palmar processes model over 12 months		–
NAVICULAR BONE	Single centre	Models until about 18 months		–
PROXIMAL SESAMOID BONES	Single centre	Outline complete about 3–4 months Enlarge until 18 months		–
CARPAL BONES	Single centre each	Fully developed about 18 months		–

Area	Centres	Notes	Closure	
PELVIS	Ilium – iliac crest and tuber coxae		Iliac crest and tuber coxae	About 10 months
	Pubis	Symphyseal branches of pubis and ischium fused at birth	Pubic symphysis	Remains open
	Ischium		Caudal portion of bone and tuber ischii	About 10–12 months
			Articular portions of pubis, ilium and ischium to form acetabulum	About 1 year
FEMUR Proximal	Femoral head		Femoral head	24–36 months
	Trochanter major		Trochanter major to femoral shaft	18–30 months
	Trochanter minor		Trochanter minor	About 2 years
Distal	Epiphysis Diaphysis	Trochlear ridges develop over about 5 months Medial trochlear ridge becomes more prominent at about 2 months	Physis	24–30 months
TIBIA Proximal	Epiphysis Metaphysis Tibial tuberosity (apophysis)		Apophysis-epiphysis Epiphysis-metaphysis Apophysis-metaphysis	9–12 months 24–30 months 30–36 months
Distal	Lateral malleolus Epiphysis	(distal epiphysis of fibula)	Fuses to epiphysis Epiphysis-metaphysis	By 3 months 17–24 months
TUBER CALCANEI		May be absent at birth, gradually ossified	Fuses to calcaneus	By 16–24 months
FIRST AND SECOND TARSAL BONES				Usually fused at birth
PATELLA	Single centre	Incompletely ossified at birth Fully modelled about 4 months		
FIBULA		Little ossification until 2 months		
DISTAL TO TARSUS: Same as thoracic limb				

Appendix B
Exposure guide, image quality and film processing faults

Area/view	RS	FFD (cm)	AWF	Grid	kV	mAs
Head						
Cranium, lateral	600	150	–	CH	65	40
Cranium (under GA)	600	150	–	CH	75/80	64
Sinus, lateral	600	150	–	–	55	12
Pharynx	600	150	–	CH	65	35
Rostral, lateral	600	150	–	CH	60	18
Cervical spine						
Upper	600	150	–	CH	68	45
Mid	600	150	–	CH	70	50
Lower	600	150	–	CH	75	64
Lower/T1	600	150	–	CH	90	90
Thoracolumbar spine						
Withers (DSP)	600	150	yes	CH	65	50
Mid thoracic (DSP)	600	150	yes	CH	65	50
Caudal thoracic (DSP)	600	150	yes	CH	75	64
Cranial lumbar (DSP)	600	150	yes	CH	85	80
Mid thoracic artic./vertebrae	600	150	–	CH	100	160/180
Sacrum (cranial)	600	150	yes	CH	110	80
Sacrum (caudal)	600	150	yes	CH	70	63
Cranial coccygeal	600	150	–	CH	70	40/50
Scapulohumeral joint						
ML, standing	600	150	yes	CH	100/105	100/130
CrM-CdLO, standing	600	120	yes	–	80	25
ML, under GA (cassette tunnel)	600	130	yes	CH	100/105	130/160
Elbow						
ML, standing	600	150	yes	CH	70	20
CrCd, standing	600	120	–	–	66	13
Carpus						
LM and obliques	150	100	–	–	63	10
DPa	150	100	–	–	65	12
DPr-DDiO	150	100	–	–	65	10
Metacarpus/tarsus						
LM and obliques	150	100	–	–	62	9
DPa	150	100	–	–	66	12
RC/T II/IV	150	100	–	–	57	10
Metacarpo/tarsophalangeal joint						
LM and obliques	150	100	–	–	62	9
DPa/DPl	150	100	–	–	65	12
L45°Pr-MDiO	150	105	–	–	60	10
Pastern						
Flexed oblique	150	100	–	–	62	10
Feet						
Lateral	150	100	–	8:1	70	22
Lateral	150	100	–	–	62	16
DPr-PaDiO, distal phalanx	150	100	yes	8:1	60	9
DPr-PaDiO, navicular	150	100	–	8:1	73	25

APPENDIX B
*Exposure guide, image quality
and film processing faults*

Area/view	RS	FFD (cm)	AWF	Grid	kV	mAs
PaPr-PaDiO, navicular	150	100	–	–	66	14
DPa, weight-bearing	150	100	–	8:1	70	22
Pelvis						
Ischium	600	130	–	2	120	160
Pelvic canal	600	130	–	2	130	250
Coxofemoral joint	600	130	–	2	135	220
Sacroiliac joint	600	130	–	2	135/140	320
Ilial wing	600	130	–	2	135	220
Stifle						
Cd60°L-CrMO, standing	600	120	yes	–	57	13
CdCr, standing	600	120	yes	–	75	20
LM, under GA	600	120	yes	CH	65	40
CdCr, under GA	600	120	yes	CH	80	64
Patella, CrPr-CrDiO	600	120	yes	–	65	13
Tarsus						
LM	150	100	–	–	60	13
Obliques	150	100	–	–	63	13
DPl	150	100	–	–	70	13
DPl, flexed	150	100	–	–	70	15
Thorax						
Caudodorsal (diaphragm)	600	150	–	CH	80	36
Craniodorsal (aortic arch)	600	150	–	CH	90	36
Caudoventral (caudal heart)	600	150	–	CH	90	36
Cranioventral (cranial heart)	600	150	–	CH	110	40
Sternum, lateral	600	150	yes	CH	85	100
Abdomen						
Lateral, standing (7 day foal)	600	150	–	CH	70	63

Notes:
RS: Relative speed rating of screens.
FFD: Focus/film distance.
AWF: Aluminium wedge filter.
Grids:
    CH – Cross-hatch parallel 12:1 ratio grid.
    2 – Two crossed 12:1 ratio focused grids.
    8:1 – 8:1 ratio focused grid, 47 lines/cm.

ALTERING THE TABLE FACTORS

The exposures above are based on a 500 kg horse of Thoroughbred type. As an approximate guide the kV should be increased by 5% for limb radiography of heavier horses, and reduced for neonatal foals both by 5kV and halving the mAs. Relative speed rating of screens and distance factors must both be considered when converting the above exposure guide.

Relative speed (RS)

Speed classification of film/screen combinations in terms of relative speed enables comparison of systems between manufacturers. Although the exposures required will be the same to produce images of similar opacity, the detail and resolution may vary. Some manufacturers use 100, 200, etc., some may use 2, 4, 8, etc., but the interrelationship is the same. Speed 8 requires half the exposure (mAs) needed for speed 4; speed 200 requires double the exposure (mAs) of speed 400 screens, etc. Generally speaking, if using only one screen from a pair (i.e. when used with single emulsion film) the speed of the system will halve, e.g. one screen from a pair rated 400 will give a speed of 200.

Distance

The distance between the source (focus) and the cassette (film) affects the radiopacity of the image produced. When the focus–film distance (FFD) is altered, the total amount of x-rays (mAs) must be increased or decreased to make a comparable exposure. The equation to calculate the exposure for a change in distance is:

$$\text{Old mAs} \times \frac{(\text{new FFD})^2}{(\text{old FFD})^2} = \text{New mAs}$$

i.e. The mAs decreases as the square of the distance.

FACTORS AFFECTING IMAGE QUALITY

There are many factors which have an effect on contrast, sharpness, resolution and opacity of the radiographic image. Choice of screen, film and grid is a major factor and needs to be carefully considered. Faster screens mean shorter exposure times can be used, reducing the risk of movement blur, but these provide less resolution than slower screens. Individual films have inherent contrast and latitude values. When x-raying structures greater than 10 cm in depth the use of a grid should be considered to reduce scattered radiation. The final choice of factors will be a compromise for any given area radiographed.

Rare earth vs. calcium tungstate screens

Rare earth screens are more efficient and require less exposure than calcium tungstate, the light conversion of rare earth phosphors being approximately four times greater. As a general rule rare earth screens produce better detail than calcium tungstate screens. Faster film–screen combinations require less exposure, which reduces the risk of movement blur, but as speed increases image detail (sharpness) decreases.

Spectral sensitivity of screens and films

Screens emit light in a specific part of the spectrum. It is therefore important to match the spectral output of the screen to the spectral sensitivity of the film. Failure to do so, in general, will result in loss of system speed and loss of information transfer. Calcium tungstate phosphors are blue emitting; rare earth phosphors may be blue, green or ultraviolet. Ensure the darkroom light filtration is correct for the type of film in use.

[717]

Single vs. double emulsion film

Single-emulsion films, so-called mammography films, offer greater detail than conventional double-emulsion films, and are used with a single screen. They do not suffer from parallax unsharpness, which is evident with double-emulsion films. They are, however, much slower and are not practical when using low-output portable machines as exposure times are too long, increasing the risk of movement. They can be used in conjunction with medium-speed screens, as opposed to specific mammography screens, to increase the speed of the system without sacrificing too much detail.

Grids

Scattered radiation has a significant effect on image contrast. This can be improved by good collimation of the primary beam. Grids can also be used to control scattered radiation to improve contrast. However, they increase the exposure required, resulting in longer exposure times and increasing the risk of movement blur. Focused grids need careful positioning to avoid grid cut-off and must be used at the correct distance for optimum results. Parallel grids have slightly more latitude when using FFDs greater than 120 cm. Whether focused or parallel grids are used they must be aligned perpendicular to the primary x-ray beam. The higher both the grid ratio and lines per centimetre, the more effective the grid is in reducing scatter, but the higher the grid factor. The grid factor denotes how much an exposure needs to be increased to give comparable opacity to a film obtained without a grid, e.g. grid factor 2 – double the mAs. If a grid is unavailable, an air gap between the object and the cassette helps to attenuate scattered radiation. An air gap will, however, increase magnification and geometric unsharpness. See Chapter 2 for guidance on grids for use with digital systems.

Unsharpness

Movement is a common cause of unsharpness of the radiographic image. This can be reduced by the use of short exposure times as well as sedation of the patient. The former can be achieved by using a shorter focus–film distance, but the shorter FFD increases geometric unsharpness (penumbra).

Penumbra is the result of the focal spot in the tube not being a point source. The amount of unsharpness increases with an increase in focal spot size. It is also increased with reduced focal–film distance and increased object–film distance.

Poor screen–film contact is another cause of image blur and usually results in only part of the radiograph appearing unsharp. This can be checked by placing a thin wire mesh on top of the cassette and making an exposure using a large FFD. Areas of poor contact will result in blurring of the image.

Focal spot size

With high-output stationary x-ray machines there is usually a facility to select different-sized focal spots. A smaller focal spot (e.g. 0.6 mm) usually

[718]

results in better resolution, but an increased exposure time is required to achieve the same mAs output. When movement is likely to be a problem, e.g. in most proximal limb examinations, a larger focal spot (e.g. 1.5–2.0 mm) should be used to reduce exposure times to a minimum.

FILM PROCESSING FAULTS

Longitudinal scratches – usually caused by the film guides on the racks of automatic processors

Films tacky from automatic processing – usually a problem with the fixer rather than the dryer

High-density marks:

Black splashes
  – developer or water splashed on film before development

Black crescent-shaped marks
  – poor handling after exposure

Black fingerprints
  – developer or water on hands when handling film before processing

Static
  – can be the result of formica workbench, dry darkroom atmosphere, man-made fabrics or loading/unloading the cassette

Localized fogging
  – black marks around the edge of film is either light leakage in a cassette or the film box has been opened in white light

Overall high density:

Overdevelopment
  – developer too hot, development time too long or developer too strong

Heat
  – 20°C is maximum temperature for 3 months' storage

Time
  – film has a limited 'shelf life'. Film fog increases with age

Safe lighting
  – bulb too strong, too close to working surface, incorrect filter, crack in filter

Background radiation
  – higher than recommended level of background radiation

Low-density marks:

White splashes
  – fixer, grease or oil on film before processing

White crescent-shaped marks
  – poor handling before exposure

White fingerprints
  – fixer, grease or oil on fingers when handling film before processing

Sharply defined marks
  – usually artefacts inside cassette on screen

APPENDIX B
*Exposure guide, image quality
and film processing faults*

Overall low density:

Underdevelopment

– developer too cold, development time too short or developer too weak or exhausted

Other processing faults:

Chemical contamination

– very patchy image with no contrast over entire film caused by the developer being contaminated with fixer

Milky white stain or image

– image has not cleared due to insufficient fixing

Brown stain

– appears after a period of storage and is due to inadequate washing

DIGITAL FILM FAULTS

See Chapter 2

DEFINITIONS (ALSO SEE GLOSSARY, APPENDIX C)

Resolution objective measurement of how much detail can be provided by a film–screen combination, measured in line pairs per millimetre. Indicates size of the smallest object that the system will record, i.e. the smallest distance that must exist between two objects before they can be seen as two separate entities.

Definition subjective impression of the amount of detail that is seen in a radiograph. This is difficult to quantify.

Appendix C
Glossary

This glossary is not meant to be comprehensive, but provides brief definitions of some colloquial terms which may differ in usage in different countries, some anatomical terms which have recently been changed or adopted, a few radiological or radiographic terms, and other words not easily found in a dictionary or standard radiology text. Explanations of many technical terms may be found in the text by reference to the Index. Some radiological terms are discussed in greater detail in Chapter 1. Some words have different meanings when used in different circumstances, but only the definition relevant to the context of this book is included.

air gap space (occupied by air) between the object being radiographed and the cassette; the air gap will attenuate scattered radiation, thus a grid is not required.

antebrachiocarpal joint formerly called the radiocarpal joint.

antebrachium the forearm.

apophysis bony outgrowth with a separate centre of ossification, such as a tuberosity or process, under tensile forces from, e.g., a ligament.

arthropathy colloquial non-specific term to describe pathological changes within a joint (e.g. steroid arthropathy).

back-scatter deflection or production of radiation back towards the source; it is of most practical importance when high exposures are used; its effect on the film can be minimized by placing a sheet of lead behind the cassette.

Birkeland fracture articular fracture of the proximal palmar or, more commonly, plantar aspect of the proximal phalanx; the term has been used to encompass fragments from a number of different locations; some of these fragments may be developmental in origin.

bucked shins colloquial term used to describe periosteal and endosteal modelling on the dorsal aspect of the third metacarpal (metatarsal) bone resulting in an acquired convex contour to the bone; it is usually preceded by obvious 'shin soreness'.

callus, external new bone formation in response to a fracture on the external side of the bone (periosteal new bone).

callus, internal new bone formation in response to a fracture on the internal side of the cortex (endosteal new bone).

carpitis colloquial term used to describe inflammation of the antebrachiocarpal and/or middle carpal joints. Synovitis may or may not be accompanied by detectable radiographic abnormalities.

centrodistal joint formerly called the distal intertarsal joint (of the tarsus or hock).

chondroid inspissated pus (found in a paranasal sinus or guttural pouch) appearing radiographically as a radiopaque mass.

chondroma tumour composed of cells closely resembling those of normal cartilage, usually appearing radiographically as a space-occupying mass with some mineralization.

Codman's triangle triangular area of new bone adjacent to the cortex which develops as a result of elevation of the periosteum associated with neoplasia, inflammation, infection or trauma.

collimator device for restricting the field covered by the primary x-ray beam.

cone method of collimating the x-ray beam.

contrast degree of definition on an x-ray between adjacent structures of differing radiopacities.

contrast medium substance used to delineate a structure or structures; a positive-contrast medium (agent) is radiopaque; a negative-contrast medium (air) is radiolucent.

cross-hatch grid grid composed of two sets of parallel lead lines perpendicular to each other.

CT compute(rise)d tomography.

definition clarity or distinctness with which radiographic image detail is seen.

delayed union failure of a fractured bone to unite within the expected period; if the cause is corrected healing should occur eventually.

density degree to which a tissue absorbs incident x-rays.

density, tissue weight per unit volume.

dental sac developing tooth.

dentigerous cyst cyst containing all or part of a tooth (or teeth); also called a temporal teratoma. All dentigerous cysts are temporal teratomas although not all temporal teratomas contain dentigerous material.

desmitis inflammation of a ligament.

detail degree of sharpness with which individual shadows appear on the radiograph.

diaphysis shaft of a long bone.

distal interphalangeal joint formerly called the coffin, pedal or coronopedal joint.

distal intertarsal joint now called the centrodistal joint.

dorsal conchus formerly called the dorsal turbinate.

double contrast use of both positive- and negative-contrast media (agents), e.g. barium and air.

dystrophic mineralization mineralization in soft tissues (due to abnormal nutrition of the tissue). Occurs in areas of cell necrosis.

edge effect or edge enhancement term synonymous with a Mach line or band; a radiolucent line which may be created by one bone edge superimposed on another.

entheseophyte new bone formation at the site of insertion of a tendon, ligament or joint capsule.

epiphysis separate centre of ossification at each end of a long bone.

epiphysitis colloquial term used incorrectly to describe inflammation in the region of a physis or growth plate, most commonly the distal radial physis.

exposure latitude degree of overexposure or underexposure that can be tolerated in a correctly developed film and still produce an image of acceptable radiographic quality.

fatigue fracture synonymous with a stress fracture: an incomplete fracture, the result of repetitive overload and microfractures.

flatness lack of contrast on a radiograph.

fluid line horizontal interface separating a radiopaque area (fluid) distally from a more lucent area (often air) proximally.

fluoroscopy production of a visual image on a fluorescent screen for diagnosis.

focal distance perpendicular distance from a focused grid to the place in space where the planes that pass through the grid would converge.

focus–film distance distance between the x-ray tube focal spot and the plane of the radiographic film.

focused grid grid with lead strips slightly angled so that if they continued they would meet at some line in space, the focal point.

graininess lack of homogeneity in a radiographic image due to a clumping together of silver particles.

grid thin plate consisting of alternating strips of radiolucent and radiopaque (lead) materials which attenuate scattered radiation.

grid cut-off absorption of excessive amounts of primary radiation by the grid (and thus underexposure of part of the film) due to an incorrect angle between the primary x-ray beam and the grid; when a focused grid is used, the x-ray beam must be perpendicular to the grid and centred on the centre of the grid and with the focal spot of the x-ray tube at the proper focus distance to avoid grid cut-off.

grid ratio ratio between the height of the lead strips and the distance between them in a grid.

hairline fracture incomplete non-displaced fracture, sometimes used incorrectly as synonymous with a fatigue or stress fracture.

intercarpal joint now called the middle carpal joint.

involucrum sclerotic bone surrounding a sequestrum.

joint mouse small bony or mineralized fragment within a joint, usually mobile.

kV kilovoltage.

kVp kilovoltage peak (generally synonymous with kV).

kyphosis abnormal flexion of the thoracolumbar spine in the sagittal plane so that the dorsum appears abnormally convex; may be congenital or acquired.

light beam diaphragm method of collimating the primary x-ray beam by use of adjustable lead sheets incorporating a light beam to indicate the surface area to be exposed.

linear grid grid in which the lead strips are parallel to each other.

lordosis abnormal extension of the thoracolumbar spine in the sagittal plane so that the dorsum appears abnormally concave; may be congenital or acquired.

luxation complete dislocation or displacement of a joint.

mA milliamperage – number of x-rays produced during an exposure.

Mach line or band synonymous with edge enhancement; a radiolucent line which may be created by one bone edge superimposed on another.

mA s milliamperage-seconds – exposure magnitude expressed as the product of milliamperage and time in seconds.

margination definition of a bone contour, i.e. well or poorly marginated.

metaphysis wider part at the end of the diaphysis (shaft) of a long bone, adjacent to the physis.

middle carpal joint formerly called the intercarpal joint.

modelling there is confusion between the histological and radiographic use of the terms 'modelling' and 'remodelling'. Histologically, modelling refers to resorption and formation of bone which is not coupled and occurs at anatomically different sites (bone drift). It is a continuous process which regulates the macroscopic structure according to Wolff's law. Radiographically, modelling has been used to describe the formation of bone relevant to the cartilage model which is being replaced, i.e. the normal formation of bone. Thus the two definitions do not agree, so to avoid confusion, strictly speaking the term 'modelling' should be used to describe the macroscopic changes in the shape of a bone as it adapts to the stresses applied to it (see also 'remodelling').

moiré lines Interference pattern seen primarily in digital radiography, caused usually by grid lines interfering with other linear patterns in the system. Literally, appearance of shot silk.

MRI magnetic resonance imaging.

non-focused grid grid in which the lead strips are parallel, perpendicular to the surface of the grid.

non-screen film high-definition x-ray film designed for exposure without intensifying screens; much higher exposure factors are required than if screens are used.

non-union cessation of fracture healing without bony union; may be classified radiographically as an atrophic non-union or a hypertrophic non-union.

odontoma tumour arising in tissues which normally produce teeth, usually solid and radiopaque.

opacity degree of whiteness of the object being radiographed.

osselet colloquial term used to describe enlargement on the dorsal aspect of a metacarpophalangeal joint which may be associated with thickening of the joint capsule and/or synovial proliferation, degenerative joint disease or an articular chip fracture. There may be mineralized tissue within the abnormal synovial tissue.

osseous metaplasia formation of bone in a non-bony structure.

osteitis inflammation of bone.

osteoarthritis synonymous with degenerative joint disease.

osteochondroma (a) benign tumour of projecting adult bone capped by cartilage undergoing endochondral ossification; (b) radiopaque body of mineralized cartilage which may be free floating or attached to synovial tissue (synovial osteochondroma).

osteolysis bone destruction and resorption seen more easily in cortical bone than cancellous bone because of greater contrast. There is a delay of at least 10 days between histologic and radiographic evidence of lysis.

osteoma solid, radiopaque tumour of bone, usually well marginated.

osteomalacia decreased bone mass due to insufficient or abnormal mineralization of osteoid.

osteomyelitis infection of a bone which has a medullary cavity.

osteopenia decrease in the radiopacity of bone due to osteoporosis or to osteomalacia.

osteophyte spur of new bone.

osteophyte, marginal or articular spur of new bone at the chondrosynovial junction of an articular margin.

osteoporosis loss of bone mass due to imbalance between bone resorption and formation.

pastern joint correctly called the proximal interphalangeal joint.

periosteal new bone new bone production, the result of elevation of the periosteum from the cortex; there is usually a lag of at least 14 days between the initial stimulus and the radiographic detection of new bone.

physeal dysplasia abnormality of development of the physis; in some cases this may be a more appropriate term than physitis for a physeal abnormality.

physis growth plate of a long bone.

physitis inflammation of the physis often incorrectly called 'epiphysitis', characterized radiographically by irregular width of the physis with or without modelling of the adjacent metaphysis. Remnant cartilage cones may be seen as triangular radiolucent areas in the metaphysis.

podotrochlear apparatus the navicular bone, distal sesamoidean impar ligament and collateral sesamoidean ligament.

podotrochleitis inflammation of the navicular bone (and/or navicular bursa).

primary cut-off absorption by a grid of the primary beam (grid cut-off).

primary radiation, primary beam radiation from the x-ray tube which is incident on the subject matter or which continues unaltered in photon energy after passing through it.

proximal interphalangeal joint formerly the pastern joint.

proximal intertarsal joint now called the talocalcaneal-centroquartal joint.

radiocarpal joint now called the antebrachiocarpal joint.

radiography practice of obtaining radiographs.

radiology study of radiographs; the science and application of ionizing radiation.

radiolucency degree of blackness of the object being radiographed.

radiopacity degree of whiteness of the object being radiographed.

rare earth screens intensifying screens that use rare earth phosphors; reduced exposure factors can be used in comparison with calcium tungstate screens.

remodelling there is confusion between the histological and radiographic usage of the terms 'remodelling' and 'modelling'. Histologically, remodelling refers to resorption and formation of bone which is coupled and occurs in basic multicellular units. This regulates the microstructure of bone without altering its shape and is a continuous process, replacing damaged bone with new bone. Thus it cannot be seen macroscopically or appreciated radiographically. The term has been used radiographically to describe the reshaping of bone to match form and function (e.g. after fracture repair), but strictly speaking the term 'modelling' should be used (see also 'modelling').

resolution objective measurement of how much detail that can be provided by a film–screen combination, measured in line pairs per millimetre. Indicates the size of the smallest object that the system will record, i.e. the smallest distance that must exist between two objects before they can be seen as two separate entities.

ringbone colloquial term used to describe new bone formation in the pastern region, which may encircle the parent bone. It is a non-specific term and its use is discouraged because of confusion caused by the prefixes high and low, true and false, articular and non-articular.

scatter radiation multidirectional radiation resulting from the interaction of the primary x-ray beam and an object; it causes loss of contrast between parts of the image on the radiograph.

scintigraphy production of two-dimensional images of the distribution of radioactivity in tissues after systemic administration of a radiopharmaceutical imaging agent.

sclerosis increased opacity of bone.

scoliosis curvature of the thoracolumbar spine from side to side; usually congenital.

secondary radiation particles (such as electrons) or photons (such as x-rays) produced by the interaction of the primary x-ray beam with matter.

seedy toe term with different usage in the USA and the UK. In the USA it describes separation at the white line seen secondary to chronic laminitis and rotation of the distal phalanx. In the UK it describes separation at the white line filled with crumbly dry material and is often of unknown aetiology. It is not generally associated with rotation of the distal phalanx. Unless white line separation is extensive there is usually no associated lameness.

sequestrum necrotic fragment of bone; a sequestrum usually is a sharply demarcated sclerotic fragment separated from the parent bone by a zone of radiolucency and an outer rim of sclerotic bone (the involucrum).

silhouette sign effect produced when two fluid opacities are contiguous and the clear outline of one is lost; the two fluid opacities thus merge into one; often used in thoracic radiology.

soft x-ray beam low-energy, low-penetrating x-ray beam made at low kVp settings.

sore shins see 'bucked shins'.

splint colloquial term used to describe (a) active or inactive periosteal new bone on a second or fourth metacarpal (metatarsal) bone; (b) inflammation of the interosseous ligament.

splint bones second and fourth metacarpal (metatarsal) bones.

standing lateral positioning technique for a lateral projection using a horizontal x-ray beam, vertically positioned cassette and standing patient.

stress fracture synonymous with a fatigue fracture.

stressed radiographs radiographs of a joint obtained with the joint passively manipulated to assess joint integrity and to detect subluxation or luxation.

subluxation partial dislocation (displacement) of a joint.

summation radiopacity created by superimposition of more than one structure.

survey radiograph (a) radiographic study of a large area; (b) plain radiograph obtained prior to performing a contrast study.

talocalcaneal-centroquartal joint formerly called proximal intertarsal joint.

tarsocrural joint formerly called the tibiotarsal joint.

temporal teratoma neoplasm in the temporal region comprising of a number of different types of tissue, none of which is native to the area in which it occurs.

tibiotarsal joint correctly called tarsocrural joint.

turbinate bone now called conchus.

ultrasonography imaging of soft tissues using the principle of echography: the variable transmission or reflection of ultrasound waves by tissues of differing densities.

valgus bent outwards: a deformity in which the angulation of the part is away from the midline of the body. Usage is confusing when terms such as carpal valgus are employed since, although the limb distal to the carpus is angled outwards, the carpus often appears 'knock-kneed', i.e. deviates inwards.

varus bent inwards: a deformity in which the angulation of the part is toward the midline of the body. Usage is confusing when terms such as fetlock varus is used: the distal limb is angled inward, but the fetlock appears to deviate outward.

weight-bearing radiograph radiograph of part of a limb obtained with the horse bearing some weight on the limb, ideally with the foot flat.

Wolff's law modelling of bone according to the stresses placed on it, to be functionally competent while using the minimum amount of bone tissue.

xeroradiography dry radiographic process in which the sensitive material consists of a plate carrying an electrical charge on the surface; when radiation interacts with the surface the charge is released; the plate is dusted with a special powder and an image is formed by the powder being attracted and retained in the charged area. Definition is high.

Index

Note: page numbers in *italics* refer to figures, those in **bold** refer to tables

Index

[747]